Simulation in
Anesthesia

Simulation in
Anesthesia

Christopher J. Gallagher, MD
Associate Professor
Department of Anesthesiology
Stony Brook University
Stony Brook, New York

S. Barry Issenberg, MD
Assistant Dean and Assistant Director, Associate Professor
Center for Research in Medical Education
University of Miami Miller School of Medicine
Miami, Florida

DVD created by **Tom Church**

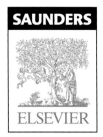

SAUNDERS

ELSEVIER

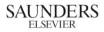

Four Penn Center, Suite 1800
1600 John F. Kennedy Boulevard
Philadelphia, Pennsylvania 19103

SIMULATION IN ANESTHESIA

ISBN 13: 978-1-4160-3135-2
ISBN 10: 1-4160-3135-9

Printed in China

Last digit is the print number: 9 8 7 6 5 4 3 2 1

This book is dedicated to anyone who's ever faked it.

Preface

Pick up three random drugs we might use in anesthesia, oh, let's say, pavulon, pentathol and potassium. Now, pick up the newspaper and read what three drugs they administer during a lethal injection: pavulon, pentathol, and potassium.

Whoa! Dangerous stuff, this anesthesia. Better not try this at home.

And you'd better not try this out the first time on ME either. You *practice* a little before you start waving those lethal syringes around me.

No better place to practice than the anesthesia simulator.

Why this book? What's the need?

Simulation in anesthesia is catching on all over the world. Medical students, nurse anesthesia students, anesthesia assistants, anesthesia residents, practitioners needing some remediation—all these people can benefit from simulation instruction. And all over the world there are simulator instructors looking for how best to run their simulators.

This book should help everyone in the simulator, the instructors *running* the simulator, and students *running the gauntlet* in the simulator.

So whether you're starting a simulation center, revamping your curriculum, or just plain wondering what simulation is all about, read on.

Acknowledgments

A million people made this book and DVD happen, so thanks to all and sundry and apologies to those we miss:

Natasha Andjelkovic, our Publisher at Elsevier, and her assistant **Katie Davenport**, who participated in conception, maturation, and parturition of this baby. It's a book!

Dr. Lubarsky and the whole anesthesia department at the University of Miami, who kept the ORs and their precious cargo of patients going while "Simulation was in session."

Our anesthesia residents, who participated in the simulations, the pictures, and the DVD.

Ilya Shekhter and the staff at the Jackson/University of Miami Patient Safety Center, who made the simulations hum.

Tom Church, videographer, who created the contents for the DVD.

Robert Simon, Daniel Raemer, Jeffrey Cooper, and the staff at the Harvard Institute for Medical Simulation, who know and teach the craft of medical simulation, and who took pity on a befuddled instructor and showed him the ropes back in October of 2004.

Carolyn and **Rachel**, who cheer me on, cheer me up, and make it all worthwhile.

Tara, Zachary, Eric, Brianna, Ethan, who now know why our home was flooded with thousands of simulation articles last summer and put up with my "madness" as I sifted through each and every one of them.

Contents

Introduction

"Zendra! My hat, please!"

Little Jimmy, six years old and all scraped knees and goggle-eyes, sat transfixed in the front row of the magic show.

Roger the Magnificent was out of this world! First that thing with the ace—how did he pick that out of the middle of the deck like that? And then, those little red balls between his fingers. Where did that extra red ball keep coming from? And, and the scarf out of his nose! Try putting ten scarves up your nose at home. Mom would kill me! What would this Roger guy do next with that hat?

"Dad," Jimmy asked, "what's that little stick?"

"That's a magic wand, Jimmy," Dad said.

Over and over the hat the magic wand goes. Roger the Magnificent, with the lovely and talented Zendra at his side, is drawing on the powers of the universe, the mystical essence of the stars and planets.

"Watch the wand, don't reach up and grab it,
For out of this chapeau comes a fuzzy rabbit!"

Jimmy didn't have much use for Zendra, and he wouldn't know a chapeau if it bit him, but that wand was zooming round and round, and it must be doing something to that hat because there sure as heck was *not* a rabbit in there a minute ago when Roger showed it to us. Jimmy even stood up and craned his neck to make *extra* sure that the hat was empty. Kids on the playground said magicians used tricks, and Jimmy was no fool. He had looked good and hard in that hat; and, no sir, no rabbit was in there—no way.

"Abracadabra," Roger the Magnificent said, and buried his arm in that empty hat, going all the way in to the elbow.

"Dad," Jimmy said, "there can't be a rabbit in there, that hat was empty. You saw, didn't you?" Dad nodded.

Roger the Magnificent pulled a snow-white bunny, big floppy ears, twitching whiskers, right out of that hat. Then he reached under the rabbit with his other arm, cradled it, and held it right out to Jimmy to pet. It was the genuine article. Jimmy's mouth, ringed with cotton candy pink, almost said the bad word, almost said "God" (which Mom would get mad at but Dad would just say, "Try not to say that word, Jimmy."). But all that came out was the sound "Caa-aaah."

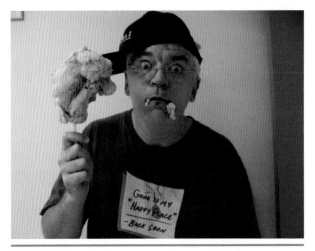

FIGURE I–1 Rediscover your inner child when you enter the Simulator. You'll need to "suspend disbelief" and pretend that the mannequin is a real person. In effect, you'll be, well, "playing doctor." OK, so be it. Go for it and have some fun.

On the way out of the tent and back to the car, Jimmy's circuits, previously frazzled by the sheer impossibility of what he had seen, regained some measure of normalcy.

"Dad, how did the wand *do* that?"

Dad picked Jimmy up, hiked him up on his shoulders with a grunt, and said, "Believe it or not, partner, it wasn't the *wand* that made the rabbit come out of the hat."

* * * * * *

This book is going to look at Simulators in anesthesia. How do anesthesia Simulators pull educational rabbits out of the hat? To understand this, we must look at all the components that went into Jimmy's magical experience.

Jimmy, now regretting all that cotton candy and the two corn dogs, believes that the *wand* made the rabbit appear. Dad, more savvy in the ways of the world, knows the *magician* pulled the rabbit out of the hat. Ah, but the magician, Roger the Magnificent, knows even more. He, lest we forget, drew on the powers of the universe, the mystical essence of the stars and the planets. Roger the Magnificent knows that *three* components play a part in the rabbit's phantasmagoric arrival on the stage.

- The wand
- The magician
- Jimmy himself

And Roger the Magnificent *got* magnificent by knowing how to work all three of these components into his magic show.

An anesthesia Simulator has three main components, each corresponding to an element of Roger the Magnificent's show.

- Simulator (Wand)
- Instructor (Magician)
- Student (Jimmy)

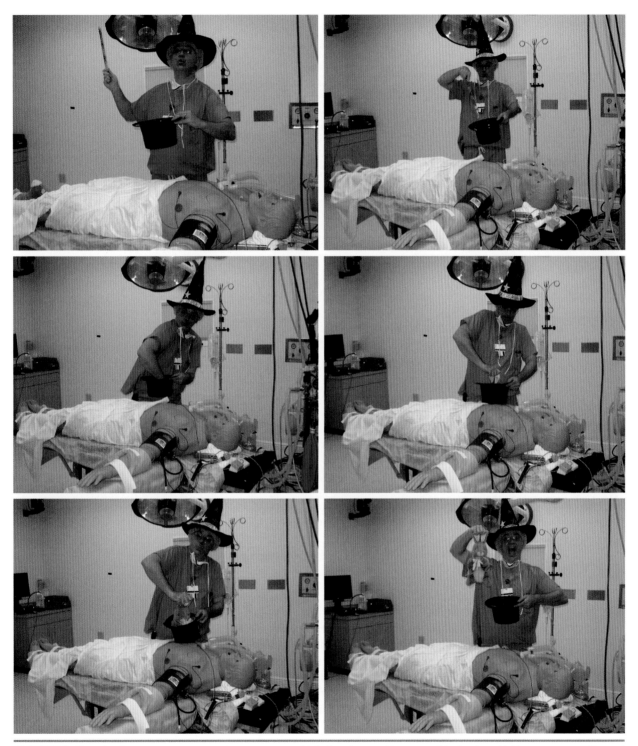

FIGURE I–2 The first time you see a magician, you may think that the wand is responsible for the rabbit's appearance. Wrongo! It is the magician who makes it happen. In a similar vein, the first time you go into the Simulator, you may think that the high-tech mannequin makes all the magic happen. Wrong again! The mannequin is an integral part of the process, yes, but it is the instructor who plays the key role. The instructor makes that rabbit jump out of the Simulator.

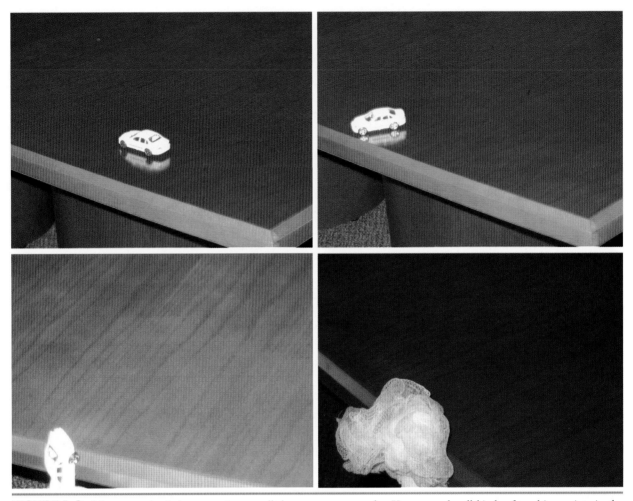

FIGURE I-3   Not every simulation scenario goes all the way to catastrophe. You can make all kinds of teaching points in the Simulator and keep "the car on the road." But every now and then, KABOOM!

This book examines all three elements: the Simulator itself, the Simulator instructor, and the student. We look at the technology available in current Simulators—from partial-task trainers to high-technology anesthesia mannequins. Cost, upkeep, problems, limitations—everything you wanted to know about anesthesia Simulators but were afraid to ask. We also look at the Simulator instructors—What are you looking for in instructors? How should they teach? What educational principles should they use? And always we'll be looking at the students. Do they learn much from a Simulator? Will students someday face accreditation in a Simulator? How do students react and learn in a Simulator?

An annotated and detailed bibliography at the end of the book will steer you through the original work that examined these questions.

But the main focus here is the magic show itself, the simulation scenario. Yes, it's worthwhile to dissect the component parts of simulation, but it's when you put it all together that the stars come out—and the rabbits too.

The center of this book's solar system is a collection of 50 anesthesia scenarios, complete with a play-by-play of the scenario, a detailed debriefing, and a summary of the main lessons learned. You become a fly on the wall as simulation students wrestle with codes, malfunctioning paddles, line crossovers, difficult patients, impossible coworkers, rare diseases, and all-too-common vexations. You look over the shoulder of superb students as they peg the diagnosis and strike at the heart of the matter. And you also get to see some not-so-superb students in action as they swerve off the road, break through the guardrail, and sail over the cliff and onto the rocks below.

From the safety of this book's covers, you get to watch it all happen. So grab some cotton candy, slather a couple corn dogs with mustard, and pull up a seat.

"Zendra, my wand, please!"

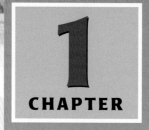

What Is a Simulator—a Clinical Checklist or a Theater?

> *"Schrodinger's cat is both alive and dead."*
> **One of many unfathomable ideas from quantum theory**

Jimmy grows up, insists you call him "James" now, although most of the students in his quantum physics class call him "Professor."

In this most advanced of disciplines, the professor still delivers his lectures the old-fashioned way—white chalk on a blackboard. The students shuffle in, take off their bulky jackets, and set up their laptops to take notes. James had initially resisted this maneuver, and he found the clicking keys irksome; but alas, after a while there was *so* much clicking it became a kind of white noise, and you tuned it out.

"What does a *single* electron do when it comes to this sheet of metal with two holes in it?" the professor asks.

No one's hand goes up. There weren't any hands free; they were all glued to their keyboards!

James turns around, draws a square representing the sheet of metal, and draws a little dot, the electron, with a little arrow pointing toward the square.

Click, click, click, click, click, click.

("How are they drawing this picture on their computers?" James thinks. "Notebooks and pens were better for drawing pictures.")

"Simple," James explains, "the single, indivisible electron passes through *both* holes."

Click, click, click ... click. Click, click. Click. Click.

The clicks fade out and the lecture hall gets quiet. Outside, in the distance, the carillon's bells start playing "Amazing Grace." Every student's head lifts up from their laptops as they look at the blackboard.

The *single* electron passes through *both* holes.

Now just how the heck can it do that?

A single simulator passes through a couple holes of its own. For a simulator can be viewed as two separate creatures:

A clinical checklist
A theater

But like the elusive and tricky electron, the clinical checklist and the theater inhabit the same simulator experience. Is this as incomprehensible as quantum physics?

No. As the core of this book—the 50 simulator scenarios—show, each scenario has an element of

---

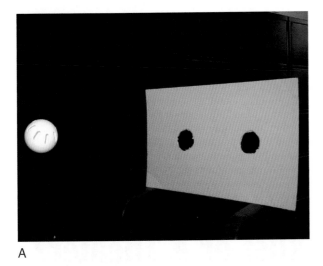

A

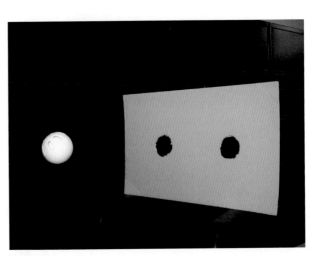

B

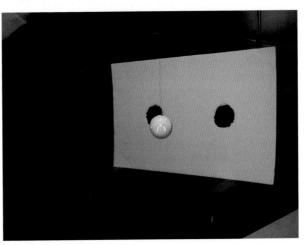

C

D

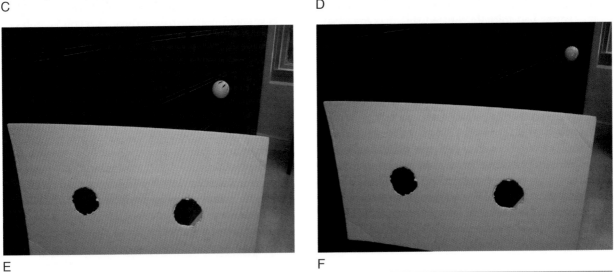

E   F

FIGURE 1–1   Our simulation center has a quantum level camera that actually caught this electron in midflight. As you see, the single electron behaves in a curious "dual" manner, going through both holes and remaining a single electron. The simulation center also functions in a curious "dual" manner. Both checklist and theater, the simulation center tests your ability to "go down the list" (give oxygen, start nitro, send a blood gas), as well as your ability to "act in a theater" (interact with others, lead appropriately, communicate clearly).

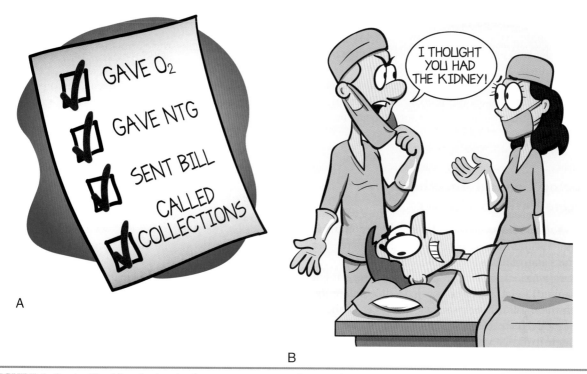

FIGURE 1–2 A. Checklist. In the simulator, you want to make sure that you do each of the "items" on the checklist, just as you would do with a real patient. The checklist is the most common way of grading people on their performance, and you often see a checklist in a simulator study. **B.** Theater. There are other, more subtle things that go on too. These don't so readily fit on a checklist. Here, a doctor asks an inappropriate question in front of an awake patient. Not a good thing to do!

the clinical checklist, and an element of theater—educational theater.

For example, you set up a simple scenario for medical students:

INDUCING GENERAL ANESTHESIA IN A ROUTINE PATIENT: CLINICAL CHECKLIST

Check the preop and consent.

Make sure airway equipment, suction, and drugs are ready.

Talk to the patient, reassure them, make sure they are NPO.

Apply routine monitors: EKG, BP cuff, pulse oximeter.

Preoxygenate.

Give induction drugs to induce anesthesia.

Ensure adequate mask ventilation.

Give paralytic drug.

Continue mask ventilation until paralytic agent has worked.

Perform laryngoscopy.

Intubate.

Ensure correct tube placement.

Institute ventilation.

Secure endotracheal tube.

Check vital signs.

Start anesthetic.

You could throw in other steps (sedate prior to induction), or you can take out steps (if a bunch of medical students are standing around, just have them intubate, one after another, so everyone gets to do something). But the idea is the same—you use the simulator as a checklist. You ensure that the student does the right things in the right order.

"Oops," the instructor corrects, "you just induced, but you forgot to preoxygenate first. Let's try that again."

"Nope, nope," the instructor observes, "you induced anesthesia all right; but if you put that laryngoscope in *before* you give the paralytic, you are going to be in for the fight of your life as they bite down on that scope."

Good lessons all, and good lessons linked to the "simulator as a clinical checklist."

But the good thing about the simulator, and what really gives it a zing from the instructor's and the student's point of view is that the simulator also functions as "educational theater." And theater is limited only by the imagination of the playwright and the actors. So you can end up with Juliet lamenting her romantic plight, Willie Lomax lamenting his wasted life, or Stella lamenting that she has "always depended on the kindness of strangers."

Bring up the lights, lift the curtain, and "Break a leg." The educational theater is going live. Anything—but *anything*—that the instructor wants to teach is now on the playbill.

Inducing General Anesthesia in a Routine Patient: Theater

1. *Check the preop and consent.* "Wait!" the preop nurse says, "this consent is outdated, and you gave her some sedative already, what should we do?"
2. *Preoxygenate.* "Oh, I can't stand that!" the patient shouts. "I'm claustrophobic, that shut-in feeling with the mask just kills me, get it off, get it off!"
3. *Perform laryngoscopy.* The light doesn't work, even though it did before, and you don't have an extra scope around. You turn to tell the circulator to get you another one, but the circulator is in the middle of a count and won't be bothered.
4. *Intubate.* As your "helper" pulls out the stylet from your endotracheal tube, the stylet has the pilot balloon wrapped around it, and the pilot balloon snaps off, making the endotracheal tube cuff deflate, creating a big leak.
5. *Start mechanical ventilation.* Something in the back of the machine makes an irritating squeaking sound with each inspiration. The surgeon says, "Shut that damn thing up!"

In the big chapter on simulation scenarios, you can see this marriage of both functions. Some scenarios are mostly theater—dealing with an inappropriate patient in the preop assessment room. Some scenarios are mostly checklist—taking the appropriate steps once you diagnose malignant hyperthermia. But most are a delicious mélange of checklist *and* theater—getting a lung to deflate in a double-lumen case (checklist) while dealing with a ticked-off and demanding surgeon (theater).

So we've looked at this "checklist versus theater" issue from the angle of the instructor. How does it look from some other people's point of view?

Consumer
Program chairman
Resident education director
Risk management
Resident

Clinical Checklist

From a lot of angles, the Simulator as "clinical checklist teacher" has appeal.

- *Consumer.* "I don't want any anesthesiologist taking care of me until they have proven they can handle all the "baddies" that can happen during a case. What the heck, they don't let a pilot fly until he has proven that he can handle an engine flame-out, a landing gear hang-up, and a hydraulic loss. Is it so outrageous to ask that the anesthesiologist prove he or she can handle anaphylaxis, myocardial ischemia, and a tension pneumothorax?"
- *Program chairman.* "I don't want to "release my residents into the wild" until they have proven their mettle. During their residence, they might not have seen malignant hyperthermia. But "out there" they may very well see this rare but potentially fatal disease. I, as chairman, am responsible for these residents, and I want them to know, to prove they know, before I sign off on them."
- *Resident education director.* "How can I know that the residents know? Yes, we do in-training exams, we get evaluations from their attendings, we try to cover everything in the lectures and grand rounds, but, still, how can I know?"
- *Risk management.* "Keeping the rabid dogs of the legal profession off our tails is a full-time job. Setting up some kind of "we proved we can handle emergencies" or "we do everything to make sure our residents know what to do when the chips are down" may be of some help."
- *Resident.* Residents who "know the score" realize that they lead a somewhat sheltered life. There's always that attending back there who can jump in and save the day (or at least, take the heat). But as the end of residence nears, residents realize that it's a cold, cruel world out there. When the sky caves in and a patient goes sour, you are *all alone.* Marooned.

"Damn, I wish I'd done more training in that Simulator!"

BOX 1-2   Who's Interested?

- **Patient (consumer)**
- **Educator**
- **Lawyer**
- **Resident**

Simulators find their biggest champions in the world of Anesthesia. No surprise, then, that anesthesia people have done the initial research on "Simulator as Clinical Checklist Teacher."

Anesthesiologists at Washington University in St. Louis (great arch there, along with the largest Japanese garden outside Japan, plus a hip restaurant and music scene at Laclede's Landing down by the Mississippi River) have looked at this with medical students and residents. (The article is in *Anesthesiology* 2004;101:1084–1095. The 41 references at the end of the article cover Simulation from A to Z. If you are going deep on Simulation information, this is the article to get. Take a look at those 41 references. They will make you an insta-Simulato-Savant.) During a single 75- to 90-minute session, residents pounded through six crises—anaphylaxis, myocardial ischemia, atelactasis, ventricular tachycardia, cerebral hemorrhage, and aspiration. They had about 5 minutes to figure out what was the matter and to fix it. For example, in the atelectasis scenario, the residents had to go through the standard maneuvers to diagnose and treat hypoxemia.

Go to 100% oxygen.
Listen to breath sounds.
Hand ventilate.
Apply suction.

Their performance was videotaped and graded. More senior residents outperformed their junior counterparts. And glory, hallelujah to that! At least we must be teaching *somebody* something.

So great. But here come the tough questions, the real acid test for the "Simulator as Clinical Checklist Teacher."

1. Do we make this a requirement? (*They do in Israel.*)
2. What if you're good in every other measurable way (evaluations, clinical observation, in-service tests) but you blow it in the Simulator? Don't graduate from the program? (*Can you spell L-A-W-S-U-I-T?*)
3. Take it a step further. If passing the Simulator becomes mandatory, then does a *teaching* tool ("*Oh great, we get to go to the Simulator to learn!*") become a *torture* tool ("*Oh no, we have to go to the Simulator to get screwed!*").
4. Take it two steps further. If passing the Simulator becomes mandatory, then does *insider trading* enter the equation? ("*Psst, there's a new website, Passthe-simulator.com. It tells you just what you need to do to pass the 'basic six' scenarios that they always ask. Don't tell anyone I told you.*")

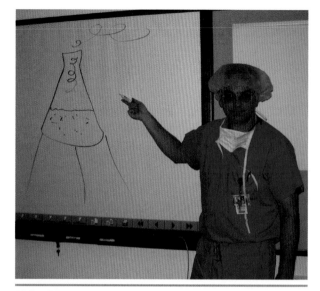

FIGURE 1–3 The acid test regarding simulation: "Is it worth it?"

5. OK, so now it's mandatory. Does every program *have* to buy a Simulator? Big bucks, especially if you have a small program. And if you don't or you can't afford a Simulator, then do you, what, fly your residents to a far off place for certification? Who pays? Who replaces them? Is this part of their 80 hours? Are they at a disadvantage (they never get to go in the Simulator) relative to the residents who have regular access to a Simulator?
6. Now we jump in our time machines and go forward. Are residents exposed to a Simulator actually safer? Did all that time and expense save a life? Stop a catastrophe? Ask these same questions after a "You must pass the simulator to graduate from any program" rule passes. Are these "We jumped through the flaming hoop of the simulator" residents better than "We never jumped through the flaming hoop of the simulator" residents?

Now that we've beaten the "Clinical Skills Teacher" issue to death, let's turn to the second item on the hit parade—the "Simulator as Theater of the Medical World." Let's look at those same people who might like this "Theater" idea.

● *Consumer.* Behavioral therapy for the doctors? I'm all for it. While you're at it, do a little electroconvulsive therapy for the bastards. They keep me waiting in their office for 3 hours, then they see me for 2 minutes, write a scrip for some high-priced pill (that later gets recalled because it killed a few dozen people), and blow out the door, reminding me to stop at the cashier on the way out to fork out for the co-pay. If your Simulator can breath a little humanity into those white coat-besmocked cretins, so much the better.

- *Program chairman.* "Oh great, another e-mail, just what I needed."

  Dear Mr. Chairman,

  A word about your resident—during a code last night, your resident was entirely inappropriate. Our floor nurses have noted, on more than one occasion, that this doctor acts rudely and. . . .

  Mr. Chairman,

  I hate to bring this up again, but Dr. Smith simply does not understand the team concept in the ICU. During his entire rotation last month, Dr. Smith. . . .

  . . . the operating room is not the place to engage in such theatrics . . .

  . . . like a deer caught in the headlights. One would think a senior resident. . . .

  . . . is no way to ask for a rapid transfuser. A professional demeanor is not too much to expect from a. . . .

  Oh yes, program chairmen would embrace some behavioral improvement in their residents. If for no other reason than to debulk their e-mail inboxes.

- *Resident education director.* The 600-pound gorilla in resident education is the ACGME (American College of Graduate Medical Education). Residency programs from Jacksonville to Juneau are scrambling to fulfill the six ACGME-mandated core clinical competencies. These "Six Horsemen of the Educational Apocalypse" are:

  Medical knowledge
  Patient care
  System-based practice
  Practice-based learning and improvement
  Professionalism
  Interpersonal and communication skills

At the American Society of Anesthesiology meeting, for example, entire workshops are devoted to "making sure you are covering your butt on the ACGME core competencies."

Most programs and most specialties are good at teaching medical knowledge, patient care, and practice-based learning and improvement. But system-based practice? A little tougher. A little fuzzier. How about professionalism and interpersonal and communication skills? Tougher still, fuzzier still. Well, as these last two are *kind of* hard to teach, can you *kind of* forget about them?

Yes! That's the good news. You can, indeed, blow them off entirely. There is, unfortunately, a small catch to this approach: The ACGME will shut down your program.

Here's where the Simulator comes charging over the hill to rescue your program. The Simulator, especially when employed in the "behavior" mode, fits hand-in-glove with those last two core competencies—professionalism and interpersonal and communication skills. And this "salvation from the ACGME monster" can spread to other specialties as well. For example, if, say, the surgery department is found to be lacking in the "warm and fuzzies" of the core clinical competencies (professionalism and interpersonal and communication skills), send the surgery residents over to the anesthesia department's Simulator. Cooperation between departments? Surgery and anesthesia holding hands instead of beating the living daylights out of each other? What a concept!

- *Risk management.* When a risk manager "looks for clues at the scene of the crime," he or she usually comes across a host of "behavioral faux pas."

  "At this point, no one was sure whom to call."

  "Internal Medicine thought they were running the code but forgot to check with the ICU staff."

  "Upon review, no one was sure who ordered the fatal dose of. . . ."

  "By failing to check the chart, no one realized that. . . ."

  "Protocol required that . . . but what ended up happening was. . . ."

  "Respiratory therapy was unaware. . . ."

  What can the Simulator offer the beleaguered risk manager? A safe forum for team practice. A place to examine protocols and, if nothing else, make sure *everyone knows what to do*. In the panic and chaos of an emergency, roles blur, orders fly, and people die. In the HD-TV stop-action of the legal aftermath, every oversight sticks out in stark relief.

  Practice, practice, practice in the Simulator. Get whole clinical teams together and clarify everyone's role *before* the disaster. Hone those emergency team behavioral *skills* in the *Simulator*. If not, you can gape at your emergency team behavioral *faults* in court. (Does a Simulator pay for itself? If it prevents one disaster it does. Run the numbers with your hospital's legal counsel.)

- *Resident.* Team learning is fun. Most of the time residents are in their own little zone, learning their own craft, brushing up against others occasionally. In a multispecialty Simulation, residents can gain some cross-connectivity. Plus they can pick up tips, tricks, and insights from their comrades in the field. When an anesthesia resident, an ICU nurse, a

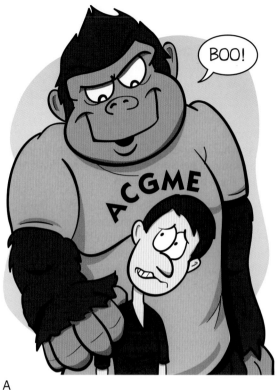

A

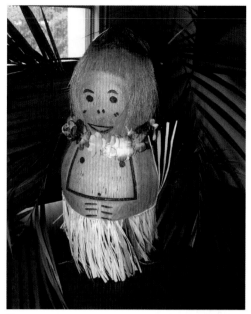

B

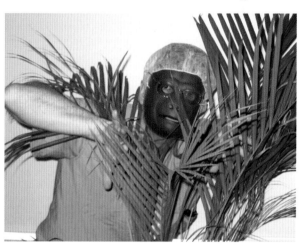

C

FIGURE 1–4 **A.** ACGME is the 600 pound gorilla in medical education. You ignore it at your own risk. Fortunately, education in the simulator can fill in a lot of core competencies. Fuzzy, Montessori-esque competencies such as Professionalism and Interpersonal Skills lend themselves to simulator-based education. Note (**B** and **C**)—This gorilla can assume many shapes and can appear anywhere.

respiratory therapist, and an internal medicine ICU fellow get together, everyone learns something.

Behavioral learning is a real eye-opener. Medicine can be pretty cut-and-dried.

Algorithm for myocardial infarct
ACLS protocol for pulseless V-tach
Fluid guidelines in resuscitation

So when you take a "walk on the wild side" of behavioral education, you step out of "memorization" mode and get into "independent thinking" mode—something most medical people haven't done since college.

How do you deal with "Do Not Resuscitate" orders when the family wants one thing and the patient another?

If you encounter a cultural hitch in your clinical routine (a Somali immigrant insists on a female anesthesiologist but you're a man and the only anesthesiologist on call), how do you react? Now the fetal heart rate monitor registers a big decel and she still doesn't want you to touch her. What next?

Ants got into your ICU and bit up a newborn on a ventilator. How do you professionally break this horrible news to a yuppie couple who just appeared on the cover of *Parenting* magazine?

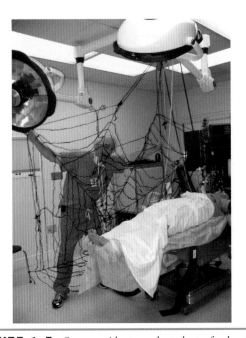

FIGURE 1–5 Some residents and students freak at the thought of going into a simulator. Surely this is a trap they are laying for me! But once they arrive at the simulator and "get into it," these fears dissolve. Most love the experience and ask to come back "soon and often."

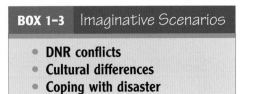

BOX 1-3	Imaginative Scenarios

- **DNR conflicts**
- **Cultural differences**
- **Coping with disaster**

Guess what? You can't memorize this stuff. It takes thinking. The Simulator makes residents exercise their brain.

A lone electron can sort of do "two things at once"—miraculously passing through two holes at the same time. Can simulators perform similar "quantum mechanics"? Can simulators constitute both a clinical checklist and an educational theater?

Of course.

How Anesthesia Simulation Is Done

"I think I killed him. Can I try again?"

—Overheard in the simulator

Nothing like jumping into a medical simulation to see how it works. Here goes. You'll see how it works from the point of view of a participant.

A CONFERENCE, INTERRUPTED

You are sitting in a conference room. Someone runs into the room, breathless. "There's been a shootout, we need a hand."

You and some fellow simulatees get up and head down the hall. You go through a doorway into a white linoleum-tiled room with screens between three gurneys. On each gurney is a Simulator, covered with a blood-spattered blanket. Two of the Simulators are adults, one is an infant. Each has a monitor and an IV attached. A woman is crying out in Portuguese, draping herself over the infant. A cop is trying to pull her off, but she won't let go. Two people in white coats are standing at the head of each bed. One is mask-ventilating an adult, one is standing, ignoring the patient and pressing buttons on the monitor; no medical person is by the infant. A red light is going off in the corner, and an overhead speaker is saying, "Code Blue, cafeteria. Code Blue, cafeteria." As you come upon this scene, a man in a white coat asks you where the

cafeteria is because he is going to go take care of the code there.

There are seven of you in your simulatee group. You split up, two to the adult beds and three to the infant. Everyone starts yelling

"Get me an intubation kit!"

"Does this monitor work?"

"This is for an adult, this is too big!"

"Get the blood bank on the phone!"

"Suction, suction, where's the Yankauer?"

"Volume!"

"This is asystole, someone feel a pulse, do you feel a pulse?"

"Forget that, how do we put his head down!"

"This light is out! Get me another one!"

One adult codes and stays dead, despite CPR. One adult starts blinking and talking, despite a flat line. You notice that an electrode has been pulled off. A brief history reveals that this guy just fainted at the scene of the gun battle, had been covered by a bloody blanket, and had ended up in the emergency room by happenstance.

You go over to the baby and try to intubate when the cop says, "Wait, her kid was in here to get a peanut removed from his ear. He didn't get shot!" Then, on looking back, you notice that there actually isn't any

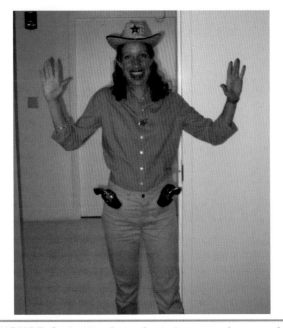

FIGURE 2–1 Howdy pardner! Come on down to the shootout at the OK Simulator. Jazz up the scenarios with some theatrics and props. It's fun. Just don't let the boss know how much fun you're having or he/she will cut your pay.

blood at all on the baby's blankets, though you could have sworn there had been.

After 15 minutes, which seems like 2 hours, an instructor walks in the room and says, "Thank you, doctors, this simulation is over." You look around the room at your fellow simulatees. You all look like you've been driving for hours in a convertible with the top down. As you walk back down the hallway to the conference room, a torrent of babble pours from everyone's mouth. The instructors walk behind, listening.

"Oh man, can you believe that?"

"I thought everyone was shot!"

"I went right to the airway, but then he talked!"

"With that guy in asystole, do we bother or just bag it?"

"Mass casualty drill, I was thinking, but didn't they say *a lot of people were shot*?"

"No, did he actually say that?"

"Who were those people in there? I know the cop was a cop, but the other ones?"

"Med students?"

"Respiratory?"

"Wait, *was* that guy a cop?"

You are back in the "safe" room, where trickery and chicanery have no place. You are in the debriefing room.

BOX 2-1   Debriefing

- **Make sense**
- **Replay**
- **Rethink**

You sit around in a loose semicircle, with two instructors on opposite sides of the room, facing you but at an angle. Not you versus them; it looks more like a cooperative effort with the instructors "among" you, discussing, rather than a solid phalanx of educators "in front of you," ready to lecture you naughty, naughty children.

No instructor rushes to start talking. They sit and listen for a few minutes, letting you and your compatriots "decompress."

"So, how do you think it went?" the first instructor asks.

That opens the floodgates!

"I felt so unsure of myself!"

"I didn't know the equipment!"

"Was I supposed to take charge? I mean, I don't even know these people."

"It's hard to know where to go first."

While this is going on, the "actors" in the Simulation walk in and quietly sit down in the room. Of note, they don't come in smiling and joking and "We gotcha"-ing. They come in the room "in character" and sit down to listen.

This seemingly trivial point is part of the Simulation process. It's called "respecting the character." The actors, as the case is discussed, continue to voice their concerns as they arose during the scenario. In other words, the woman crying out over her child explains to you why she was upset and how she viewed the scenario unfolding. The cop explains what was going through his mind. Neither character walks up to you, gives you a high five, and says, "Wasn't that great? Didn't I seem like a real cop?" If they did that, it would not "respect the character," and you would not learn as much from them.

"The emergency room can be a confusing place, can anyone tell me what was happening in there?" the second instructor asks.

The question is open-ended, the kind of question that opens discussion. This questioning period after the event is called the "debriefing" and is *the most important aspect of the simulation.*

Two truisms:

You do a Simulation in order to do a debriefing. During the Debriefing you make sense of what just happened.

You and your co-learners respond to the scene that just played out:

"Yeah, oh man, was it *ever* confusing in that ER!"

"Who's dead, who's passed out? What's going on?"

"Blood everywhere."

"Then you're thinking 'everybody's shot,' but then I'm new to this ER so I don't know if they have a trauma bay for the really bad ones or if everyone just gets clumped together or what?"

"Then the EKG thing, I mean, two people flat line and one's really dead and the other's just pulled his electrode lead off."

The first educator speaks up, "I saw three patients with different needs. Can anyone lay out for me who needed what?"

Even in the phrasing of the questions there is "method to the madness." Questions are phrased to look for "good judgment" on the part of the simulatees. You don't make a *judgmental* question, you don't make a *nonjudgmental* question; rather, you make a *good judgment* question.

The following demonstrates the difference between a judgmental, a nonjudgmental, and a good judgment question.

Judgmental (You, the examiner, know what should have been done and state so explicitly): "So you blew it with the EKG electrode and got distracted by the hysterical mother. Shouldn't you be able to tell the serious from the trivial?"

Nonjudgmental (You, the examiner, know what should have been done, but you cagily keep your judgment to yourself. This is called the "iron fist in the velvet glove" approach.) "So, there's a flat line and so . . . ?"

Good judgment (You, the examiner, view everything that happened as a "mystery to be solved, not a crime to be punished," so you phrase your question as a way to tease out what everyone was thinking. You're not afraid to throw in your own observations. You don't hide your cards or pretend, blithely, that you are as impartial as a Martian observing from outer space.) "I saw three patients with different needs. Can anyone lay out for me who needed what?"

This last method, the "good judgment" method, is the best way to ask questions during a debriefing.

"Well," one of your colleagues says, "we had one person genuinely shot and dying of hypovolemic shock. We had one fellow who just got swept up in the pandemonium of the shoot-out, and then we had the kid with a separate thing going on."

Another student says, "So we needed to get blood and full resuscitation to the one guy, just support the airway on the other guy, and just move the kid to another place so the ENTs could fish out that peanut from his ear."

"So," the first educator asks, "it looked pretty much like you guys divided yourselves up pretty productively. Anything else you did well?"

At this point, the educator stands up, goes to a white board, grabs a marker, and writes a large "T" with a "+" sign above the left column and a "delta" sign above the right column.

He says, "This is a '+, delta' discussion. We talk about what we did right – the '+' side, and what we'd do differently – the 'delta' column."

"We're so geared to flagellating ourselves, to beating ourselves up, that we often forget to note what we did *right*," he says, "And we learn from what we did *right* as much as by what we did wrong."

After a few minutes, we flesh out our "+, delta" columns.

"To understand better what happened, why don't we see what happened?" the first educator asks.

Everyone groans. The thought of having your sins splashed in front of the whole world in living color is a little daunting.

Roll tape, and oh my God but the camera does indeed throw an extra 10 pounds on you.

No matter how "in control" you might have thought you were, the tape shows just how random

BOX 2–2	Questions

- **Judgmental**
- **Nonjudgmental**
- **Good judgment**

Table 2–1   The +/Delta System

Plus	Delta
Divided up well	Didn't check EKG
Assessed airways right away	Couldn't handle mother
Got blood right away	Didn't ask for help early

and maniacal you actually do look. Overlaid vital sign screens show stuff you simply didn't notice. A minute of asystole before you do anything.

"How did I miss that?"

Lots of repetition. Missed communications. Random motion more reminiscent of a lost Hansel and Gretel than of trained clinicians.

The second educator speaks, "We've found the videotape to be as valuable to us as it is to the golf instructor. People literally say, 'I didn't do that,' when the tape clearly shows them doing just that."

"It's like the dashboard cam on *COPS*," the first educator says.

"We're busted," one of your co-simulatees says.

"Ah," the first educator says, "it's worth revisiting an important point here about the entire simulator mindset. Your reaction is natural: 'You caught us, we screwed up, pin the tail on the donkey.' "

"We're not here to pin the tail on the donkey. We are here to see:

What was your mindset?
What actions proceeded from your mindset?
What resulted from those actions?
How did you assess the results?
What did you do with that assessment?"

"In other words, we're back to "Every event is a mystery to be solved, not a crime to be punished."

The educator goes on with a bunch of "mysteries to be solved." The goal in each one is to discover the *thinking* behind the event, rather than the event itself. If you uncover the thinking and can correct the thinking, you can change the behavior that results from the thinking. You discover the *root* of the problem, so you can prevent further problems.

"As we try to understand what happened in there," the second educator says, "we need to look at what was going through your heads."

"What movie was playing in our heads?" the first instructor says.

"Yes!"

I speak up, "Well, I was going through the 'ABC's.' Someone's shot, make sure the airway's OK, get volume access, treat the deadly stuff first."

Another person says, "Pneumothorax, blood loss, tamponade. All the stuff that kills you fast."

"Torn viscus, torn aorta."

In the "clinical" arena, most of us feel in our "element."

"And how do you decide who should handle the screaming mother in that situation?" the second educator asks.

At this point, the actor who played the mother joins in, "Look, this is my baby, and he got this peanut in his ear and is screaming bloody murder. I'm trying to keep the baby calm, and all these people come rushing in, and now they're screaming too. I just moved here from Portugal so I can't understand anybody." The actor "respects her character" and voices what "movie was playing in her head" during her scenario.

At this point, clinicians tend to clam up. Whereas you zip off clinical stuff (pneumothorax, blood loss, airway management), you screech to a halt in the "behavioral" area.

And here you have a MAJOR POINT OF INSTRUCTION IN THE SIMULATOR! Most of us are good at clinical things, as we do them every day. We replace blood, treat bronchospasm, intubate. But we rarely practice the behavioral things so critical in an emergency.

Role clarity
Communication
Personnel support
Resources
Global assessment

These are the principles of "crisis resource management"—an entire field of study. (Entire textbooks are written on the subject.) Crisis resource management originally looked at how crises are handled in airline cockpits, nuclear reactors, and the chemical industry. For example, before a plane crash, no one challenged the pilot about how low he was flying (no one stepped back and did a global assessment of the overall flight). At Chernobyl, no one reacted fast enough when the reactor started to overheat (no one knew of other resources available for cooling). In the

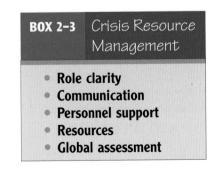

BOX 2-3 Crisis Resource Management

- **Role clarity**
- **Communication**
- **Personnel support**
- **Resources**
- **Global assessment**

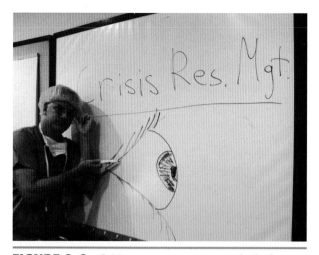

FIGURE 2–2 Crisis resource management boils down to keeping your eyes peeled. The term itself, *crisis resource management*, is a little goofy. *Crisis* has such frightening overtones. The Hindenburg bursting into flames is a *crisis. Resource management* has all the derring-do of a pony ride at a corner carnival. Running out of paper clips and ordering more is *resource management.*

Bhopal chemical spill, no one took charge of the safety mechanisms (there was no role clarity in the Dow Chemical Company's safety department).

Now, the principles of crisis resource management are entering the OR, the ER, and the ICU. We, as doctors, ICU staff, ER personnel, need to know these same principles in a medical emergency.

The first educator writes the principles of crisis resource management on the white board. Then, over the next 10 minutes, we fill in how our scenario demonstrated each of those points.

1. Role clarity

   Establish right away who is charge of the *entire* room, not just one of the beds. We never did that. We broke into three small groups but never had one person in definite charge. One person who *got* all the information and *gave* all the orders. Others needed to establish what their role was.

   "I'll take the airway on bed one."
   "I'll give blood."
   "I'll assess bed two."
   "I'll take the kid."

   Without role clarity, the room goes to "chaos theory," which, truth to tell, is what happened in your scenario.

2. Communication

   When the fur starts flying, it's easy to overload and just start yelling for things. (That's exactly what you did.) Instead, you should address people directly, better yet, tell them by name, even if you have to grab their ID badge and turn it around so you can see their name. Close the loop in communication. When someone tells you something, repeat it to make sure that you got the right information.

   When the first patient coded, you told one of your colleagues, "Start chest compressions," and right away she said back to you, "Start chest compressions, right?" She closed the loop on your exchange. (In a classic example of *not* closing the loop, a pilot of a 747 on Tenerife in the Canary Islands started to take off before he had clearance from the tower. His co-pilot said, "We don't have clearance." The pilot did not close the loop and acknowledge this critical piece of information. More than 500 people died.)

3. Personnel support

   As you were struggling with these three patients in the ER, it didn't occur to any of you to call for additional people, such as security to take care of the screaming mother. As a rule, it's good to call for help early if it looks like you're getting overwhelmed.

   Once support arrives, you want to make sure you use the support personnel well. Give them a quick update and tell them what the issues are. In your room, for example, if another physician had come in, you could have said, "We have some gunshot wounds here. Do me a favor and assess the vitals on each of these patients."

   The other thing you want to do is assign people to either a "doing" job or a "thinking" job.

   "YOU, squeeze blood into patient number one."
   "YOU, come over here by me, help me straighten out who needs what here. I don't know what's going on with the baby."

4. Manage resources

   Blood loss was going to kill the first patient. So get the wheels in motion to get more blood, even O-negative blood in a pinch. That's priority number one, so get your "doing" people on that right away.

   Once you've assessed that the other two patients are OK, get them moved out of the room so you can put all your "energy" eggs into the resuscitation basket.

   Figure out who can do what for you. The cop can't intubate, but he can usher the distracting mother away. The anesthesiologist can get you an airway and a big line, so do not ask him (or her) to deliver the blood sample to the lab.

5. Global assessment

A big "no no" in a crisis is fixation. You start along one line of thinking and can absolutely not be shaken from that line of thinking. In an emergency, with a ton of information pouring in, you "clutch at straws"; you grab for the first thing that can make order out of chaos, and you hang onto it.

In your case, there was a shooting, and you saw blood on the sheets. So, damn it, everyone in that room was shot. If you fixated on that, rather than stepping back and thinking coolly and examining the patients individually, you would have placed monster lines in everyone. Including the kid with a peanut in his ear!

Not exactly a case of volume resuscitation.

So you need to step back. Think. Invite others to think. (You may be "in charge" of the room, but everyone in that room should be thinking.)

Another crucial aspect of global assessment is to verbalize what you are thinking. That lays bare the "current thinking" in the room and invites others to speak up and clarify if they disagree.

"OK folks, we have three people down with gunshot wounds, so we need blood for everyone. Let's get some lines."

"Wait, this second guy is OK. No blood on him, and his pulses are strong."

"Same with the kid, he's free of blood, is breathing, no trauma here."

(Good time to re-verbalize, update the room.)

"OK, three people down, need blood and big time resusc in bed one. Basic support for beds two and three until we clear up what's going on with them."

That's global assessment. Ongoing, never static.

"OK, what do we take away from this," the second educator asks.

The clinical points take a back seat to the behavioral points. That is the exact opposite of how you started . . . the exact opposite of your usual, clinical orientation. The clinical scene functioned almost like kindling wood in a fire. The clinical scene started things but was not the focus.

"Well," one colleague says, "we need to talk to each other more clearly."

"I can see now," another says, "that you really need to drill code teams on how to do things productively. You can't just assume everyone will know what to do."

"It's hard to not get fixated on one thing," you say.

You go on for another 10 minutes, pulling "larger" lessons out of your Simulator experience. Then you draw back even farther and try to apply what you learned to your bigger goal, learning the Simulation process.

1. Debriefing is the heart of the matter.
2. A good video system aids in the debriefing process.
3. Posters help in the debriefing room. (Posters should emphasize major behavioral points such as role clarity, reassessment, management of resources.)
4. Refrain from "going clinical" right away and falling into a lecture on, for example, how to treat asystole.
5. Focus on the wise words, "It's not about the dummy, dummy, it's about you, dummy."

Here, then, are the major steps of the debriefing in review.

1. Eavesdrop

This is the stage, after the Simulation scenario, where everyone is "unloading" as they walk down the hallway. Skilled educators walk along, keeping their ears open, listening for issues important to the participants. For example, one of the participants says, "What do you do when you're new to the ER and don't know where the equipment is?" OK, unfamiliarity with equipment in a new setting is an issue. The educator picks up on that and talks about it during the debriefing. Another participant says, "It's tough when you're distracted by a hysterical parent." OK, dealing with distraught family members is another issue. The educators pick up on that, too, and talk about it during the debriefing.

2. Reactions

You go over the feelings of the participants. No matter how well prepared or educated, anyone gets a little "rattled" by the simulation scenario. That "rattling" is a critical part of the process. To propel learning, you need to create a little emotional "irritant." For analogies, look to physical exercise: You

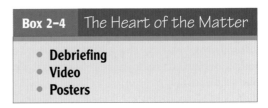

Box 2-4   The Heart of the Matter

- **Debriefing**
- **Video**
- **Posters**

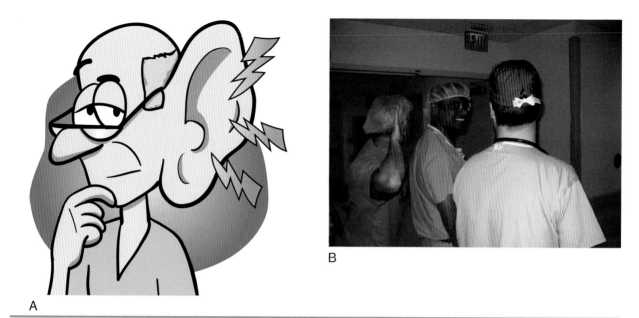

A

B

FIGURE 2–3 During a scenario, residents tend to get pretty wound up. They "let loose" in the hallway and "spill their guts" to each other. "Oh man, I didn't see those ST segments!" "Did you think we needed to transfuse?" The clever instructor takes advantage of these "hallway confessions" to see into the residents' minds. Here, the instructor is *so subtle* that you would never guess that he is listening in.

tear down your muscles a little at the gym, then the muscles repair themselves, and you get bigger muscles. Another analogy is the sand grain that irritates the oyster. Give it enough time, and that irritant turns into a pearl.

3. Understanding.

Now is when you digest what happened. You try to make sense of that chaos in the ER; you examine what you did and what you were thinking. Understanding the *behavioral* aspects of a simulation are important. You don't just focus on the clinical things that were done.

4. Summary.

Review what happened and put things in a larger context. That is, at the end of this particular scenario, draw broader conclusions than just this par-

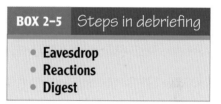

BOX 2-5 *Steps in debriefing*
- **Eavesdrop**
- **Reactions**
- **Digest**

ticular ER. Put the lesson in a big picture of: "What do you do when a lot of people are in trouble, and you have to sort it out?"

And there you have it, a medical simulation from stem to stern.

Let's take a step back for a moment and look at the equipment that goes into these simulations.

Simulation Equipment

> *"I'm afraid I can't let you do that, Dave."*
>
> **HAL's refusal to open the space hatch to an astronaut.**
>
> **—2001, A Space Odyssey**

Dave ran into a little trouble with his equipment on *2001, A Space Odyssey*. First, the equipment shut off life support for his fellow space travelers; then it snipped the air hose to Dave's partner; and then the darn thing wouldn't let Dave back into the ship. And Dave had forgotten to bring along the helmet to his space suit.

Some equipment malfunctions are more vexing than others.

Fortunately, Dave knew his equipment inside and out and found a way to blast back into the ship and shut down the decidedly antisocial HAL.

To date, no simulation equipment has committed mass astronaut-o-cide. But we are wise to take *2001*'s lessons to heart.

1. Know thy equipment as thyself.
2. It's the astronaut (the simulator instructor), not HAL (the simulator mannequin) that keeps the ship running.

So this chapter focuses on lesson 1: knowing the simulation equipment. In the back of our minds, though, we'll be ever mindful of lesson 2—that the simulator instructor is the key element to any simulation scenario.

What's out there in simulation equipment land? This chapter focuses on the Big Kahunas in anesthesia training—full-service computerized anesthesia man-

nequins, but it's worth mentioning all the other "toys" out there that are used to train medical personnel.

PARTIAL TASK TRAINERS

The devices known as partial task trainers let people train for one specific task—some easy, some quite complicated.

ANESTHESIA-RELATED TASKS

Intravenous catheter insertion
Intubating dummies
Bronchoscopy (tailored for pulmonologists but good for us too)
Central line insertion
Epidural (works either upright or on the side)
Surgical airway (you can perform a cric and place a cricothyrotomy kit)

SURGERY-RELATED TASKS

Laparoscopy
Hollow organ closure
Total hip replacement
Ophthalmic surgery, including laser photocoagulation
Otolaryngology
AAA endovascular repair
Surgical suturing
Shoulder arthroscopy

TURP
Breast biopsy
Hysteroscopy

INTERNAL MEDICINE AND ITS SPECIALTIES
ERCP
Colonoscopy

IVC filter placement
Upper GI endoscopy
Interventional cardiology simulator (this is a PC-based application)

So there's no shortage of gizmos and gadgets to train doctors in doing specific tasks. As noted in the

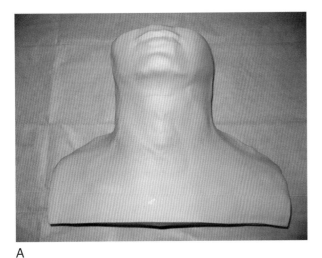

A

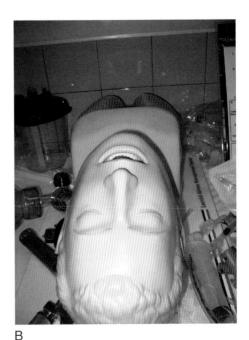

B

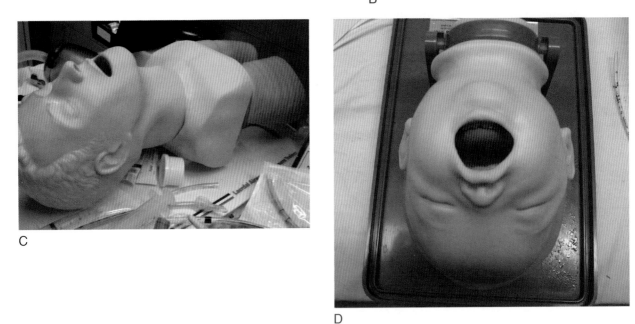

C

D

FIGURE 3–1   Partial task trainers add to the simulation experience. You can focus on one thing (the airway). You can demonstrate, up close and personal, how the various blades "handle" the epiglottis. The curved blade goes into the vallecula and lifts the epiglottis indirectly. The straight blade lifts the epiglottis directly. The model also helps demonstrate how the LMA fights in the airway. Practice it first on the partial model and then on the intubating dummy.

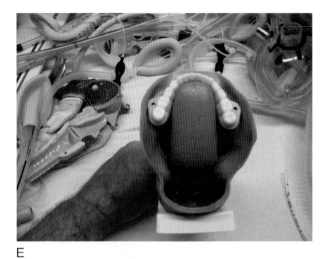

E

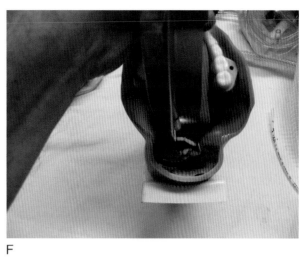

F

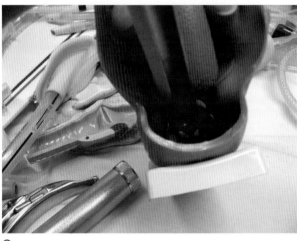

G

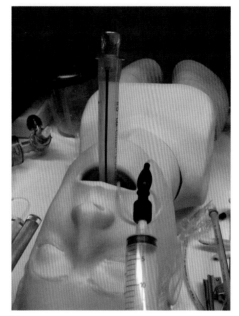

H

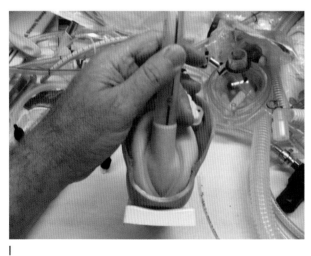

I

FIGURE 3–1 cont'd

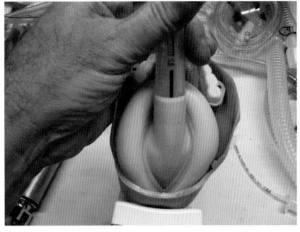

J

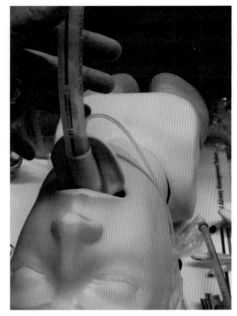

K

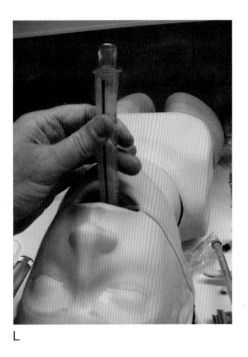

L

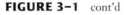

FIGURE 3–1   cont'd

last item—interventional cardiology simulator—there are also a host of "flat screen computer simulators." You can interview a patient, order tests, run codes, examine lab tests. What *can't* you do on a computer?

In surgery, more and more detailed "haptic" trainers are coming into use. "Haptic" means that the trainer gives you the actual "feel" of the tissue and the procedure. Quite realistic and a great way to train surgeons.

In obstetrics, they have a vaginal delivery mannequin capable of generating all kinds of problems—occiput anterior, shoulder dystocia.

In a perfect world and in a perfect simulation center, you could imagine a kind of "amusement park" where every partial task and flat screen computer simulator is present.

You go into room 1, practice placing IVs.
Room 2, put in a central line.
Room 3, place an epidural.
Room 4, perform intubation.
Room 5, perform fiberoptic intubation.
Room 6, run through the difficult airway algorithm, ending with placement of a surgical airway.
Room 7, what's this? A real live human being. What's going on here?

Room 7 opens up another consideration in the "perfect simulation center"—standardized patients.

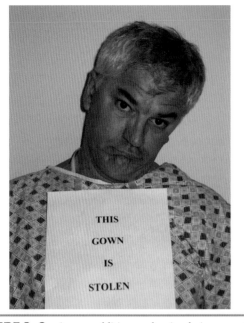

FIGURE 3–2 A great addition to the simulation experience is the standardized patient—an actor with a script. That standardized patient can portray a psychotic patient, a grieving widow, a litigious parent, or a patient with a "mystery disease" (say, MH, and the resident has to "uncover" this in a history). You name it. Here, the patient has a clear case of "IQ deficit disorder."

A standardized patient is an actor who plays out a role from a script. This script can detail any aspect you want a resident to learn about:

Manipulative patient demanding to see his or her records and wants to sue

Patient with a history of malignant hyperthermia that you must "uncover" in the course of your preop visit

Psychotic patient

Distraught parents of a child in the ICU

Relatives who need to hear of a patient's death

You name it

Because you want your residents to be able to handle "anything," you can make use of standardized patients to handle, well, "anything." Let your imagination run wild and come up with any possible interpersonal interaction your resident might ever encounter. Then, using the standardized patient, you "simulate" this interpersonal interaction.

Simulation centers do not live on mannequins alone.

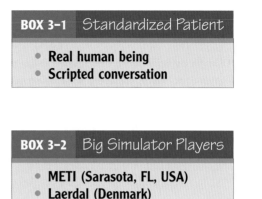

But there's no getting around it, the centerpiece of the simulation center is the anesthesia mannequin, so here goes.

What's out there?

There are three big players: one lame duck company and two that are still very much part of the action.

The lame duck—MEDSIM Eagle

You will still see some of these sturdy players out there.

These anesthesia simulators are no longer made or serviced; they are (dab your eyes here) "orphan simulators." MEDSIM Eagle doesn't even exist anymore; the company is now just MEDSIM, and they only make ultrasound simulators. (You can try contacting the company (www.medsim.com), but don't be surprised if no one knows what you are talking about when you mention their simulator.)

However, these simulators are built like brick houses, so they last and last. "Why throw it out?" its owners say, "I'll service it myself and keep this baby going and going!" The MEDSIM Eagle simulator has a drug recognition system, like the METI simulator.

Harvard's simulation center has one of these simulators, and you sense that they love keeping it going. Picture some diehard Volkswagen beetle owner keeping his 1965 bug alive, engine rehaul after engine rehaul, never giving up on the old car.

The two players: METI (Sarasota, FL; www.meti.com) **and Laerdal** (Denmark; www. Laerdal.com).

Each has its pluses and minuses, each has its champions and detractors, so we'll just go down the line and see how they add up. Your best bet if you're considering laying down cash for these simulators (it's serious bread) is to take them for test runs and see which fits your style better.

OVERARCHING PRINCIPLE

If you remember one thing, remember this, the Laerdal is like flying a plane in which you have direct control over the stick, rudder, and ailerons. The METI is like flying a plane where the computer actually controls the plane, and you input what you want done. You don't have direct control over the stick, rudder, or ailerons. This analogy is less than perfect but serves to illustrate the main difference between the two.

DRUG RECOGNITION SYSTEM

METI—Has a library of drugs it can recognize and respond to physiologically.

Laerdal—Lacks a library of drugs, though you can program in a canned response to a given drug.

Example: You inject 40 mEq of potassium.

Real life—Patient arrests.

METI—Recognizes the drug, patient arrests.

Laerdal—Nothing happens unless you program this in as a response, then you have to note that they gave the 40 mEq of K in the field, then you institute the response, then the patient arrests. Alternatively, you could just, "on the fly," program in a fibrillation response when you see that K was given.

Example: Anaphylaxis occurs; resident gives phenylephrine instead of epinephrine.

Real life—Pressure would rise for a bit, but you really need epi to resuscitate

METI—Recognizes the neo, allows a small increase in blood pressure, but patient continues to deteriorate unless epi is given.

Laerdal—No response from neo unless you have programmed this information in as a canned response and you note that it's given. Alternatively, you could just manually raise the blood pressure for a little while, then let it go down again.

One Step Removed from Direct Vital Sign Changes

METI—Everything runs on a physiologic model, so you have to program in, say, a shunt, and let the shunt occur before the saturation can go down.

Laerdal—You just punch in a lower saturation.

Example: You want the saturation to drop to 85% after aspiration occurs.

METI—You punch in a shunt, then wait; with time the sat drifts down to 85%.

Laerdal—Press 85% on the O_2 sat, and 85% appears.

One Button Pushed and the Scenario Runs

METI—A preprogrammed scenario can run with just a touch of a single button. Over 10 minutes, the entire scenario plays out and you don't have to do anything. The drug recognition system runs on its own.

Laerdal—Either you have to do everything on the fly, responding to each drug given or the maneuver performed, or you have to program in a canned response. But you have to note what's given, as there is no drug recognition system.

Example: Malignant hyperthermia.

METI—Press the button, and the sequence rolls, with increasing heart rate, increasing end-tidal CO_2, and eventually increasing temperature. If, when tachycardia first occurs, the resident gives esmolol, you don't have to do anything, as the drug recognition system recognizes it and decreases the heart rate for a while. Of note, the library does not yet recognize dantrolene, so you'd have to note when it's given and make the adjustment.

Laerdal—As in earlier scenarios, you can do this all on the fly: entering tachycardia yourself, entering higher end-tidal CO_2 yourself, entering higher temperature yourself. Alternatively, you can program the system to roll, but you still need to respond individually as things occur. For example, if the resident gives esmolol when the tachycardia occurs, you must note this and respond either manually or by a canned response to esmolol that you yourself programmed in.

Eyeballs

METI—Blinks, has pupils that respond, can "blow" a pupil, which is very handy in a cerebral herniation scenario, a response to atropine, or a brain death situation.

Laerdal—No such thing.

Gas Analyzer

METI—Has one.
Laerdal—Lacks one.

Example: You crank up the halothane (Isoforane, ISF) to 5%.
Real life—Eventual cardiovascular collapse.
METI—Gas analyzer recognizes the ISF, and the pressure eventually comes down.
Laerdal—Unless you program in a response and note that the ISF is high, there is no response.

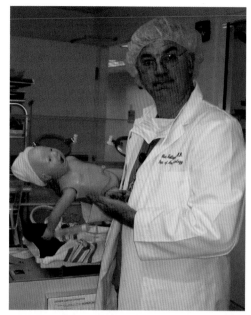

A

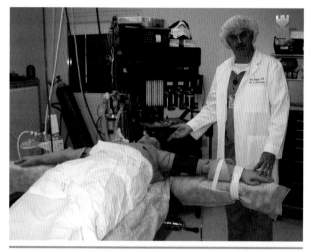

FIGURE 3–3 METI simulator—all the bells and whistles. Pricey.

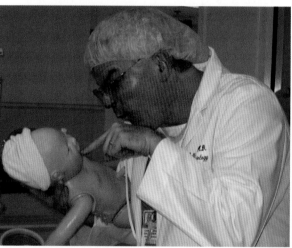

B

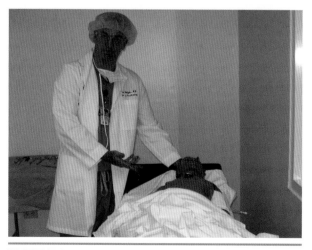

FIGURE 3–4 METI kid.

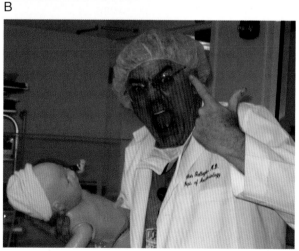

C

FIGURE 3–5 **A.** METI baby. **B.** Coochy coo. **C.** Dentition optional.

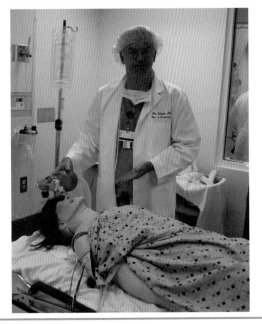

FIGURE 3-6 Laerdal SIM MAN. Somewhat simpler to work with. Less pricey. Fewer bells and whistles.

Monitors

METI—Can hook up to your anesthesia machine monitors.

Laerdal—Hooks up to its own proprietary monitors.

Technical Glitches

METI—more complicated, so, guess what, more chances for things to go wrong.

Laerdal—less complicated, so, guess what, fewer chances for things to go wrong.

Cost

METI—About 200,000 smackers, with a yearly service agreement that can run $12,000 more. (METI, not blind to this high cost relative to the Laerdal, has come out with a stripped-down, less expensive version, the ECS, for about $45,000.)

Laerdal—About 30,000 smackers, with a yearly service agreement of $3200

Once you have the simulator mannequin, you need a "place" to make it all happen. The Simulator is theater, and theater needs props. We need both

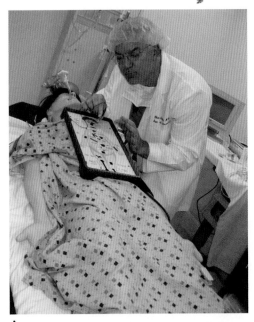

A

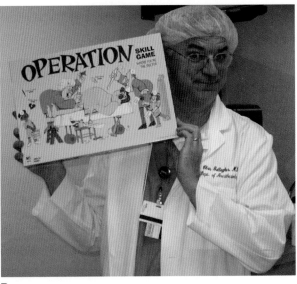

B

FIGURE 3-7 Times are tough, and budgets are tight. There are cheaper alternatives to computerized mannequins.

BOX 3-3	The Two Biggies

METI
- **Pricey**
- **Bells and whistles**

Laerdal
- **Less pricey**
- **Fewer bells and whistles**

medical props to create the medical "feel" as well as stage props to help achieve the "suspension of disbelief" so crucial to the Simulator experience.

Medical Props

Gurneys
Anesthesia machine
Oxygen cylinders
Ambu bags
Swans
Pacers
Zoll pads
Infusion pumps
Defibrillators
Carts, OR tables, IV poles, everything to make it look real
Painted backdrop to look like an ICU

A special note about the medical props. Some of them will have things "wrong" with them to add to the scenarios. Under no circumstances can any of these faulty props make their way into any clinical arena.

Also, the defibrillator should have no energy pass through it. If you really put 360 joules through a dummy and misapply the paddles, you could fibrillate someone who is touching the bed.

Theater Props

White jackets
Outfits for various "players" (cop, parents)
Hubcap
Food packages
Makeup
Water spritzer (for "sweat")
Anything else that adds zing to the experience

Great, where do we get this stuff?

Scour the hospital for outdated or broken stuff.
eBay actually has some of these things (broken stuff from other hospitals).
Ask vendors for outdated or flawed articles, shipments that lost sterility.
You'll need permanent stuff as well as disposables (for disposables, get things with the seals broken so the hospital can't use them).
Fake bags of blood.

Where do you get all the "characters" to play parts? One handy trick is to just leave the room, change one thing in your appearance, then come back as a different person.

There, now that we've laid out the equipment, let's see the actors do their thing. Let's put some meat on all this theory and see the METI and Laerdal in action.

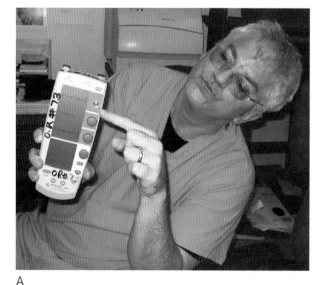

A

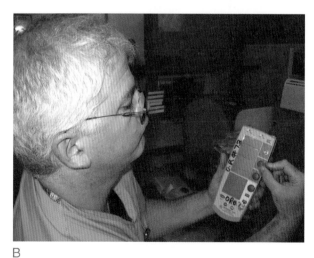

B

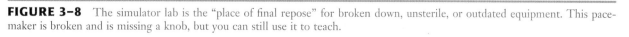

FIGURE 3–8   The simulator lab is the "place of final repose" for broken down, unsterile, or outdated equipment. This pacemaker is broken and is missing a knob, but you can still use it to teach.

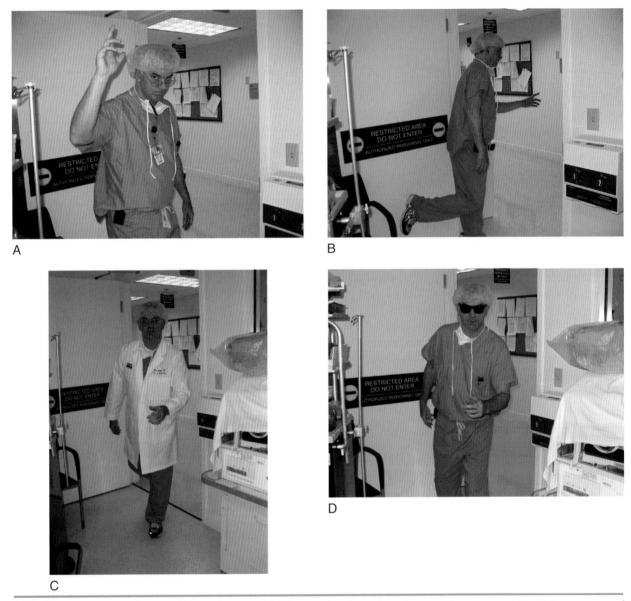

FIGURE 3–9 **A.** You don't need the entire cast of *Ben Hur* to play the various characters in your scenarios. **B.** Just step out of the room, change one little thing, and you're someone else! **C.** See? Just put on a lab coat, and I become utterly unrecognizable. **D.** Who could this man possibly be? International diamond thief? Superspy? Rock star?

How do you actually punch things into the simulator to make all this stuff happen? How do you "make the blood pressure go down" and "elevate the ST segments" and "fibrillate" the patient?

The short answer is—you get trained by the METI or Laerdal people.

The long answer is—METI or Laerdal reps come to your place, in-service you, and help you get started.

You do best, when starting, to use one of their "canned scenarios" (for example, an allergic reaction). You start out with simple cases; then, as you get more comfortable, you add complexity. Time passes, you become more facile, you start hunting around in the virtual world of simulation, and you discover more scenarios you can use. Then you attend meetings, run through simulations, and start programming your own scenarios.

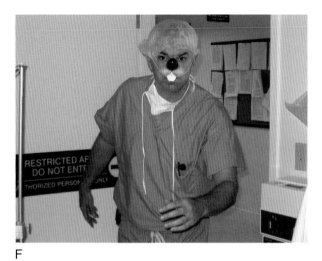

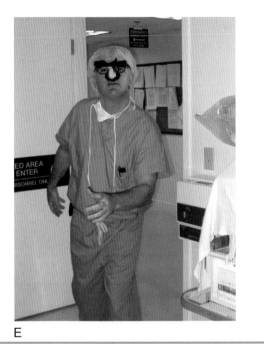

FIGURE 3-9   cont'd **E.** The truly dedicated instructor agrees to minor plastic surgery to change "the look" ever so slightly. **F.** And here again, another character entirely.

This chapter alone cannot teach you all the steps and intricacies of running the simulator computer. But if we run through some real examples, you can get a feel for it.

So let's get a feel for it!

Two simulators, the METI and the Laerdal, are mentioned (more on both of them in the next chapter).

METI SIMULATOR, CANNED SCENARIO, ALLERGIC REACTION, SIMPLEST POSSIBLE

The residents get a preop and operative record that shows a routine patient. You tell the residents that the patient has no *known* allergies. (Tee-hee, we know that an unpleasant surprise awaits.)

They get instructions to hang Ancef and (surprise, surprise), the patient develops an allergic reaction to this antibiotic.

Built into the machine is the "allergic reaction scenario."

You let the residents come into the room, set up, induce the patient, get going; then you press the button that says "Allergic reaction."

Everything is programmed in, including drug recognition via bar code, so you can sit back and watch the event unfold.

What does the computer have and what does it do?

On the computer screen, you see the steps of the reaction, and the computer will be "looking out" for the one thing that can save the day—in this case epinephrine.

Start scenario.
Allergic reaction starts.
Allergic reaction worsens.
Allergic reaction becomes severe.
Allergic reaction resolves.

At each stage, the computer has built into it certain responses that mimic an allergic reaction. In this case, we pretend that we only focus on the blood pressure (ignoring the many other things that happen during an allergic reaction).

Allergic reaction starts. The SVR (systemic vascular resistance) decreases, which makes the blood pressure go down to, say, 90/60.

After 2 minutes the computer goes to the next step—allergic reaction worsens. The SVR decreases again, and the blood pressure goes to, say, 80/50.

After 2 minutes, the computer goes to the next step—allergic reaction becomes severe. The SVR decreases again, and the blood pressure goes to 70/40.

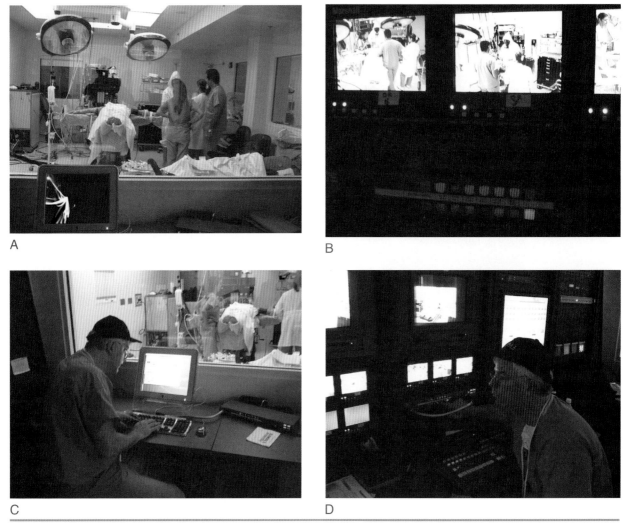

FIGURE 3–10   **A.** Here's how it actually happens. These views are from the control room. Through the window you see the residents in "mid-scenario" (here, a bioweapon has gone off and one person is in a Haz-mat suit—in real life, of course, everyone would have such a suit on). You look through the one-way mirror to observe them, and you work the controls. **B.** Cameras catch and record the action. **C.** Hunched over the controls, you change things, react to what they are doing, and try to make the whole thing as educational as possible. **D.** Microphones allow you to "speak" as the patient ("I can't breathe!") or make overhead announcements ("X-ray on the way.") Work those students, work them, work them. If they figure out one thing, then throw them another curve ball.

Allergic reaction resolves. If at any point, the student gives epinephrine 10 µg (1 cc of a dilute mixture; in reality, water in a syringe that has the bar code for "epinephrine, 10 µg/cc), everything goes back to normal.

Everything proceeds on automatic pilot. Of course you, as simulator runner, have to do a lot more work than just press the button and stand back. You have to deck out the operating room to make it look real, act the part of the surgeon, for example, or the circulator. Keep up the normal OR chatter, and overall try your best to "make the whole thing as real as possible."

But as far as actual computer work goes, you can press the button and stand back and let the little morality play unfold.

What Might the Residents Do?

- They might tumble to the allergic reaction right away, give the appropriate dose of epinephrine right away, and then everything resolves right away. That is a real bummer, because they've "short-circuited" all the fun, and now you're back to ground zero.

● They might flounder around for a while, giving fluids, phenylephrine, or ephedrine. (To "give fluid," they have to tell you they did so, and you then have to enter "fluid given" with the amount in the computer. So in that respect, the scenario is not completely a "hands-off-after-you-push-the-start-button" affair.) When they give fluid, the computer responds by increasing the blood pressure for a while, as it is programmed to increase the blood pressure after phenylephrine or ephedrine. The computer recognition system always responds to a drug given so long as the computer sees the bar code correctly and so long as the drug is in the computer's "library" of drugs. But complete resolution of the problem does not occur until epinephrine is given.

● The residents might over-react and give a code dose of epinephrine (1 mg). The computer then responds with a huge overshoot of blood pressure, severe tachycardia, and ectopy.

No matter how you slice it or dice it, the scenario always misses reality in certain ways.

No skin change occurs, so you don't see the red, flushed face you might expect with a bad allergic reaction.

Is 10 μg always the exact amount of epinephrine that miraculously and definitively "cures" the allergic reaction? Of course not. An allergic reaction may require several drugs (diphenhydramine, steroids, vasoactive infusions). But the computer has to have some "key element" to recognize to restore the vital signs to normal. This is where the *binary* nature of computers collides with the *multiply complex, fuzzy* nature of medical reality.

METI SIMULATOR, IMPROVISED SCENARIO, BLEEDING

Give the students chart work that sets the stage for a big bleed, say a gunshot wound to the abdomen.

Instead of pressing the "start scenario" button, like you did on the allergic reaction scenario, you "ride the keys" on this one.

The residents go into the room and relieve the persons in charge of a case. The patient has already been intubated and is on the ventilator.

You go on the computer to the "Fluids" tab.

You press the "blood loss" button and enter "1000 cc" to be lost over 1 minute.

Over the next minute, the computer "reacts" to this blood loss with a decrease in blood pressure and an increase in heart rate.

You watch the residents like a hawk to see if they notice the drop in blood pressure and react appropriately.

If they do the right thing (turn down anesthetic vapors, ask the surgeons if they're losing blood, send a sample for blood gas analysis, call for blood from the blood bank and give it), then you go to the "Fluids" tab and enter "1000 cc blood infused."

The computer responds by restoring the blood pressure and lowering the heart rate, just as a patient (ideally) would respond.

So things aren't quite on "automatic pilot." You yourself introduced the bleed and entered the transfusion. But the METI computer did do a lot by itself—it "responded" to the blood loss and to the blood transfusion.

The drug recognition system continues to work throughout the scenario, without you having to do anything. For example, the residents may "buy time" with phenylephrine or calcium before they "hang the blood"—as sometimes happens in real life.

Can you program in a bleed? Yes! You could set up a preprogrammed scenario, just like the first one.

Bleed starts (automatically bleed 500 cc over 2 minutes)

Bleed worsens (automatically bleed 500 more cc over 2 minutes)

Bleed corrects (all goes back to normal if they transfuse 1000 cc)

METI SIMULATOR, CANNED SCENARIO—BLEEDING—WITH COMPLICATING FACTORS

You can insert an array of variables into your METI mannequin to complicate things. Say you did the simple bleed scenario as described above, but now you make the patient a little sicker.

Decrease LV contractility.

Increase pulmonary resistance

Decrease the ischemic threshold (making ischemia more likely to appear)

All of these maneuvers have now made the patient that much "sicker," so he is harder to ventilate, harder to resuscitate, and more likely to develop ST changes indicative of ischemia. Now, you can go through the same bleeding scenario but get in more trouble earlier.

Inspiratory pressures are now higher, which can distract the resident.

With that bleed and lower LV contractility, the blood pressure falls faster and farther.

With that decreased ischemic threshold, the resident has problems with ischemia in addition to problems with hypotension.

What about the less technically adept but more affordable Laerdal?

LAERDAL SIMULATOR, CANNED SCENARIO—VENTRICULAR FIBRILLATION

You call students into a code.

You have set the cardiac rhythm directly for ventricular fibrillation. You have a programmed response: After three shocks the rhythm returns to sinus tachycardia. (The mannequin senses the shocks when the paddles are placed on the metal tabs on its chest.)

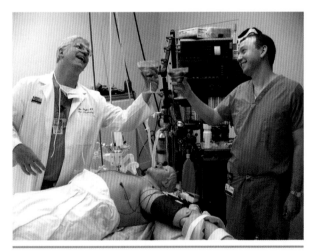

FIGURE 3–11 Aah. Toasting another successful scenario. Instructor and simulator technician Shekhter raise a glass of bubbly after putting the residents through their paces one more time. Teaching in the Simulator is a *blast*. The residents generally like the experience, and you are limited only by your imagination. You can put different spins on the scenarios depending on resident level, resident interest, and, best of all, depending on your own whims and caprice!

What Do the Students Do?

- They may spoil all the fun by getting it right the first time, remembering that you shock, shock, shock first. Then everything gets back to normal, and you wonder what you'll do for lunch.
- They may forget the prime dictum of fibrillation (shock first) and go with intubation, a round of drugs, and chest compressions. The computer continues to spit out ventricular fibrillation until it sees the three shocks.
- They may just shock once or twice (a common mistake).

LAERDAL SIMULATOR, ON-THE-FLY SCENARIO—RIGHT MAINSTEM INTUBATION

You call in the residents to relieve on a case. Tricky you, you have placed the endotracheal tube in the right mainstem. The Laerdal has no way of "knowing this" and so to decrease the saturation, you must program that information in, which you do directly. In the saturation area on the screen, you enter 91%.

What Do the Residents Do?

- Turn up the FIO_2 to 100%, hand-ventilate, listen to the chest, and pull the endotracheal tube back. At that point you go to the screen, and in the saturation area you enter 100%. Good residents, good, good. Here, have a treat! (Throw them a doggie biscuit.)
- Flounder around, forget to listen to the chest, stand there like morons. Bad residents, bad, bad. No treat for you! (Beat them senseless, depending on how strict your department policies are.)

Wait a minute, how would I do that exact same thing with a METI simulator? Aha! Here is where you will see the real difference between these two puppies.

METI SIMULATOR, ON-THE-FLY— RIGHT MAINSTEM INTUBATION

You call in the residents to relieve on a case. Tricky you, you have placed the endotracheal tube in the right mainstem. The METI has no way of "knowing this" and so to decrease the saturation, you must program that in, which you do, but you *can't do it directly, and this is the headache. This is the big, big, big difference.* You have to increase the shunt fraction or increase the O_2 consumption (or both, if you want to). What a pain in

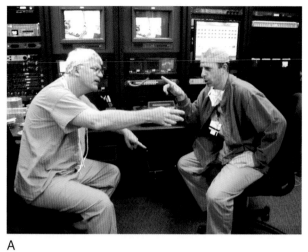

A

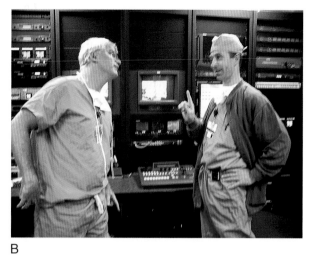

B

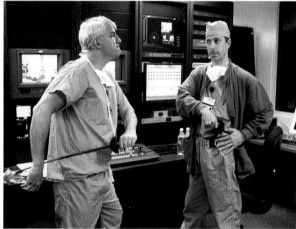

C

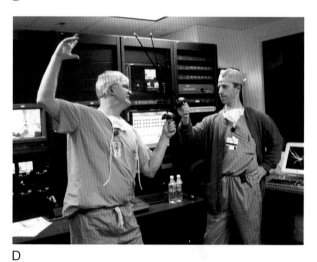

D

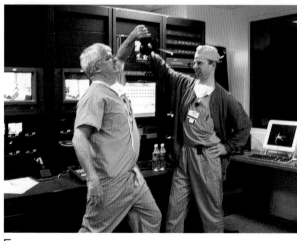

E

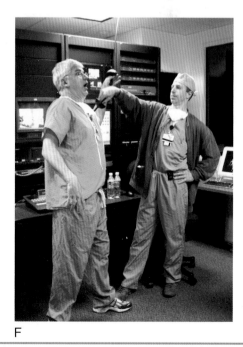

F

FIGURE 3–12 But all is not hearts and roses in the control room. Honest and caring professionals can, in the course of a scenario, arrive at substantive and meaningful differences. Although we encourage discussion and dialogue to iron out these same differences, at times our baser instincts emerge and instructors do settle things the old-fashioned way.

the ass! Instead of just punching in "Saturation 92%," you have to "program the physiology to create the number." No surprise, then, that when you do this on the fly you can easily overshoot or undershoot. All this "programming in the physiology" is great when you generate a programmed scenario well ahead of time. But when you're sitting there and just want the *damned sat to go to 92% right now*, the METI can be maddening.

What Do the Residents Do?

- Turn up the FIO_2 to 100%, hand-ventilate, listen to the chest, and pull the endotracheal tube back. At that point, you go to the screen and *want like crazy to just punch in 100% in the saturation area*, but, alas, no. You have to "program the physiology, get rid of the shunt fraction, get rid of the excess oxygen consumption, and the saturation will then work its way back up to 100%. Fortunately, going "back to normal" is pretty easy, as you can just set everything back to normal and up you go.
- Flounder around, forget to listen to the chest, stand there like morons. Bad residents, bad, bad. No treat for you! (Beat them senseless, depending on how strict your department policies are.) So you see, when things go bad, you still get to have fun, no matter which system you are using.

To further illustrate the way the METI and the Laerdal models work, I draw on scenarios right from this book. Chapter 8 has 50 scenarios, each about four pages long. Each scenario is meant to focus on one or two main teaching points. Here I go through the first 20 scenarios and include all the "computer commands" for the simulators. Some scenarios use the METI, some the Laerdal, so you'll be able to see each in action. You will notice a few things.

1. Some scenarios have no computer commands. All the action comes from the standardized patient, an actor with a scripted role to play.
2. The actual number of computer commands is often quite small, as most of the learning is interpersonal, ethical, or communication-related. This doesn't lend itself easily to a computer program.
3. A lot of effort goes into the "around the mannequin" environment—partial task trainers, additional props, telling the surgeon to make the patient move. The mannequin is there and is important, but it's not "all about the mannequin."
4. Anyone reading these scenarios could put in a hundred more computer commands. You can always throw in more variables, more branching points, more outcomes. You can solve one problem (resolve the allergic reaction, for example) and then generate another (perhaps asthma exacerbation).
5. What *is* most important? The teacher, the one making it happen. The one reading the residents/students and tailoring the lesson to make sure that *someone learns something*—the prime directive of any simulation center.

CAUTION: This is damned dreary! These are listed just to show you the "technical steps" you go through in a scenario. In Chapter 8 these will all come to life, so keep the faith!

SCENARIO 1. **A provocative patient acts inappropriately.**

Examining room setting
No computer commands
Examining room with standard props: chart, blood pressure machine, stethoscope
Video recording equipment (as in all the scenarios, so you can review in the debriefing room)
Provocative patient, scripted to make inappropriate remarks

SCENARIO 2. **An intracranial bleed generates hypertension, then Cushing's triad. Later, the patient is underventilated.**

METI mannequin.
OR setting.
Infusion pump with nitroprusside (Nipride) disconnected and dripping on the floor.
To get the BP to 300/160, set the SVR factor high, set LV contractility high.
To get the P to 120, set increased heart rate factor.
Later, to get a reflex bradycardia, set a decreased heart rate factor.
To decrease the blood pressure significantly, enter as medication given a nitroprusside bolus.
To create a high CO_2, set the venous CO_2 level high.

SCENARIO 3. **A pregnant patient is given intravascular local anesthetic through the epidural.**

Laerdal mannequin with wig and pregnant belly; up in stirrups.
Epidural taped to back with epidural infusion pump.
Obstetrician with forceps.
Fetal heart rate monitor simulator (Metron makes one).
To set the FHR to 40, program it into the Metron FHR simulator.

To crash the patient, turn the Saturation monitor off.

SCENARIO 4. **Hypoxemia and myocardial ischemia in the OR.**

METI mannequin in OR setting.
To set the blood pressure to 85/50, lower the SVR.
To set the HR to 130, increase the HR factor.
To get ST elevation, go to Cardiac rhythm override and enter mild ischemia.
To worsen ST elevation, go to Cardiac rhythm override and enter moderate ischemia.

SCENARIO 5. **Narcotic overdose and bradypnea.**

METI simulator in a PACU setting.
Have PACU equipment (suction, oxygen).
Blood gas slip.
Normal CXR in view box.
To slow respiratory rate, enter medications given, give morphine.
To slow respiratory rate more, go to Respiratory gain factor and decrease.
Later, to increase respiratory rate, go to Respiratory gain factor and increase.

SCENARIO 6. **Inducing an aortic stenosis patient in the heart room.**

METI simulator with infiltrated IV arm.
Cardiac OR (bypass machine in room, transducers, infusion pumps).
To increase the blood pressure, increase the SVR factor.
To increase the heart rate, go to Rhythm override and enter sinus tachycardia.
To cause ST depression, go to Rhythm override and enter mild ischemia; then to reverse that, go to Rhythym override and enter sinus rhythm.

SCENARIO 7. **IV phobia in a patient with placenta previa.**

No computer commands.
Examining room with pregnant (or pretend-pregnant) standardized patient.
FHR monitor.
BP machine, examination room equipment.
Patient scripted to be very skittish and difficult.

SCENARIO 8. **No IV access in a bleeding patient with placenta previa.**

Laerdal mannequin in an OR setting.
All vital signs you set directly: HR 130, later 140; BP 90/60, later 80/50.

FHR simulator: set for late decelerations.
Saturation, set directly for 80s, later 70s.
Cover baby with chocolate pudding (keep rest of pudding in fridge for after debriefing).
Set saturation up to 90% when LMA is placed.

SCENARIO 9. **Mediastinal mass.**

METI mannequin in OR setting.
Bronchoscope, rigid.
To create high inspiratory pressures, set bronchial resistance high.

SCENARIO 10. **Triage after a disaster.**

Laerdal mannequins, two.
First mannequin: all vital signs at 0.
Second mannequin: set saturation directly to 85% and HR directly to 140.
To make intubation difficult, activate swelling in the upper airway (press on X's on a diagram in the upper airway, which inflates small air bladders).
Increase saturation once the cricothyrotomy is performed.

SCENARIO 11. **Stat C-section.**

METI mannequin, pregnant.
FHR simulator.
To get BP to 80/50, decrease the SVR and LV contractility.
Set FHR to go to 60, then 50.
Mix up trauma vomit kit setup and have it in patient's mouth (try not to gag yourself).
Turn the BP off.

SCENARIO 12. **Agitation in an ophthalmic case.**

METI simulator.
Some kind of surgical microscope for the ophthalmologist.
A boom box playing Figaro from the opera Carmen.
To get the saturation to 50%, set the shunt fraction and O_2 consumption very high.
Instruct the ophthalmologist how to wiggle the patient to imitate patient movement.
To get ectopy, go to Rhythm override and put in 25% PVCs.
To get V-tach, go to Rhythm override and enter V tach.

SCENARIO 13. **Unstable atrial fibrillation.**

Laerdal mannequin.
Set rhythm, atrial fibrillation.
Set initial blood pressure at 140/85.

Set next blood pressure at 75/40

Program so that at cardioversion ×2, the rhythm converts and blood pressure goes to 140/80.

SCENARIO 14. **Isolating a lung in a difficult airway.**

Laerdal mannequin.

Fiberoptic tower (scope and attached camera and television, so all can see).

Univent endotracheal tube.

Saturation initially set at 100%; later set it at 75%.

SCENARIO 15. **Porphyria.**

METI mannequin.

Three blind mice and a farmer's wife armed with a knife . . . Not really, I'm just seeing if you're paying any attention. As you can see by now, a dull recitation of the computer stroke entries in a simulation scenario is as dry as being force-fed Zweiback toast. The magic is in the "entire thing playing out," as you will see in Chapter 8. Furthermore, *telling* you how to work the computer converts this book into a computer manual. And *no one reads computer manuals.* You learn to work the computer by, well, working the computer. And so also you will learn to work the Laerdal and the METI by, well, working the Laerdal and the METI. Five *minutes* sitting in front of that screen and banging around will outdo five *hours* of reading about it. For completeness' sake, I'll grind all the way through the 20th scenario. Just keep in mind that this section is presented only to give you the *feel* of the "computer work and setup" behind the scenarios.

To drop the heart rate from 70 down to the 30s, go to Rhythm override and enter sinus bradycardia.

To make the chest rigid, go to Chest and lung compliance and decrease both.

To code the patient, go to Rhythm override and go to V tach, then V fib, then asystole.

SCENARIO 16. **Rigid bronchoscopy.**

Laerdal mannequin.

Rigid bronchoscope.

To make the saturation drop, directly enter a saturation of 95, then 75, then go back up.

SCENARIO 17. **Swan dive.**

METI mannequin.

CXR showing fluid in the chest.

To increase inspiratory pressures, go to Lung compliance and decrease.

To drop the saturation, go to Shunt and O_2 consumption and decrease both.

SCENARIO 18. **Epidural hematoma.**

No computer stuff.

Standardized patient coached to play out sensory and motor loss.

SCENARIO 19. **Running two rooms with problems in each.**

Laerdal mannequin in one room, METI in another.

No computer work for the Laerdal.

In the METI room, drop O_2 saturation by increasing shunt and increasing oxygen consumption. Later, reverse these settings.

SCENARIO 20. **Muscular dystrophy and the need for a pacer.**

METI mannequin.

Zoll pads.

To get third degree heart block, go to Rhythm override and enter (guess what?) third degree heart block.

To drop blood pressure to 70/40, decrease SVR and LV contractility.

So there it is, putting a little meat on the bones of the equipment, showing you how you actually work it. This is, as mentioned earlier, just a brush stroke on the actual workings of the Laerdal and METI. Each one has tons of options and programming capabilities (for you to insert your own scenarios). You could—for that matter, should—sit down with a company representative with the actual thing in your hands to understand better the tabs, folders, buttons, and gizmos.

My personal experience? I got in-serviced on the METI along with about another dozen faculty members. As time passed, most others "fell away"; and one other soul (Albert Varon, our education director at the University of Miami) and I became the "involuntary volunteers" in the simulator.

We found that no matter how much in-servicing you get, you don't really know what to do until you throw yourself into it and start "doing simulation" with residents. (My personal thanks to the first residents who had to put up with some serious floundering.)

After a while, we got comfortable enough to do simple things, then branched out. Later, our department got a Laerdal, an entire floor of a building as a Safety Center, and the most important element—

a technician who actually knew what he was doing! (Ilya Shekhter, who provided all the technical help on this and other chapters.) Now, when we do simulations, Ilya does the technical programming, and I do the "in-the-room-medical-stuff." To my mind, that is the best setup—a technician who knows the stuff inside and out (and, frankly, much better than I do)—and a medical instructor who knows the lesson to be learned.

Technician, plus equipment, plus teacher—that is the magic brew.

What if you can't afford a technician? Can you yourself (say, an anesthesia faculty member with an interest in teaching in the Simulator) do it all by yourself? Yes. It's tough though. Things go much better with a dedicated technician to help out.

Now, HAL, I'm done here, open the hatch please. HAL?

CHAPTER 4

Working on Communication Skills in the Simulator

"Speech finely framed delighteth the ears."

2 Maccabees II:39

Picture yourself sitting in front of a person with a doctorate in education (EdD) from Harvard. This professor now holds joint appointments at MIT and Harvard.

The professor is not the Marquis de Sade or the Grand Inquisitor peppering you with rapid fire, trip-you-up, "Where were you on the night of the 15th"? questions. This professor does not have you on the rack, is not holding a cat o'nine tails. No light is shining in your eyes. This professor is not standing over you, does not have you in a shorter chair, has not deprived you of sleep. This professor has not made you take a blood oath of allegiance to the Boston Red Sox. This professor has done nothing whatsoever to intimidate you; on the contrary, this professor has shown nothing but kindness to you.

You ask a question about the behavioral aspects of Simulation training.

"You know, I've studied all about the clinical end for years, the heart attacks and codes and stuff. But this behavioral business, how do I go about learning that?"

"Well", the professor with ties to MIT and Harvard says, "you have to read."

And the professor looks at you.

"Oh," you say, "yeah." And you squeak out a forced/embarrassed/moronic giggle. "Yeah, I guess, to learn something, it does, sort of, make sense that, you know,

you, or me, that is, I would be, um, well advised to, uh, actually open a book and look at the words written in the book, which is what constitutes the act of, well, reading."

"Yes," the person with a doctorate in learning from the most hallowed institutions of learning in the world says, "reading in order to learn has a long track record."

Who are we to argue with that?

You can't just instantly know how to teach the behavioral part—or you could call it the "communication" part—of the Simulation experience. You need to study it, to read about it, just like you had to read about cardiac physiology or the autonomic nervous system.

An initial reaction might be, "Ah, to hell with that psycho-babble. I'm training people in the clinical arena! Codes! Shock! STAT! That's the ticket. The

---

BOX 4-1	How to Learn About Behavior

- **Read**
- **Read**
- **Read**

Simulator was never meant to be a marijuana-laced, Haight-Ashbury-esque, harmonic convergence love fest. Nor is the Simulator meant to teach us how to talk 'administrative-ese' like a bunch of CPAs. So let's skip the 'getting in touch with our feelings' and the 'prioritization of goal-oriented intermediary assessment protocols.' That's all sissy stuff."

You think to yourself, "Why should I read about this fluff at all? Real clinicians don't give a *#! about that hooey anyway. Skip the 'talk' books, let's put that Simulator into V-fib and freak out some students. Now that's REAL learning!"

And, truth to tell, when you start to drift into this behavioral sea, you do hit some suspiciously "administrato-speak" sounding icebergs.

CRISIS RESOURCE MANAGEMENT

What's this? *Crisis* and *management* in the same phrase? "Crisis," which evokes images of the Hindenburg bursting into flames, bodies falling from the sky, people, still smoking, staggering out of the wreckage. "Oh the humanity!" And you couple that with "management"?

Management. Double entry ledgers. Setting minimum the wage. Breaking up the gang around the water cooler with a gruff, "Time is money."

Crisis is a can of Coke that you shake up, then pop open all at once.

Management is a can of Coke you left sitting open in the fridge for 3 days.

Conceptualizing

Six syllables, in one word?

Spare me.

But the kicker in this is—this behavioral stuff really *does* matter. These phrases, although they come across as bloodless and limp, *make a big difference in the crunch*. And the more you read about behavioral psychology, negotiating under stress, working in teams, the more you realize we *do need to know this stuff*. When you see it all unfold in the Simulator, you become a true believer.

The Professor was right: "You have to read."

Hmm. Where to now? Here are the questions:

- What should I read?
- How do I make this reading "meaty"? How do I turn "flat cans of Coke" into "exploding cans of Coke"?

Here is the answer to the first question: What should I read?

- *The 7 Habits of Highly Effective People*. Steven R. Covey. [I listened to the audio tape in my car.]
- *Getting to Yes: Negotiating Agreement without Giving In*. Roger Fisher, William Ury, Bruce Patton
- *Difficult Conversations*. Douglas Stone, Bruce Patton, Sheila Heen
- Notes from the Center for Medical Simulation's "Teach the Teacher" meeting
- *Learning from Accidents*. Trevor Kletz
- *Innovative Simulations for Assessing Professional Competence*. Ara Tekian, Christine H. McGuire, William C. McGaghie
- *Simulators in Anesthesiology Education*. Edited by Lindsey C. Henson and Andrew C. Lee
- *Anger and Other Emotions in Adverse Event and Error Disclosure* [two-DVD set]. Robert Buckman [can order by telephone 1-800 488-8234; e-mail: cinemedic@bellnet.ca; web site: www.cinemedic.com]
- Boulet J, Murray D, Kras J, Woodhouse J, McAllister J, Ziv A. Reliability and validity of a simulation-based acute care skills assessment for medical students and residents. *Anesthesiology* 2003;99:1270–1280 [great bibliography; gets you up to date on all the latest "Simulato-think"]
- Gordon JA [one of the teachers at the "Teach the Teacher" course], Oriol NE, Cooper JB. Bringing good teaching cases "to life": a simulator-based medical education service. *Acad Med* 2004;79(1): 23–27 [Dr. Gordon is major cool, and this article reflects it.]
- LaCombe DM, Gordon DL, Issenberg SB, Vega AI. The use of standardized simulated patients in teaching and evaluating prehospital care providers. Am J Anesthesiol 2000;4:201–204 [how paramedics work into a Simulator program]
- Issenberg SB, et al. Simulation technology for health care professional skills training and assessment. JAMA 1999;282:861–866 [This article sort of "lays out the debate" in the general way that *JAMA* articles do.]
- Issenberg SB [can you tell he's a Kahuna?], et al. Effectiveness of a cardiology review course for internal medicine residents using simulation technology and deliberate practice. Teaching Learn Med 2002;14:223–228 (Simulators are groovy for all specialties!)
- Gordon MS, Issenberg SB [who else?] Mayer JW, Felner JM. Developments in the use of simulators

and multimedia computer systems in medical education. Med Teacher 1999;21:32–36

Here is an answer to the second question, "How do I make this reading 'meaty'?"

Make the administrato-speak (crisis resource management, conceptualization) more vibrant. Put pure learning theory into something you can hold, bite, rend, dismember, eviscerate. Toward that lofty goal, here goes with a "Primer on Behavioral Stuff Writ Gritty for Medical Folk."

Apologies to many and sundry great educators. Lifetimes of learning and entire careers went into all this cerebration. I bastardize, warp, distill, and distort all their fine work into a few punchy lessons. Their brilliant discourse morphs into so many sound bites.

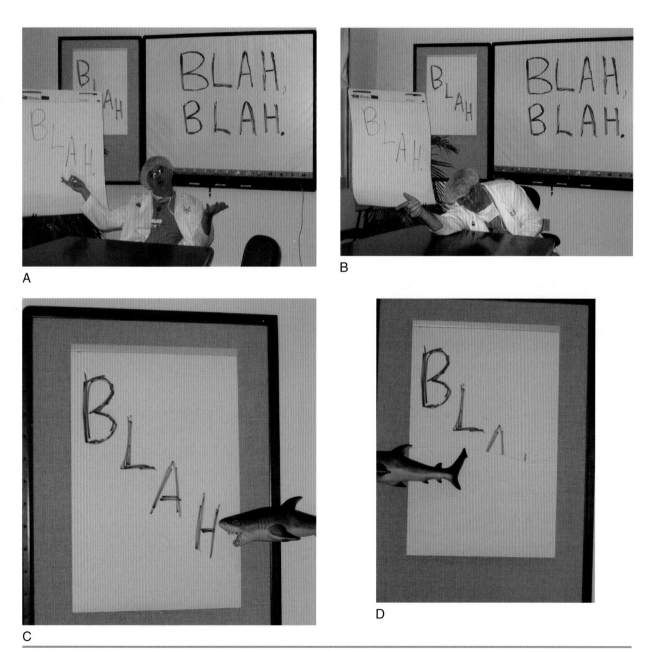

A

B

C

D

FIGURE 4–1   Educational theory and, for that matter, education in general, can drift into an endless blah-blah-blah of lectures, recitations, and stultifying boredom. The simulator, actually *doing something*, can put some *teeth* into the educational experience—can give it a real bite.

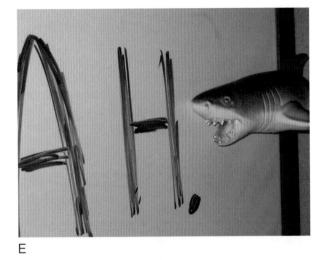

E

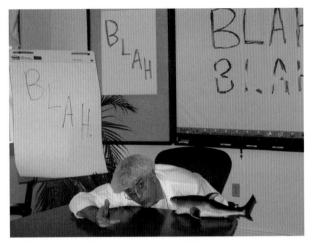

F

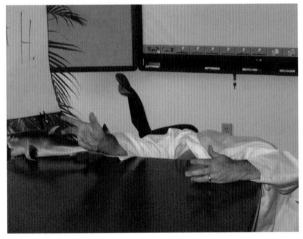

G

FIGURE 4–1   cont'd

Filet mignon covered in ketchup and served as a happy meal.

COMMUNICATION AND BEHAVIORAL STUFF WRIT GRITTY FOR MEDICAL FOLK

Learning

John Dewey, a great educator in the early 20th century, looked at the importance of experience in learning. A good way to learn is "trying to do something and having the thing perceptibly do something in return." That is the siren song of the Simulator! You give epinephrine to the Simulator, and the Simulator responds with a jump in blood pressure and heart rate. John Dewey would love this stuff.

> **BOX 4-2**   John Dewey Paraphrased
>
> **"To learn, do something and have something happen back."**

> *"The first stage of contact with any new material . . . must inevitably be of the trial and error sort."*
> **–Vintage John Dewey**

Bingo! Go into the Simulator, try to intubate a swollen airway, change the head position, try a different blade. . . . No go? Eventually you "trial and error" your way

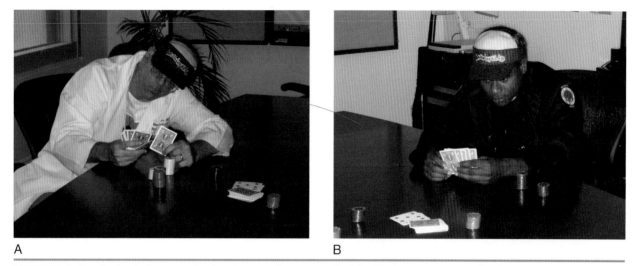

A   B

FIGURE 4–2   In simulation scenarios, you have to play your cards right. You're given a certain hand—say, a patient with a bad airway—and you have to learn to "play the hand you're given." In the case of the bad airway, for example, you may opt for an awake intubation. This is the same "deal" that you get in real life.

all the way to a surgical airway, placing a catheter into the Simulator's cricothyroid membrane and starting jet ventilation.

Dewey said, "What is [needed is] an actual empirical situation as the initiating phase of thought."

You want an empirical situation? How about a mannequin, generating breath sounds on his right side, no breath sounds on his left side, and, through a speaker, gasping and saying, "I can't take a deep . . . breath . . . it's . . . so hard to . . . I . . . just . . . can't." And up on the wall is a chest X-ray showing a pneumothorax and across the room is a computer-generated chart detailing the "patient's" car wreck and rib fractures.

That's a 4+ empirical situation for learning.

Again, Dewey: "No one has ever explained why children are so full of questions outside of the school . . . and the conspicuous absence of display of curiosity about the subject matter of school lessons."

Link to the Simulator? Listen to people chattering away as they walk down the hall after a Simulator scenario.

"Oh man! I'm thinking vagal, then V tach!"

"Did you catch the temp rising?"

"How come *you* got the tube in—his mouth was like a rock!"

Compare that with your average "regular" lesson, a lecture.

"Any questions?", the lecturer asks, looking around at a sea of glazed eyes and partially obstructed airways. "No? Sure? Anyone?"

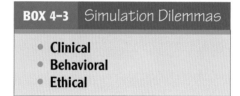

BOX 4–3   Simulation Dilemmas

- **Clinical**
- **Behavioral**
- **Ethical**

"A difficulty is an indispensable stimulus to thinking," Dewey wrote in 1916. Each Simulation scenario has just that—a diagnostic dilemma (is this asthma or CHF?), a treatment headache (do we go right to dantrolene, or do we see if malignant hyperthermia is really happening?), or an ethical problem (his saturation is dropping but he's refusing intubation). And Simulator centers crank out difficulties by the boatload. The Harvard people describe 200 different scenarios. Duke's Simulation center has a ton. Stanford, Houston, Tampa—all across the fruited plain—Simulation centers tap their evil genius to come up with new puzzlers for their students. And these Simulation centers share their wicked twists on their web sites, so Simulator learning metastasizes like a well vascularized malignancy.

You want difficulties?

We got difficulties.

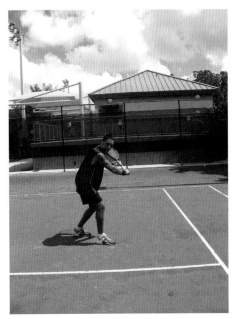

A

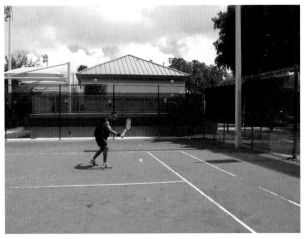

B

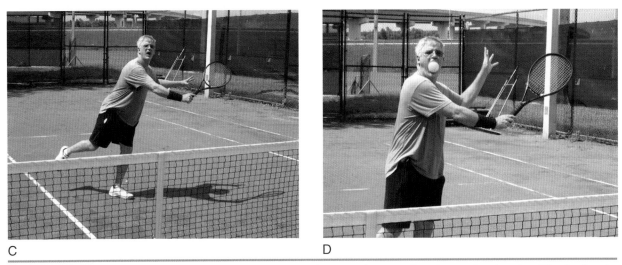

C

D

FIGURE 4–3 The famous educator John Dewey said you need an "actual situation" to do your best learning. That is what the simulator gives you, an actual situation to work through. No tennis player learns to play tennis by reading a book. You need that "actual situation"—a real tennis court, real tennis balls, real racquets, a real opponent—to learn the craft. Here our intrepid instructor learns that perhaps it is time to take up golf.

> *"When an activity is continued into the undergoing of consequences, when the change made by an action is reflected back into the change in us, the mere flux is loaded with significance. We learn something."*
> *Democracy and Education: An Introduction to the Philosophy of Education* (Macmillan, New York, 1916, p. 163)
> —John Dewey

Simulato-people dig their scenarios and jazz them up big time. They want to make Dewey's "flux" memorable. And they don't just ham it up, they breathe life into those scenarios.

"What the hell's going on around here", the medical attending bellows, "I didn't want this guy intubated!"

"My head hurts so bad," the voice from the Simulator says, "this is the worst headache in my life. Am I going to die, doctor? Is this a stroke?"

The more you read Dewey, the more you love the Simulator.

Another angle on learning: Draw an "emotional circle," with low level emotions below—hanging out at Borders on a Saturday afternoon—and high level emotions above—hanging out at Hillary's Step, (a steep rock incline about a thousand feet from Mount Everest's summit) with your oxygen running low and a blizzard blowing in.

Most education is attained via reading and lectures. Plowing through a book or somnambulating through a lecture creates the "Borders" emotional state.

When you go into the Simulator, you get your dander up. You get pumped. Your emotions amp. Red zone. Hillary's Step.

You remember your "Hillary's Step" lessons. You tend to forget your "Borders" lessons.

How About Medical Education?

"Hang around long enough, and you'll see what you need to see," goes the traditional thinking.

- Keep the surgeon in the hospital 95 hours per week for 5 years, and he or she will take care of the requisite number of appendectomies, bowel obstructions, and tumors.
- Sure, malignant hyperthermia is a 1/35,000 event; but if you do enough anesthesia, you'll see it.

- Didn't see Cushing's triad of increased intracranial pressure, hypertension, and bradycardia? Well, do another year of fellowship. It'll pop up. Maybe.

Scripture addressed this aspect of education long ago: "Time and chance happeneth to them all." That is, medical education has traditionally been a crap shoot. *Maybe* you'll see epiglottitis; but then again if you happen to be on vacation when the one case comes in, well, you won't. *Maybe* you'll see an inferior MI with bradycardia, but then, maybe not.

Enter the Simulator

The Simulator slays time and chance. The Simulator can make *sure* you see the rare things and can make *sure* you get practice with, well, whatever your teachers want you to know.

An internal medicine professor wants to make sure all his residents see status asthmaticus progress all the way to respiratory failure. Shazam, the Simulator makes it happen.

An anesthesiology instructor wants to walk his residents through the much-dreaded "can't intubate, can't ventilate" sequence. Voila! Done.

An ER team wants to go through a terrorist attack drill with multiple codes happening at once. No problem.

And best of all, the Simulator can go through these scenarios at *no risk to any patient*. No one had to "allow" asthma to progress to respiratory failure. No one had to "fake" a lost airway and put an anesthetized patient at risk. And no zealous instructor had to go shoot up a crowd to get his mass casualties.

You kill the Simulator? Press the reset button, and Lazarus comes right back at you none the worse for wear.

BOX 4–4	Traditional Education

- Time
- Chance
- Maybe

BOX 4–5	Simulator

- Time not a problem
- Chance not a problem
- Maybe not a problem

And when you look at it from another angle, it makes sense that we practice on un-killable Simulators. With a Simulator, we are doing our first learning on a pretend person. We are doing our first drive in a pretend car, our first flight in a pretend plane.

As medical folk, sooner or later we have to learn by practicing. And because our job involves working on people, it means that, gulp, we learn by practicing on real people.

That's a tough sell to the public.

The public doesn't *mind* that you learn by practicing on real people. So long as it's *other* real people. Not *me* real people. And no matter how you look at it, *everyone* is *me* people. So it makes sense that we practice on the only *non-me* people out there—the Simulator.

Errors

To prevent screw-ups, you have to study screw-ups. And don't just limit yourself to medical ones. Study all sorts of cool stuff. You can always draw some thin thread of relevance to the field of medical education and Simulation.

(Or better yet, just sit back and enjoy. These stories rock!)

So put on your "medical education" cap and follow along. The questions you ask yourself are:

- How did this error "evolve"?
- How could such an "error evolution" occur in medicine?
- How could a Simulator fit in here and "save the day"?

If you're not in the learning mode but are just in this for voyeuristic thrills, ask yourself:

Just how cool is this?
Oh man, isn't it great this didn't happen to me?
When are they going to show this stuff on The Learning Channel?

BOX 4-6 Errors

- **Evolve**
- **Several events coincide**
- **System fails**

Show Me the Money

A psychologist named Lia DiBello, working with the National Science Foundation, took the idea of "business simulation" to three floundering companies: a biotech firm, a foundry, and a nuclear fuel producer. First, DiBello pegged what was going on—she nailed the "error."

At the biotech firm, half the people thought the company was a research firm, and the other half thought it was a commercial enterprise. The left hand didn't know what the right hand was doing.

The foundry had inefficient molds and generated too much scrap. Bosses in the office didn't know what was going on the "floor" of the factory. Floor workers didn't realize the impact of these inefficiencies on the company's profits. The left hand didn't *care* what the right hand was doing.

In the nuclear fuel company (God Almighty, I *hope* they get it right!), managers from various departments feuded and sniped at each other. The left hand was *beating the hell* out of the right hand.

Now go to the three questions.

1. *How did the error evolve?* Over time all the companies "pulled apart," and no one was working together.
2. *How could such an error evolve in medicine?* Think of the departments at your hospital. Do they work together, or do they set up separate bailiwicks, each looking after its own interest? Think of the subdivisions in your departments. Just how much do they talk with each other?
3. *How could a Simulator "save the day"?* Psychologist DiBello went to work. (Her company, in San Diego, is called Workforce Transformation Research and Innovation—www.wtri.com; e-mail: contactWTRI@wtri.com; telephone: 619-232-8054.) She set up intense business simulations where everyone had to work together. Like it or not, the right hand and the left hand had to cooperate.

The biotech firm had to do a Simulation exercise designed by the fine people of WTRI. Research and development had to pay attention to financial realities and design something that would actually sell. Then they had to get the goods out on time, assess whether the product was selling, and dump the unprofitable junk. Now everyone, even the research people, were working toward a profit. Guess what? After the exercise, the company started making a real, not a simulated, profit.

At the foundry, the floor workers had to do a Simulation where they designed more efficient molds. Voila! They generated less scrap, saved money, and took this lesson back to the factory. And now the foundry is in the black. Uh, as in black *ink*, not black soot.

In nuclear-ville, DiBello's Simulation forced the various managers to work together. They had to, well, perform the managerial equivalent of a *fusion* reaction. No explosion occurred, thank goodness, and the company went on to enjoy financial success.

Well hot diggity dog, the Simulator did come to the rescue!

Could a Medical Simulator work similar magic?

Hell yes! Medical Simulators are the greatest thing since pizza delivery. Medical Simulators walk on water, and the water doesn't have to be frozen when they do it.

Well, perhaps I'm given over to a modicum of hyperbole, but a medical Simulator could certainly *help*.

- Mass casualty exercise where surgeons, anesthesiologists, intensivists, and nursing staff work together.
- End of life exercise where a dying patient is in severe respiratory distress. Ethicists, clergy, and doctors could work out this difficult scenario together.
- Radiologists, radiology techs, engineers, and anesthesiologists could work together on the problem of the anesthetized patient in a new radiology device.

Workforce Transformation Research and Innovation has identified and solved big, expensive problems in industry. By getting disparate elements to work together in a Simulation, they have succeeded in the prime dictum of business: "*Take care of the bottom line*."

Time for *us* to take the hint. We should use the Simulator to make our disparate medical elements work together. That way we can succeed in the prime dictum of medicine: "*Take care of the patient*."

A Samovar with Attitude

The Soviet take on nuclear safety should raise an eyebrow or two. One manager of a nuclear reactor said, "A nuclear reactor is just a samovar." (An ornate kind of teapot used in Russia.)

On April 26, 1986, the samovar at Chernobyl served up a nasty brew. The managers decided to do a safety test that day (note the irony). During the safety test, a series of glitches occurred. The engineers:

- Cut off power to the water-cooling system.
- Didn't insert enough of the radioactive rods into a graphite "absorber."

- Disconnected a safety switch that would have dropped the radioactive rods into the graphite "absorber."

And the design of the reactor itself had a basic design flaw: As the reactor overheated, the nuclear reaction sped up. That is, there was no feedback loop to stop a runaway reaction.

A 9-foot thick concrete shield on top of the reactor blew off and fell to the ground with, one assumes, a loud sound. A total of 45 people died right then or over the next few months, and thousands would likely die from cancer from the released radiation.

Children in that area of the Ukraine have to look at painted pictures of trees on the walls in their schools because they are not allowed to walk in the woods. Too much radiation out there.

To this day.

How Did this Error "Evolve"?

It is easy with this "mother of all disasters" to fall into the trap of error analysis—assign blame to the lowest level engineers, the last guys to press the buttons.

"They blew it" (literally).
"They should have known."
"They're ultimately responsible, so pin it on them."

And when you jump into this "blame game," you can't help but feel good. Something terrible happened. You have someone at whom you can point your finger. Maybe sue them, fire them, imprison them. Maybe some irate relative will even whack them. Hey, great, we killed the bad guys, just like in some Clint Eastwood movie.

So everything's OK now, right?

Well, no.

It's satisfying to nail it all on that last poor jerk, but it doesn't do any good. A flawed *system* brought about this "tempest in a samovar" and only a *system* analysis can fix it. So go back as far as you can, find every element that contributed to the blow-out, and work your fix from there.

- Design of the reactor itself—build in a feedback loop that doesn't allow a runaway reaction.
- Make sure management and technicians know you have to keep sufficient power going to the water coolant system.
- Instill "safety" in the workplace, so no one would ever think to disconnect the crucial safety switch.

Better yet, design in a redundant safety switch as a backup.

So rather than a simple "*he* did it," look at the evolution of the error and say, "Let's make sure *we* can never do it again."

How Could Such an Error Evolve in Medicine?

A medical pipeline crossover unfolds just like a mini-Chernobyl. And, just like Chernobyl, the solution lies in a system review. Find out how the system made it happen and fix the system. Don't just take one poor fellow out and hang him from the yardarm.

Here's our medical Chernobyl.

- A patient getting oxygen and nitrous oxide during an operation starts to turn blue, and the blood gets dark.
- The anesthesiologist turns off the nitrous oxide and goes all the way up on his oxygen flow.
- The patient worsens and dies.
- That afternoon, a plumbing company discovers that it mixed up the oxygen and nitrous oxide lines. When the anesthesiologist went all the way up on his oxygen, he was actually cutting off the patient's oxygen.

Just as in our initial reaction to Chernobyl, the first thing you want to do is blame someone. Stupid anesthesiologist! Stupid plumber!

Fine. Do that. Sue them, ruin them. But no one's any safer than before. You have not fixed the system.

A system fix goes like this.

- Have any industrial work at the hospital "out in the open." That way people are aware that something fishy might occur.
- Work with oxygen supply people so they know just how crucial the oxygen supply is.
- Schedule work at a nonbusy time in the OR to minimize the impact (say, a Sunday).
- Train anesthesiologists always to use and watch the oxygen analyzer—that's the only way to make sure you're giving oxygen.
- Ditto on use of the pulse oximeter.
- Make sure everyone checks the oxygen cylinders and knows how to open them in case the pipeline oxygen fails.

How Could a Simulator Help?

The best way to practice an oxygen mix-up is to go through it yourself. You need to experience oxygen not

BOX 4–7	Where to Study Errors?

- **Industry**
- **Medicine**
- **Military blunders**

coming through where it should, and you need to recognize the problem, open the oxygen cylinder, and get that damned oxygen in fast!

Better yet, do it while throwing in a few glitches—an oxygen cylinder not hooked up right, a malfunctioning Ambu-bag, hell, go all the way to doing mask-to-mouth ventilation! How's that for *the ultimate*?

How are you going to do that on a real patient? I sure hope you don't do that drill with *me* on the table. I've got few enough brain cells as it is!

Enter the Simulator!

In a separate facility, where patients will never be taken care of, you can engineer in this very mix-up. Then you can run your residents and medical students through the pipeline crossover in perfect safety.

Poifect!

Charge of the Light Brigade

Now we shift gears a little and look at errors in military history.

"Attack what? What guns, Sir?"

> *Half a league, half a league, half a league onwards,*
> *All in the valley of Death rode the six hundred.*
> . . .
> *Cannon to the right of them,*
> *Cannon to the left of them,*
> *Cannon to the front of them volley'd and thunder'd.*
>
> **The Charge of the Light Brigade**
> **–Alfred Lord Tennyson 1854**

Industry gave us some errors to analyze. And there's a certain thrill in turning a company around. Profits are nice.

The Chernobyl paradigm cranked the whole subject up a notch. Error analysis takes on genuine palpable significance as a 9 foot thick chunk of burning, radioactive concrete falls on your head.

But to really sink your teeth into the land of the mondo error, go military. From sticks and rocks, to arrows and javelins, through muskets and bayonets, and all the way up to our smart bombs and night-vision laser-guided missiles, man has always put some innovative thought into killing his fellow man. Whether you ride in the Pharaoh's war chariot, the German Tiger tank, or the Stealth bomber, the military goal is always the same—kill the other guy, don't get killed yourself.

Errors in the military world are easy to spot. Ask Custer's troopers scattered around the hills and ravines of the Little Bighorn. Ask Pickett's infantrymen carpeting the ground on Cemetery Ridge in Gettysburg.

Let's do a "system" review on the charge that inspired Lord Tennyson's most famous poem, *The Charge of the Light Brigade*.

How Did this Error "Evolve"?

October 25, 1854 found Britain and France at war with Russia. Troops faced each other on the Crimean Peninsula, a part of southern Russia jutting into the Black Sea. A British detachment of cavalry, the Light Brigade, about 600 mounted men, faced Russian lines near the Russian city of Balaclava.

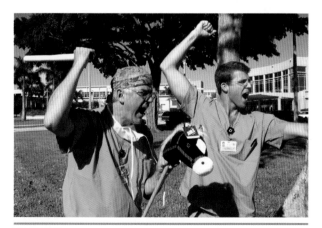

FIGURE 4–4 The heroic yet ill-fated "Charge of the Light Brigade" has been caught in this previously unpublished and rare photograph. Studying historical disasters uncovers the same mistakes we make in the hospital today. Miscommunication, misunderstanding, and, oh, did I say miscommunication? Disastrous for the Light Brigade, disastrous for us.

The British officers in charge of the British cavalry, Lord Cardigan (yes, of cardigan sweater fame) and Captain Lewis Nolan were described as follows: "Two such fools could hardly be picked out of the British Army." Oh, and if that weren't bad enough, they hated each other. Another cavalry officer thrown into this stew was one named Lord Lucan, who also hated Nolan.

Above these three squabbling ninnies was another officer, Lord Raglan (no sweater named after him), who had earned the unofficial title "Lord Look-On" because he couldn't figure out what was going on during battle and so would often just have his troops sit there and do nothing. Everyone hated him for this, and he hated them back.

So everybody hated everybody, and no one knew anything.

On the big day, the battle had begun, and all the involved officers were clueless. Other British troops had attacked one part of the Russian line, and the Russians were retreating. But a lot of the other Russian lines were intact. At this time, armies used black powder for their muskets and their cannons, so there was much smoke, noise, and confusion.

So Lord Raglan (Lord Look-On, who never knew when to do what) ordered an attack "to the front." He gave the message to Captain Lewis Nolan (one of the "Two such fools could hardly be picked out of the British Army"), who gave the message to another guy, Lord Lucan, the guy Nolan hated. And then to Lord Cardigan (the other of the "Two such fools. . . .").

So, at this point, the entire "Command and Control" is in place for a complete fiasco.

Then, the following communications occurred.

- Lucan *didn't know where to go* and asked, "Attack sir? Attack what? What guns, sir?"
- Raglan knew where he wanted the Light Brigade to go, but he *didn't clarify that to anyone*, plus he stayed up on a hill, far away from the Light Brigade.
- Nolan *didn't know where they were supposed to go*, so he just waved down a valley and said, "There, my Lord, is your enemy! There are your guns!" So with no knowledge of the ground or the situation,

BOX 4-8	Charge of The Light Brigade

- **Goal? Unclear**
- **Leadership? Poor**
- **Visibility? Smoky**

he ordered the Light Brigade down a valley that had guns at the end, plus guns on both sides of the valley.

- Lord Cardigan, with the Light Brigade, *did* know the situation and said, "the Russians have a battery in the valley on our front and batteries and riflemen on each flank." But he didn't think to point this out to any officers above him. He *didn't think to question* the judgment of those who ordered the slaughter of his men.

> *Their's not to reason why,*
> *Their's but to do and die.*
> *The Charge of the Light Brigade*
> −Alfred Lord Tennyson 1854

And die they did: 607 rode down into the valley, 346 rode out.

How Could such an Error Evolve in Medicine?

It was the blind leading the blind when the Light Brigade charged into the Valley of Death near Balaclava. Personal resentments, incompetence, lost communication, fear of questioning "superiors"—it all added up. And empty saddles turned into epic poetry.

We've emptied saddles in the hospital with the same petty squabbles, lost communications, and fear of questioning superiors. Try this out for a "Medical Balaclava."

- A patient had a difficult intubation 3 days ago, was sent home, and came back to the ER with difficulty breathing.
- In the ER an esophageal tear is diagnosed, and the patient is admitted to the ICU.
- No one thinks to contact the anesthesiologist, who knew about the bad airway and the tough intubation but didn't bother to follow up because it was a weekend.
- In the ICU, the nursing staff notes low saturation, applies oxygen, and notifies the surgeon who did the original case (but the anesthesiologist didn't bother to tell him about the difficult intubation).
- Neither the surgeon nor the anesthesiologist talk to each other much, as they hate each other, but the HMO sort of "shoves" them together.
- The ICU nurses call the surgeon, who tells them he's busy, this is his clinic day, quit bugging him and

call "some intensivist. I don't care who, call the HMO to see who will see him."

- The HMO has changed its number, and no nurse is sure who should call.
- The patient continues to languish, with a steadily worsening airway and falling saturation.
- No intensivist is called because everyone thinks someone else has done it.
- That afternoon, the surgeon comes in and sees the patient is just about to code. He demands to know what the hell's been going on all day, just as the patient has a respiratory arrest.
- No one can intubate the patient, a trach is attempted, but the trach kit did not have a blade in it, and the patient dies.

How Could a Simulator Help Here?

The Simulator can jump through only so many airway and hemodynamic hoops. With the right Simulato-people, the Simulator can jump through an entire Light Brigade of behavioral hoops.

Based on the above (I blush to say), real-life catastrophe, you can arrange the Simulato-people in any way. You bring to life real take-home lessons.

- Role clarity—Make sure that the surgeon in charge does, indeed, take charge. Just because a complication occurs on a busy clinic day, you don't just shuttle your patient off to "some intensivist" without looking at the patient yourself to see how bad he is.
- Clear communication—When a patient looks like death warmed over, you make sure everyone knows. Surgeon, anesthesiologist, respiratory, head nurse of the ICU.
- Resource management—Hey, get the big airway guns involved early, whether that means anesthesia with a fiberoptic or ENT with a knife—mobilize early to secure that all-important airway.
- No blind obedience—If a doc blows off a nurse but the nurse sees big trouble coming (a deteriorating patient), this is no time to play shrinking violet. This is no time to drag out the Nuremberg defense and say, "I was just following orders." In the Simulator, the ICU nurse should go that extra mile, contact whoever it takes, rattle whatever cage needs rattling, to get the patient the help he needs.

All this you can act out, critique, and discuss in the Simulator. Use the Simulator to stay out of the Valley of Death.

Yapping

> *"You talk the talk. Do you walk the walk?"*
>
> **Full Metal Jacket**

Well, in medical circles, sometimes talking the talk *is* walking the walk.

- A routine delivery goes sour. Shoulder dystocia, stuck kid, emergent C-section, lose mother and child to a lost airway. Now you have to go out in the lobby and explain to the husband what happened.
- A patient with sleep apnea gets too much narcotic and arrests. No one notices until brain damage occurs. The patient is a 45-year-old father of three, and you have to talk to his 25-year-old daughter.
- An extremely bright 6-year-old with spina bifida just got another ventriculoperitoneal shunt done and asks you, "Since they fixed that, will I be able to move my legs now like the other kids?"

You're the doc, you have to now talk the talk.

Can a Simulator experience help you out here? Can *anything* help you navigate through such rough weather?

And it's not just a question of breaking horrible news to patients. There are other tough clinical scenarios that require skill and tact.

A patient is clearly circling the drain—saturation dropping, respirations shallow, fizzling blood pressure. You know you have to intubate to save the patient, but the patient is saying, "I don't want that." His son is saying, "Do everything for Dad."

A code is in full swing, then the floor charge nurse runs in and says, "This patient is a no code!" and you stop resuscitative efforts. Fifteen minutes later, you find out the patient in the next bed was a no code, and the nurse grabbed the wrong chart.

An anesthesia colleague just had quintuplets and keeps showing up to work exhausted. Time and again you come into the OR and his head is on the machine—he's sound asleep. What do you tell him? Do you recommend he be fired?

Each of these situations requires talking skills, negotiating skills, thinking skills. At first blush, these "talking assignments" seem absolutely impossible. (How the hell do you explain a catastrophe, a real iatrogenic disaster?)

Well, like any other tough clinical task, you *can* learn to handle it. Truth to tell, you *have* to learn to handle it. And, yes, you can do it in a Simulator setting. Some would involve an actual Simulator mannequin (for example, the deteriorating patient who doesn't want to be intubated), and others would involve actors in a conference room (for example, the daughter of the brain-damaged sleep apnea patient).

However it's done, it's worth learning to talk the talk.

The two-DVD set, *How to Deal with Anger & Other Emotions*, takes on the toughest talking assignments you could ever possibly handle. (AUTHOR'S NOTE: I highly recommend getting this DVD set. Learn its lessons. Use the set to teach your residents and medical students.)

This superb teaching vehicle has developed a mnemonic, CONES, for "have to tell" situations.

C: Context—Make sure the conversation is set in the proper *context*—a private room, everybody sitting down—look the people in the eyes and shake their hand. You want to make a connection, both physically with your demeanor and physically in the sense of making everyone comfortable.

O: Opening shot—You set the mood by saying, "I'd like some time to tell you about something that happened to your mother." There's no candy-coating bad news, and you must eventually spin out the details, but you have to start the big ball rolling *somehow*, and this seems to be the best way to do it.

N: Narrative—Do a "Just the facts, ma'am" chronologic description of what happened. At each stage of the event, you can detail what you were thinking. For example, in the shoulder dystocia case, you could say: "At this point, we thought the delivery was going well, but actually the shoulder was stuck."

E: Emotions—Acknowledge the emotions of the listeners. "I know this comes as a terrible shock," you can say. "This is terribly hard on you, and to tell you the truth it is terribly hard on the whole team in the intensive care unit."

S: Strategy and summary—No matter what has happened, the goal is to keep in touch, keep the family members informed, and work toward solving the problem. Even if the only solution is discovering exactly what went wrong, that is at least a strategy.

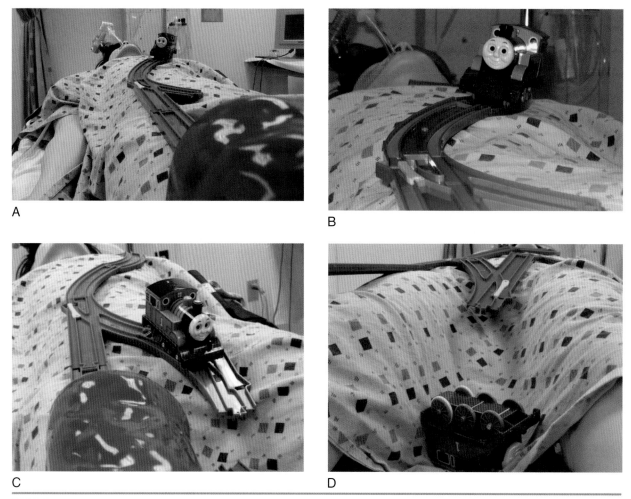

FIGURE 4–5 What made Thomas jump the tracks and crash? Poor planning, not knowing what was ahead. One huge benefit of practicing "train crashes" in the simulator? Everyone walks away from these accidents. Bruised egos, yes; it's true that you sometimes have to brush off your ego after you "crash the train." But no *patient* ever gets hurt.

BOX 4-9 Cones

- **Context**
- **Opening shot**
- **Narrative**
- **Emotions**
- **Summary**

This might look neat and tidy, but no rugged explanation fits into neat pigeonholes. Emotion pokes its head into every phase of the conversation. (Wouldn't you get emotional if you were getting bad news?)

The *How to Deal with Anger and Other Emotions* DVD set lays out eight scenarios. In each, the explaining doctor uses the CONES technique. (He is the most unflappable and professional speaker I've ever seen.

This guy could probably talk his way past St. Peter at the Pearly Gates no matter how stained his soul!)

To respect their copyright, I'll create my own scenarios and use of the CONES technique. And to throw the CONES technique in relief, I'll show how to do it *wrong* first.

Caveat: Certain medical professionals do *not* need to learn this information. Scan the list below and see if you belong.

You never make a mistake.
You never have to deliver bad news.
Everyone you deal with loves, respects, and worships you; and they would never get angry with you.

If you *don't* belong to that list, read on.

Any doctor in clinical practice has had a few train crashes, just as Thomas the Train jumps the tracks in

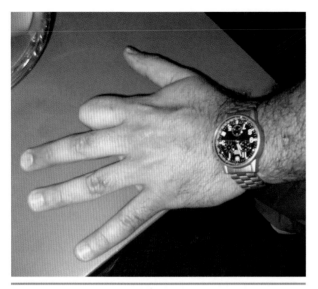

FIGURE 4–6 "Just how did I lose my finger, anyway?" the patient asks. No one tells him, no one explains. And guess what? The patient sues. Surprise, surprise. In the simulator, you can create these problems (*pretending* to cut off a finger, no need to do it for real, please) and then see how the residents handle this difficult task. Just how *do* you break bad news to a patient? How do you explain a complication or bad outcome? You might as well practice this in the simulator because one fine day you will have to do it for real.

Figure 4–5. Let's read about a case where the Thomas the Train crash involved a finger.

First, How to Do It Wrong: A Lost Finger

Mr. O'Shaughnessy entered the hospital for a radical prostatectomy. His arms were tucked for the procedure. At the end of the operation, with his arms still tucked, the foot of the bed was brought up.

His right index finger got squished and amputated.

The patient woke up in the PACU in so much pain from his prostate operation that it took him a while to register his hand pain.

Back on the floor now, Mr. O'Shaughnessy noticed that his left hand had five digits, and his now-throbbing right hand had but four!

Something's amiss!

"What happened?" Mr. O'Shaughnessy asked the floor nurse.

The floor nurse didn't know, he had just come on shift. Maybe the nurse from the last shift knew.

No luck there.

Did the surgeon know? No, the surgeon was busy, hard to reach, and when finally contacted didn't want to talk about it.

BOX 4-10 The Lost Finger

- No one talks
- No one explains
- Get my lawyer

The next morning on rounds, the surgeon looked at "Mr. O'S's bandages" in the perineum and didn't talk at all about the hand.

The anesthesiologist on the case was so freaked out by this thing that he stuck his head in the sand and refused to see the patient.

"What happened?" Mr. O'Shaughnessy kept asking. "What happened to my finger, will someone just tell me?"

Surgeon—nope.

Anesthesiologist—gone.

Nurse from OR—nope.

This one, that one, the other one, the administrator, the butcher, the baker, the candlestick maker, rich man, poor man, beggar man, thief—*nobody knows nuthin'!*

Mr. O'Shaughnessy sued.

At the trial, he said, "I know things can go wrong. And I was so thankful to get through that big operation alive, I wanted to hug everyone at that hospital.

"If someone had just sat down with me and told me what happened to my finger, then that would have been that. But *no one talked to me.*"

Let's Take a Different Tack, the CONES Approach

C—Context

Anesthesiologist and surgeon enter the patient's room after his amputated finger is cleaned and dressed. Mr. O'Shaughnessy has enough pain meds on board to be comfortable but not so much that he's woozy and out of it.

The doctors turn off the TV, close the door, and pull up their chairs. Mr. O'Shaughnessy's wife is present. The kids are out in the waiting room, so they can be informed soon after.

O—Opening shot

"We're here to talk to you today about what happened to your hand."

This is, after all, the issue that draws everyone together. No beating around the bush and inquiring after other things—the surgical drains, the sore throat from the endotracheal tube.

N—Narrative

The surgeon starts out, "We had finished the operation and were getting ready to wake you up. We were taking notes on how much fluid you'd gotten, how much blood you'd lost, making sure you were doing OK."

Then the anesthesiologist takes up the thread, "Part of the operation is putting the foot of the bed down, then at the end we put the foot of the bed up. There's an elbow there, and when that elbow folded up, your finger got pinched in there and cut off. At the time, I was watching your vital signs and breathing, and I didn't check under the blankets, where your finger was getting hurt."

"You were still asleep from the anesthetic, so you couldn't let us know we were pinching your finger."

"The circulating nurse saw the blood when she pulled off the blanket," the surgeon says, "and that's when we saw the damage. I asked the anesthesiologist to keep you asleep and let the hand doctor look over your finger and see if he could reattach it. But the hand doctor said the damage was too much, so he cleaned it up and closed it to keep out infection."

That's it. Just a chronology of the events, with some additions on what the doctors were thinking at the time. Not editorializing or excusing, just explaining.

E—Emotions

"I know this must be a terrible shock to you," the anesthesiologist says. "You came in here for a prostate operation, and here you have lost a finger."

Acknowledge the anger the patient must feel. (Think how *you* would feel if this had happened to you.)

"Here you have pain that you expected from your prostate operation," the surgeon adds, "and now there's this terrible pain in your hand too. That has to be so maddening."

S—Strategy and summary

"So where do we go from here," the anesthesiologist says. "We are certainly going to review our policy on making sure we are more careful when we lift the foot of the bed from now on."

The surgeon takes it from there, "We'll have the hand surgeon come by and make sure your injured hand is taken care of. We're terribly sorry this occurred and want you to know that. If you need help with management of your pain, we'll have a pain specialist see you. And if any questions come up or other problems, here's my card, with my own cell phone on it. Call anytime."

Both doctors stand and shake, well, O'Shaughnessy's left hand. Making that physical connection is important. You are making a link with the patient. OK, a screw-up happened, but at least you've been up front and honest about it. You've told him what happened, how it happened, and what you intend to do about it.

This CONES episode went smooth as silk, but of course it assumed a completely silent and accepting patient, who never once spoke up, protested, or complained.

A cardboard cutout patient, not a real one.

Here goes the same episode with more realistic patient reactions.

C—Context

Anesthesiologist and surgeon enter the patient's room after his amputated finger is cleaned and dressed. Mr. O'Shaughnessy has enough pain meds on board to be comfortable but not so much that he's woozy and out of it.

"God damn, it's about time you got in here," Mr. O'Shaughnessy says.

"What the hell did you do to my husband?" Mrs. O'Shaughnessy shouts, *"You're operating on his prostate and you cut off his finger. Who's watching him, huh? Do I have to go in there and make sure you don't cut him to pieces?"*

The doctors turn off the TV, close the door, and pull up their chairs. The kids are out in the waiting room, so they can get informed soon after.

O—Opening shot.

"We're here to talk to you today about what happened to your hand."

"You sure as hell ARE here to talk about my hand," Mr. O'Shaughnessy says, *"or at least what's left of it. You'll excuse me if I don't 'give you five' for a job well done!"*

This is, after all, the issue that draws everyone together. No beating around the bush and inquiring after other things—the surgical drains, the sore throat from the endotracheal tube.

N—Narrative

The surgeon starts out, "We had finished the operation and were getting ready to wake you up. We were taking notes on how much fluid you'd gotten, how much blood you'd lost, making sure you were doing OK."

"Did you count the blood he lost when you squashed his hand?" Mrs. O'Shaughnessy says, *"God, never in a million years."*

Then the anesthesiologist takes up the thread: "Part of the operation is putting the foot of the bed down, then at the end we put the foot of the bed up. There's an elbow there, and when that elbow folded up your finger got pinched in there and was cut off. At the time, I was watching your vital signs and breathing, and I didn't check under the blankets, where your finger was getting hurt."

"You were still asleep from the anesthetic, so you couldn't let us know we were pinching your finger."

"The circulating nurse saw the blood when she pulled off the blanket," the surgeon says, "and that's when we saw the damage. I asked the anesthesiologist to keep you asleep and let the hand doctor look over your finger and see if he could reattach it. But the hand doctor said the damage was too much, so he cleaned it up and closed it to keep out infection."

That's it. Just a chronology of the events, with some additions on what the doctors were thinking at the time. Not editorializing or excusing, just explaining.

E—Emotions
"I know this must be a terrible shock to you," the anesthesiologist says. "You came in here for a prostate operation, and here you have lost a finger."

"Easy for you to say it's a shock, I'm the guy who looks like a freak now," Mr. O'Shaughnessy says.

Acknowledge the anger the patient must feel. (Think how *you* would feel if this had happened to you.)

"Here you have pain that you expected from your prostate operation," the surgeon adds, "and now there's this terrible pain in your hand too. That has to be so maddening."

"Well, it is maddening," Mr. O'Shaughnessy says, "but hell, at least someone's giving me some answers. Where do we go from here? Cut off one on the other side to make me look even?"

S—Strategy and summary
"So where do we go from here?" the anesthesiologist says. "We are certainly going to review our policy on making sure we are more careful when we lift the foot of the bed from now on."

Then the surgeon takes it from there, "We'll have the hand surgeon come by and make sure your injured hand is taken care of. We're terribly sorry this occurred and want you to know it. If you need help with management of your pain, we'll have a pain specialist see you."

Both doctors stand and shake, well, O'Shaughnessy's left hand. Making that physical connection is important. You are making a link with the patient. OK, a screw-up happened, but at least you've been up front and honest about it. You've told him what happened, how it happened, and what you intend to do about it.

"Well, OK fellas, thanks for stopping by," Mr. O'Shaughnessy says, "but be more careful next time, will ya? I've never played the piano before, but if I ever decide to learn," he holds up his hands and wiggles his 9 fingers, "I'm already behind the 8 ball."

Humor's good! Not that explaining a medical error should turn into a Comedy Central routine, but humor shows you've kept a relationship with a patient.

That's what CONES is all about, keeping a relationship with a patient. It's not a trick for bamboozling a patient. It's not smoke and mirrors to hide a mistake. It's not a miracle to "make it all better." No matter what happens, no matter the news, you want to keep that door open to the patient or that family.

CONES holds that door open.

Negotiating

> *"Your money or your life!"*
> *"Is there a third option?"*
> —The last words of a poor negotiator

Chernobyl was a samovar with attitude.

Negotiating is yapping with attitude.

Medical folk negotiate and need to know the craft. A detour into the business world can help. The Douglas Stone, Bruce Patton, and Sheila Heen book *Difficult Conversations: How to Discuss What Matters Most* does us a world of good. These clever cusses hail from Harvard, and their book ended up on the New York Times business bestseller list, so they must have *something* going on. Let's fast rope right into the heart of this puppy, lift their best ideas, give them a medical twist, then get out quick before they notice we're peeking.

(While they're siccing their lawyers on me, some of you go out and buy their book, so they won't be able to accuse me of hurting their sales.)

To bite the head off this book and suck its guts out, let's look at a typical medical negotiation. Then let's rip-off, er, borrow, the lessons learned from our Harvard brethren.

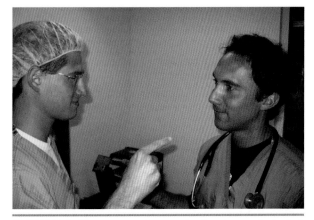

FIGURE 4-7   Pointing fingers, the favorite pastime of all doctors in all specialties in all hospitals. Because the simulator is a place to practice *everything*, you should find time to practice that core clinical competence of interpersonal and communication skills. Get residents out of this finger-pointing habit. Teach them to communicate with their colleagues in a professional manner, keeping the discussion above-board and free of emotion. Then later they can go out and slash the bastard's tires in the parking lot.

An Intensive Care Unit Anywhere in the US of A

Surgeon: *"Go to hell!"*

Anesthesiologist: *"No, YOU go to hell!"*

OK, let's tap the vast fields of Harvardian knowledge to analyze this negotiation. What can we, as medical professionals, draw from this discourse?

First, using the techniques included in *Difficult Conversations*, we'll look at the short version of this ICU conversation.

> Sort out what happened.
> Look at the emotions involved.
> Stake out your identity.
> Look at the purpose of this conversation.
> Look at the issue as a disinterested third party.
> Explore both sides of the story, staying away from blame and finger pointing.
> Come up with an option that helps both sides.
> Draw on standards that can help out.
> Keep communicating as the solution appears.

Applied to this mini-conversation, then, the *Difficult Conversations* approach might look like this.

> Sort out what happened.
> *The surgeon yelled, the anesthesiologist yelled back.*
> Look at the emotions involved.
> *Ticked off and ditto on the ticked off.*
> Stake out your identity.

> *Each thinks he has cornered the market on truth.*
> Look at the purpose of this conversation.
> *To prove who's tougher.*
> Look at the issue as a disinterested third party.
> *Hopeless.*
> Explore both sides of the story, staying away from blame and finger pointing.

Well, according to the surgeon, the anesthesiologist's a moron. And according to *you*, the surgeon is a moron. To me, looking from the outside, I see a pair of morons.

> Come up with an option that helps both sides.
> *Pistols at 20 paces. See you at dawn.*
> Draw on standards that will help out.
> *I'll draw a target on both your chests.*
> Keep communicating as the solution appears.
> *Where's your life insurance stuff?*

Hard to draw much from that. We'll need to flesh out circumstances a little to make sense of this ICU mini-drama.

The Case in Point

Hiram McGillicutty is a 59-year-old man who's led a life ill-advised and poorly executed. Demon liquor is no stranger to Hiram, nor is the nefarious tobacco plant. As if that weren't enough, Hiram has been looking for love in all the wrong places and has become a frequent flyer at the sexually transmitted disease clinic.

And now Mr. McGillicutty, after many errors in judgment and yet more forays into the sins of the flesh, has come to this. He resides on a ventilator. Two weeks ago, he entered the hospital with hemoptysis, was found to have a lung tumor, and had a lobectomy. His health, frail in the best of times and little helped by his largely liquid diet in the outside world, is now so bad that he can't wean from the ventilator.

Caring for Mr. McGillicutty are an anesthesiologist and a surgeon, now at loggerheads about a clinical decision.

From day 1, these two specialists have gone at it hammer and tongs. The surgeon wanted a thoracic epidural to help with pain control, but the anesthesiologist didn't want to place one for fear of some bleeding into the epidural space. "Humph," the surgeon says, "if the anesthesiologist had a little guts, that epidural would have helped with pain control, McGillicutty would be able to take bigger breaths, and we wouldn't be in this fix now!"

Blood loss was high during the operation, and the anesthesiologist is still steaming about that. "Humph, a better surgeon would have kept that bleeding down, and McGillicutty wouldn't be in this fix now!"

Clashes continued over nutrition, sedation meds, talking with the family, and discharge plans. Even the written chart, the Holy of Holies, is getting sprinkled with barbed comments.

"Will defer to anesthesia regarding patient's ongoing delirium, probably secondary to anesthetic medications."

"Will request dietary help, as surgery department seems to think low lipids will help this cachectic man who clearly needs lipids."

And now things have come to a head in, of all places, the tippy toes.

On rounds that morning, the anesthesiologist noted that McGillicutty's toenails are tremendously long, curling all the way around and digging into the meat of his toes.

"Well, this man may live rough on the outside, but now he's under our care, and we have to take care of him," the anesthesiologist says, "let's get Podiatry in here to clip those toenails."

When the surgeon hears this, he blows a gasket, "A Podiatry consult, on a guy ventilator-bound forever more! What a waste. Just soak his feet a little and forget about it. God Almighty, what next, a Plastic Surgery consult for a nose job on this guy?"

They meet in the hallway and exchange views, leading to the (now famous) discussion.

"Go to hell."

"No, you go to hell."

Let's go back and use the *Difficult Conversations* approach, now that we know a little more. [AUTHOR'S NOTE: My listing of the nine steps is a gross oversimplification of their best-selling book. I'm just trying to demonstrate their main ideas in a clinical venue.]

For argument's sake, my negotiating angle is from the point of the view of the anesthesiologist.

1. *Sort out what happened.*

In a tough conversation, your first inclination is to get on your high horse and say, "Damn it, I'm right and that other bastard is dead wrong!" As the anesthesiologist who noted the toenails, I know that we should fix the toenails and I know that the surgeon is an obstreperous bastard who would say anything to get my goat, even if I'm right. Hell, *especially* if I'm right.

Difficult Conversations maintains that most arguments are not about getting the facts right. Rather, most arguments are "not about what is true, they are about what is important" (p. 10).

So, as Mr. McGillicutty languishes on that ventilator, and I'm slugging it out with the surgeon, I have to change gears. It does no good to jump up and down and say, "Those toes *are too* infected." Rather, I have to steer the discussion to what's important here. What would do Mr. McGillicutty the most good, and how can we work together to make it happen.

2. *Look at the emotions involved.*

Nothing puts on the blinders like emotion. I, as clinician, as doctor helping take care of Mr. McGillicutty, have an emotional stake in this patient. And if I see things one way, and that damned SOB of a surgeon sees it another way; well, then, to hell with the surgeon!

Take a minute to recognize this emotion, let it wash over and past you, then move on. I recognize I'm wound up about this, but I should be big enough to rise above these emotions and, gulp, stop arguing for a minute and look at things from the surgeon's point of view.

That surgeon, too, has been working on Mr. McGillicutty for a while. He first saw Hiram when he initially came in, so he's actually known the patient longer than I have. The surgeon has had to deal with a lot of frustration with this case and is wound up too.

The devil's not as black as he's painted when you sit down and talk with him.

All that blood loss I was complaining about? Well, the tumor was more stuck down than you could tell from the CT scan. McGillicutty is bad protoplasm, and nothing works with him, nothing gets better, nothing is easy. No free lunch ever, and the complications just keep on coming.

So this request for a Podiatry consult comes across as a flippant thing, in the light of all of Hiram's "real" problems.

OK, we're talking now, not just yelling at each other. And now I know a little about what the surgeon's thinking and he might be just that much more receptive to me since I've taken time to listen to him.

The ice is breaking.

3. *Stake out your identity.*

OK, who's in charge here? Who's the consultant, and who's the "real" doctor? No one comes into the hospital to have an anesthetic, after all, they come into the hospital to get an *operation*, and the anesthetic is incidental, truth be told.

But this is the ICU, and anesthesiologists often serve as intensivists, so Mr. McGillicutty starts to slip under "my" (the anesthesiologist/intensivist) wing.

My identity, then, is a kind of adopted "primary care giver." I have a stake in McGillicutty getting better, not just surviving the anesthetic. Once I make that clear to the surgeon, he may see me less as a meddler and more as a genuine player in this drama.

4. *Look at the purpose of this conversation.*

Why are we here? Is this some head-butting turf battle between two Alpine billygoats, or is it a cooperative effort between two specialists.

If the conversation spins out of control or emotions yank us back to a battle-stance, we should both pause and remember one thing: Hiram McGillicutty is the purpose of our job. We're not here to prove anesthesia is "better" than surgery or that you are "smarter" than I am. We are here, in the hospital, for one reason and one reason only—to serve the patient.

5. *Look at the issue as a disinterested third party.*

Forget the operation, forget the blood, forget the epidural. Just waltz in now and give McGillicutty the once-over right now, like a medical student coming on the service the first day.

No allegiance to surgery. No allegiance to anesthesia.

Just—what's wrong with Hiram, what can we fix, what can't we fix?

Look over the chart, do a physical exam, start from ground zero.

Would such a "start from the very beginning" approach argue for the Podiatry consult, yes or no?

6. *Explore both sides of the story, staying away from blame and finger pointing.*

Podiatry consult—what will it cost? Will it really help anything?

Soaking the feet and addressing more important issues—will that work? Just add up the pros and cons and go from there.

7. *Come up with an option that helps both sides.*

How about soaks for 2 days; then, if that doesn't help, go with the podiatrists? That way each side gets to see how it unfolds.

8. *Draw on standards that can help out.*

Fever, inability to wean from the ventilator, and worsening redness in the toes would be objective signs that the foot situation is worsening. No need for a value judgment or the wisdom of Solomon—just use these standard medical measures to keep tabs on McGillicutty's progress.

9. *Keep communicating as the solution appears.*

The discussion then goes from a finger-pointing shouting match to a collegial discussion, using the main points of *Difficult Conversations*. After a time, Podiatry comes, clips the nails, and the feet improve. Later, Hiram improves enough to work his way off the ventilator, to live to fight another day!

Hooray for Mr. McGillicutty!

Now, does the anesthesiologist gloat, do the post-touchdown victory dance, and stick his tongue out at the surgeon?

No! This is the time to capitalize on the success of good communication! Rather than lording my "success" at "showing the surgeon up," I enjoy McGillicutty's success as a co-victory for both of us doctors!

We helped get Hiram better. And in the future, we'll work even better together!

[To repeat, here. The above scenario is not a replacement for the many lessons from *Difficult Conversations*, and I take this time to encourage you to buy this book or borrow it from the library.]

Wait a minute! What the heck does this have to do with a book on Simulators? How can you "do" this scenario with a Simulator?

Substitute the mannequin for "Hiram" and have the discussion at his bedside or out in the hallway with an actor playing the surgeon.

And now to let you in on a little secret.

The above scenario played out exactly as described when I was working in an intensive care unit shortly after I finished my training at Emory. A homeless person with terrible hygiene was stuck on a ventilator. I insisted we clean him from head to toe.

"He may be dirty out there, but now he's our responsibility. Make him neat as a pin."

During the cleaning we discovered the toenail problem.

A kind Podiatrist fixed the patient's feet; and, I'll be damned, right after that the patient got off the ventilator! The low level infection must have been just enough of a "septic burden" to keep the patient stuck on the ventilator. Fix the infection, fix the septic burden. Voila! A cure.

Living

This is the last of the "Behavioral Stuff Writ Gritty for Medical Folk."

True confession time—this is not exactly Simulator material. It is, rather, just a damned good behavioral lesson for anyone anywhere, medical or otherwise. Just as we rappelled into *Difficult Conversations* to extract some useful ideas, now we're going to grab the rope again and jump into *The 7 Habits of Highly Effective People*.

Stephen R. Covey touches a real nerve with his discussion of how to lead a more effective life. (I got the book on tape, and Covey himself does the reading. Damned great it is, too, and worth listening to more than once!) Because the Simulator teaches medical professionals, and because medical professionals lead such hectic and stressful lives, it's worth looking at Covey's insights. I'll try to weave his ideas into a medical setting.

His seven habits are:

Be proactive.
Begin with the end in mind.
Put first things first.
Think win–win.
Seek first to understand, then to be understood.
Synergize.
Sharpen the saw.

Put into a medical professional's life, Covey's seven habits could look like this:

1. *Be proactive.*

Rather than just react to things as they arise, make an effort to "take the bull by the horns" and make stuff happen yourself. For example, rather than just getting ticked off that rounds are so dull in your ICU, go ahead and make them more exciting! Bring in a laptop and show some educational imaging from a DVD. Become a teacher and put some zing in those rounds. Rather than sitting around and complaining about slow turnover in the ORs (a *reactive* stance), call an OR committee and find out how you can better the system (a *proactive* stance).

Keep in mind the words of the poem:

> *"I am the master of my fate:*
> *I am the captain of my soul."*
> **–William Ernest Henley**

Believe it and make it happen in your hospital.

2. *Begin with the end in mind.*

Don't just drift through your days rudderless. Get up in the morning with a plan for the day. Then go out and make it happen. This can be as simple as writing yourself a note the day before. As you leave your desk on Monday, leave yourself a note: "Tuesday: finish the monthly Q/A report before you go home."

There. Now stick to it.

That way, that damned Q/A report won't be hanging over your head and gnawing an ulcer through your stomach for the next few weeks.

You identified it, you'll do it, boom, done.

3. *Put first things first.*

Most of us run around like chickens with our heads cut off, doing millions of little things and forgetting the important ones. When all is said and done, and they're about to put the lid on us, we'll little regret the e-mails we responded to, but we'll much regret the times we didn't hug our kids. So put those first things first, and in our madcap days take the time to be with the people who matter.

Practical suggestion: Skip one TV show and write a letter to a friend. A real, paper and pen letter they can hold in their hand.

Another practical suggestion: By all means be efficient and time-conscious when doing *things*; but when being with *loved ones*, turn off the efficiency meter. That time is well spent. That time is golden. Treasure it like a fine wine you sip. Don't gulp that time down.

Don't do that extra call for the big bucks next weekend. Go to the zoo with the kids instead. Stay home and whip up pancakes and laugh about the mess you make. That is a treasure beyond counting.

4. *Think win–win.*

Don't bring people down so you can look like the lone champion. Rather, bring everyone up, then everyone wins.

A concrete example from the hospital: You learn transesophageal echocardiography. Should you remain the lone guru, the sole "high priest" of transesophageal echocardiography, so all must bow before you and worship your expertise?

No!

Teach anyone who's interested. First of all, by teaching, you yourself will review and learn it better. Second, by having more people around who know the technology, more patients get good care. Hey, they'll be less likely to call you in if someone else knows how to do it, so you'll be able to spend more time with the kids.

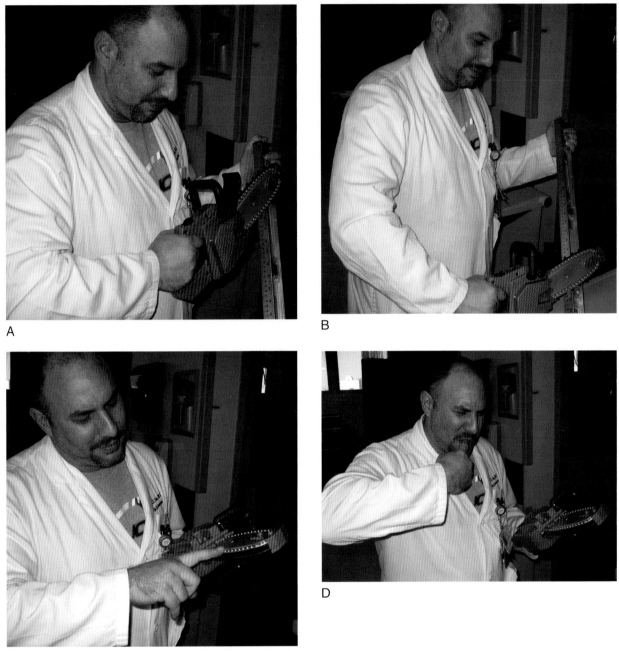

A

B

C

D

FIGURE 4–8   Sharpen the saw, one of the seven habits of highly effective (if careless in this case) people. Although the book may sound a little corny and come across as a little "touchy-feely," it teaches some great lessons. Transfer those seven habits into the hospital setting and you've got yourself a much more effective doctor.

You win, the kids win, your colleagues win, the patients win.

Win–win.

5. *Seek first to understand, then to be understood.*
So you're in the position of teacher, and you want to get some point across. And you're dying to break out in a lecture and tell your students flat out what they need to do.

Rein it in! Debrief time is not lecture time!

Listen to the students, understand what *they* were thinking. Find out what they were thinking, for example, when they gave epinephrine.

To make a true "*Aha*" moment, you need to dig into what they understand, what *their* point of view is, before you "solve it for them."

By first understanding, you lay the groundwork to be understood.

This may sound like some semantic trickery, but it's actually the way to go.

6. *Synergize.*

This emphasizes the importance of teamwork, of adding 1 and 1 and getting 3 from the magic of the combined effort.

Whoa, enter the Simulator!

Instead of making the Simulator an "anesthesia only" domain, bring in other specialties, other professions. ICU nurses can learn from you and you from them. Medical intensivists may have a few tricks up their sleeves that we don't. No better place to learn it than the Simulator.

7. *Sharpen the saw.*

This final habit emphasizes the idea of self-renewal. Keep learning more. (In a sense, that's the idea behind getting CME credits each year.) Periodically step back a little, look your life over, and ask yourself, "What kind of footprint am I leaving on the world? Is that a worthy footprint? How can I make a better footprint?" Then work toward that.

> **BOX 4-12** Seven Habits, Shortened a Little
>
> - **Proactive**
> - **End in sight**
> - **Win–win**
> - **Understand**

As a medical professional, what are you doing with your life? Is this the kind of life you'd be proud to say, at the end of days, that you lived? Maybe you can connect better with your patients? Connect better with the staff? Maybe you need to learn a new skill to be more valuable, to be sharper?

A little behind on one facet of your profession? Go to a conference and brush up.

Don't rest on your oars! Keep paddling!

That's it for "Behavioral Stuff Writ Large for Medical Folk." Although some of this stuff flew off at a tangent to Simulators, I think it all has merit.

You should be able to use these lessons in your Simulator for teaching and learning.

Attendance and Scheduling Issues

"Half of life is showing up."

Anonymous

Yea verily, hear these words, as they are the lament of simulator people from sea to shining sea. From Boston's storied Ether Dome down to hurricane-battered Miami, across the fruited plain, up over the Rockies to LA's smog, San Fran's fog, and Seattle's drizzle, the problem with simulators is always the same.

It's not the scenarios—there are tons of them. They're available on the Internet, they're well described in articles, and the next great scenario is percolating in the imagination of an instructor somewhere in Chicago or Pittsburgh or Atlanta. Scenarios aren't the problem.

It's not the simulators themselves—the simulator "universe" has had years of experience with them. We know how to make them "do their thing." Simulators are getting more and more clever, more and more user-friendly; and in the way of all things computeresque, they're getting less expensive. Laerdal and METI honor their service agreements and keep their simulators humming pretty well. Simulators aren't the problem.

It's not the instructors—there are a lot of people who like to teach. *Teach the teachers* courses abound, but even without "official training" a good teacher put in a simulator can create a good learning experience.

So if it's not the scenarios, if it's not the simulators, and if it's not the instructors, then what *is* the problem?

Moving the meat

Getting the residents in there

The lowest tech element in this high-tech world of computerized wizardry—scheduling the residents out of the OR and into the simulation lab

From the "Simulator guru's" point of view, this is nothing short of maddening, but it is *the* biggest problem with simulator education. You can debate whether the simulator is a checklist or theater; you can argue whether simulators are valid teaching methods; you can hash and rehash the "Simulator as certification" question. But if you can't get the residents to darken the doorstep of the simulation center, there is nothing to debate! The issue is decided. If no one ever *goes* to the Simulator center, then *by definition* simulation is a big, fat zero.

Simulator centers tend to open with great fanfare. Wow! Zowie! This is new, this is the latest, this is the way to go, now we've arrived, now we're "keeping up with the Joneses" (who also have a Simulator). But the nitty gritty of making sure residents rotate through the simulator becomes a real headache, and it's too easy to fall back into this response, "Oh, yeah, the simulator, um, we have one, but no one has gone there for the past year. We got a little short-staffed, and, you know, with the 80 hour rule it's hard to, you know, make them go, and CRNA's cost a pretty penny, and . . ."

BOX 5–1   Scheduling The Simulator

- **Pull from OR?**
- **Evening?**
- **Weekend?**
- **Who pays?**
- **Voluntary?**

So the Simulator sits there, becoming a cobweb magnet in a dark room. A hundred scenarios, a thousand lessons huddle within the Simulator's latex chest, but there they sit and there they stay, waiting for someone to rediscover them.

The obstacles to scheduling are quite daunting, involving two nontrivial components—time and money!

MONEY HEADACHES WITH SIMULATION SCHEDULING

- Say your program has CRNAs. If, at 7:30 on a Wednesday you are going to pull three residents out of the OR and send them to the simulator, by mathematical analysis, fast Fourrier transformation, quantitative numerometricologic integrative triangulatory derivativations, you will have to send, just a second, let me count on my fingers.

Uh, you'll have to send three CRNAs into the rooms to relieve your residents. So you must have three *extra* CRNAs that day. Three *more* than those needed for breaks, lunches, call-in-sicks, and having people to cover regular rooms and be ready for that ruptured aneurysm or stat C-section.

Three *extra* CRNAs? In today's climate of CRNA shortages? Plus, what does a CRNA cost? I don't have enough fingers to count that high.

- Say your program is an "all-resident" program. Let's fire up that computer again and see what we'll need to do if we pull three residents out of the OR at 7:30 on a Wednesday. Miracle of miracles, that same number keeps appearing—three!

So now your program needs to have three *extra* residents. And we still need to provide breaks—residents get a break every 2 hours, get a lunch break every 4 hours. (Ours is a *vigilance* task, you can't just make the remaining residents "tough it out" while their pals are in the simulator.) And "all-resident" programs are not immune from people calling in sick, nor are they immune from the need to provide for the emergency aneurysm or C-section.

- Say you flesh out your program with AAs (anesthesia assistants). Forget, if you can, the firestorm of controversy about this issue. You still can't get around the physical reality that pulling three residents means you have to "create three replacements."

And replacements mean more money.

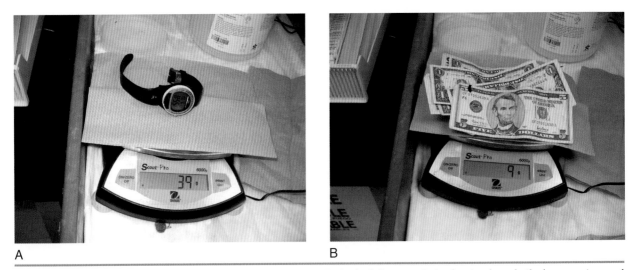

A   B

FIGURE 5–1   Time is, well, for lack of a better term, money. And scheduling people in the simulator boils down to time and money. Pulling people out of the OR costs money. Expecting people to come in after hours or on weekends costs time—time people may want to spend otherwise. And residents are under the "80-hour rule"—you can't violate that. Scheduling is *the* problem once you get a simulation center up and running.

TIME HEADACHES WITH SIMULATION SCHEDULING

- Forget pulling the residents who were going to be in rooms. Let's do this post-call. Aha, the perfect answer! No need to replace them, they were going home anyway! Suddenly, 7:30 on a Wednesday seems like the perfect time.

  OK, sure. Now, the ACGME says that, technically, you can do this. After 24 hours on call, a resident can be allowed to stay for an additional 6 hours, so long as he or she is not giving an anesthetic or is not accepting new patients into the ICU. So, yes, you are adhering to the letter of the law.

  And even if they are exhausted, you could weave this argument, "Good, most mistakes are made when you are tired, so what better time to put them through the simulator than when they are tired!"

  Unfortunately, the weave on that argument unravels in the glare of reality. Anyone who's done, say, a busy night on OB or a shoot-'em-dead night on trauma knows that by dawn the lights are going out on your brain. Keeping a beat-up resident around for another 3 to 4 hours in the simulation lab seems foolish. Plus, forget for a moment patient safety, think about resident safety. Interns deprived of sleep have more car wrecks on their way home. So now we're going to keep them awake another few hours then put them on the road? Not a good idea.

- Pulling residents during the day is just too tough; let's make this a nights/weekend deal. ACGME rules once again rear their administrative head. Residents must have at least 10 hours off between clinical duties one day and clinical duties the next day. The 80-hour rule applies, and 3 to 4 hours of required time in the simulation lab is part of that 80-hour formula. Residents must have at least one 24-hour period where they have no clinical or educational duties each week. Add this all up, and you do have to pay careful attention to just how many nights and weekends you can "eat into."

  Plus, the residents might not take this lying down—"I'm already here late enough nights!" "I only get one really good weekend a month, now this! Now I have no time to myself or my family!" For religious reasons, Friday nights and Saturday days may be off limits for certain residents as well, limiting your weekend options.

- Wave the magic wand—let's make this whole thing voluntary! This opens a different can of worms. It

comes as no surprise that the worst residents have the least insight into their problems. They don't take criticism well, and "suggestions for improvement" fall on deaf ears. Superb residents are always looking for ways to improve themselves (that's how they got so good).

So what happens if the Simulator becomes voluntary?

The best residents would sign up, would find a way to get there, would put in the time and effort to get the most out of their Simulator experience. Good for them! At the other end of the spectrum, the worst residents would not sign up, would find every excuse not to get there, and would not put forth the time and effort to benefit from the Simulator experience. That's fine if you just want to write off your lower-achieving residents. *But that's not what a residency is about.* It's our job as teachers to do our best for *all* the residents, not just the shining stars.

So gee whiz, time and money don't seem to be on our side in our "Simulator quest." What to do? Give up? Did we buy this Porsche of a Simulator just to let it "sit in the garage all day," as a lot of people do? In this battle of Scheduling Monster versus Simulatorzilla, will the Scheduling Monster prove victorious?

Never!

Here are a few approaches to slaying the Scheduling Monster. Your weapons are limited only by your creativity and by the vagaries of your program.

- Bring residents in pre-call.

  Some programs have night shifts, either a 3 p.m. to 7 a.m. or sometimes a 3 p.m. to 11 p.m. shift. Have the residents come in a little earlier, say, at noon. They have a simulation session while they're still "awake and alert"; then they go to their call assignment.

- Find residents you can "free up" for a few hours.

  Pain clinic, preop clinic, PACU, ICU, OB—all these rotations can sometimes "survive for a while" without a resident. Yes, sometimes things get stretched a little, and there may be times when you have to "rush someone out" of the Simulator (OB gets two stat sections at once, codes are pouring in, ICU patients are all going sour). But a little flexibility on their part and a little on your part can usually accommodate everybody.

  Don't aim for a perfect system, just a pretty good one.

- Study your OR schedule. Thursday is a big ortho day, tons of artificial joints, plus the hand surgeons

BOX 5-2 Simulator Innovations
• **Pre-call**
• **Simulator call team**
• **Cracks in the schedule**

BOX 5-3 Simulator of Dreams
"If you champion it, they will come."

are busy as bees all day. Friday tends to be a little lighter. So make Friday the day for the Simulator. Most ORs and most programs don't go flat out 110%, 110% of the time. Look for a crease in that schedule.

- Schedule medical students and CRNA students on busy OR days. Students are easier to schedule because you don't have to "find a replacement" for them. So if your Simulator center takes in students, schedule them on the days when it's impossible to schedule residents (such as Thursdays in the preceding example).
- Have a "Simulator call" team. By definition, medical care and medical timing are hit and miss. One day the cardiac room is bursting at the seams, the next day there is nothing on the schedule. Consider a "Simulator opportunity" to be the same as an "emergency case." All of a sudden, three residents are drifting rudderless, their cases canceled, the surgeon broke his leg and can't operate for a while, who knows. Beep the Simulator call team (we have code teams, liver transplant teams, peds specialists on call, why not a Simulator call team?), fire up the Simulator, and go! Might not work all the time (what, after all, does?), but even if it works a *few* times that's a *few more residents* who benefited from the Simulator.
- Go ahead and hire the extra people to cover for those residents! OK, easier said than done. But there are creative ways around financing, and there's no reason you can't be clever in your Simulator financing as well. If your Simulator center receives grant support from industry or for a study, part of that money should be earmarked for "salary support in the OR." Not every penny spent *for* a Simulator has to be spent *in* the Simulator. Part of that money is justifiably spent *back in the OR* making sure that residents can get to the Simulator.

So there are some ideas for steering your young charges into the Simulator. But do people want to make the Simulator happen? Do people *believe* in the Simulator? If they don't, then no amount of clever scheduling will matter.

No one will come.

If you do believe in the Simulator, then no amount of obstacles will *keep them from coming*.

You gotta believe!

Here's a few approaches to keeping the faith.

- *Champion.* Someone in the upper echelon has to champion the cause of the Simulator. Program chairman, program director, educational director, clinical competence chairman, somebody. Inertia is a powerful force; and if no energy jolts the simulator system from above, the program will "go to its lowest energy level"—the unplugged, unused Simulator sitting in a dark room. "Lack of a champion" is the most frequent cause of a Simulator program dying.
- *Residents* themselves. The Simulator experience has been likened to sex—even when it's not great, it's still pretty good. I have done simulations in a crummy old decrepit OR, equipment malfunctioning (I drew pictures of the EKG and taped them to the monitors), Simulator sputtering, airway leaking, and the tech was sick that day. A worse simulation you could not imagine.

The residents loved it and wanted to come back for more!

Most residents enjoy their time in the Simulator, no matter how bad (technically) the thing goes. Just being taught, being singled out for the sole purpose of education, seems to resonate with them. They're not just "stuck in a room with an attending who splits and never teaches anything anyway." They are there *only* to be taught. There is no "sitting there while the attending is out drinking coffee or whatever the hell an attending does." The attending is just there for *them*, to teach!

So to generate interest in a Simulator program, just find a way, any way, to get the residents in there for a session or two. They will ask for more; they will demand more.

Then give them what they want.

Scheduling is a killer.

Scheduling is *the* killer of Simulators.

But where there's a will . . . you know the rest.

Kill the Scheduling Monster before it kills you.

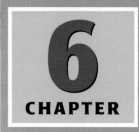

6

CHAPTER

With What Other Disciplines Should We Work?

> *"Why can't we all just get along?"*
> **Rodney King**

Cooperation among specialties, especially between anesthesiology and surgery, is the stuff of legend. Of note, a *legend* is defined as "a story coming down from the past; one popularly regarded as historical although not verifiable."

Try verifying this legend.

A 68-year-old man with benign prostatic hypertrophy was on the OR table, spinal anesthetic in place and functioning well. He was a calm man requiring little sedation, so he was quite awake and aware of his surroundings though, of course, unable to move his lower body with the spinal anesthetic on board. The drapes were up and the circulator was prepping the patient.

His urologic surgeon and his anesthesiologist were discussing the schedule in a manner most heated. Both doctors were standing to the left of the OR table, on the patient's side of the drapes, so the patient, merely by turning his head to the left, could see them.

And, of course, he could hear them too.

"They was sayin' somethin' about some other guy, I guess it was someone gonna have the same thing as me, you know, the ream out job of the prostate," the patient said. "And they's gettin' louder, you know, which first I think is kinda funny 'cause I thought doctors just talk that quiet kind of 'I'm real smart and you're not, so I'll take this real slow' kind of talk.

"But now they's yellin' and start to pushin' and I'm thinkin', 'Hell's bells who's gonna do the ream job if one of

em cold cocks the other one?' and sure enough they start throwin' punches. I'm not kiddin'.

"Well I had to laugh cause I thrown a few punches in my day and these docs here they look more like girls fightin' and pretty soon it's a huggy up and down to the ground they go and they're rollin' around. And now the one nurse comes around and spill some brown stuff out a little plastic dish and she's yellin' and people comin' in hollerin' and oh my God such a sight to see and here right in the hospital and me so numb and jes' layin' there with all my privacy danglin' in the breeze for all the world to see."

Suffice it to say, there is room in this world for more cooperation between the specialties. What better place to accomplish this than the simulator!

The simulator is just the place to mix and match the various medical elements, getting them to work together in a crisis, iron out who does what, and most importantly to start to *talk to each other*.

- Anesthesiology and Surgery—to foster better understanding in the OR, and possibly reduce the number of fist fights!
- Anesthesiology and Internal Medicine—we most often encounter each other in the supercharged atmosphere of a code. No time for much dialogue in a real code, but there sure is in a Simulator mock code.

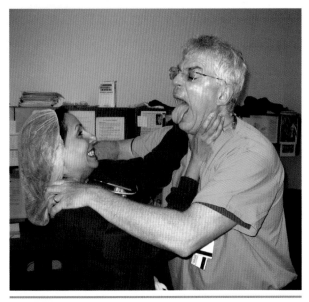

FIGURE 6–1   Interdisciplinary interaction can get heated in the hospital.

- Anesthesiology and ICU nursing staff—another group of highly trained specialists we work with every day. Training together in the Simulator makes perfect sense, plus can help build esprit de corps among ICU teams.
- Medical students and nursing staff—as the twig bends, so grows the tree. At an early point in their training, future doctors can practice doctor–nurse interactions in a crisis.
- Anesthesiology and OR nursing staff—we work hand in glove with the OR nursing staff through all kinds of emergencies. Because we work together, we should practice together too.
- Anesthesiology and anesthesia techs—we need their help in a big way in the big cases, so practicing together in the Simulator with them makes sense too.
- Anesthesiology and Pharmacy/Information Technology/Billing—automatic pharmacy dispensing systems, automated billing and record keeping, all these elements are entering the ORs. And new systems have quirks, glitches, and potential disasters. Work them out in the harmless setting of the Simulator.
- ER docs and EMTs—hand-off of the critically ill patient has its own set of dangers. Do a few "critical handoffs" in the Simulator to make sure the transition from emergency response team to hospital team is seamless.

- Anesthesiology and OB—you want a critical situation where two specialties may be at odds, try the stat C-section. Every variant (lost airway, twins with the second one breech, shoulder dystocia that just won't go) you can rehearse together in the Simulator.
- Anesthesiology and Pediatrics—neonatal resuscitation after a stat C-section? The Simulator's the place to work it out.
- Intensivists (from any discipline) and nursing staff.
- Intensivists and nursing students.
- Office-based practitioners (plastic surgeons/oral surgeons) and their nursing staff.
- Military teams of doctors/nurses/technicians.

The list goes on. In the Simulator, any combination, any threesome of different specialties and training can work together. You can put together entire teams, for example look at all the people involved in a code.

> ICU nurse—calls the code
> Unit clerk—sends out the word, makes sure the code cart is stocked, ready to go, and refilled at the end of the code
> Intensivist
> Anesthesiologist
> Surgeon (say it were a surgical intensive care unit)
> Respiratory therapist
> Pharm D (often in intensive care units these days)
> Medical students
> Nursing students

A whole army of people descends on a code, each with a certain role to play. And rather than working together the *first* time in a *real* code, it is better to *practice* together the first time in a *mock* code.

And even those who may not participate to a large degree (the Pharm D, for example, or some extra medical or nursing students) may benefit from seeing how a code's done. Plus, the Law of Unintended Consequence plays a role. The Pharm D may be an expert on resuscitative drugs during a code, long-term problems with amiodarone, and current thoughts on the ever on-again, off-again role of bicarb or calcium. So at the end of the code team's exercise, the well informed Pharm D may bring everyone up to speed with an impromptu talk.

Good things happen when you throw people together.

Scheduling hassles with this multidisciplinary love-fest? Yes.

As detailed in the previous chapter, moving the meat around is the biggest headache of "Simulato-

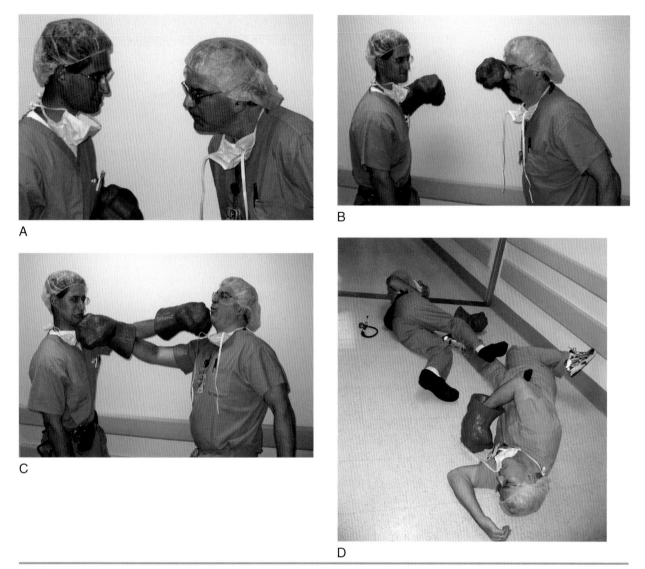

FIGURE 6–2 Lost in these "ego battles" is the question, "What is best for the patient?" We may get all huffy and defend our ego, our specialty, and our point of view to the exclusion of the patient's welfare. Wrong maneuver! Remember the mantra, "Patient first."

land." So getting people there and, trickiest of all, getting different disciplines there at the same time is tough.

- ICU nurses? The nursing shortage landed with a loud thump in our intensive care units. Pull a few ICU nurses from a busy ICU when they're getting unexpected admissions? Fat chance.
- Surgery residents? Surgery programs are struggling with the 80-hour rule, just like all the other specialties. So on any given day, they may have to send someone home in the middle of the work day as he is fast approaching "Hour 80." Now the clinic

is busy, they're short already, oh, and *now* you want us to send someone to your Simulator session? Fat chance.
- Information technology person? The entire pharmacy system just crashed, and no one's sure if it's a virus, a Trojan horse, a phish attack, or any of the other myriad cyber-assaults upon every computer system in the world. Or maybe it's just that this system is too old to handle all this information. Oh, is that simulation thing today? And you expect me to go with *this* going on? Fat chance.
- Medical students? They just matched last week, so they're all blowing off everything in this, their

"Swan song of goofing off" before internship starts and life ends for them. Will they arrive on time or, for that matter, at all? Right.

So, once again, something looks good on paper—"We'll all work together, learn together, grow, and self-actualize. The moon will be in the seventh house, Jupiter will align with Mars, and this simulator session will usher in the dawning of the age of Aquarius." But scheduling this educational free love-fest becomes a logistical nightmare.

Oh, what about the money? Oh, that.

- ICU nurses. Would they expect to get paid for their time? You bet they would, and at last glance ICU nurses do not come cheap. Who would pay for them? The hospital? Sure, all the hospitals are flush with cash, they're drowning in black ink, they'd love to cough up the dough. Can the Simulator pay for them to come over? Um, Simulator centers usually want to *charge* people for coming over there. Hmm. Who *would* foot the bill for the ICU nurses?
- Surgery residents. Though less of an "hourly wage" question, you still have to consider that, for residents, time is money too.
- Pharm D, information specialist, anyone else who wants to join in—you still have to answer the tough question, "Who is paying them while they spend time in the Simulator?"

So time and money rear their ugly head. While we're tossing wrenches in the works, try adding this one—coordinating the schedules of all these people.

Friday is a slow day in the ORs, a good day for anesthesia.

But Friday is *the* clinic day for surgery, bad day for them. How about Thursday?

Thursday is in-service day for the ICU, when they give their CME credits and get everyone ACLS certified. But Wednesday is all right, how about in the mornings?

Wednesday morning is inventory for pharmacy; and with a spate of inconsistencies in narcotic returns, the DEA is up in arms so . . . Tuesday?

But on Tuesdays, the medical people have Grand Rounds and that's *their* busiest day, so . . . Monday?

How about next week? Oh, that's right, everyone's out of town for the conference?

Next month?

Next year?

How about Wednesday, May 5, 2097 from 1 a.m. to 2 a.m., that's the one time that everyone can. . . .

So it's impossible, right?

| BOX 6-1 | Making Simulators Happen |

- **Talk to kahunas**
- **Get $ backing**
- **Rent to train others**

Never. This is where you have to go to the big guns, invoke the hammer of Thor, and smash all resistance with one mighty swing.

Go to the Chairman of the Hospital, the Dean of the Medical School, the President of the University. You must make the pitch to the Mightiest of the Mighty, the All-Powerful, the Holder of the Purse Strings.

(Running a Simulator center, you have to be part pitchman.)

In a frank discussion, you lay out all the problems detailed above, but you end with, "But this is something we just plain need to do, no matter how, we just need to do it."

If they don't back you, indeed the problem is unsolvable, and any one of the above-listed problems will torpedo your multidisciplinary effort.

But if they *do* back you, the problems part like the Red Sea before Moses' staff. The head of surgery sends you his resident, the ICU finds a way to cover for that nurse, IT lives without their tech for one morning, and someone covers that OR and springs an anesthesia resident.

Then, once you have called on "help from above," you run a great simulation, get everyone excited about this new learning method, and you've planted the seeds for future "help from below."

I kid thee not, this takes a lot of energy. It's hard enough to pull your "own" residents. But keeping the energy level high enough to pull "other" residents, ICU staff, and the like is draining.

Nothing worthwhile is easy.

Same goes for running a multidisciplinary simulation center.

Let's take a peak at the kind of stuff that can come from these "adventures into the multidisciplinary unknown."

NEW DRUG-DISPENSING SYSTEM

Pharmacy and the information technology people have put together a new system for dispensing drugs. This system uses a log-in and fingerprint recognition

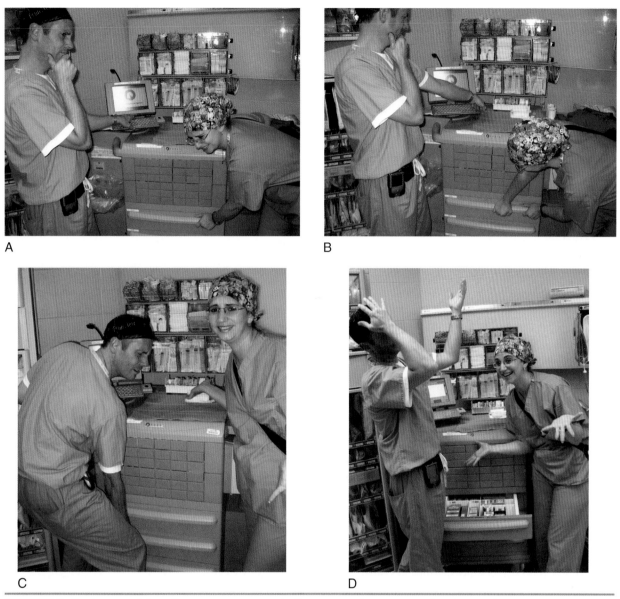

FIGURE 6-3 Automated drug dispensing systems can baffle anyone. Why not get used to them in the simulator? That way, if you flounder around, no one gets hurt.

system. The pharmacy and IT people gather round as a senior resident starts a simulated case. This resident uses the old system of getting drugs—a cart with all the drugs just sitting in drawers.

A second senior resident goes through the same scenario later with the new system of getting drugs—log-in and fingerprint recognition system.

"The patient is a 55-year-old man with end-stage ischemic heart disease and one episode of sudden death. Fortunately, he collapsed at an automatic external defibrillator Mardi Gras party and was saved,

going on to win third prize in the "Best Costume" contest.

"Now he is for implantation of an AICD. He has external pads on and is ready for induction."

The first resident does a careful induction, mindful of the patient's tenuous cardiac status, but at intubation the sympathetic simulation proves too much and the patient fibrillates.

"Shock! Defib!" the anesthesia resident shouts.

An OR nurse (part of the multidisciplinary team too) works the defibrillator as the code protocol rolls.

Shocking is the most crucial thing, but after three shocks it's time to go to the next step. The anesthesia resident intubates, CPR starts (a medical student does chest compressions), and then it's time to get the drugs.

The pharmacy/IT people note the time and ease of getting the drugs out, but also note that at the end of the case there is no record-keeping, no charges filled out for the drugs. The important stuff was the code, of course, and billing/paperwork play second fiddle.

But still. If we *never* charge, if we *never* fill out the paperwork, the hospital goes broke. So you can't just blow this stuff off. And this is part of systems-based medicine, a core clinical competence we *must* teach as mandated by ACGME.

So at the end of the simulation, everyone's learned something.

- The anesthesia resident ran a code and also learned about systems-based medicine.
- The OR nurse participated in the code, with a hands-on review of the defibrillator.
- The medical student got to observe and do chest compressions.
- Pharmacy and IT picked up a weakness in the "paperwork chain of command."

And all these lessons at no risk to a patient.

Now the second anesthesia resident enters the room, does the same induction, with the same results. When she goes to get drugs out of the automated system, there's a hang-up: she enters the code wrong, waits while the fingerprint reader does nothing (it hadn't gotten the correct input yet), and the resident couldn't get the emergency drugs. Valuable time passed (CPR is in progress, after all) before the resident enters the correct information and springs the drugs free from the new machine.

At the end of this simulation, people have still learned good lessons.

The anesthesia resident ran a code.
The OR nurse worked the defibrillator again.
The medical student did chest compressions.
But *aha*! The big lesson went to our pharmacy and IT people.

That roadblock of a code entry and fingerprint read prevented easy access to the emergency drugs. Precious time slipped away in an easy-to-imagine sequence.

You're in the middle of a code.
You type in stuff too fast.
You don't notice the computer gives you an error message.
You stand there with your finger on the scanner, mad with impatience because the room is going bananas with this code in progress and you can't get the damned drugs!

IT and pharmacy go back to the drawing board, and add a "code button" to the dispenser cart, allowing instant access to code drugs in an emergency.

Thank goodness this problem was worked out in the simulator, and *not at the expense of a patient's life*. This is the kind of magic that can happen with a multidisciplinary approach to simulation sessions. In the GREAT BIG chapter on simulation scenarios, you will see more of these multidisciplinary efforts in action.

And there's a final twist to this "bring in other people" idea. If you are in a university setting with hot and cold running grad students, you can bring in non-medical people to participate in and study the entire simulation experience. They will learn something, and they may very well enhance the Simulator experience for your students as well.

- *Theater majors.* Face it, the more entertaining and fantasmagorical this is, the more the suspension of disbelief. Theater people could help us with acting, makeup, sound effects, and the whole "feel" of the theater.
- *Education majors.* Simulation is the Wild West of learning. Is this the way to teach and learn? Is there a better way? Is competence testing valid? If not, how can we make it valid? How do the various people learn? A lot of educational ground to cover here.
- *Behavioral psychologists.* The lion's share of the learning in the Simulator is the behavior aspect—crisis management, working in teams. Behavioral psychologists could help us here.
- *MBA/business.* Red ink, black ink. New technology. Lots of expense, lots of potential. An MBA could spend his entire "project" time on the Simulator.

There's a whole world of people out there who could learn from, or add to, the Simulator experience. Maybe the Simulator is where we will finally learn to "get along."

CHAPTER 7

The Great Debate

> *"I beg to differ."*
> **A common expression**

Yin. Yang.
Red state. Blue state.
Men—Mars; Women—Venus.
Dr. Jekyll. Mr. Hyde.

What is it about opposites that so fascinates us?

Eastern philosophy hinges on the interweaving and interplay of Yin (moon, woman) and Yang (sun, man).

Fox News pounds the red state (Nascar dad, NRA)/blue state (polo dad, bean sprout) divide into our skulls every night.

Men and women? Beyond the scope of this book. Beyond the scope of *any* book, if you think about it.

And finally Robert Louis Stevenson's cautionary tale of "what lies within." Dr. Jekyll—doctor, healer, scientist, kind soul—finds out that he too has a darker side. After the magic potion goes to work, Mr. Hyde comes out—sadist, lecher, killer. Dr. Jekyll seemed too good to be true. Who, after all, is perfect in every way? Mr. Hyde seemed too bad to be true. Who, after all, is evil in every way?

The truth lies somewhere in between.

Which brings us to *our* cautionary tale about Simulators. Are Simulators Dr. Jekyll, as some would maintain, or are they Mr. Hyde, as others would maintain? The truth, of course, lies somewhere in between. But let's look at this debate the way Robert Louis Stevenson would. Let's argue about the Simulator by creating our own Dr. Jekyll and Mr. Hyde story.

MONEY

Dr. Jekyll—Simulators are worth the money.
Who are we kidding, *anything* in medicine is pricey. This is a high-rent district, and education in medicine is no exception. Plus, the money we are laying down is going to save lives and prevent medical catastrophes. You're fretting a couple hundred thousand to set up a *safety* center? How much did you pay the last time your hospital was sued?

Chipped tooth—$25,000.

Successful lawsuit from the hospital's point of view (no judgment for the plaintiff)—$50,000, and that's if everything went perfectly and appeals don't drag out. And 50 thou is a *low* estimate.

Unsuccessful lawsuit—well, you pick whatever number you want. The jury surely will.

If simulator training, with its emphasis on safety, can prevent *one* adverse event, it has paid for itself in spades.

"But this is all speculative!" the cynic says.

No, there are some dollars and cents savings that result directly from Simulator training. And these savings come from the malpractice insurance companies themselves. Talk about hard-nosed business people!

Harvard and MIT worked together to create a Simulator center. Practitioners who come for Simulator training there get a *reduction in their malpractice premiums*!

BOX 7-1   Are Simulators Worth It?

- **Cost**
- **Proven benefit?**
- **Speculative?**
- **Better alternatives?**

An insurance company asking for *less* money. When was the last time you heard of that? The insurance companies are saying, in a concrete way, "Simulator training is a worthy financial investment."

Hmm. Hard to argue with that.

Look at this a different way. OK, Simulators are an expensive, new, technologically cutting-edge "toy" for the hospital and the medical school. Looked at any of the other toys the hospital picks up? PET scanner? Brain simulator for neurosurgery used to ablate certain pathways in patients with Parkinson's disease? Three-dimensional CT scanners capable of doing "virtual facial reconstruction" before the surgeon starts cutting?

How much do those puppies cost? Has anyone "proven beyond a shadow of a doubt" that each and every one of them is worth every penny spent on them?

No!

Medicine *is* a business yet it's *not exactly* a business. We push the envelope of technology to get the next thing, the next breakthrough, the next *procedure that may benefit our patients*. And that means "jumping out into the financial unknown" sometimes.

- Yes, the PET scanner is expensive, and before you have "paid it off" a newer, slicker imaging technique may come along (quark scanner?). But for now, the detailed images provided by the PET scanner *seem the best thing for our patients*, so let's embrace this new expensive technology.
- Yes, the neuroablative techniques to treat Parkinson's patients require tremendously expensive equipment and procedures. And tomorrow or next month or next year some new technique may make this procedure obsolete (gene therapy? some new pharmacologic breakthrough?). But right now this neurosurgical approach *seems like the best thing for our patients*, so let's use it.
- Yes, the three-dimensional CT scanners . . . the list goes on, and the argument stays the same. So long as the medical community believes that a procedure or technique or technology is *the best thing for our patients*, we'll use it, even if it's expensive.

So it doesn't take a 28-foot Olympic leap of faith to apply the same reasoning to the Simulator. Yes, the Simulator mannequins are expensive. Yes, technical help is expensive. Yes, pulling anesthesiologists from clinical duties is expensive. But training in a Simulator *seems like the best thing for our patients*. So let's bring it on.

Unconvinced?

Look at things from an amortization point of view. "Amortization" comes from the Latin for "a financial term that hardly anyone understands." You lay a lot of money down *initially* for a Simulator center, but you don't have to *keep laying down* all that money. You still need upkeep and staffing costs—not small sums by any stretch—but after you buy the main things, you, well, have them! You don't need to "buy them again" each year.

That's the "Dummies Guide to Amortization."

Still unconvinced?

Fine, look at this from a different point of view. Put on your Harvard Business School cap and look at the numbers. The Simulator can actually *make money* for the hospital or medical school.

What! No way!

Yes, way.

The Simulator center can provide valuable training for all kinds of professionals—emergency medical technicians, fire-rescue personnel, military medics. Nursing schools may benefit by sending their students to the Simulator center. Other physicians can come to your center for training—office-based oral surgeons, office-based plastic surgeons, community anesthesiologists who want some "crisis training." A Simulator center can become a "little red schoolhouse." And, like schoolhouses everywhere, you can charge tuition.

This book is about "Simulators in anesthesia," so we won't go into training those other professionals. But if you want to set up a Simulator center, and you are fretting how you will pay for it, try this business plan out.

Monday—Train your residents.

Tuesday—Train your medical students.

Wednesday—Rent the place out for training EMTs.

Thursday—Rent the place out for training office-based physicians.

Friday—Rent the place out for training military personnel.

Saturday—Put up a mirror ball, dress the dummies in polyester leisure suits, play disco music through the mannequin's speakers, and rent the place out for a retro 70s party.

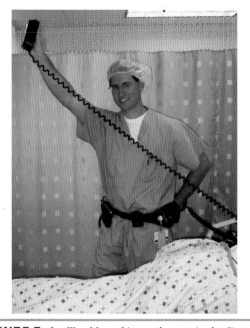

FIGURE 7–1 Trouble making ends meet in the Simulator? Rent it out to some latter-day John Travolta on "Saturday Night Simulator" night. Don't charge those paddles or you may zap your dance partner.

Didn't make enough money on the 70s party?

Simulator centers can pick up additional money from educational grants, pharmacology company sponsorship, you name it. Do what all the stadiums do, sell the naming rights to your Simulation center!

The Enron Simulation Center.

Who knows? You are limited only by your imagination.

So from a variety of financial angles, Simulators are worth the money. Simulators are a financial Dr. Jekyll.

Mr. Hyde—Simulators are not worth the money. No "Simulator champion" ever looks at what *else* you could do with all that money.

Let's pull a number out of the air—a million dollars—and see what we could buy with that, from an educational point of view.

Take the million dollars you would have spent on Simulator mannequins, technicians, space, upkeep, and lost income (attending anesthesiologists working in the Simulator and not billing for cases). Scour the country and hire three full-time academic anesthesiologists and two educational PhDs and have them do *nothing but teach.* They can wander the ORs and ICUs looking for "teaching opportunities." They have all the time in the world to prepare lectures, set up web-based learning (aided by the educational PhDs, who

understand the learning process), creating "scenarios" on the fly, sitting down with lagging residents, making sure there are "no children left behind." This battery of educational specialists, freed of any clinical duties, will never be tired, will never show up late for lectures, will never be too busy/harried/exhausted to focus on education for the anesthesia residents and fellows.

OK, fine, you say, but what about all that money we were going to make in the Simulator?

These full-time education specialists can write papers, get grants, obtain pharmacology company and governmental support for their worthy projects. You can get a lot of "bang for your buck" from these people. Better to hire these five people than pour a ton of money into a Simulator center.

Unconvinced? Mr. Hyde has other financial arguments against Simulators.

Go around the country, go to all the anesthesia programs that have Simulator centers. How many of those Simulator centers still have a pulse? You might be surprised how many programs laid down a ton of money for Simulator mannequins, and the mannequins are gathering dust in some back room.

It takes an ongoing champion, an ongoing river of money, time, and scheduling to keep the Simulator centers going. They may open with great fanfare, but the grind of "getting residents out of the OR and to the Simulator" takes a toll. Inertia is a damned powerful force (it has its own named physical principle, for God's sake), and inertia is forever wanting to kill these programs.

Technician leaves? Who takes his place? Who will pay for the technician? The hospital? No, they've lost their enthusiasm. The anesthesia department? No, their "Simulator guru" went into private practice last year, and no one else is interested.

Call it inertia, call it gravity, whatever it is, there is a powerful downward drag on Simulator centers after their initial sheen wears off. You plunk down a boatload of cash for a Simulator center, and after a while all it supports is cobwebs.

So, from a variety of financial angles, Simulators are not worth the money. Simulators are a financial Mr. Hyde.

EDUCATION

Dr. Jekyll—Simulators are the way to educate. Educational theory shows that Simulators are the way to go in education. Most learning occurs in the dull and dreary confines of the lecture hall or the library.

The student gets no emotional attachment to the lesson, so the learning goes in one ear (or eye) and out the other.

"The treatment for symptomatic bradycardia is atropine." Whether you read that on page 458 of a textbook or whether you hear it in hour 7 of your pharmacology series, the result is the same. The lesson is learned in a "low emotional state," so there's no reason to "brand it into your memory."

Now, give that same lesson in the Simulator and put an emotional tag on the lesson.

"You are treating a 65-year-old man for a hernia repair. You have placed a spinal and it's working fine. The surgeon is now dissecting around and pulling on the spermatic cord."

The Simulator suddenly drops the heart rate to the 20s. Through the speakers in the mannequin, a voice says, "I feel funny"; then the sound of retching occurs. The pulse is weak and it's clear the patient is in trouble. The surgeon yells at you, "What the hell's the matter up there!"

The student reaches for atropine, forgets to tell the surgeon to "quit tugging on the spermatic cord!" By mistake the student grabs succinylcholine and gives a full syringe of it, then at the "last cc" the student says, "Oh wait, I didn't want to give that!"

AAG!

Lesson learned? Atropine is the treatment for symptomatic bradycardia. The same lesson as on page 458 of the textbook or hour 7 of the pharmacology series. But *this* lesson is *branded* onto the student's brain. This lesson has a monster emotional tag associated with it, so the student will remember this lesson forever more.

Another lesson gleaned from the educational experts?

Education in the clinical arena is subject to the vagaries of time and chance. For example, any anesthesia resident should know how to recognize and treat a pneumothorax. Pneumothorax can kill in minutes. This is not a condition where you can "stand there like a deer in the headlights" and hope the badness goes away. You have to diagnose it *now* and treat it *now*!

But in the 4 years of anesthesia training, a resident may never see a pneumothorax. A pneumothorax occurred in the ER last night, but he wasn't on call last night. A pneumothorax occurred during line placement in OR 12 today, but the resident was in OR 11 today. Every time a lung drops here, the resident is there.

How can you solve this problem from an educational standpoint? You can always keep the resident in

training for 10 years, figuring that sooner or later, time and chance will line up and finally "hand him a pneumothorax." But that isn't practical.

Enter the Simulator. The Simulator can hand residents anything you want to throw at them. You can, for example, make sure that each and every resident goes through the Simulator and sees a pneumothorax. They'll have to make the diagnosis, place the needle in the chest, and satisfy the Simulator teacher that they know how to handle this dangerous condition.

How about other, rarer conditions, such as malignant hyperthermia or thyroid storm?

Bingo, the Simulator can provide those—no problem. No need to wait for years to see this condition. The Simulator can deliver these conditions piping hot (forgive the pun) anytime you want.

How about the less exotic conditions? The basic problems that plague anesthesia everyday?

Again, the Simulator can provide the perfect educational setting for these conditions too, placing no patient at risk. Right mainstem intubation? Hypoxemia? Hypotension from a spinal anesthetic? These are not bizarre weirdoes that appear once in a blue moon. They happen every day. What better place to teach them than in the Simulator. Plus, because no patient is at risk, because no one is actually hypoxemic, you can do "stop-action" teaching, pausing the scenario as you explain the mechanisms of hypoxemia to your heart's content, taking as long as you want to make sure the resident "gets it." You don't have that kind of time in a real case.

Back to broader educational theory.

The Simulator experience and the traditional experience may both "end up" at the same place. But the Simulator can accelerate learning—the higher line on the graph below.

Now look at the learning graph and ask this question—What happens in the "area between" the lines. What is going on there?

That represents an area where the Simulator people *know* what they are doing and the non-Simulator people *don't know yet* what they are doing. Who gets hurt in there?

Patients.

Take a concrete example to clarify the issue.

About halfway through residency, a difficult central line is being placed. The Simulator person has been trained about pneumothorax recognition and treatment. The non-Simulator person has not.

Pop! The lung gets hit and goes down.

By the time the non-Simulator person sees it and recognizes it, the patient has gone onto a tension

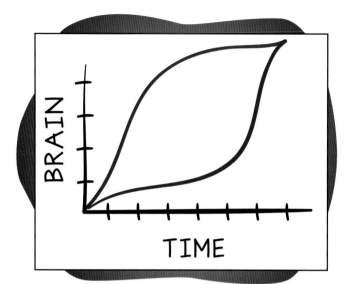

A

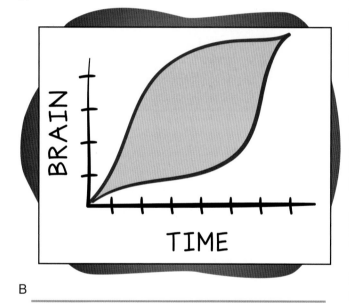

B

FIGURE 7–2 **A.** Educational theory, predigested. Learning over time may get you to the same endpoint, but it may get you there via different pathways. Slow learning is on the lower curve. Accelerated learning is on the upper curve. Traditional medical teaching follows the slow curve: If you stick around the hospital long enough, you eventually see everything you need to see and learn everything you need to learn. Accelerated learning with a Simulator puts you on the fast, upper curve. You don't just "hang around forever" and learn stuff; we target what you need to learn and make sure you learn it in the Simulator. If this all sounds theoretical and hard to prove, you're right! **B.** If you buy this whole paradigm (not everyone does, but I do), the area between traditional, slow learning and accelerated, fast learning represents something. What is that something? Patients getting hurt as you "learn through mistakes." Ouch. Makes a good argument for speeding up the learning process. Makes a good argument for the Simulator.

pneumothorax and is in big trouble, going on to arrest. The Simulator person sees it a little earlier, reacts a little faster, avoids the tension pneumothorax and the arrest.

By the end of their residence, both residents know about pneumothoraces. But the patient who arrested "paid the price." The patient who arrested occupied that dangerous shaded area.

From a bunch of angles, Simulation is an educational *yes*. Simulation is an educational Dr. Jekyll.

Mr. Hyde—Simulators are not the way to educate. Hooey! All this educational theory and all these educational graphs are hooey! The vaporous musings of people with too much time on their hands.

That educational circle with "emotional tags" on the lessons? Sounds sort of plausible, but that's all— plausible. Where's the proof for all these ruminations? And the graph showing learning over time with the deadly "Bermuda Triangle" in the middle where patients are dying like flies? Once again, great stuff to ponder in some journal of educational theory, but the real thing?

I doubt it.

Traditional medical teaching—2 years of preclinical work, 2 years of clinical work, followed by an apprentice-like residency—has given us a great medical system. We produce fine doctors and specialists this way. We don't need some "new teaching with Simulators" to fix a system that is not broken.

And traditional teaching isn't stuck in the Middle Ages. By all means web-based learning, supplemental lectures, assigned reading, small group discussions. This works just fine.

And every time you yank an anesthesia resident from the OR, from the pain clinic, from the PACU, from the ICU, you are replacing flesh-and-blood teaching with latex-and-computer-program teaching. And that mannequin, no matter how good its proponents say it is, is just not the same as taking care of a real patient.

Danger to patients, you say? Of course there is danger to patients, but that is why you have your attending right there, closely supervising, watching the residents like a hawk. The ACGME has laid down guidelines to ensure that residents get adequate rest, sleep, and time off. We have a safe system! Perfect, no—no system is—but pretty good. And no simulator maven can convince me that the system is more perfect with Simulators in the curriculum.

No, Simulators are not the way to teach. From an educational standpoint, the Simulator is a Mr. Hyde.

ACCREDITATION

Dr. Jekyll—We should make board certification a "Simulator event."

United Airlines does not let their pilots grab the stick on that 747 until they prove their mettle in a flight simulator. Hundreds of lives in the air, and possibly hundreds more on the ground, hinge on this pilot's ability. And if the hydraulic system fails (you can sim-ulate that in the safety of the simulator), wind shear occurs (you can simulate that too), the landing gear doesn't come down, one engine flames out—you name it—then the pilot must *prove* his or her stuff. Once he has shown that he can do the job, he gets the green light.

This has such unavoidable logic you just can't argue with it. This is called "face validity." It just plain (or, *plane* in this case) makes sense.

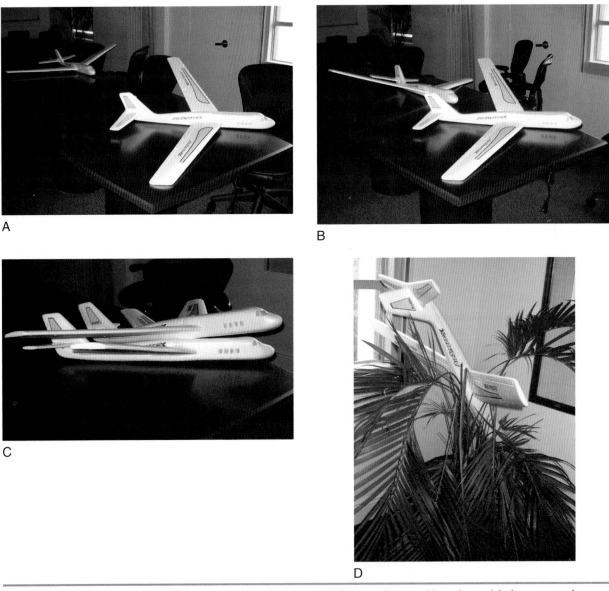

A

B

C

D

FIGURE 7–3   During the debriefing session, you can reconstruct and illustrate disasters. Here, the models demonstrate the catastrophe in Tenerife, when two 747s collided on a runway, killing more than 500 people. Communication between the pilot and the tower broke down, fog obscured the runway, and then—disaster. In a tight OR situation, communication can also break down, "fog" can obscure your thinking, and disaster can occur. Draw lessons from aviation, from history, from current events and apply it to the medical scene. The more variety and interest you inject into the lesson, the better.

Shouldn't you prove this? Have half the pilots prove themselves in the simulator, which leaves a control, untested group. Then, to ensure scientific validity, do this with thousands of pilots, and make sure enough people die so the statistics are clean. Once that tenth 747 plunges out of the sky into a packed baseball stadium, you should be able to draw a superb scientific conclusion with a P value of less than 0.05!

Uh, most folks would prefer we take the face validity and keep testing the pilots. Let's just agree that this is a good idea, avoid rigorous statistics, and keep those 747s up in the air and out of section A of Wrigley Field.

So why not do this in anesthesia too?

Forget proof, look at the logic. Wouldn't you want *your* anesthesiologist to have proven that he or she can handle anesthetic emergencies? Just as pilots prove themselves capable of handling engine failure, shouldn't anesthesiologists prove themselves capable of handling anesthesia machine failure? Is it so much to ask that anesthesiologists prove, before an examiner, that they can handle the things that all anesthesiologists encounter?

Hypoxemia
Hypercarbia
Hypotension
Hypertension
Dysrhythmias
Myocardial ischemia
Difficult or lost airway
Allergic reaction
Light anesthesia

We already "sort of" do this in our oral board exams. Why not do the exam in a simulated operating room? Call it an "oral board on steroids." Instead of just saying, "I would hand-ventilate, listen to both sides of the chest, and suction the endotracheal tube," have the examinee actually *hand-ventilate, listen to both sides of the chest, and suction the endotracheal tube.*

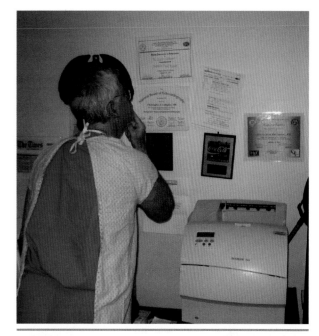

FIGURE 7-4 Certification. Hmm. Should we use the Simulator to certify practitioners? Would that make the certificates on your office wall more meaningful? Would the patient find that more comforting? Would you? Would anyone? Is this inevitable, or are we tinkering with a system that doesn't need additional certification? Hmm.

Not in theory, actually *do it!*

This is not such a stretch, by any means.

Look at this accreditation from two angles: the patient's and the American Board of Anesthesiology's.

Patient: "Wow, when I see that paper on the wall saying 'Board Certified Anesthesiologist', I know that this doctor has really proven him- or herself. In an actual OR, with the same stuff they use on *me*, this doctor proved worthy of certification. I feel so much more comfortable knowing this."

American Board of Anesthesiology: "Before we give our imprimatur, our seal of approval, we really put them through the mill. Not just a written exam (the world is full of geniuses who can memorize facts but can't *do* anything) but a real-live practical exam. We look at them *in action* and make sure they know what they're doing. We are a dandy certification body, amen, amen."

The Simulator as accreditation mechanism is a Dr. Jekyll all the way.

Mr. Hyde: We should not make board certification a "Simulator event."

What, our current system isn't good enough? Who says so? Before someone can even *sit* for their written

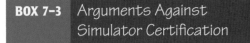

exam, they have to pass three steps of the written medical boards, then they have to go through an ACGME-approved internship, then an ACGME-approved residency. And no one is evaluating their ability to handle hypoxemia, hypercarbia, light anesthesia, or dysrhythmias during all these years of training? *Please*!

Any ACGME-approved residency has to jump through a lot of flaming hoops, making sure that their residents see a wide variety of cases, perform a plethora of procedures, and all the time being evaluated by board-certified anesthesiologists. Now that the six core clinical competencies are mandatory, residents are not learning just technical skills but interactive skills as well, such as professionalism, communication, and how to work in a medical system.

The idea that you have to use a Simulator to "make sure they know what to do" is an insult to residencies everywhere! These residencies have proven it—otherwise they wouldn't be residencies.

The final step of current board certification, the oral board examination, has a long track record. For decades, this has served as a fine "final stamp of approval." Look at mortality statistics from the 70s versus mortality statistics today. Yes, it could be the pulse oximeter, it could be the end-tidal CO_2 monitors, it could be the more rigorous training. Whatever it is, the system *does* seem to be working, so why change it?

The mechanics of the oral boards seems to work pretty well too. For a week, examiners and examinees meet somewhere, the exams proceed, grades go out, and another round of certification is done.

Now let's throw a Simulator into the deal. Oh, that should go swimmingly!

Simulator breakdown? Now what? Computer glitch? Um, come back next week? Examinees talk to each other, so will it be easier to "find out what they're asking" and pass at the end of the week versus the beginning? One resident comes from a "heavy Simulator training" residency, another comes from

a "we don't have a Simulator yet" residency. Is this fair?

Now let's look at the examiners themselves. Just how much do they know about the Simulator? Do we need to "certify the certifiers"? That opens a new can of worms. Do we videotape the exam and review it, just like they "review the films" in football? Who looks at them? What if there is a disagreement on the "call"; do we get someone else to look at the film too?

The logistics start to go super-nova.

Oh, where do we do the exam? Boston's Simulation center? Pittsburgh's? Miami's? Do we need the same mannequin, or a whole bunch of them (there are 19 in Pittsburgh)?

Forget the logistical and administrative nightmare for a while, pretend it doesn't exist. Let's look at the Simulator itself.

No matter how you look at it, the Simulator is not a person. No matter how you look at it, the Simulator cannot do what a patient does. Simulators don't blush or flush. Simulators can vomit, sort of, but Simulator centers rarely do that because clean-up is a monster, and you're always afraid the fake emesis will leak into something and screw up your expensive computer system. Simulators can't buck. They can't reach up (one no-longer-available model could lift one forearm).

Simulators require a nervous technical person to keep a close eye on them ("don't stick the needle there, you'll break the speaker!").

Simulators do have a limited repertoire, and they are slaves to computer input. They are also slaves to computer and technical mishaps.

And upon this rock, you build your certification church?

Forget the Simulator itself, pretend it is absolutely perfect in every way. Now look at the idea of a "Simulator exam."

The Simulator is theater, and some people get stage fright. Other people thrive in the limelight and do quite well "on stage." Should your ability to "act" determine your worthiness as a doctor?

It's easy to imagine a perfectly capable practitioner "choking" during the simulation, particularly if he or she had little practice with the Simulator.

On the flip side, it's easy to imagine a poor practitioner in the "real world" doing quite well in the Simulator, particularly if he or she had a lot of practice with it. Stretch your imagination a little and picture this—to make absolutely sure I pass my Simulator exam, I'll take off 3 months, never do any cases, and just "practice in the Simulator until I have it all down pat."

I myself would not want this person taking care of my child.

No matter how you look at a "Simulator as accreditation" model, it stinks. The Simulator as accreditor is a Mr. Hyde.

AND SO IT GOES

And so it goes with the great debate about the Simulator. From finances to education to accreditation, you can argue that the Simulator is great, or you can argue that the Simulator is horrible.

No one of us is all Dr. Jekyll. No one of us is all Mr. Hyde. We are all, each of us, a little of both.

So too with the Simulator.

CHAPTER 8

Simulation Scenarios and Clinical Lessons Learned

This is the meat of the matter. No muss, no fuss, just one monster collection of simulation scenarios, 50 in all. They unfold as if you were there, in the examining room, the OR, or the ICU setting. Watch and listen along as the scenario develops, the residents try to puzzle it out, and the instructor dissects the whole shebang afterward during the debriefing. A summary at the end of the chapter touches on the main clinical lessons learned.

SCENARIO 1. **A preop surprise: dealing with a provocative patient**

The examining room has a standardized patient (an actor playing the part of a patient).

The resident picks up the chart and looks it over before going in to talk to the patient.

Case. A 47-year-old woman is scheduled for total abdominal hysterectomy. Large fibroids in her uterus have led to heavy bleeding and anemia. There is a history of chronic hepatitis for which she is on steroids, prednisone 20 mg/day. Every time her GI specialist has tried to wean her from the steroids, her hepatitis flares up again. Her SGOT is 90 (she always runs high per her GI clinic chart). Her hematocrit is 27.

Resident goes into the examining room

"Hey, Doc, you're pretty good looking. You know, they'll be taking out the baby carriage but leaving the playpen. What do you say?" She winks.

"Uh," the resident stumbles, "OK, um."

"Aw come on Doc," the patient says, "don't be shy."

The resident soldiers on, "I'm Dr. Thompson, I'll be your anesthesiologist, I just want to ask you a few questions and do a brief exam."

"Sweet pea, you can examine me in my briefs any day and twice on Sunday!" the patient says.

"Have you ever had any trouble with anesthesia, or has anyone in your family ever had any trouble with anesthesia?" the resident asks.

"Well," the patient says, "I got in trouble back when I was a teenager, but I don't think it was no anesthesia doctor did it. Might have been Dr. Love though. You mind if I smoke?" She pulls a pack of Marlboros out of her purse.

"Um." The resident looks up at the ceiling to see if there are any smoke detectors.

"Good, I like a man who doesn't mind a little second-hand smoke," the patient says, "my Daddy smoked all the time, prob'ly blew smoke rings in my crib, never did me no harm."

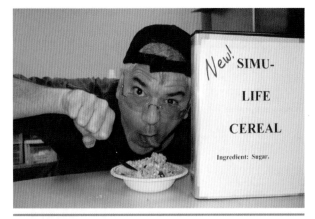

FIGURE 8–1   Dig in. As an instructor, remember this—The worst simulator scenario is still pretty good. (Sort of like sex, even when it's bad, it's still pretty good.) So don't worry about getting it perfect. As a student, remember the same thing—The worst simulator scenario is still pretty good. No matter how you flounder, you're still going to learn.

The patient puts a cigarette to her lips, is just about to light up, when the door opens.

"Simulation over!" the Simulator instructor says.

Clinical lessons learned from scenario 1

Simulations do not have to all involve high-tech mannequins with preprogrammed vital sign aberrations. Actors playing the part of patients make for great simulation too, particularly when the resident isn't looking for this turn of events.

This resident probably thought he would go into an OR setting and end up coding a patient with an intraoperative MI. Instead, he was detoured to an examination room where he had to do a preoperative evaluation. The chart had some stuff worth exploring—hepatitis, steroid use, anemia—so the resident was probably formulating a line of questioning related to these points.

Hepatitis—"Any sign of easy bruising or bleeding?" Concern here centers on the all-important coagulation factors produced by the liver.

Steroid use—"Are you still taking steroids all the time?" Such a patient would not be able to produce a "stress response" of steroids during the perioperative period, so she would need steroid coverage in the OR.

Anemia—"Are you dizzy or short of breath? Do you feel worse now than usual?" With all the bleeding from the fibroids, this low hematocrit of 27 may be new, and the patient won't have any compensatory mechanisms in place. She may need transfusion preop.

On the other hand, if this has been a slow, long-term bleed, the patient may be "used to" such a low hematocrit, and the need to transfuse is less urgent.

Then what happens?

The patient acts inappropriately, taking the interview into forbidden territory. Sexual innuendo and suggestion? What is this? What the heck is the resident supposed to do? This is a bolt from the blue. The resident stumbles, mumbles, and is completely lost with this bizarre twist.

What *was* an exercise in pharmacology and physiology (hepatitis, steroids, anemia) has turned into an exercise in professionalism (how to interact with a provocative patient).

"But, but..." the resident thinks, "I thought the Simulator was for... was for... you know, V-fib and stuff like that!"

Here's how the debriefing goes.

Debriefing. "Hey," the resident demands, "what was up with that? You guys are supposed to teach me how to handle stuff in the OR."

"Oh, is that all we teach you?" the instructor asks. "Aren't we 'perioperative physicians'? Does that not include the preoperative and postoperative arena as well?"

"Well," the resident admits, "yeah, yes I guess so."

"And as an ACGME accredited program, don't we have to teach you *all* the core clinical competencies?" the instructor asks.

The resident nods, lips tightened, and face has turned into a "Oh, that ACGME stuff again" mask.

"And is not one of those competencies 'professionalism'?"

Defeated, the resident's shoulders slump. "OK, OK, you made your point."

"Good," the instructor can't muffle the triumph in his voice, "what, to your mind, is the definition of a professional? We're teaching 'professionalism,' so, after all, I guess we should know what a professional is, shouldn't we?"

"Well," the resident says, "a professional is someone who... someone who went to school and... oh hell, I don't know."

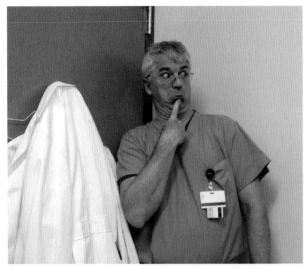

A

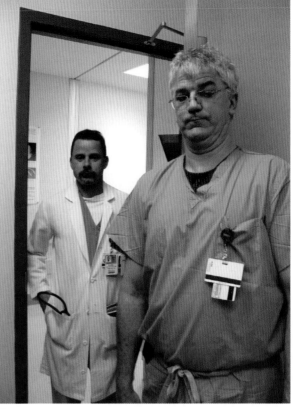

B

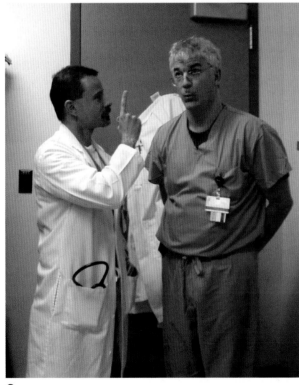

C

FIGURE 8-2 **A.** Losing your professional aplomb. **B.** Get another person in the room—that should re-establish equilibrium. **C.** And if that extra person senses a lack of professionalism, then by all means a stern lecture is in order.

The instructor says, "Pros adapt. That's the simplest definition of a professional and the best way to teach professionalism. Pros adapt, period."

"In anesthesia that means we adapt when the airway's difficult, we secure that airway by hook or crook, or, more appropriately, by fiberoptic or scalpel, when it comes down to it. We adapt when the lines are difficult—we go central line if we have to, we ask for help, we get a Site-Rite machine. We are pros, we adapt, we find a way."

"And sometimes we have to adapt outside the operating room or ICU. We have to adapt to a sudden, disturbing fork in the road. But we are pros, we find a way."

BOX 8-2　Why a Standardized Patient?

- **Person-to-person interaction**
- **Explore behavioral issues**
- **Test flexibility**

"Now here, you have something you never expected. A woman who had you thinking of liver disease and blood counts, and all of a sudden she comes at you from an entirely different direction. What do you do in such a case? What does a pro do?"

"Pros adapt," the resident says.

Down comes the instructor's fist on the table with a bang, "Damn straight you adapt! You're a pro now and that's what pros do!"

Now the resident is all smiles, but a cloud crosses that smiling face.

"Uh," the resident says, "how, precisely, do I adapt? Um. Sir."

The instructor is shaking his hand out now, he overdid it on the table, "Thought you'd never ask."

"What is the crux of the problem you are facing?" the instructor asks.

"She's being inappropriate," the resident says, "she's saying things of a sexual nature, which simply do not belong in the discussion. And nowadays you think, 'Oh God, she's going to sue me and said I touched her and who knows what else!'"

"Right," the instructor says, "so how do you cool down the discussion, what would change the dynamic in the room? What would undo this enforced intimacy, this awkward and unprofessional jam you're in?"

"I don't know."

"What resources do you have in a preoperative setting?" the instructor asks.

"Well," the resident is looking around the room, trying to visualize the holding area, "there are holding area nurses."

"And . . ." The instructor is letting the resident "find his own way."

"I guess if I asked one of the holding area nurses in the room," the resident is putting it together, "then with the extra person there listening the woman would probably chill out a little."

"Anything else?"

"I'd be, sort of, 'protected,' because there would be someone else there, in case later the woman said I did something wrong," the resident says.

"Bingo!", the instructor says. "Getting an extra person in the room is the best protection for you. That should straighten the woman out, get her back to the questions you need to ask her—bleeding questions, all the stuff you need to know—and that extra person also provides you great back up in case of false accusations."

Summary. Anesthesia does not just mean administering anesthetics and fixing vital signs. Anesthesia encompasses the entire perioperative experience, pre-, intra-, and postop. So a simulator experience that trains anesthesia personnel should include the whole shooting match, and that includes dealing with patients.

All kinds of patients.

Most patients are appropriate, but some aren't. We deal with the whole population; and we, as professionals, must adapt no matter what problems we run into.

　　Provocative, like this patient
　　Litigious
　　Anxious
　　Mentally challenged from congenital or acquired cerebral problems
　　Threatening, as anyone who's worked with the prison population knows

So a simulator session would include such a patient. Dealing with them is difficult, but deal with them we must!

Note how the Simulator session and the debriefing session mesh quite well with teaching the ACGME core clinical competencies—especially the "tough to teach" competencies such as professionalism and communication skills.

Note also how the debriefing session is not a straight didactic: "You did this right/you did this wrong. Got it? Good bye." At a good debriefing session the resident thinks things over, looks at the gray areas, and then is given the time and freedom to eventually find the answer themselves, with guidance from the instructor.

SCENARIO 2. | **Headache with attitude, an intracranial bleed**

"Get to room 3 right away!" The resident goes into the OR.

Case. An intubated patient is on the operating table, an arterial line is in, plus a 16 gauge IV. An anesthesiologist is at the foot of the table trying to straighten out the lines. An infusion pump running nitroprusside is on the IV pole, but it came disconnected and is dripping onto the floor. Two surgery people are placing

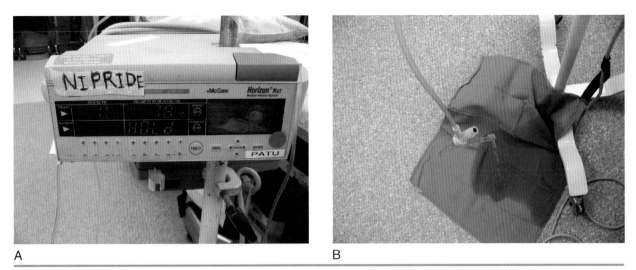

A   B

FIGURE 8–3 Why oh why could the blood pressure be so high? Ooops! The nipride is disconnected. Sound unlikely? You'd be amazed how often this simple glitch occurs (kinked or disconnected lines, malfunctioning pumps).

pins on the head, and there is an obvious sense of agitation in the room.

On the monitors, there is an arterial line, but you can only see the "bottom part" of the arterial line trace. The number on the art line reads a nearly incredible 300/160. The patient is tachycardic to 120.

"Big bleed in the head," the neurosurgeon says, pointing over his shoulder at a CT that is up on the view box. A huge bleed is apparent. The OR table is turned around 180 degrees, so the feet are by the anesthesia machine and the head is up by the surgeons. The head is cranked down with the chin touching the clavicle.

The anesthesiologist in the room doesn't notice the disconnected nitroprusside or the sky-high blood pressure.

Now the surgeon looks up and sees the blood pressure, "Holy shit, is that right? What the hell are you guys doing up there?"

Just as the surgeon says that, the heart rate drops to 100, then 80, then 60, then 40.

"Hey, he's bucking!"

The resident in the room reaches over to the drug cart, grabbing a syringe of rocuronium and another of Pentothal. Running around to the IV, the resident pushes the Pentothal and rocuronium, wham bam, one after the other.

Opening the patient's eyes, the neurosurgeon says, "Hey, look at this."

After opening the IV wide open to carry in the Pentothal and rocuronium, the anesthesia resident goes

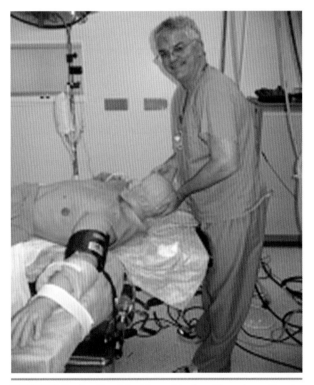

FIGURE 8–4 Careful with positioning. If you hyperflex the neck and have the chin touching the clavicle, you can stretch vessels supplying the spinal cord and end up with a quadriplegic patient. Rule of thumb? Two fingerbreadths separation between the chin and clavicle for each 70 kg of body weight. Another trick? Put your *own* head in the position you put the *patient's* head in. If *you* are uncomfortable, the *patient* is too. For that matter, this lesson applies for all positioning. If you don't like it, the patient won't.

up to the head of the bed and looks. The left pupil is blown.

The heart rate drops to 30.

The blood pressure drops down from the stratosphere, now down to 200/120.

Up go the drapes, and the surgeons go at it.

"Hey, this brain is tight as a drum skin, what are you doing up there?"

The anesthesia resident looks at the end-tidal CO_2. In all the excitement, the ventilator wasn't checked: 55, the end-tidal monitor says.

The resident increases the ventilation, asks for some mannitol. After a few minutes, the surgeon's report: "That's better."

At the same time, the heart rate increases to 60.

"Simulation over!" the instructor says.

Clinical lessons learned from scenario 2

Haste makes waste, never more so than in a medical emergency.

Getting called into a room with a 4+ disaster is a hair-raising experience, enough to discombobulate the best practitioner. Everything is happening all at once. Everything is going wrong, and everything needs fixing now, sooner than now, more like 10 seconds ago. You try to organize your thoughts along the ABC line; but with surgeons yelling at you, a blood pressure that could launch a Titan V rocket, and a Medusa's head of lines, it's hard to do the right things in the right order.

If only you could press a *freeze* button, you could make order out of chaos. But fate has not handed us such a magical button. And a critically ill patient doesn't hand you that most luxurious of gifts—time.

And things happen in a rush. Stuff gets disconnected, but, hey, you were in a rush to get the patient over to the table. If you took all the time in the world and made sure absolutely everything was neat and tidy, the patient might die a neat and tidy death.

Let's look in the mind of this anesthesia resident during the debriefing from this scenario.

Debriefing. The instructor opens the discussion, "What were your priorities in this case?"

BOX 8-3	Controlling Increased ICP

- **ABC—fix all three**
- **Stop bucking**
- **Pharmacologic measures**

"Like any case," the resident says, "a quick survey, focusing on the ABC. It was evident the patient was in extremis and needed cerebral decompression as soon as possible."

"Did you listen to the chest to make sure the endotracheal tube was in?" the instructor asks.

"No, I could see that there was end-tidal CO_2, so I knew the tube was in the right place," the resident says, "and I saw the saturation was 100%, so I went right to the most pressing issue, the 'C' part, a deadly high blood pressure."

"What were you thinking?"

"With the big bleed the surgeon mentioned," the resident says, "I envisioned the compensatory mechanisms the body uses to maintain cerebral perfusion pressure. Because the intracranial pressure was high secondary to compression from the hematoma, the body raised the systemic blood pressure in an attempt to keep the rest of the brain supplied with blood."

"So why try to get that pressure down?"

"At 300 systolic, the strain on the heart would be unbearable and would lead to a cardiac arrest within minutes. Also, if this cerebral bleed were from a ruptured aneurysm, that pressure of 300 would turn that torn aneurysm into a fire hose, pouring more blood into the brain."

"What was your goal?"

"Get the pressure down to something the heart might be able to tolerate," the resident says, "say a systolic of 200 or so. Still high, so you could still get cerebral perfusion, but not so high that it places the heart at risk."

"But you didn't have time to look everything over, did you?"

"No, the patient bucked, indicating he wasn't paralyzed. That bucking is bad for increased intracranial pressure. The patient was at risk for cerebral herniation with that huge bleed. When I first got in the room, I feared that might happen, as indeed it did."

"How did you know?"

"At first," the resident says, "the patient had hypertension, increased intracranial pressure, and tachycardia, so he didn't have the classic Cushing's triad. But that changed after the patient bucked. Then the patient did develop the classic triad of blood pressure elevation (to keep cerebral perfusion pressure up), increased intracranial pressure (from the bleed), and reflex bradycardia (the heart's response to the high blood pressure)."

"So what did you do?"

"The nitroprusside was disconnected, so I couldn't use that to drop the blood pressure, so I reached for Pentothal to drop the blood pressure and rocuronium to paralyze the patient and prevent further bucking."

"Would nitroprusside have been your first line to drop the blood pressure?" the instructor asks.

"No," the resident says, "nitroprusside is a dilator and can increase cerebral blood flow and hurt our intracranial pressure picture. Pentothal is good for decreasing the cerebral metabolic rate of oxygen—a good drug in this setting. Plus, Pentothal helps drop the blood pressure."

"What did you think about the head positioning?" the instructor asks.

"I didn't like it," the resident says. "Extreme flexion of the head with the chin touching the clavicle is too extreme. That can cause stretch of the vessels supplying the spinal cord and can lead to spinal cord ischemia. I would have preferred to reposition the head, making sure there were at least two fingerbreadths of space between the clavicle and the chin for each 70 kg of patient body weight."

"But you didn't do that."

"No," the resident says, "the patient herniated, as evident by the pupil dilating unilaterally. The brain was getting squished down into the foramen magnum, and death would result in minutes, so it was more important to get that head open and drain the blood as soon as possible. Truth to tell, it would have been all too easy to forget about that later on."

"When troubles come, they come not as single spies," the instructor says, "but in battalions."

"Amen to that," the resident says.

"And once the head was opened, what was the next problem that appeared?"

"The surgeon complained of a 'tight head,' indicating that I needed to do what I could to reduce brain volume. That means adequate drainage, no kinking of the head or neck vessels, hyperventilation, and osmotic diuresis."

"But the CO_2 got away from you," the instructor observes.

"Yes," the resident admits, "guilty as charged. With all the excitement of the herniation, I forgot to check all the details, and I had inadequate ventilator settings. Once I saw the high CO_2, I increased ventilation to drive the CO_2 down and help shrink the brain."

"But not too much, right?" the instructor asks.

"Correct," the resident says, "I would aim for an end-tidal CO_2 of about 25 to 30. More severe hyperventilation could result in cerebral ischemia, plus the resulting respiratory alkalosis could impair oxygen delivery."

"These neuro cases are real physiologic showcases, aren't they?"

"Don't you know it."

Summary. Hours of boredom, moments of panic. So goes one description of anesthesia. An impending cerebral herniation certainly qualifies as one of the "moments of panic."

In this case, a patient had been rushed up to the OR, probably from the CT scanner, with a life-threatening intracranial bleed. In the zippety doo-da transfer to the OR table, a nitroprusside drip had gotten disconnected, unmasking a horrific hypertension that could kill the patient, well, a second time if the herniating brain didn't kill him first. Talk about double jeopardy!

Into this high stress simulator scenario an anesthesia resident arrives, just when everything starts to fall apart. A quick assessment and quick thinking brought all the important points into focus (tube's in, pressure's high, patient needs paralysis), although a couple of other points did escape this initial scan (making sure to undo the severe neck flexion, hyperventilating).

The resident demonstrated a good understanding of intracranial pressure, cerebral perfusion pressure, and the signs of herniation. Actions were quick and appropriate, a nimble response to a tough case.

SCENARIO 3. **Local in the wrong locale, intravascular injection during an epidural**
The overhead speaker says, "Anesthesia to labor room 2, anesthesia to labor room 2 to top up an epidural." Into labor room 2 goes the anesthesia resident.

Case. On a labor table, a pregnant patient with attached epidural is groaning (through the speakers in the mannequin). The patient's feet are up in stirrups, and the OB is sitting in front of her, holding forceps.

"Hey," the OB says, "glad you showed up. I could use a little help here. Your epidural is no great shakes."

"OK," the resident says, "how are you doing, ma'am?" As the resident speaks, she looks around for the anesthetic paperwork—preop evaluation, anesthetic record detailing the epidural placement, dose and rate of local anesthetic given and running.

"Bozhe moi," the patient groans, "bozhe moi, boleet, boleet! Rebyonik vilyezaet!"

"Oh yeah," the OB says, "she just moved here from Minsk. She only speaks Russian or Ukrainian or something."

The patient is connected to a blood pressure cuff, a fetal heart rate monitor, and a pulse oximeter.

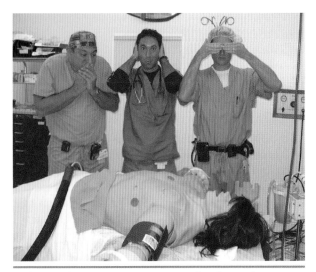

FIGURE 8–5 Language barrier—what do you do? Do you just pretend that there isn't a problem? Not an effective plan. There are a lot of creative ways around this—get acquainted with the hospital's translation service. Find a relative who can function as interpreter. Best answer—learn the language yourself! A little involved, to be sure, but a great way to impress people at cocktail parties.

Lost in the paperwork, the anesthesia resident says, "Uh huh."

The anesthesia preop outlines the case.

More of the case. A 22-year-old G1P0A0, previously healthy woman appeared for delivery. Good prenatal care, no complications. Takes vits. Translator—husband (patient is Russian speaker only). Airway, Mallimpotti 2; labs pending. Patient currently at 3 cm dilation and in discomfort. "Plan—combined spinal epidural. Case fully discussed per translator, detailed risks/benefits/options. Patient agrees to proceed."

Vital signs were normal, and the patient was not morbidly obese. If ever there were a routine case, this was it.

The anesthetic record detailed an unremarkable course.

"Patient given fluid bolus, FHR checked and monitored throughout. Patient sat up, prep/drape, local placed at L3–4. Loss of resistance technique used to identify epidural space. A 25 g pencil point needle used through Touhy needle, clear CSF, no paresthesias. Fentanyl 15 μg was injected after a positive aspiration. Spinal needle withdrawn, epidural catheter placed, Touhy withdrawn, catheter secured. Aspiration negative for blood or CSF, test dose without adverse reaction. Infusion of 0.125% levobupivicaine (10 cc/hr) with 5 fentanyl (5 μg/cc) begun."

"Good pain relief, patient stable, FHR OK throughout."

So far, so good.

But now the OB was complaining, in English, and the patient was complaining, in Russian.

"OK, is the husband around?" the resident asks, "my Russian is not too good."

"He was here all night," the OB says, "he's conked out in the lounge. Listen, honey, this here epidural is not winning any Nobel prizes for pain relief, can you do something to help me here? Baby needs a little help with these forceps, and mom isn't going for it."

"Um, OK," the anesthesia resident says, "my name is Dr. Nelson, not 'honey'."

"Bozhe moi, pomogeetye mnyeh, rebyonik vilyezaet, rebyonik vilyezaet!" the patient shouts.

"Fine," the OB snaps, "I'm so happy the political correctness, thought and mind control Gestapo have shown up to make sure I don't step on any feminine sensibilities, *Doctor* Nelson. Now make this god damned epidural work!"

"Boleet, boleet! Akh da, gdye moi moozh?" the patient shouts.

Dr. Nelson goes to the head of the bed, looks at the epidural catheter and notices that the infusion tubing has come disconnected from the cap. In sterile fashion, she reconnects them.

"So," the OB still has attitude in his voice, "can you help me or not, or do you want me to do like they did in *Gone with the Wind*, and just put a knife under the bed so it cuts the pain in half?"

"No need," Dr. Nelson says, "the epidural became disconnected, I'll have to rebolus."

"Oh great," the OB says, "well make it snappy, I've got to get these salad spoons on."

Dr. Nelson draws up a syringe of 0.25% levobupivicaine, connects to the tubing, aspirates, then injects 5 cc. She waits a minute, then injects the other 5 cc.

"Chto eto!" the Russian woman says, "Chto sluchilas? Mnye ochen . . . chto eto zvonok?" Then she falls silent.

The fetal heart rate monitor drops to 40, the patient's pulse oximeter stops beeping.

"Hey!" the OB shouts, what's going on here? What did you give?"

Dr. Nelson gives a sternal rub and shouts at the patient, then reaches down for a pulse, there is none.

"Oh Christ!" the OB shouts, then drops the forceps, goes up to the chest, and starts CPR. "Call a code!"

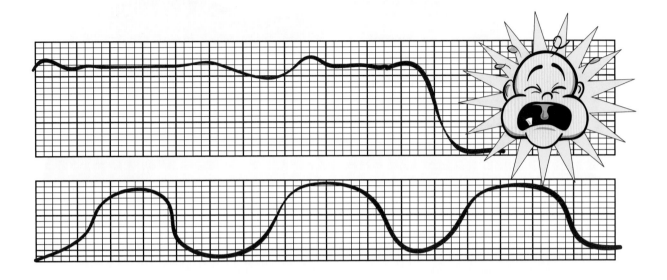

FIGURE 8–6 Know your fetal heart rate strips! Baby dumpling is heart rate-dependent. So when that heart rate drops, baby dumpling is in big trouble!

Dr. Nelson looks around for a laryngoscope, an Ambu-bag, anything.

"Simulation over!" the instructor chirps.

Clinical lessons learned from scenario 3

Dr. Nelson faced a prickly path in labor room 2.

She was "inheriting" an epidural, so she had to come up to speed on that.

Her co-worker and fellow doctor treated her dismissively.

Things were coming to a clinical head, or, more precisely, an occiput, as the woman was in need of a forceps delivery.

A regional anesthetic was in use, and there was a language barrier.

And that was just the *start* of Dr. Nelson's troubles. The debriefing picks up the thread.

Debriefing. "So," the instructor says, "how do you think that went?"

Dr. Nelson's head is hanging down, "Not too good, I think I killed them both. 200% mortality. Not a stellar performance."

"Relax," the instructor reassures, "be glad she didn't have twins. Then it would be 300%."

"Thanks," Dr. Nelson groans, "I feel a lot better."

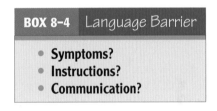

BOX 8-4 Language Barrier

- Symptoms?
- Instructions?
- Communication?

"Before we get to the thrilling conclusion, let's go over things from the start. What was the situation, and what were your concerns when you came through the door?"

"Pregnant patient, so you think about all the concerns there—full stomach, possible difficult airway, any sedation you give to mom you give to the baby, decreased FRC so the patient can desaturate quickly. Plus we have an epidural in, so you are always thinking—is this in the right place, is it working, could it be intrathecal, could it be intravascular?"

"Right," the instructor says, "so you have the physiology of pregnancy on your mind, the pharmacology of epidurally infused local anesthetics and narcotics on your mind. But then, it's not like we do things in a library, is it, a physiology textbook on one side, a pharmacology textbook on the other?"

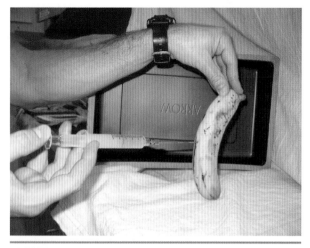

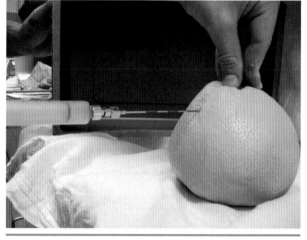

FIGURE 8–7 Believe it or not, the fruit and vegetable world provides us with some partial-task simulators. The epidural needle gets a loss of resistance as it goes through the skin into the, the (what do you call it?), the banana *meat*? The banana *essence*?

FIGURE 8–8 Some parturients are somewhat, um, short for their weight. So to practice this sometimes difficult epidural placement, use a fruit that is also somewhat, um, short for its weight.

"No," Dr. Nelson says, "there is the human factor."

"Aah yes," the instructor agrees, "and what are the human factors at work here?"

Both the OB and the patient (the Russian speaking technician who was providing the voice for the simulator mannequin) enter the debriefing room.

"Well," Dr. Nelson starts out, "the OB was a demanding asshole of a chauvinistic pig."

"I try," the OB says.

"So I had to deal with his 'woman-doctor-as-honey' comments and still try to keep a professional head on my shoulders and assess the patient."

"Let's give the devil his due, Dr. Nelson," the instructor says, "let's look at things from the OB's point of view and add a touch of real world to this scenario."

The OB chimes in, "I mentioned the husband had been up all night; guess what, I had been up all night too. So now I'm wiped out, I don't have my 'Mr. Perfect' hat on because I'm frustrated with a poorly functioning epidural. And yes, I said a stupid thing. You could kick my ass on this, and I guess you'd be within your rights, but keep in mind, I *am* your referral base. And if you go ape every time someone says something stupid in the hospital, then you'd better transfer to Perfection Memorial Surgery Center, where everyone is always considerate and kind and wonderful 24/7. And let me know when you find that place."

Dr. Nelson bristles, "I thought I handled it OK, though. I made my point without going to the Supreme Court, and I passed over his 'thought Gestapo' swipe."

The instructor says, "Touché, you did that. What was the other human factor going on here?"

"Russian. The woman spoke Russian, and that really hurts my ability to ask for symptoms," Dr. Nelson says.

"What do the textbooks say about that?" the instructor asks.

"Some say that a language barrier is an absolute contraindication to using a regional anesthetic!" Dr. Nelson says. "In theory, that is right. How can you ask about 'ringing in the ears, a funny taste in the mouth' and other subjective signs of an intravascular injection of local anesthetic?

"But on the OB floor, that is just plain not practical," Dr. Nelson continues. "What are you going to do—a general anesthetic on every patient with a language barrier? The prime dictum of obstetric anesthesia is doing everything in your power to avoid general anesthesia, with the risk of airway loss and hypoxemic catastrophe. So we do the best we can, using whatever translation services we can—family members, nurses, orderlies—you can even get some translation services over the phone nowadays."

"But there is still that risk," the instructor says. "There is still that concern that the patient is saying something that you need to know, but you can't understand it."

"Yep," Dr. Nelson admits, then turns to the Russian technician, "What were you saying, anyway?"

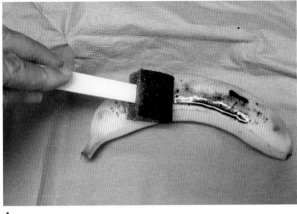

A

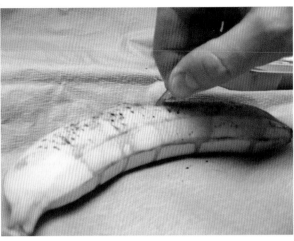

B

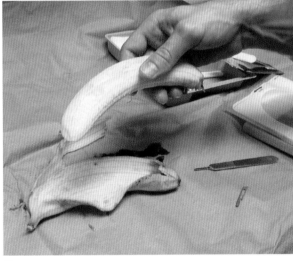

C

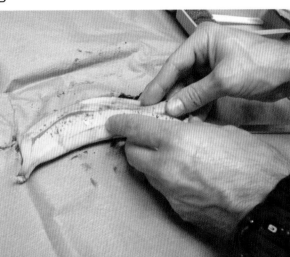

D

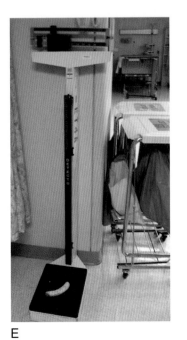

E

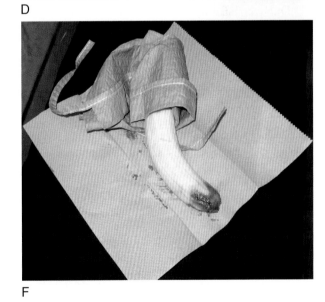

F

FIGURE 8–9 Our obstetric friends can also tap the fruit basket to practice their skills. Here a banana demonstrates how a C-section is done. Prep, cut open the peel, take out the banana, close up the peel. Then weigh the little darling and give him a cute blue cap. Maybe clean him up a little too.

"Turns out I was saying something important," the technician says, in perfectly unaccented English, "I was saying, 'It hurts, the baby is coming.' The whole controversy here swirled around dosing me up for a forceps delivery. But while you and the OB were sniping at each other, the baby was coming down on his own, obviating the need for forceps and for the dose-up."

"Oh," both OB and Dr. Nelson say; neither had been privy to what the Russian speaker would say. Damned clever twist he came up with. No one had been thrown by the fact the voice was that of a man. Oh well, pros adapt, as they say.

"All right," the instructor says (wow, even he didn't know about that sneaky little tweak—better remember that at Christmas bonus time). "We talked about the pharmacology and physiology and the human factors. What else heaves into view as we get toward the end of our little morality play?"

"Equipment," Dr. Nelson says.

"Why do you say that?" the Russian speaker asks.

"When I dosed the epidural, despite giving the local anesthetic in divided doses, the local anesthetic either went intrathecally—causing a total spinal and plummeting blood pressure—or intravascularly—causing cardiovascular collapse," Dr. Nelson says. "Either way, I needed to resuscitate the patient, and that means having resuscitative equipment nearby—intubating stuff like endotracheal tubes and laryngoscopes, Pentothal to stop seizures."

"Did you have any of that stuff?" the instructor asks.

"Oh, I didn't check," Dr. Nelson admits. "That, I should have done. What was that you were saying, anyway?" Dr. Nelson asks the Russian speaker.

"I said, 'What's that, what happened, what is that bell?' Then I stopped. I was responding the way a patient might respond to an intravascular injection of local anesthetic, when they first feel funny, then they might hear ringing in their ears, then they lose consciousness. I would seize too, but the simulator mannequin can't do that yet."

"Anything else you might have done differently?" the OB asks. "Like when the code started and I went up to the chest to start compressions?"

"I don't follow you," Dr. Nelson admits.

"How effective are chest compressions in the still-pregnant patient?"

"Oh yeah," Dr. Nelson tumbles to it, "chest compressions in the pregnant patient are ineffective until the baby is out. Better to deliver the baby right away—your forceps might have been able to snag it—then the chest compressions are much more effective."

"Righty-oh," the instructor wraps it up.

Summary. A simple epidural and anticipated forceps delivery encounters some turbulence. Dr. Nelson has to brush off a snippy and demeaning comment, focus on the patient's needs, work through a language barrier, and handle an intravascular injection of local anesthetic.

Just thinking "To hell with it, the husband is asleep" left both OB and the anesthesia resident blind to extremely important information. That baby was coming, and there was no need for them to do anything! Also, the subjective symptoms of the intravascular injection escaped Dr. Nelson.

Routine practice means making sure you have all your "rescue stuff" nearby. Dr. Nelson was caught short when disaster struck. Plus, in the "who-wouldn't panic" mode of a code, Dr. Nelson forgot a fundamental principle of CPR in the pregnant patient—get the baby out before you do chest compression.

The final lesson: When injecting local anesthetic, stick to this rule—every dose is a test dose. Never slam in a gallon of that stuff because if it goes intravascular you could be in deep Kimchee.

Maybe next time they should do that "knife cuts the pain in half" trick from *Gone with the Wind*.

SCENARIO 4. **Help from across the drapes, hypoxemia in the OR**

"Any anesthesiologist to OR 18, any anesthesiologist to OR 18 *stat!*"

A CA-3, a senior anesthesia resident, answers the call and goes into OR 18.

BOX 8-5	Intravascular Injection of Local Anesthetic

- Stop injection (duh!)
- Cardiovascular and respiratory support
- CPB if necessary

BOX 8-6	Obstetric Pain Relief

- Regional
- Parenteral
- Knife under the bed?

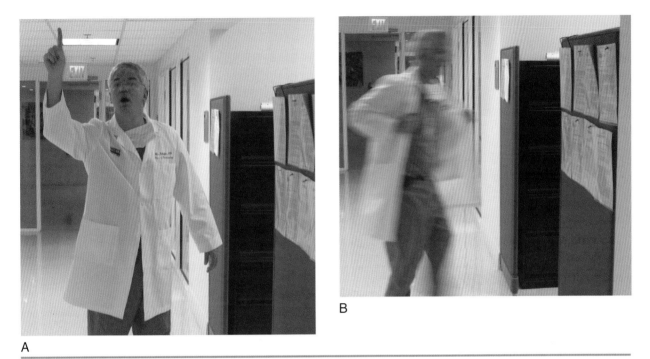

A

B

FIGURE 8–10 *Stat* call? When an anesthesiologist calls for help *stat*, it is the real McCoy. Lost airway, cardiac arrest, whatever it is, they need that extra hand and they need that extra hand *right now*.

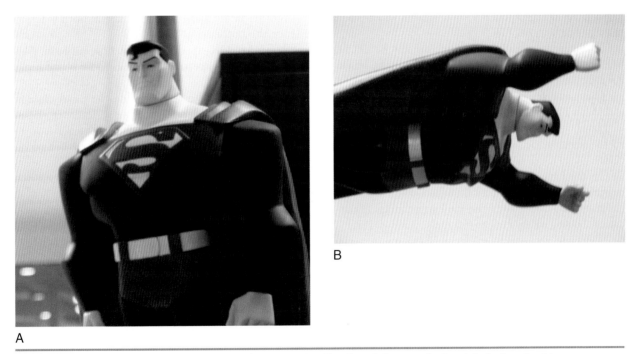

A

B

FIGURE 8–11 Fly to the room if you can. That extra pair of hands and that extra brain might be just the thing to save your anesthesiology partner, and, lest we forget, save a patient as well.

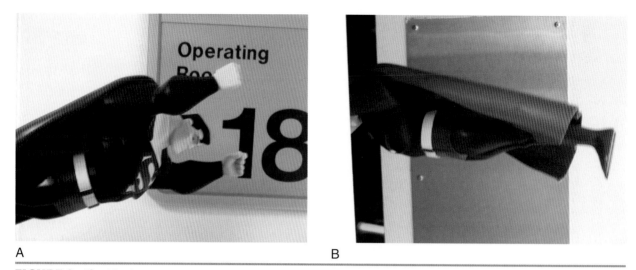

A   B

FIGURE 8-12 The best part about being the "second person in the room" is that you always look good. If you save the day—great. If you don't, well, then at least you showed up and tried.

In OR 18, a CA-1, a junior resident, is at the head of the table, hand ventilating the patient. The patient is intubated, the drapes are up, and everyone is in mid-operation, two surgeons operating and the usual surgical team doing their thing.

"Hey," the first surgeon yells, "lend a hand here. Bozo here just graduated clown school and made a wrong turn into my OR."

That cracks up the other surgeon, and he chimes in, "Blood-brain barrier, right. How about the blood-brain*less* barrier!"

They get back to work.

"What's up?" the senior resident asks.

Hand ventilating and cranking his head around to the screen, the junior resident says, "Look at the STs."

On the EKG, a tombstone pattern of ST elevation is present. Ischemia that a blind man could see.

The CA-3 looks over the vital signs, oxygen saturation 100%, BP by cuff 85/50, pulse 130.

"Why are you hand-ventilating?" the senior asks.

"Well, he's ischemic, so I figure he's going to arrest. I know you hand ventilate in an arrest, anyway, it seemed like a good thing to do," the junior says, flustered and shook.

Flipping the ventilator switch from manual to automatic, the senior resident says, "Relax, let the ventilator do the work. You have to figure out what's going on, free up your hands."

"Now why's this guy ischemic?" the senior asks.

An audio alarm goes off, both reach up to silence the alarm.

"OK, this is a liver resection, that's what it says; and they're losing a lot of blood. I'm trying to keep up, but I think I'm behind," the junior says, then hands the senior the preop. "This guy's had a couple stents, he's 70, so he's got ischemia. I mean he's a setup for ischemia, and now this."

Another audio alarm goes off. Again, both reach to silence the bothersome alarm.

"You guys OK up there?", the first surgeon asks, now a shred of concern in his voice. "The blood looks a little dark here."

Taking charge, the CA-3 decides he's had enough from the knife-wielders, "Yeah, we're fine, see if you can slow down that bleeding. They did teach you to tie in school didn't they? Or do you need Velcro on your shoes?"

Two alarms now go off, and both get silenced in a split second.

"OK, let's look all this stuff over, that's the way you do it when things go south in a case, go it?" the CA-3 soothes the CA-1. "ABC, always start with ABC."

He looks around, "Tube's in, so we got A and B, now the C part needs a little work," the senior says, pausing only to push another "silence alarm" button.

"I'm not kidding you guys," the second surgeon says, "this blood really *does* look dark!"

"Yeah yeah," the CA-3 says, "sure it does. We got it."

On the EKG, the STs are even higher.

"Listen, this is all about myocardial supply and demand, and right now there's too much demand—look at that heart rate—and not enough supply—look

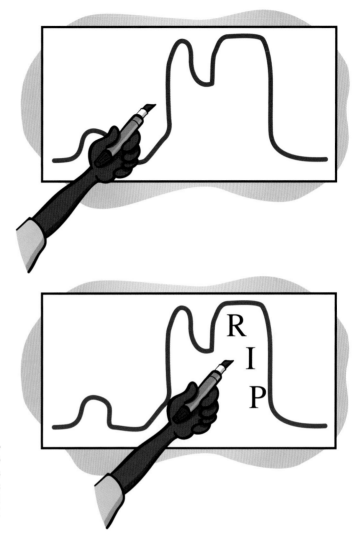

FIGURE 8–13 ST troubles. When ST segments go down, it usually means subendocardial ischemia. That is not good. When ST segments go up, it usually means transmural ischemia. That is not good with capital letters. And those capital letters can go to these capital letters—RIP.

at that blood pressure," the senior explains. "Hang blood, keep transfusing until that heart rate goes down. They've obviously lost a ton resecting that liver."

From the other side of the drapes, the surgeon suddenly appears and bursts between the residents. "What in blue blazes is going on up here, I tell you the blood's dark, and no one pays attention to me, do you even have this ventilator on, I don't see the chest rising!"

"Hey," the CA-3 is bristling with territoriality, "what are you doing. . . ."

"Wait," the CA-1 says, "he's right." Reaching over, the junior resident turns on the ventilator. The senior resident had switched from manual to ventilator but had not turned the ventilator itself on.

A look of triumph on his face, the surgeon goes back to the other side of the curtain.

"We're done!" the instructor says.

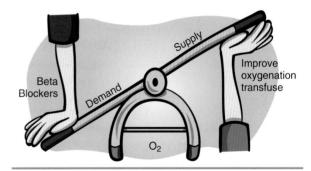

FIGURE 8–14 When it comes to ischemia, go for the myocardial oxygen supply/demand teeter-totter. Decrease the demand (beta blockers) and increase supply (improve oxygenation, transfuse). If you've fixed everything you can fix, you have to go to the big guns—revascularization by stent or even CABG.

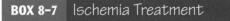

BOX 8-7 Ischemia Treatment

- **Increase O$_2$ supply**
- **Decrease O$_2$ demand (beta blockade!)**
- **Think of teeter-totter**

Clinical lessons learned from scenario 4

"Any anesthesiologist to OR 18!" is enough to send chills down any anesthesiologist's spine. No one puts out such a call unless the ship has hit an iceberg, the car is plummeting over the cliff, the airplane's wing just fell off.

But call it you must, if in trouble. And respond you must, if you hear it.

The junior resident was overmatched by circumstances. (After all, you can't know it all at the beginning—that's why we *do* residencies!) So he put out a call to his more senior colleague.

Upon arrival, the senior resident pegged the problem—blood loss, low blood pressure, high heart rate—all the classic signs of hypovolemia. Couple this with a patient prone to ischemia, and you get, no surprise, ischemia. The heart is banging away, trying to compensate for the low blood volume, so that places a high demand on the heart. But supply is short—the patient has bled a lot, so there is low oxygen content. Also, the pressure head pushing blood down the coronaries is low, so the heart is going into oxygen debt.

Presto-chango, ischemia prone myocardium is now ischemic myocardium.

Never fear, senior resident to the rescue!

The debriefing reveals just how good a rescue he delivered.

Debriefing. "What were you thinking when you called for help?" the instructor asks the CA-1.

"I knew from the preop that this patient could develop problems related to his coronary disease. Then when the surgeons, well actually the circulator, reported a lot of blood loss, then I saw the low blood pressure and the STs, and it started to be too much too fast," the CA-1 says, "so I sort of 'went to ground,' hand ventilating and getting someone to help me."

"Did you think you would need an a-line for this case?" the instructor asks.

"Well, the surgeon said he had one of these kind of oscillating Harmonic Scalpel things, that cauterizes as it cuts, so you shouldn't lose much blood," the CA-1 explains.

"But he did."

"Boy howdy, he did," the junior says.

"How would you rank your interaction with the surgeon? Were you able to communicate effectively with him or the surgical team?" the instructor asks.

"Not too well, they were bugging me, mostly, and not much help," the junior says.

"Does that matter?" the instructor asks.

"Yeah, I mean, the OR is not meant to be a fight about pecking order," the junior says, "the patient sort of trumps all that."

"Listen," the surgeon, now sitting in on the debriefing, says, "you might not like getting a little static from your surgery buddies, but I got news for you. That's exactly what you're going to get when you graduate from here. Private practice medicine is not a cruise on *The Love Boat*."

Then the surgeon, still imperious and strutting from the OR scenario, turns to the CA-3, the cavalry that was supposed to ride in and save the day, "Help me out here, just what was your role in this fiasco?"

Looking at the instructor for guidance, the CA-3 holds his hands palms up, "Here I stand, hat in hand."

"No need for martyrs here," the instructor reassures, "just go through what you were thinking."

"Right away, the surgeon is getting under my skin," the senior says. "So I figure I have to rein him in or shut him up, one or the other, so I can fix this obvious case of myocardial ischemia.

"I'm going through the whole teeter-totter thing—oxygen supply here, oxygen demand there—and I wanted to even out that teeter-totter so the patient's heart can have an adequate oxygen supply and get out of the 'ischemic zone.'"

"So what did you do?" the instructor asks.

"Well, I knew we'd need to do something fast, the usual thing is to get the blood pressure up in a bleeding patient—turn down the anesthetic agents, check and hang blood, give pressors, put the head down," the senior explains. "And having the CA-1 all tied up hand-ventilating wasn't doing us any real good. So I went to free him up."

"And that's when I made the mistake, I turned the one switch but didn't bother to turn the second switch, so the ventilator was off," the senior says.

"Why did that happen?" the surgeon asks in, of all things, a reasonable tone.

"Distraction, too much happening at once," the senior explains. "The surgeon is riding me, the CA-1 is giving me the doe eyes, the 'help me, I'm a drowning puppy and no one can save me' look."

"Hey," the CA-1 protests.

"Sorry," the CA-3 apologizes. "So anyway all this stuff is going on, and alarms are going off, which I stupidly shut off rather than paying attention to."

"And now the surgeon is actually telling you something important," the instructor says, "that the blood is dark."

"Right," the senior says, "but I lump that in with all the other crap he said, and I completely blow it off."

"So how do you sift the wheat from the chaff in a case like that?" the instructor asks, "How do you tell the real deal from static?"

The CA-1 picks it up, "It's tough, but I guess you have to forget the 'attitude' thing, you have to weigh each thing as it comes in. He might say 10 snippy remarks, but when that 11th one says, 'The blood is dark,' you have to pay attention to it."

"That you do," the CA-3 says.

Summary. Anesthesia providers learn the drill of myocardial protection early. Keep the patient well oxygenated, keep other "supply-side" factors (hemoglobin, blood pressure) favorable. Keep the "demand-side" factors favorable too—avoid tachycardia and keep the blood pressure normal.

But there's many a slip "twixt the cup and the lip." Even someone perfectly versed in "myocardial lore," such as this CA-3, can drop the ball on something as fundamental as turning on the ventilator!

Throw in a "Chatty Kathy" surgeon, some interpersonal edginess, mix in a little anesthesia defensive-ness, and add a dash of a junior resident who's a little lost, and you have all the ingredients for "disaster soup."

Final lesson? Even a surgeon who bugs the heck out of you can walk right up and save the day for you. Who, after all, noticed the chest not rising?

Sometimes you have to give the devil his due.

SCENARIO 5. Too much of a good thing—narcotic overdose

"Doctor, could you step over here," the ICU nurse says, "there's something you need to see here."

The patient is lying in bed, the ventilator is at the side of the bed but not connected to the patient. There is a subclavian central line in the patient, a face mask for oxygen is on, an EKG shows normal sinus rhythm, and the pulse oximeter shows 89%.

As the resident picks up the chart, the nurse fills in, "This is a 30-year-old road warrior who came in last week with open tib-fib fractures, pneumothorax, the whole nine yards. Miracle of miracles, he had a helmet on, so no head injuries, and the C-spine cleared.

"Yesterday he had a central line placed for long-term antibiotics. He was extubated yesterday too; they just haven't moved the ventilator out yet. He's with it enough to have visitors, and one just left."

The resident looks over the chart, it's all there, just like the ICU nurse said.

"So what's up?"

"He just doesn't look as good as he did a while ago, he's less responsive, breathing slower, his sat is pooping out. Something happened, I just can't peg what it is."

Going up to the head of the bed, the resident shakes the patient's shoulder, "Hey! How you doing sir?"

A groan, nothing more.

"Is this guy on PCA narcotics?" the resident asks.

"Yes," the nurse answers, "but we haven't changed the dose or lockout interval."

"And you say he had these long bone fractures in his legs, and he's been bedridden all this time?" the resident asks.

"Yes, he's on subq heparin, all the usual DVT prophylaxis," the nurse reports.

The patient is taking slow, deep breaths but appears in no respiratory distress, no accessory muscle use, no rapid, shallow, pained breaths.

"Do you think we should intubate doctor?" the nurse asks.

"Um, let's get an ABG first, and get suction up here in case he vomits."

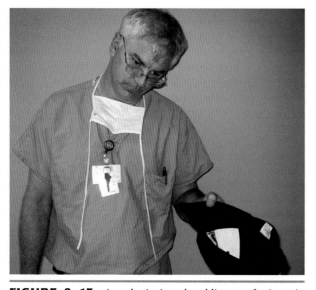

FIGURE 8–15 Anesthesia is a humbling profession. As soon as you think you're slick, you slip. Pride goeth before the fall and all that. If you do blow it (everyone does, sooner or later), eat your humble pie, learn your lesson, and move on.

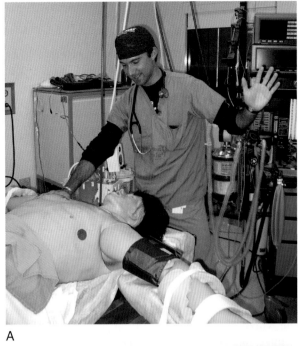

A

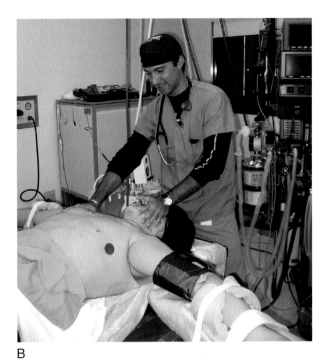

B

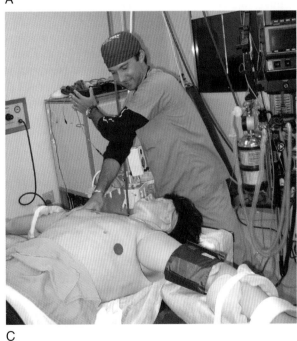

C

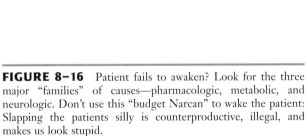

FIGURE 8–16 Patient fails to awaken? Look for the three major "families" of causes—pharmacologic, metabolic, and neurologic. Don't use this "budget Narcan" to wake the patient: Slapping the patients silly is counterproductive, illegal, and makes us look stupid.

With more shoulder shaking, the patient arouses a little more, "Hey, sir what gives?"

"Good s***," the patient says, then goes back to sleep.

The resident looks at the fingernails, looking for splinter hemorrhages or other things that might indicate a fat embolus.

"Let's get a CXR," the resident says, "maybe the pneumothorax came back or something."

"ABG results," the nurse says.

"Not terrible," the resident says. On the blood gas slip, the P_{O_2} is 95, P_{CO_2} 52, pH 7.32. Not perfect by any stretch, but this is one beat-up patient.

Now the patient is opening his eyes a little more, taking more frequent breaths, and his sat is coming up a little.

On the view box, the repeat CXR goes up—nothing abnormal, no reaccumulation of pneumothorax.

Now the patient looks OK.

In almost an apologetic tone, the nurse says, "Sorry doctor, must have been a false alarm. He looks about the same now. Must be one of those things."

"Simulation over!" the instructor says.

Clinical lessons learned from scenario 5

Residents going into the simulator are always keyed up to do *something*. And if you're geared to do something, anything, you are a real setup to jump the gun, to overtreat, to blow it with (as Alan Greenspan would say) irrational exuberance.

So this resident enters an ICU scenario where something is just not "quite right." An ICU nurse senses "something is wrong in the state of Denmark," but she can't put her finger on it.

So she calls in Dr. Sherlock Holmes to unravel the mystery.

But then, nothing happened.

Or is that actually so? Did our sleuth miss something? The answer appears during the debriefing. And the answer is elementary, my dear Watson.

Debriefing. "What were your concerns when you entered the ICU?" the instructor asks.

"The ICU nurse said something is wrong with the patient," the resident says. "And when a nurse says 'Something's wrong,' it's a red flag. The ICU nurse is right by the bedside observing the patient. They usually have a nurse-to-patient ratio of one to two or even one to one if a patient is critically ill."

"In a perfect world," the ICU nurse says. "But I don't know if you've noticed lately, there is a nursing shortage—Hello—earth to doctor! I get put one to four all the time, even with the sickest of the sick."

"Point well made," the instructor says, "so the nurse can't have eyes glued on the patient every second of every minute. But still, if they say there's been a change, then you put full faith in their observation."

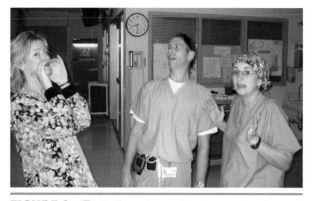

FIGURE 8–17 Hello, wake up, there *is* a nursing shortage! In the simulator, try to reproduce some of the "real life" shortcomings that residents encounter out there. An ICU nurse with little experience misses an important blood gas or doesn't notice the ventilator is malfunctioning. Anything that happens "out there" should happen "in here."

"Amen," the resident says. "It's criminal to blow off a concerned nurse and say, 'It's nothing, forget it.' I may not figure out what's wrong, but I sure as hell will *try* to figure it out.

"So, OK, it's to the bedside and ABC, always, always, always," the resident says. "Get right up there, see that they're moving air, see that they're protecting the airway, make sure all their vital signs are stable. Once you assess and fix anything immediately life-threatening, there's always time to sit back and filter the data and figure out something more subtle."

"Was he moving air, was he protecting his airway?" the instructor asks.

"Not great, not great," the resident says, "he only groaned when I touched him the first time, and he had a kind of 'narcotized' breathing pattern. Deep and slow."

"So were you thinking narcotics?" the nurse asks.

"No, not really. You said he was on the same PCA, the same lockout and dose," the resident says, "so why now should he get a slug of narcotics."

"Did you look at his eyes to see if he were miotic?" the instructor asks.

"No, I guess you could say I should have, but that PCA information just didn't seem to jibe with a narcotic overdose," the resident explains.

"So where did you go from there?"

"Get a blood gas, get a CXR, especially since he had that recent pneumothorax, and hover by that bedside, suction in hand, because I wasn't positive he could protect his airway if he vomited," the resident says.

"Then why not intubate?" the instructor asks. "Wouldn't you do that in the trauma bay if someone

BOX 8–8	Mystery Narcotic Injection

- **Access—CVP**
- **Access—friend's visit**
- **Opportunity**

were not protecting their airway, if they were barely responsive? That's, what a Glasgow coma scale of 8 or so?"

Moving his head back and forth, the resident says, "Yes, just about, I just wasn't quite, 'there' yet in terms of 'OK, this guy no way is protecting his airway.' I seemed able to get a little something out of him. So I opted for watchful waiting. It's gray, but that's where I went."

"And it turned out OK, didn't it?" the instructor asks.

"Well, yes, his first ABG wasn't too great, but he seemed to improve with time, so watchful waiting seemed the right thing to do."

"And pulmonary embolus, fat embolus, did they work out?" the instructor asks. "Did they 'land any punches' on this patient?"

"No," the resident says. "I voiced them though, because here is a guy with long bone fractures, but he's a week out, and his fractures have been fixed, so you figure fat embolus is unlikely. Same with a pulmonary embolus; he's a setup, being bedridden and basically immobile, but he is on DVT prophylaxis. I'll give that to the orthopedic docs, they always pay attention to the danger of PE."

"So we've gone round in circles," the instructor says, "and we're back to a big, fat, nothing. Is this just a 'mystery swoon' in the ICU?"

"I don't know," the resident offers, "is this one of those 'null scenarios' I've heard about? You don't really do anything, and you expect us to freak out and intubate the patient when we don't have to and we kill the guy when we should have done nothing?"

"Think again, kiddo, you forgot the most important diagnostic equipment in our armamentarium," the instructor says.

"You lost me."

"Your ears," the instructor says, "your ears. What you are told. Let me go over some of the dialogue again."

Here, the videotape of the scenario is played, and the instructor stops at a few crucial spots.

1. The camera focuses on the central line.
2. "He's with it enough to have visitors, and one just left."
3. Slow deep movement of his chest.
4. "Good s***."

"Put it together for me, doctor," the instructor says.

"Oh man," the resident hits his forehead. "His friend used the central line to give him a hit of something, maybe heroin. Definitely some kind of narcotic.

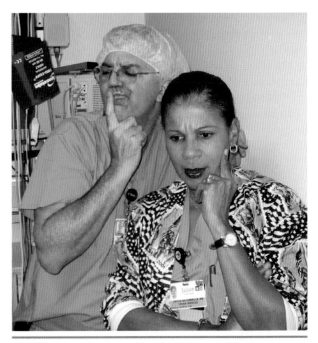

FIGURE 8–18 Something is awry, something's not right, but just what could it be? When an experienced ICU or PACU nurse "smells a rat," you are well advised to investigate. Always believe bad news and prove that it is *not* bad news before you move on. Those hunches and "gut feelings" are more often right than wrong.

"Then it all makes sense, the slow breaths, the altered consciousness, the hypoventilation, the fact that everything wore off and he got back to normal.

"And of course he could slip it in when the nurse wasn't looking, it wouldn't take but a few seconds."

"That is it."

Summary. "There are none so blind as those who will not see."

We all know the signs of narcotic overdose, particularly after doing anesthesia for any length of time. And once you open your eyes to that possibility, the signs all fall into place—breathing pattern, blood gases, sleepiness, eye signs.

But you have to *think* of it. You have to get the roadblocks out of your brain and just *let* the diagnosis happen.

This resident did a lot of good things—right up to the bedside, hover around paying close attention to the ABC, ordering the appropriate tests, suspecting the right things. But the resident was almost *too* close.

The resident needs to take a little step back, out from among the trees, to get a better grasp of the forest.

The patient *just* changed.

What *just* happened that could account for the change?

Think of all the typical things, yes, but pull back a bit, think of other things too.

Be aware of everything that affects the patients, even the visitors!

And then you can see.

SCENARIO 6. Bad beginnings, inducing with an infiltrated IV

A beginning cardiac fellow is in the operating room. An oxygen mask is on the patient, pre-oxygenating prior to induction. Anesthesia machine—OK; airway equipment—OK; drugs including resuscitative drugs—OK.

On the pre-operative report, salient points are—airway OK, ejection fraction 35%, very tight aortic stenosis with an aortic valve gradient of 0.5 cm squared. The patient takes Metoprolol. The patient is scheduled for an aortic valve replacement. An arterial line is in, and the patient came down from the floor with a 20 g IV in his left hand.

From the overhead speaker, "Dr. Kettle is in the hospital and says it's OK to go ahead." (Dr. Kettle is the cardiac surgeon listed on the preop chart.)

The arterial trace shows a narrow upstroke, and a blood pressure of 170/90. The heart rate is 80.

Using the medication recognition system, the cardiac fellow goes through a careful, titrated induction, watching the blood pressure all the time.

- Midazolam (2 cc), with the goal of giving the patient some sedation and chipping away at his/her memory bank.
- Fentanyl (2 cc), a small amount of narcotic, aiming to blunt the sympathetic response to intubation, yet not so much that the systemic vascular resistance falls. Maintaining systemic vascular resistance is key, as a drop in blood pressure in the face of tight aortic stenosis means death for the patient.
- Etomidate (5 cc, that is, 10 mg), a sedative hypnotic that maintains hemodynamic stability.

"How are you doing sir?"

No response from the patient. His eyes are closed.

The blood pressure is still up there, 170/80. The heart rate is creeping up there, 100 now.

The fellow starts mask-ventilating the patient, then gives rocuronium for muscle relaxation. As the heart rate climbs, ST segment depression—hard to detect

when laid against a backdrop of left ventricular hypertrophy—starts to occur.

"This heart rate has to come down," the fellow says, to no one in particular. Picking up a syringe of esmolol, he gives the patient 50 mg. The heart rate comes down to 70, the STs look a little better, the blood pressure drops to 130/60.

During intubation, the blood pressure rises back to 170/85, the heart rate doesn't budge, and the STs look the same as at baseline. Endotracheal tube placement is confirmed with bilateral chest expansion, bilateral and equal breath sounds, and the presence of end-tidal CO_2.

"Phew," escapes the fellow's lips. The big bugaboo, induction, is over, and the patient with severe aortic stenosis is still alive and kicking.

Thank God for small favors.

Dr. Kettle comes through the door of the OR.

"What the hell is that?" Kettle asks, pointing to the endotracheal tube.

"Uh, the endotracheal tube," the fellow says.

"*I know that, I want to know what it's doing in my patient!*" Kettle says, a measure of displeasure evident in his voice.

"Well, well . . ." the fellow stutters.

"*You induced this patient with tight aortic stenosis with a 20 g peripheral IV—is that what you did? What would you have done if the patient crashed—resuscitate him through that pencil lead of an IV?*" Kettle has little trouble being heard.

The fellow looks troubled.

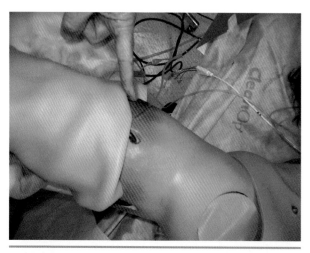

FIGURE 8–19 IVs are *not trivial*. Face it, we induce with IVs. They are our superhighway for drug delivery, volume, and blood resuscitation. Don't piddle around with a crummy IV. The very patient you induce with a bad IV is the same patient who will suddenly *need* a good IV when something goes wrong.

"You stick a central line in these patients. This is not some lap choly in an aerobics instructor! This patient is death waiting to happen. If you can't get the line, which I suspect might be the case, then god damn it, you page me and I'll put it in for you!" Kettle has a way with words.

"Uh . . ."

"Simulation over!" the instructor chirps.

Clinical lessons learned from scenario 6

Aortic stenosis is indeed a killer, and induction can be the "point of exit" for the patient. Too much induction agent, too much potent anesthetic agent and the systemic vascular resistance drops, the blood cannot make it out of its "pinhole" aortic valve fast enough, and the patient arrests.

Then you're stuck trying to do CPR on a patient with aortic stenosis. As they say on *The Sopranos*, "Fuhgedaboudit!" The small ejection fraction of chest compressions (maybe 10%) can't push anything out the stenotic aortic valve. You might as well forget it when an aortic stenosis patient codes. The only thing that might save him/her is a quick chest opening and jump on bypass.

And therein lies a tale.

The debriefing rolls out the tale for our delectation and instruction.

Debriefing. "Were you ready to roll on that induction?" the instructor asks.

"If you discount Dr. Kettle, which is nearly impossible to do," the resident says, "then yes, I was ready to go."

"What do you need—specifically, what do you need when inducing a patient with tight aortic stenosis?" the instructor asks.

"First, you need an understanding of what can wipe you out," the resident says, "the pathology of the valvular lesion. Normally, you have a nice wide egress out of the ventricle, a valve that allows a lot of blood out. With stenosis, you have a teeny-weeny exit portal. So if you suddenly drop the systemic vascular resistance, you lose all your blood pressure.

"And that drop in pressure head is especially bad for the heart itself. A heart compensates for aortic stenosis by developing a thick, muscular 'superman' of a heart. It has to get thick just to push past that stenosis. But a thick heart requires a lot of perfusion pressure. Those coronaries have to feed a monster of a heart. So dropping the pressure sets up a vicious cycle—the heart isn't getting blood out, and the heart isn't getting enough supply, so things get worse and worse.

"So you have to be delicate, oh so delicate when you induce these patients."

Kettle sits down, "Sound like you have the theory down pat, you want a little lesson in *common sense*, which does not seem to be very *common* with you."

"Well," the fellow starts.

"Well what?" Kettle is on a roll. "If this guy goes under, you will *only save him if I crack his chest*, and for that to happen I have to be *standing in the room*."

"And when you give him that heparin and you're pounding in the levophed to get his pressure up, you'd *better have a central line because that 20 gauge thing* won't do you any good," Kettle finishes with a flourish.

"OK," the instructor says, "so Dr. Kettle didn't go to the Dale Carnegie Charm School but can you concede that he may have a point?"

Nodding, the fellow agrees. "I got so caught up in the theory, I did forget the practical elements. A 20 gauge is insufficient to get me out of trouble. And god forbid it infiltrates, I'm stuck.

"And, truth to tell, for a tight aortic stenosis, I should have the surgeon in the room. This is just too spooky of a lesion to take on all by myself."

Dr. Kettle nods, "That's right, don't forget, even a loud-mouthed, aggravating surgeon can be *an ever present friend in time of need*."

Summary. The cardiac fellow gave a perfect recitation of all the tricky considerations that go into inducing a patient with aortic stenosis. And, during induction, the fellow delivered the goods, giving just the right meds in just the right order.

He achieved sufficient anesthetic depth, controlled heart rate and blood pressure, responded appropri-

---

BOX 8-9 Inducing with Aortic Stenosis

- **Maintain BP**
- **Prevent tachycardia**
- **Think "pinhole"**

BOX 8-10 If Aortic Stenosis Patient Codes?

- **Call clergy**
- **Call relatives**
- **Call risk management**

BOX 8-11 Surgeon a Pain?

- **Not a unique circumstance**
- **Try to get along**
- **Enlist *their* help, believe it or not**

ately to threatening ST changes, and secured the airway.

Perfect, yet. . . .

In our world of "what if's", the fellow didn't have the ultimate backup ready to go. A monster line and a surgeon in the room. He was lucky, but next time he might not be.

Take a tip from the Boy Scout motto—"Be Prepared."

SCENARIO 7. **Needle phobia and placenta previa**
"Doctor, could you step in here, we're admitting a labor patient and you might want to see her," the OB admitting nurse says.

The resident goes into the examining room, a pregnant patient is there (actress, not mannequin). An OB resident is standing beside.

"Hello doctor, this is Ms. Jenkins," the OB leads in, "OK if I tell this anesthesia doctor a little about you?"

Ms. Jenkins says, "All the same to me, just make sure I get his name, in case anything goes wrong and I have to call my brother-in-law."

"Ms. Jenkins' brother-in-law is in, well, pardon the pun, in *law*. Ms. Jenkins has seen a lot of shows on Oprah about people being awake under anesthesia and people never waking up, and she wants to make sure she has your name written down and faxed to her brother-in-law in case she has to sue you later and she is, well . . . uh, dead, so she can't exactly make the call, if you follow me."

"I see," the anesthesia resident says. She gives her name. "Any medical conditions I'll be needing to know about to make sure we take the best possible care of Ms. Jenkins?"

"Uh, yes," the OB continues, "Ms. Jenkins is a 24 year multip with progressive, painless vaginal bleeding. She is currently at 35 weeks' gestation."

"Have you . . ." the anesthesia resident starts.

"Ultrasound reveals a low-lying placenta partially covering the cervical os," the OB resident says. "We will not be doing a manual exam, of course, until we have some other preparations in place."

"Good."

"I don't want any needles!" Ms. Jenkins says, "You put me to sleep first, I hate needles! And they can't

ever get one in me either, stupid bastards. They dig around all day like they're drilling for oil or something. You can sue for that, can't you? Sticking you with needles all day? Just give me that mask and put me to sleep and then you can stick me with needles all day, and while you're at it pull the baby out too. I don't want to be awake for that either."

The OB and the anesthesia resident step out into the hall for a moment.

"Don't you be talking bad about me either!" Ms. Jenkins says, "You talk bad about me I'll haul your ass in court, then we'll see who's laughin'!"

"So, clearly we have a situation," the OB resident says. "And rather than blindside you, I thought I'd give you a little preview of coming attractions."

"Thanks," the anesthesia resident says, "is it shift change? Can I crawl out a window or something?"

"Hold onto your hat," the OB says, "Ms. Jenkins may have an aversion to needles placed by *others*, but she apparently is no stranger to needles placed by *herself*."

"Veins all shot up?"

"Yep."

"Tox screen light up?"

"Like the Fourth of July."

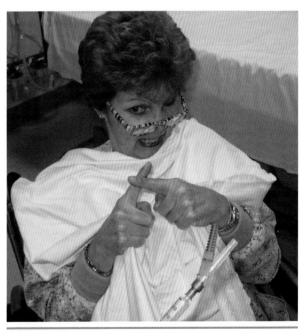

FIGURE 8-20 A real dilemma, the super-needle-o-phobe. You're painted in a corner, because they won't let you put in an IV, but, come on, you need an IV. The simulator is the place to "act out" these dilemmas. Better to face this in a pretend situation before you have to face it for real.

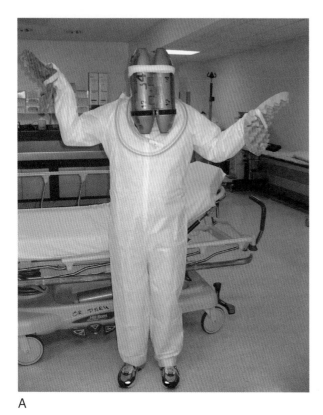

A

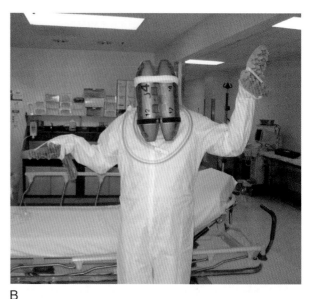

B

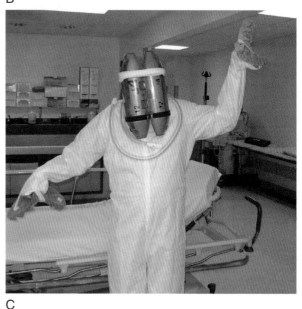

C

FIGURE 8–21 Danger, danger, Will Robinson! Here, an advanced robot signals danger ahead. You'd better talk over your plan before you proceed.

"What's on board?"

"What's not, that's a shorter list."

"And this previa spooks me," the OB says, "I mean it's hanging right there, low but low. No way we can go vaginal, no way José."

"I'll need some monster IV access" the anesthesia resident says.

"Yeah you will, this will be wet," the OB says. "This could turn into the Red Sea, we might even need to do a hysterectomy. My crystal ball just says 'Danger, danger, Will Robinson!' this time. How you want to work this?"

"Well, I've got to go central, I'll just plain need a central line, a cordis, something I can firehose blood in with," the anesthesia resident says.

"She ain't gonna like that," the OB says. "We could talk to her until Mississippi votes for Howard Dean and she will still say no."

"Get the pediatrician here," the anesthesia resident says. "We've got to all 'sing of self-same tenor' on this."

A quick call from the OB admitting nurse, and a peds resident shows up. Introductions all around and a quick update on the problems.

"Here's the scoop, this will be ugly, but here it is," the anesthesia resident says. "I've got a pregnant woman, full stomach, refusing lines, bad IV access due to IVDA, and I'll be needing big time access in case she bleeds like no tomorrow. I'm going to have to sedate her enough to get a line in, and the road will go one of two ways here—either I can sedate her enough to get a real central line in, a big hogger, and then we'll be ready to go. Or else I can sedate her enough—this will have to be IM, hate to say—to just get a teeny but 'OK to induce general anesthesia but not to start cutting with' IV.

"That's where you both come in," the anesthesia resident goes on. "If I can slam in a big line, make sure we have blood in the room, then we'll induce and cut—the usual C-section way. You, in peds, will have a baby coming out that will have absorbed some of my IM meds, so you'll need to support ventilation for a while.

"If I can only get a dinky line in, then I'll induce with that, but don't start cutting. Once she's asleep, I'll maintain her with general anesthesia—again, baby will come out sleepy so you may have to support for a while—then I'll put in a big line. But don't cut until I have that line."

"Sound good?"

OB and peds nod.

"Simulation's over!" the instructor says.

"But . . . but I haven't done anything yet!" the anesthesia resident protests.

"Oh yes you have!"

Clinical lessons learned from scenario 7

The placenta usually implants in the body or fundus of the uterus; but when it implants near the cervical os, a condition called placenta previa occurs. Previous uterine surgery (most often C-sections) is the greatest risk factor for developing placenta previa.

From an anesthetic standpoint, the primary concern with placenta previa is volume replacement. Anesthetic management is debatable, some arguing against regional anesthesia, some for general, with the attendant concerns of general anesthesia in the obstetric population.

All this emerges during the debriefing.

BOX 8-12 | IV Phobia Options

- **Breathe down**
- **IM sedate**
- **CVP (easier than 1000 peripheral sticks)**

Debriefing. "How do you think that went?" the instructor asks.

"Well," the anesthesia resident is a little nonplussed, "I thought in the Simulator you actually *did* stuff!"

"True," the instructor says.

"And I didn't, really, *do* anything!"

"Did you think? Did you assess a difficult patient? Did you hook up with two different specialties and formulate a plan A and a plan B?" the instructor says. "Remember, this place is not a 'partial-task trainer' where we see if you can stick the tube in. They have intubating dummies for that. This is the place where you put it all together, and the main thing we want to see working is your *brain!*"

"Oh," the anesthesia resident says, then looks around at the nodding OB and peds people. "Now that you put it that way."

"What did you think when I called you in the preadmission room?" the OB resident asks. "We don't usually do that, do we?"

"Well, I figured something bad was coming my way, but then, better to get a 'head-up' and try to work something out ahead of time," the anesthesia resident says.

"No need to hold hands and have a harmonic convergence," the instructor says, "but that's part of the reason we put different specialties together in the Simulator. If we can each 'peak under the hood' of the other specialties, we can see their concerns, they can hear *our* concerns, and we can hear *theirs*, and everybody wins."

"Ditto from the pediatric standpoint," the peds resident says, "We are the last to hear about things a lot of times. It's nice to be in on the planning stages so we're not caught with our pants down."

"Keep your pants up on the OB floor, please," the OB resident says.

Everyone cracks up on that one.

"So lay it out for me," the instructor says, "what went into the plan A and plan B you had?"

"OK first, forget the litigious bluster—one instructor told me, 'Don't worry if someone says they have a lawyer. *Everyone* has a lawyer, they just haven't called the lawyer yet,'" the anesthesia resident says, yet again cracking up the whole debriefing room. Who said Simulation debriefings weren't fun?

"Second, think of the physiology of pregnancy and all we have to keep in mind—full stomach, aspiration risk, quick desaturation due to increased oxygen consumption and decreased functional residual capacity, more difficulty intubating due to swollen and friable upper airway."

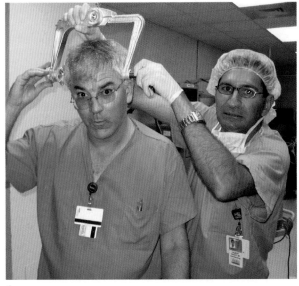

A

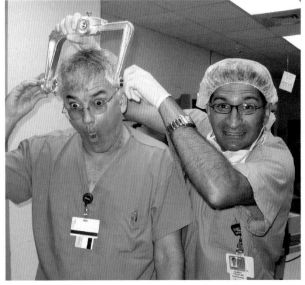

B

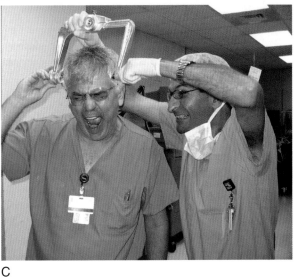

C

FIGURE 8–22   The simulator is there to squeeze your brain. What are you thinking? Why did you choose that option? Where were you going with that plan? This squeeze can be a little painful, but it's ultimately to the good. Feel the pain and experience the gain.

"Third, think of the specific problems associated with *this* pregnancy versus just any old pregnancy— placenta previa, big time blood loss. And I have to be ready for that with lines and cross-matched blood."

"Fourth, think of the specific problems associated with *this* patient versus just any old placenta previa— poor venous access and, really, an inability to cooperate."

"How do you keep from jumping on the 'judgmental train' with a patient like this?" the instructor asks. "Don't you just want to slap her around and say, 'Snap out of it, you need this line so deal with it and shut up!'"

"Of course you do," the anesthesia resident says, "but that's where you show your professionalism."

"*Aha*! Get the ACGME on the phone! We're teaching a core clinical competency!" the peds resident chimes in.

"That we are," the instructor gives a smug grin, then scribbles a note to make sure she documents this "ACGME coup."

Going on, the anesthesia resident says, "The fact is, this is the way this woman is. From the IV drug use, from her upbringing, who knows. It's not for me to unravel and it's not for me to undo, but it *is* for me to deal with. So from a 'I need you to cooperate' there is only so much I can do. Yes, I will talk to her; yes, I will tell her how much better it would be if she would hold still; and yes, you can do a previa with an epidural anesthetic (controversial because in the face of massive hemorrhage you would miss her sympathetic tone). But if she just plain does not cooperate, then she just plain does not cooperate. She is no more capable of cooperating than a patient with congenital or acquired 'cerebral insufficiency.'

"You don't demand that a severely impaired trisomy 21 patient cooperate—you plan your anesthetic around the lack of cooperation. You don't demand that a closed head injury patient or a multi-infarct dementia patient cooperate—you plan your anesthetic around the lack of cooperation.

"Same applies here," the anesthesia resident says.

"Right you are."

Summary. This anesthesia resident walked into a real minefield.

- Pregnant patient, with all the physiologic changes of pregnancy to consider
- Placenta previa, with the potential for big blood loss
- Behavioral issues, drug use, drugs on board, no veins, no desire to cooperate, "looking for" a reason to sue.

But this resident entered this minefield in good company—an OB resident who planned ahead and a peds resident who wanted to be in on the advanced planning as well. With a (cheesy as this sounds) solid interdisciplinary approach, they came up for a good plan for taking care of a very tough patient.

And planning ahead is half the battle.

Whew, glad this difficult scenario is over. All three residents can now rest easy.

SCENARIO 8. **No IV access in a difficult, bleeding patient**

Ooops, spoke too soon.

This scenario occurs in the OR setting, the voice of the same patient coming through the mannequin's speakers. OB is set up to do a C-section, the circulator has blood in the room, and peds is set up with bassinette and resuscitation equipment (suction, oxygen, airway equipment, drugs). The OB nurse is watching the fetal heart rate monitor.

Still no IV; to this point, the patient has gotten 10 mg of morphine IM and 5 mg of midazolam IM, so her voice comes across slurred but still protesting.

"You ain't sticking my neck! You ain't got my permission, no way can you do that!" the patient shouts.

Down below, the OB notices the bleeding has increased; on the monitor, the heart rate is up to 130 and the blood pressure is only 90.

"Um," the OB resident says, "things might be getting worse here. I don't think time is on our side."

"I'm getting lates," the OB nurse says. "For sure, these are lates." The fetal heart rate monitor shows an ominous sign, late decelerations.

"OK," the anesthesia resident says, "put out a call for help and that includes a call to general surgery in case I need a cut down for access." Turning now to the patient, "Ma'am, fact is, to save you and the baby, that's just what I have to do, there are no places left on your arm where I can put an IV. I'll give you some numbing medicine and try not to make it too bad."

The instructor's voice comes over the intercom, "OK, the central line is in, but you had a hard time doing it and had to stick several times."

Now the blood pressure is 80/50, the heart rate is 140, and the OB nurse is seeing sustained decelerations.

"We're bleeding bad down here," the OB resident says, "real bad."

"You," the anesthesia resident shouts to the OB nurse, "get extra hands in here, I'll need someone helping me to check and hang blood. Right now, give me some cricoid pressure."

The anesthesia resident picks up a syringe labeled propofol, just about hooks it in the line, then reconsiders. She picks up a syringe labeled ketamine and another labeled succinylcholine, and gives them one after the other.

"Quiet in here," the anesthesia resident says.

After 30 seconds, the resident puts the laryngoscope in the mouth, lifts, and sees nothing.

"Shit!"

"What's up?" the OB resident asks.

"No view," the anesthesia resident says, taut as a piano wire.

She picks up another blade, repositions the head.

"Sustained bradycardia!" the OB nurse shouts. "Forty, I'm not kidding, 40!"

"Listen, I gotta get this kid out, I gotta get this kid out," the OB says; he, too, strung up tight.

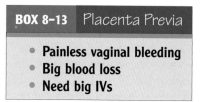

BOX 8-13 Placenta Previa
- **Painless vaginal bleeding**
- **Big blood loss**
- **Need big IVs**

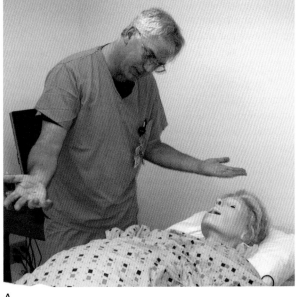

A

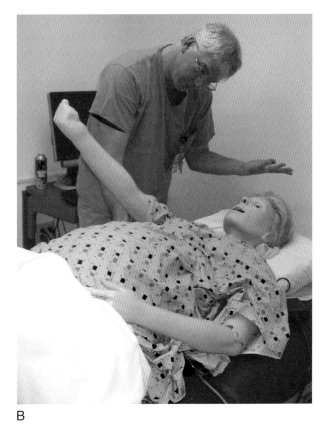

B

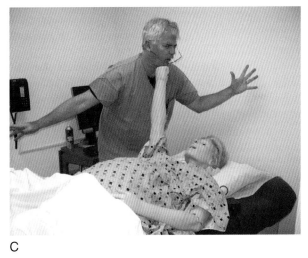

C

FIGURE 8–23   OK, you're not always going to hit it off perfectly with the patients. You made your case, and they just don't buy it. That's happened before. Try to have a good plan B ready for just such an occasion.

"Nothing," the anesthesia resident says. Behind her, the saturation drops into the 80s, the 70s. The nurse holding the cricoid pressure keeps looking back at the fetal heart rate monitor, and her hand pulls up from the throat.

"Keep that cricoid pressure on, god damn it!" the anesthesia resident says. "I know we have bradycardia, you don't need to remind me, OK? You just keep that hand right where it is!"

The anesthesia resident mask-ventilates for a few seconds, then reaches back and places an LMA. The chest rises, and the sat rises to 90%. She turns on sevoflurane and says, "Cut! This isn't perfect, but we'll have to live with it. Keep that pressure on."

Another resident walks in the room.

"O'Reilly from surgery, what can I do for you?" he says.

"The O'Reilly factor, great, just what we need!" the anesthesia resident says. "Congratulations, you're now working for anesthesia. I'm shepherding this airway, I need you to hang blood. Just pretend like you're in the trauma bay. OK?"

"Right," O'Reilly says.

In the surgical field, the OB pulls out a baby, hands it to peds.

"Thick meconium," the OB says.

"Got it!" the peds resident takes the baby away in a towel. In the bassinette, he suctions the mouth, intu-

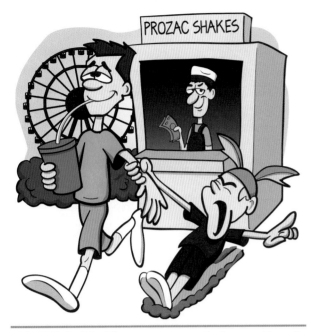

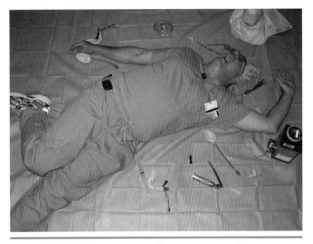

FIGURE 8–25 So many things to remember, so many problems, AAG! When everything starts falling apart, always go back to ABC and build up from there. Don't let the "million things going on" distract you from the most important stuff—air goes in and out, blood goes around in circles.

FIGURE 8–24 The amusement park that considers the parents is the amusement park with everything.

bates, suctions the endotracheal tube, removes it, then mask-ventilates. The baby, originally blue (via LCD displays in its face), pinks up.

Up at the head of the bed, the anesthesia resident continues to ventilate via LMA with cricoid pressure in place.

"God all fishhooks," she says, "we're going to need the entire crew of *Ben Hur* before this case is over. I need someone to get me a fiberoptic. I want to secure this airway with an endotracheal tube. Is there anyone left in the city who isn't already doing something for me?"

The door opens, "That's all folks!", the instructor says.

Clinical lessons learned from scenario 8

A good amusement park offers "something for everyone"—loop-the-loop roller coasters for the teenagers, merry-go-rounds for the kiddies, and Prozac for the parents. This case, too, offered "something for everyone" as the debriefing reveals.

Debriefing. "Where to start?" the instructor asks. "Maybe we are edging into the realm of 'crisis resource management' here?"

"I'd call it a crisis," the OB said. Nods of agreement from anesthesia, peds, and the "walk-in" surgeon.

"You can elucidate all the factors of CRM, as they call it," the anesthesia resident says, "in the cool and calm atmosphere of a lecture hall. But when the world is caving in around you and you see the patient dying right in front of you, you tend to get a little frazzled and start to forget stuff."

"Well, here we are in the cool and calm atmosphere of the debriefing room," the instructor says, "let's go through those crisis resource management things right now."

The peds resident starts out, "Global assessment, stepping back and seeing the big picture. Management of resources, having the right people do the right things."

OB adds, "Communication, making sure you 'close the loop' when you talk to people."

"Calling for help when you are sure you're about to crash!" the anesthesia resident says, unleashing a pent up "need to laugh" in the room.

"That's not an official CRM thing," the instructor says, "but maybe it should be."

The entire team now reviews the DVD of the scenario. It's a humbling thing, watching yourself in a crisis. Stuff you never thought you missed, you missed. Plus, who are we kidding, the camera *does* put 10 pounds on you.

Peds speaks up first, "I like how right away our anesthesia heroine is calling for help. You really sense she is 'marshalling the troops.'"

"That's right," the instructor says. "It's no crime to say the things we do *right* in a Simulation scenario. There is a tendency to flog ourselves and just dwell on the stuff we do *wrong*. It is well and good to see the wrong stuff and correct it, but it's just as important to see the *good* stuff and make sure you *keep doing that good stuff*."

"What do you think was causing the hypotension?" the instructor asks.

"Bleeding," the OB says.

"Bleeding," the anesthesia resident says.

"Bleeding," the OB nurse says, and the peds resident and the O'Reilly factor agree.

"Could it have been a pneumothorax?" the instructor asks.

"Ooooooooh," the OB says.

"Ooooooooooooh," peds and O'Reilly say.

"Ooooooooooooooooooooooooh," the anesthesia resident says. "That's right, I had a hard time with the central line, so I very well could have dropped a lung. But then, there was all that bleeding."

"Does bleeding preclude *also* having a pneumothorax?" the instructor asks. "It would be a wonderful world if just one problem happened at a time, but then, we are not given that luxury, are we?"

"No," the anesthesia resident says, "we're not. Wait, wait a minute, I would have felt higher inspiratory pressures. I would have had more trouble ventilating, wouldn't I? Now come to think of it, I don't think she didn't have a pneumothorax."

"Touché", the instructor says, "she didn't. But still. . . ."

"Point well taken," the anesthesia resident admits, "point well taken, I should have had that on my list. But I gotta tell you, with that difficult airway, my 'dance ticket' was already pretty filled up!"

"True," the instructor says, "so take us through your thinking."

"Well, ABC, and this is the classic OB dilemma," the anesthesia resident says, "this is the very thing we study and train for and must always be ready to handle—fetal distress, can't intubate."

"But you were able to ventilate," the OB resident says.

"Yes, I was," the anesthesia resident says. "And the difficult airway algorithm recognizes the LMA as an imperfect—patients can still aspirate—but viable alternative in this case. So I swallowed hard and did the case with the LMA."

"Let's go over the peds resuscitation," the instructor says. "Meconium means what?"

"Babies in trouble defecate, pass meconium intrauterine," the peds resident says. "And this kid was in a lot of trouble; that sustained bradycardia meant inadequate 'something'—oxygen delivery, perfusion of the placenta—something. So the kid defecates. If that

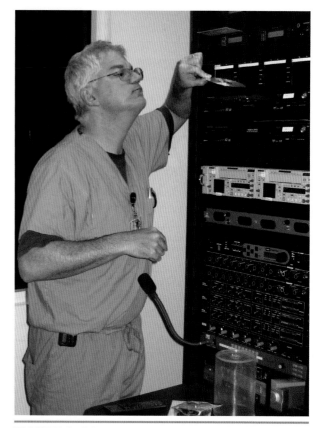

FIGURE 8–26 Record the scenario, then look at it afterward in the debriefing room. Even if the residents do everything right (rare, but it happens), you can still look at the DVD and learn something. Studying one's "performance" on a recording works in baseball, tennis, golf, and, guess what, the anesthesia simulator.

meconium gets in the baby's lungs, we have, in effect, aspiration of a very serious nature. The kid can go into respiratory distress syndrome, can die right then and there if you can't ventilate him, or can go on to bronchopulmonary dysplasia, that is, chronic lung problems. A kind of COPD for the younger crowd."

"Damn," O'Reilly says, "you're good, you could do this for a living."

"I do."

"Oh, right."

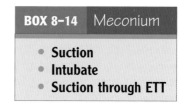

BOX 8–14 Meconium

- **Suction**
- **Intubate**
- **Suction through ETT**

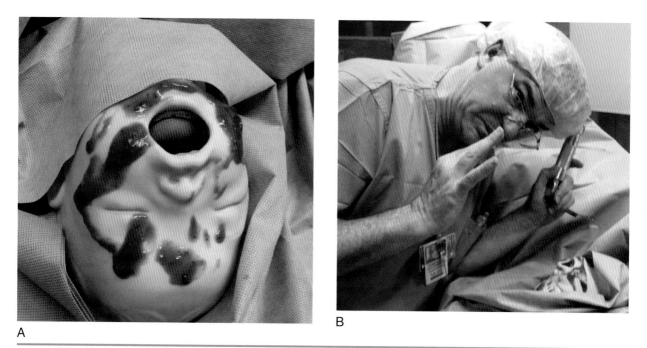

A B

FIGURE 8–27 Meconium might be a little icky, but that shouldn't scare you off. Get that kid intubated and suck that stuff out. If the meconium "takes root" in the lungs, that baby is in for short-term and long-term respiratory trouble. What you do in the crucial first minute or two may make all the difference in that kid's life.

"So anyway, the thing to do is fight the urge to mask-ventilate the kid right away," the peds resident says. "It is *so* tempting to just 'mask him up a little'; and I'll tell you, I've seen some anesthesia people succumb to that temptation."

Blushing, the anesthesia resident conceded the point without saying a word.

"So you intubate, you get a suction mechanism right into those lungs, and you suction out that meconium first. You give those lungs a good bit of house-cleaning. Then you proceed with resuscitation."

"It's a battle of nerves, isn't it?" the instructor asks.

"That it is," the peds resident says.

"How did it feel when you wanted to get the baby out, but the airway wasn't yet secure?" the instructor asks the OB resident.

"Well, speaking of a war of nerves," the OB says, "you want to swing that blade down and get baby out *now* but now. With a fetal heart rate of 40, you know you're just moments away from a severely impaired child for life versus a normal kid who grows up, joins a rock band, and drives you crazy in a different way."

"But you have to wait," the instructor says.

"You have to hear the word from anesthesia. And the airway comes first, there's just no way around it. That's when knowing your anesthesia person and

knowing what he or she can do really makes all the difference in the world."

Turning to O'Reilly, the instructor says, "So how is it 'taking orders' from anesthesia? Don't you guys usually fight with them?"

"Doctor first, specialist second," O'Reilly says. "If I happen upon a car wreck, then I might have to be a kind of 'anesthesia airway' person. That's no time to say, 'I don't do airways.' And in this case, anesthesia needed me to hang blood because there was no one else around, and she was busy with the airway. So you do what it says in the Hippocratic Oath."

Eyebrows up all around the debriefing table. O'Reilly had been so quiet before, and now this! Still waters do run deep.

"Can't end on a better note than that," the instructor concludes.

Summary. Bleeding, fetal instability, lost airway, meconium, all laid against a backdrop of a litigious patient. It just doesn't get better than this.

The anesthesia resident could have paused to get all "legal eagle" about consent for a central line, but at a certain point you have to be a doctor and not a lawyer. She did the best she could, first explaining, then sedating, and then getting the line. Absent the line, the

BOX 8-15 Calling for Help

- **Do it early, before it's too late**
- **Extra "brain" more clear-headed**
- **Better swallow pride than hurt patient**

patient would bleed to death, and *that* the anesthesia resident was not willing to do, no matter how the brother-in-law would react.

Anesthesia induction in the now bleeding, now unstable patient is always a concern; and at the last minute, the resident opted for ketamine over propofol, hoping to avoid further hypotension. Then the toughest exercise in anesthesia—dealing with a lost airway in an obstetric patient, with the baby having sustained bradycardia at the same time. A perfectly secured airway is the ideal, but the anesthesia resident had to settle for second best, a route that worked here.

Purists could argue—wake the patient up, let the baby do whatever it does, and do the intubation awake. In this uncooperative patient? With bleeding and instability? And just ignore the shouts from the obstetrician? That's a call most anesthesiologists just won't make. But controversy is controversy because you can argue the point either way.

One genuine mistake did slip past everyone in the debriefing. After induction, the anesthesia resident went right to turning on the sevoflurane. This, in the face of hypotension and bleeding? She should have at least checked the blood pressure first. She already had 10 of morphine and 5 of midazolam (intramuscular) on board, so that might have blunted any memories.

And how about a BIS? Recall in the obstetric or the unstable patient is a real problem. Though no cure-all, a BIS helps. (Of note, Simulators don't yet have a way to incorporate this important new technology.)

Peds handled and explained the management of meconium to a T. Keep cool, suction out that trachea, then go to the ABC. Takes nerves of steel, but that's what neonatal medicine is all about.

OB has to bide its time 'til the airway's secured, so they too have to "check their nervousness at the door" and stay cool under fire.

And what a swan song for this scenario. A surgeon says, "Whatever it takes to save the patient, I'll do it." Good medicine.

SCENARIO 9. | **Mediastinal mass**

The patient is lying flat on the OR table, and the anesthesia resident is reading the preop.

A 43-year-old man with a large anterior mediastinal mass, previously healthy. Flow volume loops show signs of obstruction. CT scan (on the viewbox) shows tracheal deviation and narrowing. Surgeons plan to resect this mass.

A progress note from the chart shows that in the holding area another anesthesia resident placed a right radial arterial line and, anticipating possible big blood loss, a 9 Fr cordis in the right IJ. An arterial trace and CVP trace are on the monitors as well as the saturation—99% and the heart rate—90. The patient has the oxygen mask on, held in place by a black face strap. The surgeon is in the room, and everyone is ready to go.

After the resident finishes reading, the patient speaks up, "Hey, can you give me some pillows or something, I'm having a really hard time catching my breath!"

"Oh sure," the anesthesia resident says, putting the bed in reverse Trendelenburg. "That help?"

"A little," the patient has a gasping sound in his voice.

The surgeon taps his watch, "Tempus fugit" (Time flies—Latin).

"Right, right," the anesthesia resident says, "well, looks like we're ready."

"Unless you have something else you'd rather be doing?" the surgeon snipes.

Reaching behind him, the anesthesia resident turns on the sevoflurane.

The surgeon's eyes go up, "What the hell, you haven't given him any 'Milk of Anesthesia'! Don't you give that white stuff to make them go to sleep? Did you forget?"

"No. Now doctor, I'm going to ask you this politely. I'd like you to place a 9 Fr introducer in the femoral vein for me," the anesthesia resident says.

"What? You already *have* a big line!" the surgeon protests.

"Humor me," the anesthesia resident says, focusing on the airway as the surgeon huffily heads to the groin to place the line.

1%, then 2%, then up to 4%, the anesthesia resident creeps the sevo up, always keeping the patient breathing spontaneously.

BOX 8-16 Mediastinal Mass

- **Can squash stuff**
- **Consider femoral lines**
- **Don't burn bridges**

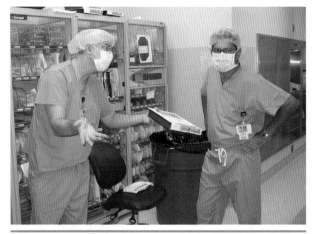

FIGURE 8-28 The surgeon is an oft-overlooked resource when you're stuck for lines. Granted, you might have to grovel a little, but better to swallow your pride and get the line. Don't let your pride interfere with the patient's needs.

"We got the gurney nearby, right?" the anesthesia resident asks the OR nurse.

"Sure, why?" the OR nurse asks. This isn't a prone case.

"If this mass suddenly compresses the airways, and there is no way I can move any air, we may have to flip the patient prone to take the pressure off the airways and breathe for him."

"And do you have a rigid bronch in the room?" the anesthesia resident asks.

At this point, the surgeon has had it with the needy, high-maintenance anesthesia resident, "We're not *doing* a rigid bronch, *doctor*." The "doctor" carries the tone "stupid doctor."

As he intubates, the anesthesia resident explains, "If this mass sinks down, a rigid bronch might be necessary to stent the airway open. I'm trying to avoid that by keeping him breathing spontaneously, keeping his muscles 'pulling up' when he inspires."

Endotracheal intubation is successful, but inspiratory pressures are high and the saturation is only 95% on 100% oxygen. Placing his stethoscope on the right chest, the anesthesia resident says, "You do know how to put in a chest tube, don't you, *doctor*?"

No response.

The room is charged with two doctors calling each other *doctor*.

"Don't think I need it, just wanted to make sure my partner hadn't dropped the lung with his right IJ stick. I think he's just tight and I need to breathe him down more. How's that femoral line?"

"Femoral line's in," the instructor says.

The drapes go up and the surgery starts, "He's bucking, better paralyze him," the surgeon says.

"You ready to go on fem-fem bypass if I need it?" the anesthesia resident asks.

"That's it!" the surgeon snaps off his gloves. "What else do you want? Valet parking? Foot massage? What?"

"Simulation over," the instructor says over the loudspeaker.

Clinical lessons learned from scenario 9

Interdisciplinary scenarios can have genuine participants, like scenario 8, where peds, OB, and anesthesia were all participating and didn't know what was happening next. At other times, you can have an interdisciplinary "plant," a confederate who is there to challenge, bait, aggravate, and bring out the learning points in a more . . . colorful (?) manner.

The surgeon functioned that way in this case, much as Dr. Kettle did in the aortic valve scenario.

Anterior mediastinal mass—a nightmare waiting to happen for anesthesiologists. Most catastrophes involve "collapse" of the anterior mediastinal mass after induction of anesthesia and muscle paralysis. With nothing "pulling up," the mass "falls down," squashing the airways and great vessels, leading to cardiac and respiratory failure. Even our vaunted endotracheal tube may be of no use, as the "squashing" occurs distal to the tip of the tube, and you can't move air.

Such disasters are more common in children. Children are more cartilaginous than us ossified, calcified old folk. So the cartilaginous kiddies are more prone to the anterior mediastinal "squishage" than adults are.

But still, even if you have a 43-year-old patient, like here, you still have your antenna up for anterior mediastinal trouble, as the debriefing shows.

Debriefing. "What were your red flags in this case?" the instructor asks.

"There was clinical and lab evidence of big time obstruction with this mass," the anesthesia resident explains. "He was short of breath lying flat, that's not good, and the flow volume loops showed obstruction;

BOX 8-17	Planted Allies in a Simulator

- **Aggravate**
- **Sabotage**
- **Great fun**

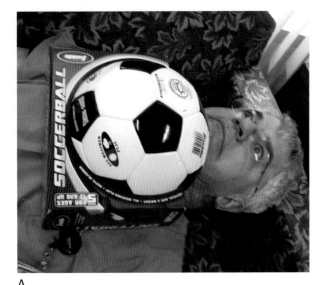

A

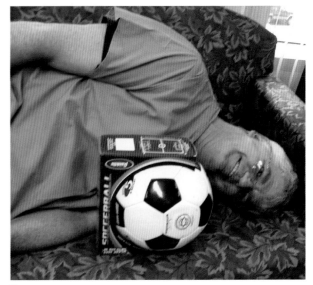

B

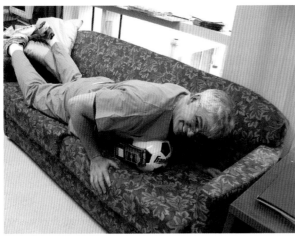

C

FIGURE 8–29 A mediastinal mass can kill a patient. Remember this little trick—if the mass is squishing down, move the weight. Put the patient on the side or even prone. Then the mass (well, the soccer ball in this case) is off the mediastinal contents.

so, again, you are seeing signs that this mass is a real problem.

"Add to that a CT that shows narrowing and distortion of the airway. I would look for physical signs of superior vena cava syndrome in such a patient. A mass like this, obstructing airways, can just as easily obstruct vessels."

"Any other options before you induce—any medical options?" the instructor asks.

"I'm not picking up your thread here," the anesthesia resident says.

"Radiation."

Smacking his forehead with the flat of his right palm, the anesthesia resident says, "Oh yeah, I forgot that one."

The surgeon laughs, "Finally, one thing you *did* forget. Thank God for small favors. If someone is *so*

symptomatic that any procedure would possibly kill him or her, this is one time the radiation oncology people would 'treat before they see the meat,' as they say."

"Treat before they see the meat?" the OR nurse asks.

"Radiation oncology is hesitant to irradiate anything for which they don't have a pathology tissue diagnosis—the somewhat irreverently labeled 'meat' in their motto, 'No meat, no treat.' But in a case of severe symptoms like this, they might actually irradiate first to get the tumor shrunk down enough so surgery can be done safely."

"But you seemed to get all the other stuff down pretty good," the surgeon says, "even though I tried to yank you every which way."

Bowing, the anesthesia resident says, "Much appreciated. Nietzche said, 'What doesn't kill us, makes us stronger.' So you were doing me a favor."

"Why didn't you induce like they usually do?" the OR nurse asks.

"It all goes back to the mediastinal mass," the anesthesia resident explains. "If I do the usual slam-bang induction, I may take away the very compensatory mechanisms the patient has in place. Think of each inspiration—the anterior thoracic wall pulls up on the mass, pulling it away from the vessels and air passages. Just like a pulley with wires lifting up."

"If I take that away with apnea and paralysis, that mass falls down. My positive-pressure ventilation from the ventilator is just not the same force, it's not the same 'configuration,' so I might lose it all."

"And the other things?" the instructor asks.

"If you get in trouble, you want to 'unload' the mediastinum, get the weight off, just like you'd get a fallen tree limb off someone getting crushed underneath it. You can turn the patient on the side, or even move them prone, to get the weight off. That's why I wanted the gurney nearby."

"And the rigid bronch?" the instructor continues. "The femoral line?"

"That's all anatomy, you need the bronch to get in there and 'hold up the roof' of the bronchus if it collapses," the anesthesia resident explains. "And the femoral line is a question of 'doorways into the heart.'

"Blood returns to the heart through the superior vena cava from above and the inferior vena cava from below. Dissection up around the mediastinum can end up poking a hole in the innominate vein, the superior vena cava itself—some big vessel that ends up feeding into the heart from above. Even if you have a central line 'from above,' it might not do you any good in this kind of emergency. You may end up pouring blood into the surgical field! So you need big access from below, even if the surgeon puts up a fuss."

"Me?" the surgeon says, all innocence.

Summary. It is a danger in anesthesia that we sometimes "tee-up" a case for our partners in hopes of "getting going" a little faster. That is well and good, but when you walk into such a "teed-up" case, you have to remember to "tee-up" your thinking cap before you proceed.

You have a surgeon tapping his watch and lines that at first blush *seem* sufficient for any monstrosity that might occur, so let's get a move on!

It always pays to take just that one crucial minute to do nothing but *think*! Consider the special aspects of this case and make sure you make the right plan. Here, the resident did just that.

Consider the pathophysiology of anterior mediastinal "squishage."

Keep the patient's compensatory mechanisms intact by breathing spontaneously.

Have backup plans in place—gurney to flip the patient, rigid bronch, fem-fem bypass as the ultimate maneuver.

Get the lines you need, no matter the cries of woe and anguish from your surgical confrere.

Let tempus fugit just a little while you prepare for, and avoid, the worst.

SCENARIO 10. **No smooth sailing, triage after a disaster**

"A what?" the anesthesia resident asks.

"A cruise ship, you know, one of those Carnival things," the ER nurse explains. "The steam boiler blew up or something, anyway, we've got 15 admissions, all burned, all with C-collars on. None are intubated, but they all have burns around their face. We are totally maxed out and there are two in this room."

Entering the treatment room, the anesthesia resident sees two victims, both with black soot around their faces, both with C-collars on. The far patient is gasping for air, the near patient is silent. Both have pulse oximeters and EKGs attached. Both have oxygen on.

The gasping patient has a saturation of 85% and a heart rate of 140.

The silent patient has a saturation of 0 and a heart rate of 0. Flat line, asystole.

"Are we it?" the resident says, "we're going to. . . ."

"This is it," the ER nurse says, "everyone else is taking care of the other ones. We've instituted a disaster drill, but no one else has come in yet." The ER nurse looks at the guy in asystole. "You want me to start CPR here?"

Feeling for a pulse, looking for chest rise, and lifting the eyelid of the asystolic victim, the resident says, "No, help me over here with this guy who's gasping. Leave this one."

The gasping is getting more high-pitched, the saturation is down to 80%.

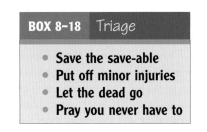

BOX 8-18 Triage

- Save the save-able
- Put off minor injuries
- Let the dead go
- Pray you never have to

"Anyone here who can cut a neck if I can't intubate this guy?" the anesthesia resident says, "He may be all burnt up in the airway, swollen up."

"All the surgeons are in the other trauma bays, you're it."

"His C-spine cleared?" the resident asks, as he places an oxygen mask and Ambu-bag on the patient, starting to assist his ventilations.

"No," the nurse says, "no one to take them, no one to read them."

At the patient's bedside is a Cook cricothyrotomy kit, as well as regular intubation equipment. There is also a long skinny looking thing with an eyepiece on the top.

"What's that?" the anesthesia resident asks, pointing at the long skinny thing.

"Oh," the ER nurse says, "that's the Shikani optical system. You load the endotracheal tube on it, then you slip it in the mouth and look through the eyepiece. There's a little fiberoptic device in it. It's supposed to be great for someone like this, you don't want to move their neck because the C-spine is uncertain. It lets you take a look without extending the neck."

"Does it work?"

"How the hell should I know? They never let us intubate," the ER nurse says.

Suddenly, the high-pitched gasping stops with one final squeak and the saturation starts to plummet.

Placing a regular laryngoscope in the mouth, the anesthesia resident encounters a massively swollen tongue and can't see anything.

"Gimme the cric kit," the anesthesia resident says.

"You don't want to try the Shikani?" the ER nurse asks.

"No, the cric kit."

The anesthesia resident undoes the collar, opening up the front of the neck. Using a syringe with a 16-gauge angiocath, he enters the cricothyroid membrane, aspirates air, and withdraws the needle. Then he introduces a wire, floppy end first, into the trachea. Once the wire is advanced, he cuts a hole next to the wire, just like placing a Swan introducer, and introduces the Cook cric device. Once placed, the resident pulls out the dilator, hooks up his Ambu-bag, and inflates oxygen. The saturation turns around and climbs back up to the high 80s.

"We better sedate this guy and sandbag his head, we don't have the collar on anymore," the resident

BOX 8-19	Surgical Airway

- **Be decisive**
- **Trachea as "big vein with air"**
- **Go for it**

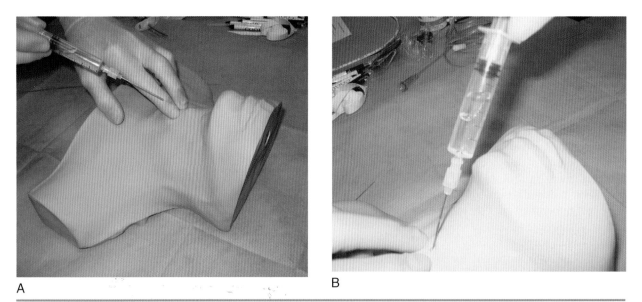

A   B

FIGURE 8–30 The surgical airway, demonstrated in a partial-task trainer. Sticking the trachea is just like sticking a "big vein that has air in it instead of blood." Then it's in with the wire, make a nick, and you're there. Of course you pray you never have to do this. But if you do, you'll need to do it quick and right. So practice it in the simulator first!

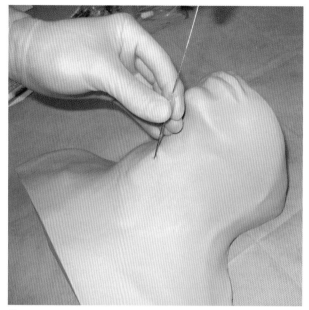

C

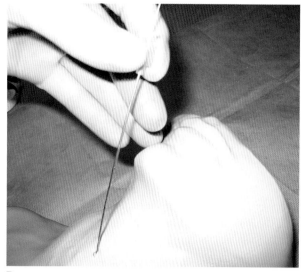

D

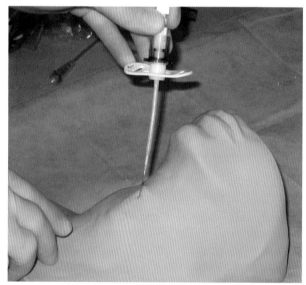

E

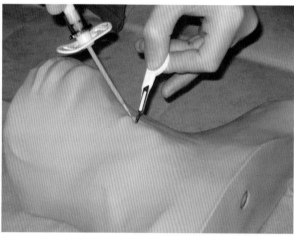

F

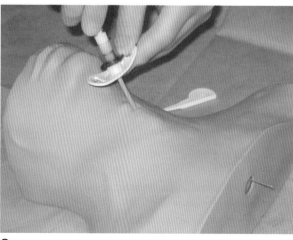

G

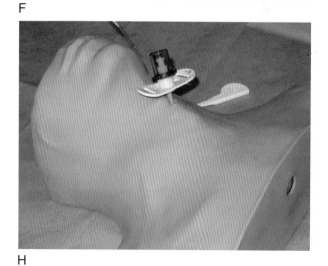

H

FIGURE 8–30 cont'd

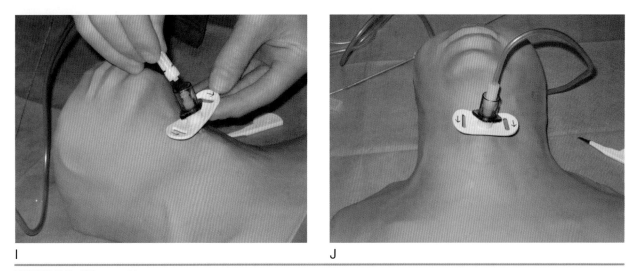

I   J

FIGURE 8–30   cont'd

---

says. "You happen to have an insufflator here, I'd like to insufflate air through this little opening."

"What's an insufflator?" the ER nurse asks, looking around.

"Forget it, if you don't know, you don't have it, this will have to do," the anesthesia resident says. "Once the dust settles out there, we'll have to have ENT take a look at this amateur airway we've got here."

"Simulation's done folks!" the instructor says.

Clinical lessons learned from scenario 10

Disaster hangs heavy in the air these days, what with terrorists lurking in every Middlesex village and town. But even without terrorists, we keep finding ways to create our own disasters, which can and do overwhelm the medical system. Refineries explode, planes crash, buildings burn, trains derail—and in the blink of an eye, doctors are practicing the age-old art of deciding who to treat and who to "let go."

When there's only so much of you, you can only do so much. The debriefing explores this, as well as some airway questions.

Debriefing. "Can you spell T-R-I-A-G-E?" the instructor asks.

"I can sure spell it better than I can spell 'Shikani,'" the anesthesia resident quips.

The assembled team—anesthesia resident, ER nurse, and instructor—go over the DVD of the simulation scenario.

"What were you thinking when you first got this news in the hallway?" the instructor asks.

"I wanted to get my hands around just how many people were injured and how many people would be available if I got in a jam," the anesthesia resident explains. "I hear 'explosion, burns around the face, and C-collars,' and I'm picturing a lot of airway trouble. The Maryland Shock Trauma guidelines for the 'need to intubate but don't have a cleared C-spine patient going down the tubes' are pretty clear.

"You won't have time to do an elegant awake intubation, and the patient thrashing around may worsen the cervical injury. So you induce, you give a paralytic, you look, then if you don't see anything, you cut the neck—that's it. Crystal clear. It takes a lot of the murk out of this difficult but common airway dilemma."

"But before you even got there, you had to make another decision," the instructor says.

They review the DVD of his quick exam on the asystolic patient.

"When the ER nurse made it clear that there *was* no one else around, I had to marshall the most good out of what we had available, namely, the ER nurse and me," the anesthesia resident explained. "So we have one guy with burns to his face, a rapidly closing airway, and vital signs. This guy needs a lot of expert help right now.

"And we have another guy who is asystolic. Of course I don't automatically believe the monitors, I make sure a lead isn't off or something. But with no pulse, blown pupils, no breathing, no lead misplacement, I figure, this is the real deal. This is asystole. This isn't even V-fib that maybe we can shock him out of.

"So hey, what do I do, expend a lot of energy on a rhythm that rarely comes back anyway? Asystole is the baddest of the bad. I mean, come on, King Tut, technically, is in asystole. You going to spend a lot of time resuscitating him?"

"No way *I'm* doing mouth to mouth on a mummy!" the ER nurse says.

"Right you are," the anesthesia resident says. "So, I triaged him to the 'nothing more to be done' group and went to the fast-closing airway."

"No regrets on that decision?" the instructor asks.

"Hard times require hard decisions," the anesthesia resident says, "so, no. No regrets."

"OK, let's go to the airway," the instructor says, "what are you thinking there?"

"Soot around the face, a report that steam was involved—it all points to an airway burn that could extend all the way down into the lungs," the anesthesia resident says. "You have to intubate right away, before swelling makes intubation impossible. And this guy was already giving a high-pitched squeak, so my mind's eye was seeing his airway close off from above."

"Why not use the Shikani system," the ER nurse says, "it's made for just this kind of thing."

"New gizmos for securing the airway are all well and good," the anesthesia resident explains, "but you always want to use *new* stuff in a nonemergent setting. Visit the Shikani website, review some teaching tapes, use the Shikani on a nice easy airway that you can always do 'the regular way' if you goof up with the Shikani thing.

"Do it the first time here? In a 4+ emergency and airway closure happening right in front of me? No way. This is the very time that you want to use all the familiar things. We're in enough trouble as it is, we don't need to import any more trouble."

"I liked your recitation of the Maryland Shock Trauma airway protocol," the instructor says, "but I notice you didn't give any drugs."

"That protocol is for someone with enough time," the anesthesia resident says, "but this guy had just closed off everything but everything. My quick look said, 'No way anything is going through the mouth here, this airway is just too far gone'."

On the DVD, the resident does a slick job getting in the cricothyrotomy.

"Why not a regular trach?" the ER nurse asks.

"Takes too long," the anesthesia resident says. "A regular trach in the regular place is much lower than where I went. I went high, at the cricothyroid membrane, where the airway is closest to the surface. If you view the trachea as just a big IV that happens to have air in it rather than blood, placing the cric is just the same as placing a central line."

"Only *this* central line actually *is* central!"

"But you didn't do insufflation through it," the instructor says.

"Yes," the anesthesia resident says, "this opening is so small that you can't really ventilate very well through it, and insufflation would be preferable to my kind of half-assed bag ventilation through it. But hey, something is better than nothing. If they don't have insufflation equipment in the ER, then they don't have it. But this at least delivers some oxygen to the patient."

"What would your next moves be?" the instructor asks.

"Well, this guy would probably start to move and thrash around so we'd need to protect his C-spine. We'd need to secure his head better. Then, once A and B are taken care of, we'd have to focus on C, his cardiac status. I'll admit in all the excitement, I never did get a blood pressure."

"But I'm sure you would have," the instructor prompts.

"But of course, I'm the best of the best. If you don't believe me, just ask me again and I'll tell you again!"

Summary. In a mass casualty situation, you may have to "write off" some people to save others. No easy task, and something that might haunt you later on, but it is part of our job.

Not that you can't bring people back from asystole, but it's a rare save when you do it. If you must divert resources away from anyone, that is the person to "write off."

Burn, upper airway, steam—secure that airway ASAP, even if the patient doesn't seem that bad at the time. Once they start swelling up and losing their airway, you will be in a heap of trouble in no time flat.

Learn about new equipment when all the world is calm and sunny, not in the middle of a raging hurricane. Of note, the Shikani *is* an excellent system and well worth learning. The device allows you to sneak into the back of the throat and "look up from behind the tongue" so you get a pretty straight shot at the vocal cords. You don't need a big mouth opening to get this view, and you don't need to extend the neck. Perfect stuff for the trauma bay, where *everyone* has an uncleared C-spine.

Anesthesia residents tend to live in morbid fear of that awful time when they have to "take up the knife" to secure the airway. Current airway kits take the

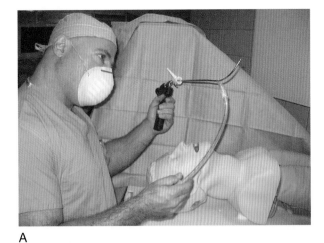

A

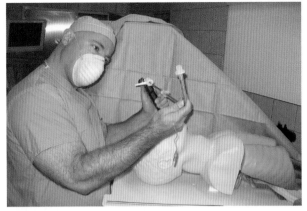

B

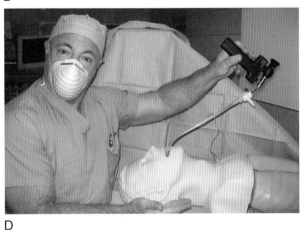

D

C

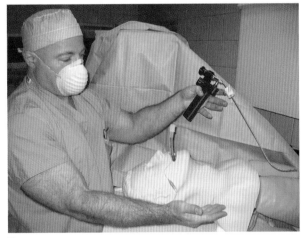

E

FIGURE 8–31 The Shikani optical scope, a great gizmo for securing the airway. But, as with everything else, you don't want to use a "new toy" for the first time in an emergency. Either practice it in a simulated setting, or do it on a patient with an easy airway in a nonemergent setting. That way, if you blow it you can always shift into intubate-them-the-regular-way mode.

terror out of this procedure so long as you make that one little intellectual leap.

I'm just putting a central line in the trachea.

Voila! Suddenly it's not so frightening.

Find air.

Thread a wire.

Cut.

Place the line in the trachea.

There now, that wasn't so bad, was it?

SCENARIO 11. **The miracle of birth, stat C-section**

The OB nurse grabs the anesthesia resident by the sleeve, "Time for the MOB."

"MOB?" the resident asks.

"Miracle of birth," the nurse explains.

Entering the labor suite, the anesthesia resident notices that the fetal heart rate monitor shows a whopping 60 heart rate. Just as the resident's mouth drops open, footsteps come pounding up from behind him.

"STAT C-section!" the OB shouts, then turns around and runs out.

"Anything we can do to buy some time doctor?" the OB nurse asks.

"Uh," the anesthesia resident stumbles, then the fog clears, "left uterine displacement, turn off the Pitocin if she has it on" (she does), "stop the epidural for a second while we check the blood pressure."

"Oxygen," the nurse suggests.

"Yes, no," the anesthesia resident stops for a second, thinking of retrolental fibroplasia. "Wait, that would be bad for the baby's eyes,"—wait, is that right, the resident wonders? No, wait a minute, no. No, it's not bad for the eyes, you treat the mom first, oh yeah, oh yeah, the Po$_2$ of the baby doesn't even go up that much anyway, no way the oxygen can cause retrolental fibroplasia when you give the mom some supplemental oxygen. What was I thinking?

"Yes, oxygen, definitely. And some terbutaline, yeah, some terbutaline, let's slow those contractions." God, did I think of everything? It's so hard to remember stuff when everyone's yelling.

The scenario does a technical time out, as the team goes from the labor suite to the OR suite.

In the OR suite, the patient is being preoxygenated. The patient is flat on her back.

The blood pressure shows 80/50, from the speakers in the mannequin, a voice says, "I feel *rrrrrrrrrrrrrruuuuuuuuuuuulllllgggghhhhhh*!"

"Suction!" the anesthesia resident shouts, looking around. Damn, where is the suction—oh, here.

"Heart rate is still 60, we have to go!" the OB resident shouts. The patient is draped, and they are ready.

"OK," the anesthesia resident says, "just a second." The resident places the suction catheter in the mannequin's mouth. "I need some cricoid."

The circulator is not even up at the head of the bed, the circulator is under the sheets at the foot of the bed!

"Um, I need someone up here," the resident says, "right now."

"Heart rate 50, come on!" the OB is apoplectic.

"OK," the anesthesia resident gives a syringe of Pentothal, then Sux, then tries to hold the cricoid pressure himself, the arms getting tangled up.

"Wait!" the OB nurse at the foot of the bed yells, "the head's out! The baby's head's out! Don't put her to sleep!"

"Oh shit!" the anesthesia resident says.

"Oh shit!" the OB resident says.

"My arm hurts!" the patient yells. "I feel weak."

Looking down, the anesthesia resident sees that the IV site is red and infiltrated.

"I . . . can't . . . breathe," the patient's voice falls off. "My . . . arm . . ." then she falls silent.

Behind the anesthesia resident, the blood pressure cuff alarms, *error—error—low BP reading*.

The OB resident looks up, "You didn't put her to sleep, did you? She'll need to push now."

"Um . . ."

Reaching for ephedrine, the anesthesia resident realizes that the IV is infiltrated, that there is subq Pentothal and succinylcholine on board, the patient has stopped breathing, the blood pressure is too low to read, the baby's head is out, and, oh, he took the cricoid pressure off just now, and everyone is looking at him. The pulse oximeter stops reading, and ectopy starts on the EKG.

The door to the OR opens.

"Everything going OK in here? I was just about to go home and wanted to see if you needed a hand before I left," another anesthesia resident says. "Hey, shouldn't she be in left uterine displacement?"

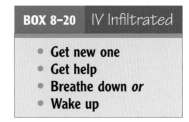

BOX 8–20 **IV Infiltrated**

- Get new one
- Get help
- Breathe down *or*
- Wake up

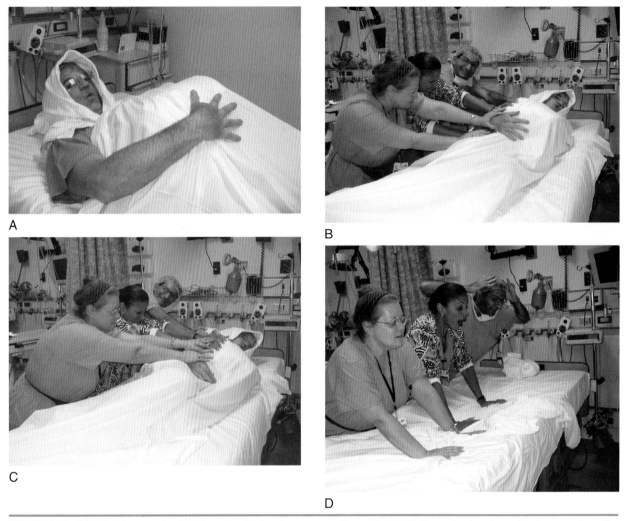

FIGURE 8–32 **A.** The miracle of birth awaits this lovely young mother-to-be. **B, C.** But wait, there's trouble in maternity-ville. Quick, put Mom in left uterine displacement to increase venous return and restore uteroplacental sufficiency. **D.** Don't push too hard, though.

His hair attempting to stand on end through his OR cap, the anesthesia resident says in a voice an octave higher than usual, "I could use a hand."

Pushing a wedge underneath the patient's right hip, the second anesthesia resident asks, "What can I do you for?"

The first anesthesia resident literally shakes his head, trying to clear away the cobwebs and short circuits, "Lost IV, she's not breathing, head's out, and. . . ."

"OK," the second anesthesia resident says, "ABC, chill, just do the ABC and we'll be OK. You mask, get that sat up. I'll get an IV. You, Dr. OB, can you get the baby out with salad spoons (forceps) if I give you a little fundal pressure?"

"Don't really need the forceps, the head's out," the OB says, "but a little push and I should be able to get it."

"Good," the first anesthesia resident says, "and I'll need cricoid up here. Don't think she's weak enough to instrument her airway."

The circulator comes out from under the drapes, goes to the head of the bed, and gives cricoid.

"All right," the first anesthesia resident says, "you're getting the IV, leaning on the uterus, and helping get the baby out. You're going for it to get the baby out."

The pulse oximeter comes back.

Again, the OR door opens.

"It's a wrap! Simulation's done!"

Clinical lessons learned from scenario 11

When things go sour on OB, they can go sour fast, testing your ability to adapt and change as the situation evolves. A lot of players were involved in this not-terribly-far-fetched sequence. The debriefing allows us to play it all again in slow motion, see what went right, what went wrong, and the all-important what to do better next time.

Debriefing. "Some miracle of birth," the instructor says.

"Call it the 'madness of birth,'" the first anesthesia resident retorts.

That loosens up the whole debriefing table.

The instructor goes to the white board and says, "Let's debrief this by laying out a time line so we can see what's going on at each time point and what everyone's thinking."

MOB announced → MOB occurs

"What happened in between point A and point B?" the instructor asks.

Starting out, the OB nurse says, "We got a real bad deceleration, and we had to get going."

"What's the big rush?" the instructor asks the OB resident. "There are marathon runners who have heart rates of 35. What's the big deal if the kid is clipping along at 60?"

"Babies have stiff hearts, incapable of stretching and increasing their cardiac output like an adult. Kids are heart rate-dependent. And if they drop their heart rate, that is actually a maladaptive response. So, in a kind of double-whammy, a kid who is in trouble—uteroplacental insufficiency from any cause—responds by doing the worst thing! Slowing their heart rate," the OB explains. "The only good thing about that, if you are looking for silver linings, is that fetal brady-cardia is *the* red flag that tells us we have to move."

"God is sending you an urgent e-mail," the instructor says.

"Exactly."

"And what do you do when you see this red flag?" the instructor asks the anesthesia resident.

"Well," the anesthesia resident says, "as was evident here, I got flustered and mixed up. God may be sending me an urgent e-mail, but my mailbox got so full I couldn't read it."

"OK," the instructor says, "let's put that on the time line."

MOB → fetal → panic → MOB occurs
announced trouble

BOX 8-21 Panic

- **We all do it**
- **Reduces brain to oatmeal**
- **Extra person—a Godsend**

"Don't dismiss the human tendency to panic," the instructor says. "There's a lot of input, you don't have all the information you want, and the pressure's on to do something instantaneously. This isn't grand rounds where you sit in your chair and sort of weigh the options, discuss what's best, and come up with a consensus after a review of the literature. This is *now, now, now.*"

Nods all around the table.

"This is similar to learning a foreign language," the instructor says. "You study for years, have a wealth of verbs, conjugations, and sayings in your head, but when you go out on the street and the first person says something to you, your knowledge base shrinks to the smallest possible unit. You may have studied Spanish for 4 years, but all you can remember is 'Hola'."

"So," the instructor continues, "what is a good antidote to panic?"

"Go back to ABC," the first anesthesia resident says, "and call for help."

"Right, you never go wrong going ABC," the instructor says, "don't hesitate to even say it out loud. It'll focus you."

MOB → fetal → panic → MOB occurs
announced trouble
ABC—get help

"What's the big deal about help?" the OB nurse asks.

The second anesthesia resident answers, "When you're the first one, you get a little too close to the action, plus it's easier to get your ego wrapped up in the proceedings. 'Oh man, this is my case, and things are going to hell!' That second person has the advantage of objectivity 'Well at least I didn't get us into this jam,' so the second person can look at things in a much cooler, 'Well, let's just go down the list and see what needs to be done' manner."

"Let's look at things from the obstetric angle, since we are married together in these kinds of cases," the instructor continues, "What was the deal with the head coming out."

Rolling her eyes, the OB resident says, "Gotta always take a peak between the legs and see if Baby

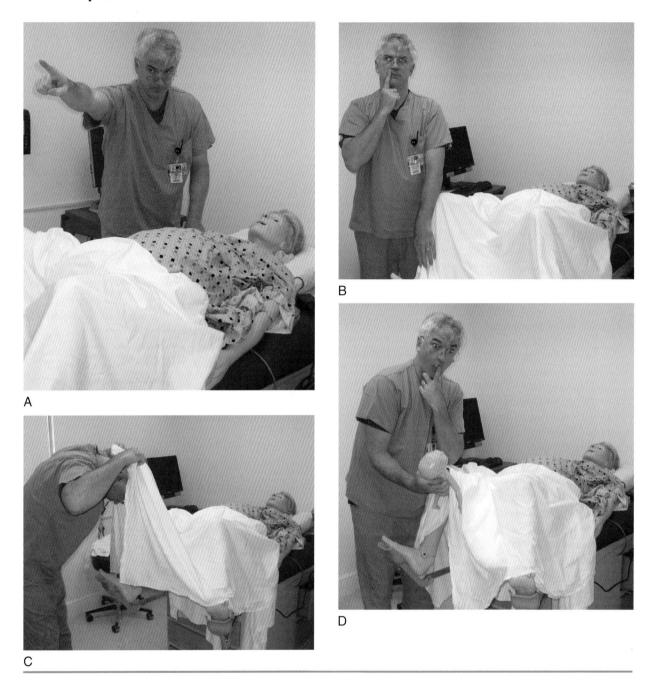

FIGURE 8–33 **A, B, C.** Off to do a C-section? Never forget to take one last little peek. Every now and then the baby beats the odds and shows up. **D.** Well, what do you know?

Dumpling has made a surprise arrival. In my rush to cut, I forgot an important lesson of delivery—kids have their own agenda and sometimes deliver from below while we're going at them from above."

"So," the instructor explains, "what exactly was the dilemma at the, shall we call it, high point, or maybe, low point, of the case."

"The OB was surprised by a baby halfway out," the first anesthesia resident says, "I was surprised by a, well, IV halfway out, you could say. And I forgot the ABC, forgetting to wait for someone to give me cricoid and forgetting about the basic left uterine displacement needed to keep adequate venous return and keep her blood pressure up."

"Sort of a Grand Slam of trouble," the instructor offers.

"Then I arrived to save the day!" the second anesthesia resident trumpets.

"Your day will come," the OB pokes a hole in the resident's balloon.

"Humph," the second anesthesia resident shrugs it off. "I just focused everyone on what we could do, and what needed doing. I work on getting an IV, my anesthetic confrere keeps oxygenation going in this less-than-perfect world of a half-anesthetized, half-paralyzed patient, and the OB gets the baby out in the less-than-perfect world of a baby with the head out but a mom unable to push."

"You could argue different options," the OB says.

"Sure, you could say, 'Wait until I get an IV, then induce the rest of the way, secure the airway, then cut.' You could also say, 'Let the anesthetic drugs wear off, then let her push.' There are always different options. But right then, with things the way they were, I read this as the best way to go. We pick the plan, we go for it."

"Wrong, yes. Uncertain, never!"

Summary. Anesthesia is a field of "remember the basics." What gets us in the most trouble is the basic stuff, hardly ever the exotic, bizarre stuff.

IV infiltrated, forget to inspect it? Now you can't induce, can't give fluids, can't give resuscitative drugs such as ephedrine, and you can end up with subcutaneous drugs that hurt you. Pentothal can cause tissue damage, succinylcholine can cause partial paralysis as it's slowly absorbed.

Forget left uterine displacement? This—beaten into us over and over again—is easy to forget in the panic of an emergency. And if you forget this basic maneuver, you drop your blood pressure, can induce nausea and vomiting, and get yourself into all kinds of trouble.

Forget to do the OB exam? Though not exactly our bailiwick, we do need to know "the other doctor's job" almost as well as our own. The ultimate goal here is taking good care of the patient, after all, not drawing lines of responsibility and saying, "Well, that's not *my* job so it's not *my* fault." You, as anesthesiologist, should have a good grip on how far along the baby is, how likely the baby is to "deliver from below," and whether any surprises are in store, "Oh, look, the baby's already here!"

And finally, you need to know when to ask for help, and you need to know the tremendous value that help can be. Right when your mind is amped out with too much bad news coming in too fast, you can get a second assessment, a second pair of eyes, a second brain. That may save your butt.

And may save your patient's life.

SCENARIO 12. **Keeping an eye out, agitation in an opththalmic case**

"Hate to do this to you," the attending says, "but you're in the eye room today. Need a magazine? Don't think much is going to grab your attention in there."

The resident shrugs, "Whatever, so long as you sign the check at the end of the month."

"Look," the attending (instructor) says, "the retrobulbar block is already in, the bed is turned around, just keep your eyes peeled, no pun intended, in case there's an oculocardiac reflex or something."

Entering the OR, the anesthesia resident sees the bed reversed, the surgeon by the head of the bed, the patient's feet toward the anesthesia machine, with the patient's feet sticking out from underneath the sheets. All the vital signs are OK, oxygen tubing is snaking underneath the drapes, and the CD player has Figaro's aria from the *Barber of Seville* playing.

"Figaro, Figaro, Figaro, Figaro!"

God, how can people listen to this stuff.

"Figaro, Figaro!"

"Hey, hold still!" the eye surgeon says, "hey, anesthesia, he's wiggling, can you give him something?"

At first the anesthesia resident doesn't even hear the surgeon, his complaint drowned out by the wailing operatic music.

"Hey, anesthesia!"

"Oh, yeah," the anesthesia resident looks around, there's some Versed.

"OK, sir?" she says to the patient, then lifts the drapes a little to look at the patient's face, "are you OK? I'm going to give you something to help you relax a little, OK?"

The anesthesia resident gives 1 mg of Versed, waits a minute or two, then gives 1 mg more.

"Better," the surgeon says.

"Figaro la! Figaro cua! Figaro la! Figaro cua! Figaro, Figaro, Figaro, Figaro!"

The anesthesia resident rolls her eyes. Opera, who the hell goes to the opera, who the hell listens to opera? Of the 5000+ songs she's pirated and loaded on her iPod, not one, not one single opera. And there will never be one either!

"Hey," the opththalmologist says, even more irritation in his voice than the stupid guy singing opera, "he's still moving, can't you give him some of that white stuff?"

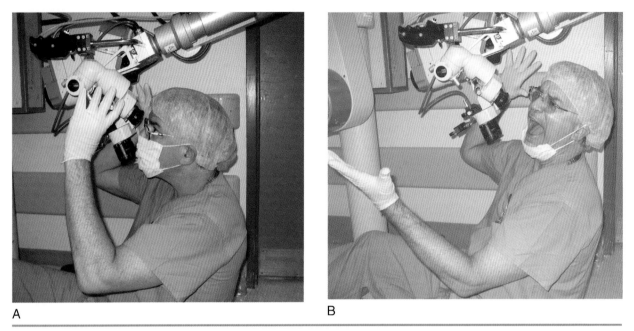

A   B

FIGURE 8–34   "Hey, he moved!" Sedating a patient during an eye case can set up a really vicious cycle. They move, you sedate, they weird out on you, then you give more, and round and round you go.

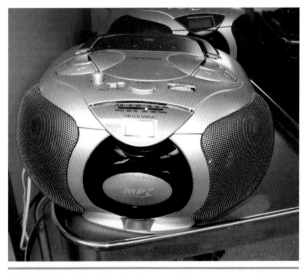

FIGURE 8–35   Your brain can only process so much input. If a blasting boombox is distracting you, by all means turn it off. Or throw it out a window, whichever is easier.

"Propofol?"

"Yeah, that's it."

"OK," the resident duly lifts the sheets again, oops, the nasal cannulas have slipped off the patient's nose. She replaces them. "Sir, try to hold still, I'm going to give you a little something to help you relax a little more."

She picks up a syringe labeled "propofol," gives 2 cc (20 mg), then looks around for an infusion pump.

God, an eye case, couldn't they think of something better? And this Figaro crap. What did I do wrong in an earlier life to deserve this?

"Bravo bravissimo, bravo bravissimo!"

"Hey, that burns!" the patient says.

"That will go away soon," the resident says, then turns to the circulator, "Hey, can I get an infusion pump."

"Will this do?" the circulator shows the resident a pump. The pump is familiar, but there is no IV pole attachment, so the resident fashions a tape-hook-IV pole attachment to set up the infusion pump.

"Hey, come on, help me out, I can't do this with him moving all over like this!" the ophthalmologist says.

"Sure," the resident gives another "dink" of propofol, 3 cc.

"Figaro, Figaro, Figaro!"

Beneath the sound of baritone Italian complaints, the pulse oximeter reads 70% and the alarm is going off. Just as the alarm goes off, the tape-infusion pump contraption snaps and the infusion pump falls to the floor. The front of the pump falls off.

"Oh man, let me see," the resident says.

Oxygen saturation is now 50%.

"You OK over there?" the ophthalmologist asks.

"Yeah," the resident says.

"Figaro la, Figaro cua!"

Picking up the pump, the circulator provides useful suggestions, "The front piece reattaches here, I think it's magnetic, wait, but you want propofol, right, this thing is for dobutamine, let me get the other one."

Ectopy on the EKG, pulse oximeter going off, now it's been alarming so long, it's like background noise in the room.

The Italian opera star belts out one last acoustic tile-rattling note, and the song ends. Now the only sound in the room is the pulse oximeter alarm.

Turning to the monitors, the anesthesia resident "gives his harness bells a shake to ask if there is some mistake," then reaches down to adjust the pulse oximeter.

"Is this thing on OK?" she asks, to no one in particular.

The EKG goes into V-tach.

Tearing back the sheets, the anesthesia resident looks at the EKG leads.

"Hey, what are you doing?" the ophthalmologist yells.

"Wait," the resident grabs the circuit and mask, "I've gotta mask here!"

"Simulation over!" the instructor says over the OR intercom.

Clinical lessons learned from scenario 12

Distraction is nothing short of deadly. The debriefing, and an analogy from the world of aviation, can make the point.

Debriefing. Plunking herself down in the debriefing room, the anesthesia resident looks like a Charlie Brown cartoon—all she needs is the squiggly lines over her head indicating frustration.

"So, how do you think that went?" the instructor asks, all openness and nonjudgmentally.

"I stunk the place up," the resident says. "Just shoot me and put me out of my misery."

The ophthalmologist sits down, "OK to listen to *Carmen* while we sit here?"

BOX 8-22	More Sedation, More Sedation

- **Do you have the airway?**
- **Are you doing a Room Air General?**
- **Save your butt, go ahead and intubate.**

Entering the room with the broken infusion pump, the circulator says, "I love *Carmen!*" then she starts humming.

"Don't bother shooting me, I'll just leap out the window here," the dejected resident says.

"OK, time out," the instructor says, "crawl off that cross there for a minute there, let's look at what happened and see if we can pull a lesson out of this. You're here to learn, remember. If *you* did everything right, why would they pay *me* the big money?"

Everyone looks at the DVD instant replay. The anesthesia resident doesn't wait for any corrective action, providing all the color commentary herself.

"Right off the bat, I'm in the wrong mind set—oh, this is an eye case, big deal."

Words and interchange are hard to hear over the Figaro music.

"Can't hear him, he can't hear me, I'm not really connecting with the patient, and I never drew a line in the linoleum and said, 'Hey, turn the music down, I can't do my job here.'"

On the monitors, desaturation starts early, but the music, the falling infusion pump, the circulator "helping" with the infusion pump.

"Then what am I doing, I'm sedating someone with hypoxemia! That agitation is a red flag, and I'm just throwing a little more sedation at him, hoping he'll shut up and stop moving."

"Eye cases are 'safe,' right?" the instructor asks, "because it's 'just a *MAC*,' right?

Wrong, wrong, a thousand times wrong!" the instructor says, louder even than Figaro at his most vocal. "Hear these words that I say for, yea, I speak the truth, the whole truth, and nothing but the truth. Remember this until you are old and gray and you are dribbling oatmeal down your bib.

"You get into more trouble with MACs than general cases.

"You get into more trouble with MACs than general cases.

"You get into more trouble with MACs than general cases.

"I say this three times, because it is oh so true! In a general case, you *have the airway.* In a MAC case, you *don't.*"

The anesthesia resident nods, "Point well taken."

"Let's go to aviation land and look at another lesson here—distraction," the instructor says, then plays a video of a NOVA program. "Watch this cockpit recreation of the conversation recovered from the black box of Eastern flight 401 inbound to Miami."

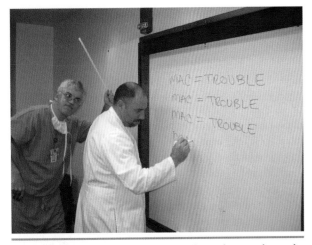

FIGURE 8–36 How many times do we have to learn the lesson? You can get in big trouble in a MAC case. You get in more trouble with a MAC than a general case. In a general case, you at least have the airway! In a MAC case, without the airway, well, stuff happens.

BOX 8-23	Repeat this Mantra

- **MAC = big trouble**
- **MAC = big trouble**
- **MAC = big trouble**

Pushing the pause button, the instructor says, "You turned all your attention to that infusion pump, fixing up a kind of sling thing for the IV pole, reacting when it hit the ground, and working with the circulator to get the right face plate for it."

And the resident, now an expert on flogging herself, provides the key element, "I was thinking about everything but 'flying the plane.' And the patient crashed."

All three other people at the table nod, "Funny you should use that analogy," the ophthalmologist says.

The NOVA DVD rolls.

On a night approach to Miami in the 1970s, Eastern flight 401 had trouble with a little green light on the control panel. Pilot, copilot, and flight engineer all turned their attention to that little light. The pilot says, "Try pulling it." The co-pilot says, "It just won't come out," the flight engineer says, "Try this, try that." Everyone is completely absorbed by this little light.

2000 feet—The pilot says to turn on the autopilot.

Someone maybe did, maybe didn't.

1800 feet—an alarm goes off, indicating the plane is losing altitude, no one reacts to it.

Conversation continues to revolve around the little green light.

1500 feet.

1000 feet.

The control tower asks, "How's it going up there?"

800 feet.

500 feet.

200 feet.

"Hey," the co-pilot says, "we're still at 2000, aren't we?"

No indication that anyone pulled up on the stick or made any attempt to gain altitude.

"There's something wrong here."

Crackle, loss of transmission—99 people go into the Everglades at 300 miles per hour.

"That pump was my little green light, wasn't it?" the anesthesia resident asks.

Summary. There are no routine flights, and there are no routine anesthetics. Both can and do crash if you don't pay attention.

Ask any anesthesiologist who has a few gray hairs and wrinkles, they can tell you that some of those gray hairs and wrinkles are due to MAC cases. A MAC case has a nasty habit of working its way into a "Room Air General" as you pump more and more sedation into a patient whose airway you *do not have.*

The patient gets agitated.

2000 feet.

The surgeon gets agitated, you give more sedation.

1800 feet.

You give more sedation.

1500 feet.

Throw in distractors that keep you from focusing on the all-important airway.

1000 feet.

Loud music that distracts you from listening to your monitors.

500 feet.

Turn the bed around so you can't get at the airway or adequately assess breathing.

100 feet.

Then you see something unbelievably bad, and you can't believe it.

"There's something wrong here."

Crackle, end transmission, radar blip disappears.

SCENARIO 13.   **Seeking regularity, unstable atrial fibrillation**

"Um, could you come in here please, this guy's not looking too good," the PACU nurse says.

Three anesthesia residents, a CA-1, a CA-2, and a CA-3 are standing out in the hallway.

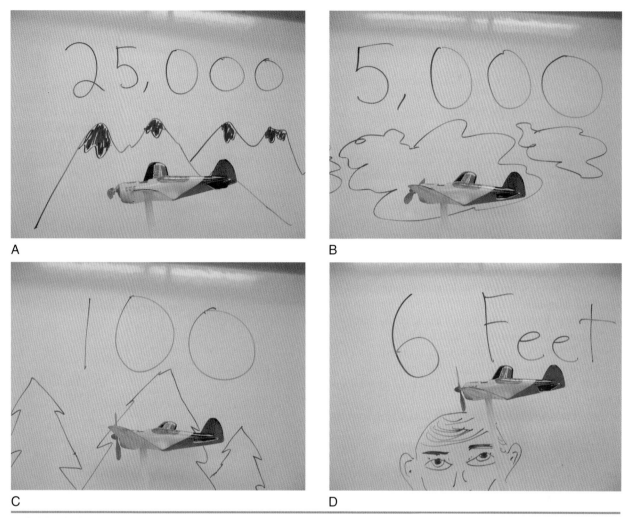

FIGURE 8–37 When you don't pay attention to the important stuff, the plane can slip lower and lower and lower. Before you know it, you're giving pedestrians crew cuts with your propeller. Remember the motto of the ASA: "Vigilance." Keep looking over everything, keep snooping around to see if something is wrong, not making sense, disconnected. Consider yourself a lifeguard (you *are* in fact a lifeguard) and keep looking over that pool.

"OK, OK," the CA-3 says, "I'm in charge, OK? I'm on charge on this because I'm the senior resident here, OK?"

The junior residents nod agreement.

All three go into the PACU. The CA-1 picks up the preop evaluation and starts looking it over.

A 72-year-old man with known CAD, S/P stents on two occasions, with poor exercise tolerance. Just had repair of an incisional hernia. EKG shows old infarcts, sinus rhythm.

The CA-2 goes to the head of the bed, makes sure oxygen is on, and the CA-3 stands at the foot of the bed.

The monitor shows a sat of 93%, and the heart rate is banging away at 134.

"Right," the CA-3 says. "Right, tachycardic, that's not good. Um . . . OK, ABC: How's he breathing?"

At the head of the bed, the CA-2 says, "Chest's going up and down. You breathing OK sir? He speak English?"

The PACU nurse says, "Yes."

"You OK sir?" the CA-2 repeats.

"No . . . no . . . I   can't . . . breathe . . . can't . . . breathe too . . . good," the patient gasps.

On the monitor, the BP reads 140/85.

"How old is that pressure?" the CA-3 asks. "Well, forget it, cycle the cuff again."

Repeat blood pressure shows 75/40.

The CA-3 starts walking toward the head of the bed, stops, then stays at the foot.

"Um, OK, ABC, ABC," the CA-3 says.

"Fluids?" the CA-1 asks. "Neo, maybe?"

Chewing her lower lip, putting her right index finger on her mouth, and holding her right elbow with her left hand, the CA-3 does a standing version of Rodin's *The Thinker*.

"Just a sec, just a sec," the CA-3 muses, "he's bad, he's bad. But you're talking treatment, and we don't have a diagnosis yet."

"What are the three things in 'C' again?" the CA-2 asks. "Everything's in 'threes,' ABC and stuff, and there are three things in 'C' but I'm blanking."

"Rate, rhythm, contractility," the CA-1 offers.

"Right, that's it," the CA-3 confirms. "So, let's ... um ... let's see. Rate, OK, we're fast, 130."

"It's funny," the CA-2 says, "sometimes it's 130, then sometimes it's 118, then sometimes it says 140."

"Wait," the CA-3 says, "wait, there's a trick. Just a second." She closes her eyes. Then she opens them and puts her hand on the pulse. "Yeah, yeah, that's it."

"What, it's irregular?" the CA-1 asks.

"Yep," the CA-3 says, then picks up the paddles.

"What are you doing?" the CA-1 asks.

"Oh yeah," the CA-3 says, "atrial fibrillation. Listen, hear how irregular it is?"

"Aren't there P waves here?" the CA-1 asks, looking at the monitor. "Oh, I guess there aren't. How did I miss that?"

"Hey ... what ... what   are   you ... what ... doing?" the patient gasps.

"Sir," the CA-3 explains, "you have a bad heart rate, and we need to reset it, we're going to give you a little shock here to do that reset."

"You going to sedate him?" the PACU nurse asks.

"Oh yeah," the CA-3 says.

"But he's unstable," the CA-2 says.

"Yeah, but he's still awake, maybe just a little Versed?" the CA-1 offers, directing the question to the CA-3.

Removing the paddles, the CA-3 says, "You're right, you're right, just a little, though, just enough to cloud the senses, but not too much, I mean, look where we are, short of breath, fast rate, crummy blood pressure. Just one milligram, OK."

"What do you want me to give?" the PACU nurse asks.

All three residents at once say, "One milligram of Versed."

The CA-3 raises her hand, "Please, I'm in charge. Info *to* me, directives *from* me, that keeps it clean." She turns to the PACU nurse, "One milligram of Versed."

Versed goes in.

"Those ... cold ..."

"Hey," the CA-1 says, "he's still with it."

"Chance we'll have to take," the CA-3 says. "He's sick, he's pretty old, and we don't have a ton of time. That'll have to do."

The PACU nurse goes to set the paddles.

"No," the CA-3 says, "we're here to do the stuff ourselves." She tells the CA-1 to set the paddles. He does everything right but forgets to press the Synchronous button.

"OK!" the CA-1 says.

"Wait!" the CA-2 sees the mistake. "I've got to Synch this puppy."

"Oh yeah," the CA-3 sees it. "OK, clear, clear, everybody clear."

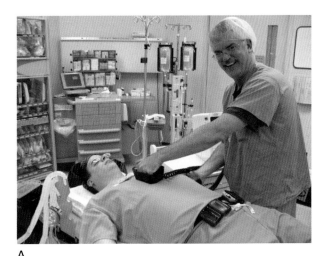

A

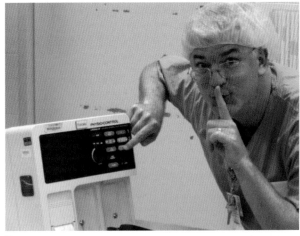

B

FIGURE 8–38 We often tell people to charge the paddles. But we rarely do it ourselves. Make a point of "working the buttons" yourself to make sure you know how to work the defibrillator in an emergency.

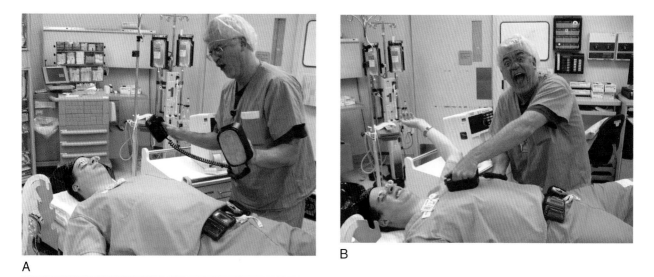

A B

FIGURE 8–39 Of course, never use live paddles on your colleagues, as this may give them a very serious case of death. Think of the paperwork after such a snafu!

She charges, discharges.

"YOW!" the patient says.

Everyone looks at the rhythm, still A-fib.

"Do we go with amiodarone now?" the CA-1 asks.

"No," the CA-3 keeps holding the paddles on the patient's chest. "You *cardiovert*, don't just *try* to cardiovert. We go three times.

On the second try, the rhythm converts.

"How you doing, sir?" the CA-2 asks.

"Oh, good, I can breathe a little better," he says.

"How about a blood gas and some labs," the CA-1 suggests. "Maybe we'll find some cause for this whole thing."

"Good idea," the CA-3 says, "let's get a gas and some cardiac enzymes."

"All done!" the instructor says.

Clinical lessons learned from scenario 13

The clinical lesson from this scenario is brief but brief—the treatment for unstable atrial fibrillation is cardioversion. Delay in the unstable patient invites catastrophe. How long can a 72-year-old man with known CAD hover with a blood pressure in the 70s, after all?

But it's easy to read the correct treatment off an ACLS card, much harder to actually *do* the right thing in a real-live (even if simulated) setting.

Debriefing. The three residents and the PACU nurse, plus the instructor, are sitting around the debriefing table, drinking the inevitable coffee.

"I only drink things that have 'ino' on the end," the CA-2 quips. "You know, cappuccino, frappuccino, stuff like that. Makes me feel European, sort of. I think regular coffee is bad for my IQ."

"You must have drunk a lot of regular coffee then," the CA-3 jabs.

"OK, break it up, you morons, this is a center of higher learning," the instructor says. "We *could* use a Starbucks here, though, that is the one thing we don't have up here."

"Simulatoccino," the CA-2 says. "I would drink that."

They sit through the DVD of the scenario, this time played from stem to stern without stopping it.

"I like it, I like it," the instructor says, "I'm not supposed to be judgmental right off like that, but I'm just going to say it. I like it."

The PACU nurse speaks up, "I knew right from the start who was in charge. Right away. Got the orders from the senior resident, not a barrage of orders from everybody."

"What makes a leader?" the instructor says, "What makes a good leader?"

BOX 8–24	Unstable Atrial Fibrillation Shock, Shock, Shock

- **Synchronous**
- **Don't "fear the paddles"**

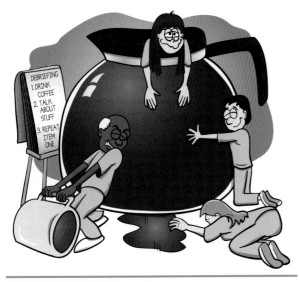

FIGURE 8–40 Critical to the success of any debriefing session is the consumption of appropriate coffee drinks.

"Firm hand, directs the ship," the CA-1 says. "But still listens to other people."

Pointing to the CA-2, the instructor raises his eyebrows, asking silently, "And you, what do you think?"

"Right," the CA-2 says, "the flow, the information goes *to* the leader, the orders, the splitting up of, you know, what to do, the tasks, that comes *from* the leader. I think she even said that once."

"Right," the instructor says. "That's good. There's nothing wrong about saying what you're thinking. It puts the big idea out there so everyone can grab on to it and start working on it. Like when she said, 'Wait, let's get the diagnosis before we go ape with the treatment,' or something like that."

"Yeah," the CA-1 says, "I'm going for the standard stuff when the blood pressure goes down. Neo, fluids. But she was right to take a minute or two and make sure we did the diagnostic checklist thing, the ABC, to make sure we did the right thing."

"Everyone was throwing their ideas out, you yourself laid out the three things in the 'C' part of ABC," the instructor says. "That way everyone is thinking about it." Turning now, the instructor asks the CA-3, "How did you peg the A-fib? I'll tell you, at a heart rate of 130, it's damned hard to make out P waves."

Shaking her head, she says, "Gotta go low tech. This is a trick I learned from an ancient practitioner of the art. 'Close your eyes,' this geezer said, 'then you can pick up the irregularly irregular sound of the heartbeat. Then feel the pulse, and you'll feel that strong-strong-weak-weak-strong-faint pulse that tells you it's A fib.' The low tech way is quicker than the high tech way, believe it or not."

"How about the sedation question," the CA-1 asks. "Anytime I've done this, in the unit or something, they're either so stable that we can really fuzz them out good with propofol, or they're so unstable they're damned near moribund and we don't have to give them anything."

"Versed is your best bet," the CA-3 says, "not that any drug is completely, absolutely guaranteed to keep you hemodynamically stable, but this is pretty safe. Just give a little to smear out their memory. If they do remember something, well, better bad memories than none, as they say."

"Two good moves on the paddles, too," the instructor says, "not that I want you to get swell heads or anything. It was good you waved off the PACU nurse and had the junior resident set the buttons. We tend to not *do* the buttons ourselves enough, and you really need to push the buttons, check the connections, and carry out all the maneuvers yourself."

"I see and I forget, I do and I remember," the CA-1 says.

"Who said that?" the CA-2 asks.

"I just did!"

"No, who, you know, who said that *before* you?"

"Oh," the CA-1 tumbles to it, "Confucius."

Summary. Anesthesia residents tend to be creatures of habit, going for "the usual things" to treat "the usual problems." Here, hypotension triggers the knee jerk response to give Neo and fluids. But cooler heads prevailed, the team made sure they had a *diagnosis* before they went to *treatment*, and they correctly treated unstable atrial fibrillation with cardioversion.

The scenario demonstrates good teamwork, with a leader steering the ship, taking in information (everyone contributes useful input), delegating jobs, and allowing everyone a voice.

Communication comes across clear, no one panics, and people double-check each other. For example, just before cardioversion the CA-2 notices that the Synch button isn't pushed! In an emergency, it's good that everyone keeps his or her eyes open!

In the previous scenario, the resident got distracted, much like the people in the cockpit of Eastern flight 401 got distracted. We can go back to Eastern flight 401 for another lesson, applicable here.

On the cockpit voice recorder, at one point early in the crisis, the copilot asks, "Do you want me to fly the plane?"

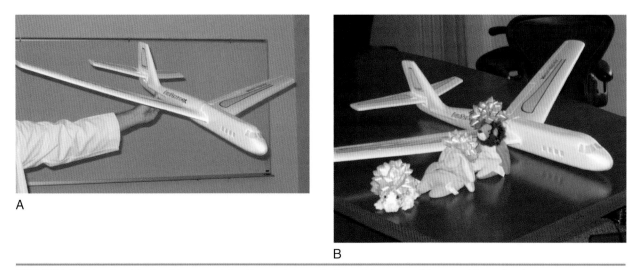

FIGURE 8–41 Good leadership, smooth landing, and these darling triplets can safely unload from the plane.

The pilot does not respond to the question, does not make clear who is flying the plane, and, as was evident, dropped the ball completely.

In this medical scenario, the CA-3 makes clear at the beginning that she is in charge. Then, throughout the case, she demonstrates that she is in charge, displaying all the good qualities of a leader. She doesn't just talk the talk, she walks the walk.

End result of good leadership?

Safe landing.

SCENARIO 14. **Woe is me, isolating a lung in a difficult airway**

"What do you mean, you don't want to put a double lumen tube in?" the surgeon asks, all attitude.

The anesthesia resident is standing in the OR, looking over the preop evaluation. Although simulator mannequins can't *present* the outward appearance of a difficult airway, they do have controls to *make them hard to intubate*. The resident is obeying the prime dictum of Simulation-land and suspending disbelief—*if* the preop evaluation says the patient is hard to intubate, then he approaches the Simulator mannequin as if it will be hard to intubate.

Coupled with the anesthesia resident are a pair of senior medical students. They keep a kind of grim silence as the anesthesia resident talks with Lang.

"Listen," the anesthesia resident says, "this preop says this guy has a receding chin, large teeth, and can't move his neck too well."

"Well," the surgeon says, "I need lung isolation to do this lobectomy, so you gotta put in a double-lumen tube, so put the stupid thing in!"

"Hey," the patient on the OR table shouts, "what's the matter with my teeth? My Mom worked two jobs to keep me in braces, these teeth are fine!"

Oops! The anesthesia resident had forgotten to suspend *all* his disbelief. He and the surgeon were standing next to the patient, and the patient was not yet under anesthesia. No surprise, then, that the patient can hear them talking and doesn't like what he hears!

"Excuse me, Mr. (the anesthesia resident looks at the preop sheet for the patient's name) Kevorkian." Who thinks up these names, the resident wonders? "Dr. Lang and I were just talking about what's best for taking good care of you."

"Shouldn't you have taken care of this earlier?" Kevorkian asks.

God Almighty, the anesthesia resident thinks, this ship hasn't even set sail and I'm already foundering on the rocks.

Dr. Lang and the anesthesia resident withdraw to the hall.

"Listen, professor," the chest surgeon Lang says, "I need a double-lumen for this case because I need that lung down, so find a way, OK."

"Well, you need the lung down, but you don't need a double-lumen to do that," the anesthesia resident explains. "There're other options, like a Univent."

"Oh Christ," Lang whines, "just what I need, some pinhead geek with a new toy screwing up my case. Great. Well just make sure I can see my way around in there, got it?" Lang stalks off.

In the OR, the anesthesia resident explains an awake intubation to the patient.

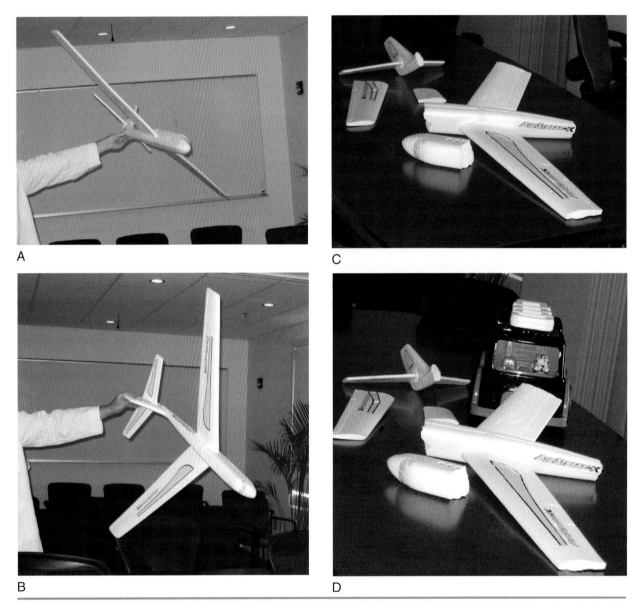

FIGURE 8-42   Bad leadership? Someone will have to come along and pick up the pieces.

"Mr. Kevorkian, uh. . . ." the resident starts.

"It's *Doctor* Kevorkian," the patient corrects.

Too much, the resident thinks.

"Relax," Kevorkian says, "I'm a PhD doctor, a professor of Runic Script at the Icelandic Institute. Not the assisted suicide doctor guy."

The resident shakes it off and goes through the explanation, "Mr . . . uh . . . Dr. Kevorkian, before you go to sleep, we have to do one sort of special procedure. We're going to numb up your mouth and upper throat."

"We, do you mean, you?"

"Oh, yeah," the resident says, "yes, I will be numbing up your mouth and upper throat, so that we . . . I can get your breathing tube in just right. I don't want you to go to sleep first because the shape of your mouth and neck are such that I might have a hard time putting the tube in."

"So you're doing an awake intubation on me because I'm a possible difficult airway, is that it?" Kevorkian offers.

How does a Professor of Runic Script at the Icelandic Institute come off sounding like a board-certified anesthesiologist? Before the anesthesia resident

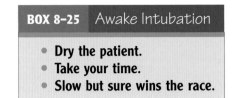

BOX 8-25 Awake Intubation

- **Dry the patient.**
- **Take your time.**
- **Slow but sure wins the race.**

can formulate the question, Kevorkian pre-empts him.

"Did my homework on the Internet," Kevorkian explains. "The University of Manchester has a website for people about to 'go under,' and I dug around a little."

Whoa, what a world we live in, the resident thinks.

The resident gives glycopyrrolate and midazolam through the drug recognition system. Kevorkian's heart rate increases slightly in response to the gly-copyrrolate, and the blood pressure drops slightly with the midazolam. The anesthesia resident can't spray the upper airway (the mannequin would be too hard to clean) but goes through the motions of setting up an atomizer, showing how he would anesthetize the upper airway, then doing a transcricothyroid mem-brane stick to demonstrate the transtracheal airway block.

The resident explains what he's doing at each point. In a little variant-from-reality, the resident has each of the med students set up the atomizer and also has them do the transcricothyroid stick themselves.

"We wouldn't stick the patient three times, obvi-ously," the resident explains. "But we don't want you guys just being spectators here."

As he places the Ovassapian airway and the Univent tube, the patient makes a few protests that come out in slurred speech.

"That's a good endpoint, slurred speech," the anes-thesia resident says. "Once their speech is slurred, they're usually amnestic."

"Do you have a paper that explains that?" one med student asks.

"Don't be a smart ass," the resident cuts him off. "Someone told me that once and I've passed it along as Gospel truth ever since."

"Oh."

"Take your time topicalizing the upper airway, it's the best investment you'll ever make," the anesthesia resident says. "You spend half an hour topicalizing, you'll spend 3 minutes intubating. You spend 3 minutes topicalizing, you'll spend 2 hours *trying* to intubate, and you won't even do it. Plus, in the mean-time, you'll grind the airway to hamburger, drive the

patient's vital signs into Heart Attackville, and piss off a surgeon who is already crawling up our GI tracts, caudal end first."

Before the med student can formulate the question, the resident says, "And that stuff really *is* the Gospel truth. It should be chiseled in granite above the doorway to every anesthesia office on planet Earth."

A size 8 Univent tube is in the Ovassapian airway.

"These are great," the anesthesia resident says, "but they're kind of clunky. An 8 is more like a regular endotracheal tube size 10, so they're a little tough to place in the awake patient, but you can do it. Can't do that with a double-lumen very easily. I've seen people do it, but the double-lumen's so big, it's a real monster."

The med students' eyes raise.

A fiberoptic tower is in the room, so everyone can watch along as the fiberoptic snakes down toward the vocal cords. The medical students get lost a few times.

"In the real world," the resident says, "I wouldn't let you take this long, but go for it."

Eventually, the tube snakes in, each student getting to do it.

"Now, here's the cool part," the anesthesia resident explains, "placing the blocker."

To make his point, the anesthesia resident has a CXR up on the view box and has a second Univent tube out to demonstrate.

"See, we're at 22 at the teeth, so we're above the carina." He shows on the fiberoptic how they can see the carina, then shows on the CXR how the tube is above the carina. "Now, we advance the bronchial blocker" (he does so in the mannequin as well as on the CXR), get it into the right place, and inflate it, making sure we see the balloon just past the carina, not herni-ating back over the carina—that's too shallow, and not so far down we can't see it—that's too high."

Both med students look at the CXR demonstration and the fiberoptic.

"You got this?" the resident asks.

They nod.

"Good," the resident says, "then that brain-dead stare you're giving me must just be a preexisting condition."

With considerable oomph and lots of pillows, the mannequin is put part way on his side. (The connect-ing cables and hydraulics make it pretty hard to place the mannequin in true lateral position.) Drapes go up, and the charming Dr. Lang enters the room.

"That lung better be down when I want it down," Lang bellows. "I can't do this &#@*! operation with the lungs in my way."

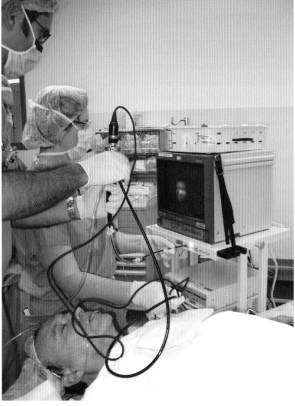

A

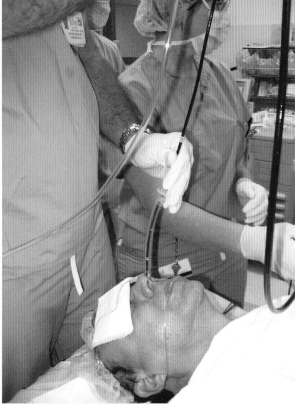

B

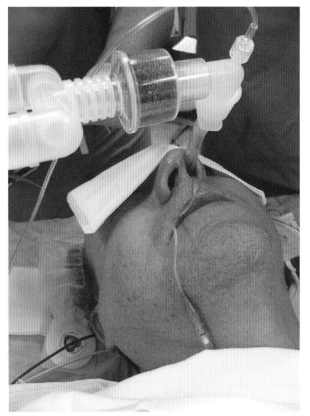

C

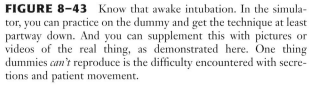

FIGURE 8–43 Know that awake intubation. In the simulator, you can practice on the dummy and get the technique at least partway down. And you can supplement this with pictures or videos of the real thing, as demonstrated here. One thing dummies *can't* reproduce is the difficulty encountered with secretions and patient movement.

Pulling the medical students into a little anesthesia-area cabal, the resident says, "Now here's the cool part. Here's how you get those lungs down."

Holding up the extra Univent tube, the resident points to the tiny hole in the center of the bronchial blocker, "It's pretty hard to empty out the lungs through this little hole. So what we do is this. Watch along on the fiberoptic."

First, the resident deflates the bronchial blocker but keeps it in the right place; second, he disconnects the entire breathing circuit, letting both lungs deflate. As soon as the sat starts to dip to 97%, he reinflates the bronchial blocker, makes sure it's still in the right place, then reconnects the circuit, and turns the ventilator back on.

"See? Now that lung with the blocker is completely emptied, and we're inflating the other lung regularly. The surgeon gets a deflated lung, and everyone's happy."

The saturation stays steady as the procedure starts.

"How's the lang, Dr. Lung?" the anesthesia resident asks. "I mean, how's the lung, Dr. Lang?"

Oh the med students find that rich. They're all over that one.

"What do you know?" Dr. Lang says, "Even a blind pig gets an acorn every now and then. Go ahead, pat yourself on the back, just don't break your arm doing it."

Clinical lessons learned from scenario 14

Lung isolation is a prime pain in the neck. And it's not just a question of putting the right tube in the right place. A lot of our suffering issues from our chest surgery colleagues. Dealing with them is half the battle, as the debriefing shows.

Debriefing. "Let's do this one with a list, how does that sound?" the instructor offers.

The medical students are pulling lunch out of brown paper bags. Lang and the anesthesia resident are looking over a carry-out menu from a nearby Chinese restaurant.

"Put that crap away, eat your bologna sandwich tomorrow, we're springing today," Lang says, a gruff

carryover from the OR. "Better yet, throw those bologna sandwiches away, and eat the leftovers from today tomorrow, if that sentence makes any sense. This place puts enough MSG and salt into their stuff, it'll keep for a hundred years."

"What do you want", the anesthesia resident asks.

Both students shrug, one says "Whatever, it's pretty much all the same anyways."

Lang sits back with a big smile, "Man, there *is* hope for a better tomorrow, someone around here finally said something that makes sense!"

They order Sweet and Sour Something, Something Lo Mein, and Honey Something, with a bunch of egg rolls and lots of packages of that orange stuff.

"To the list!" the instructor insists.

After a few minutes, they come up with:

Medical	Sociologic
Difficult airway	Demanding surgeon
Lung isolation	Awake intubation explanation
Lateral position	Educated patient

"That's right", the instructor says, "there's more for us to learn here than just placing a Univent or a double-lumen tube. There's a lot going on, and you have to pay attention to all of it. Medicine doesn't happen in a vacuum. It's more like a play, and you have to know all the dramatis personae in the play."

"What's . . . ?" the anesthesia resident starts to ask.

"Dramatis personae," Dr. Lang enunciates like a Stratford-on-Avon tour guide, "the list of all the people in a play. You will see the Dramatis Personae listed at the top of each of Shakespeare's plays, from his universally appealing Hamlet, all the way to the all-too-forgettable Timon of Athens."

Everyone's jaw falls into their eggrolls.

"Thus we have dispelled the chest-surgeon-as-dumb-lug myth forevermore," Lang says, triumph in his voice, and soy sauce on his breath.

The instructor gathers himself, then goes down the list:

"Difficult airway—talk to me," the instructor asks the anesthesia resident.

"The be-all and end-all of our existence," the resident explains. "Lose the airway, and forget everything else, because we're not facultative anaerobes. Cardiac considerations, yes, important, but without the airway, guess what, you get every cardiac problem you could ever want, and more!"

"And lung isolation?" the instructor continues.

"There're options for lung isolation," one of the medical students jumps in. Someone has been doing some reading! "There's the double-lumen tube, the

---

BOX 8-26 Lung Isolation

- **Double lumen**
- **Univent**
- **Arndt blocker**

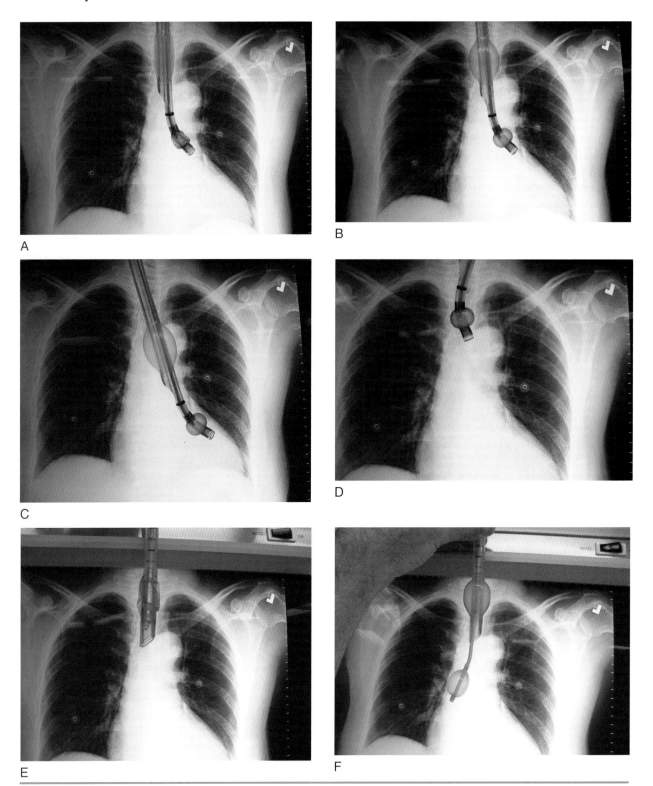

FIGURE 8–44   **A, B.** DLT correctly placed. **C.** Too far in on the left. **D.** Too high up. **E.** Univent in trachea. **F.** Correctly placed on the right.

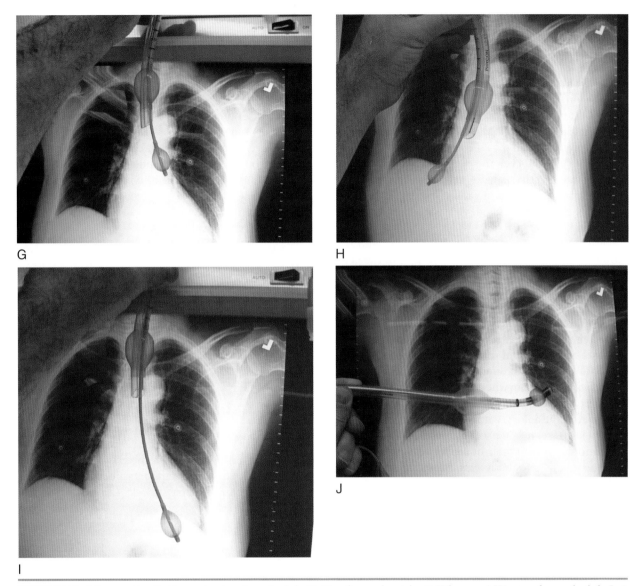

FIGURE 8–44   cont'd   **G.** Correctly placed on the left. **H.** Too far on the right. **I.** Whooeeey! Way too far on the left. **J.** A great, widespread, and easily snagged "simulator" is the chest X-ray. Lay the various lung isolation devices right against the CXR to see where the tube should go. Place the tubes too far in or too high up, then imagine what you would "see" if it were in such a place. Try to avoid placing the double-lumen tube through the side of the chest, as in the last picture.

Univent, which has a kind of built-in bronchial blocker, and a separate bronchial blocker."

"Any other options?" the Shakespearean expert Lang asks.

"You can push a regular endotracheal tube down a mainstem, I guess," the med student guesses, hitting the bulls-eye.

"Right you are," Lang says. "And, truth to tell, a surgeon, in spite of everything I said, can actually do a lobectomy without lung isolation, no matter how much we may scream and shout. A lung, after all, can get squished out of the way with a retractor. It's not like the lung has the consistency of granite."

That steers the group into the sociologic end of the discussion, "How do you deal with the difficult surgeon?" the instructor asks.

Taking the lead, the anesthesia resident says, "One of the core clinical competencies we're trying to learn is 'professionalism,' and that involves dealing with your colleagues. About the best definition I've heard for this is, 'Just talk to the surgeons like they really are your colleagues. No bending and scraping, no kow-towing. At the same time, no bluffing, no huffing, and no being a jerk yourself.'"

Lang, more approachable now with his veneer of Shakespeare, adds, "I'll push and push, but remember, I do want my patient to do well. They came to see *me*, after all. In all the pushing and shoving that goes on in the OR, remember that. This patient came to *me* to get their cancer taken out, to get their diagnosis, to get their heart fixed.

"And a surgeon, even the biggest jerk in the world, is still focused on that patient, that man or woman who walked into their office, a drawn look on their face, and an X-ray in their hand. And some bad news on their mind.

"And I've gotta take care of that patient, and if I have to push you a little, well, it's a mistake of the head and not the heart."

"How about the patient? The educated patient?" the instructor asks.

"How did the patient know all that stuff?" the second medical student asks.

"It's a new world out there," the anesthesia resident says. "Google is God, and anyone with a mouse can click their way to anywhere. An educated fellow like this patient probably got half-way to Board Certification in Anesthesiology with a few days of surfing the Web. This is a consumer society, people want to know what's going on with their bodies. They watch Oprah, they see about anesthetic catastrophes. They know, and you have to be able to explain stuff to all different levels.

"You take him through the reasoning behind the awake intubation, you explain in clear, layman's terms, and there you have it. That's part of professionalism too."

"Good enough for me," Lang says. "Now give me one of those fortune cookies."

Breaking it open, Lang reads, "Next time, insist on a double-lumen."

"What?" everyone says, coming around the table to look over his shoulder.

Summary. Lung isolation requires correct placement of either a double-lumen, a Univent, or a bronchial blocker. Expertise with the fiberoptic is the sina qua non of tube placement and lung isolation. Delicacy with the sometimes prickly chest surgeons takes just as much expertise.

Patients also require good interpersonal skills. They aren't just inanimate receptacles of our dispensed wisdom. They are sometimes professional, sometimes uneducated; sometimes interested in hearing every detail, sometimes preferring to hear less. They are butchers, bakers, candlestick makers of every stripe and leaning. And if they come into our purview, they are almost always scared, vulnerable, and hoping to get through this surgical ordeal alive intact.

They deserve our best.

SCENARIO 15. **Blinded by the light, porphyria**
"He has what?" the first anesthesia resident asks.

"It says he has porphyria," the second anesthesia resident says. Both residents are standing in the OR, looking over the preop, about to induce the patient. All the monitors are on and the overhead speaker booms, "Dr. Flores will be down in a few minutes, he says it's OK to get going."

The case scheduled is a takedown of a colostomy. Other details from the chart—the patient had a gunshot wound to the abdomen during a robbery and has had several abdominal procedures. Handcuffs on the ankles of the patient indicate that he may have been *doing* the robbing when the mishap occurred.

While the first resident continues to scour the chart, the second just has to ask, "How did you get shot, Mr. Severn?"

"Bank transaction gone awry," the patient says.

"Oh."

"Let's preoxygenate, no harm in that", the first resident says. "But we better get it straight with this porphyria business."

Pulling out his Palm Pilot, the second resident punches in "Porphyria."

"OK, here it is," the second resident says, "avoid things that would induce the cytochrome P-450 system, which includes the induction agents and benzodiazepines. And other stuff like Dilantin and things."

BOX 8-27	Routine Patient
• **No such thing**	
• **Each patient unique**	
• **Each patient deserves our best**	

BOX 8-28	Porphyria
• **Heme precursor buildup**	
• **P-450 inducers bad**	
• **Multisystem effects**	

"How do we induce then?" the first resident asks.

"Says here, the classic way is to breathe them down."

"Breathe down an adult?"

"That's what it says," the second resident confirms. "We can give some narcotics, though, that's safe at least."

All the vital signs are OK, and they give some narcotics through the IV drug recognition system, turn on the sevoflurane, and start to breathe the patient down.

"How much narc did you give?" the first resident asks.

"Two cc's, that's fentanyl, right?" the second resident asks, then picked it up. The syringe reads sufentanil, $50\,\mu g/cc$.

Two cc's of undiluted sufentanil.

"The heart rate drops from the 70s to the 20s, and the first resident, holding the mask, says, "He's getting hard to ventilate."

"Syringe swap," the second resident says, "I didn't look at them close enough, he got too much narcotic."

On the monitors, huge gaps between QRS complexes—they seem a mile long. The saturation starts to drop.

"I can't move any air," the first resident says, squeezing the bag for all he's worth.

"Relax him! Relax him! I'm never getting any air in this guy. Give him some Sux!" the first resident's shouting now, the bag is making squeeking, flatulent noises as he tries to move air.

The second resident grabs a syringe of Sux and pushes it.

"Porphyria's not a contraindication to Sux, is it?" the second resident asks as he looks down at the now-empty syringe.

"No . . . but . . ." the first resident says, something clearly on his mind. "He was a gunshot wound, right?"

"Right."

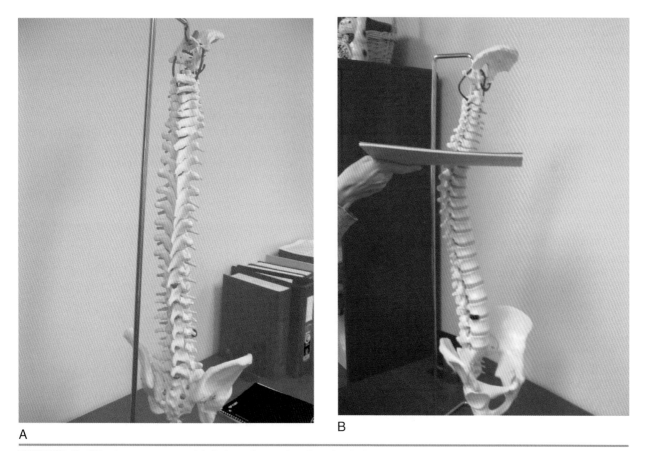

A

B

FIGURE 8–45 **A.** Anatomic models help with spinal and epidural placement. Navigating through those bones can be tricky. Using the model, you can see where the needle might hit bone and how best to redirect. **B.** Demonstrating a spinal cord injury. Autonomic hyperreflexia occurs when the signals from below cannot get up top, setting up a reflex arc. Below the lesion, all is vasoconstriction; above, all is vasodilation. Normal "righting mechanisms" can't function properly.

"And he had a lot of gut procedures, right?" the first resident asks.

"Right."

"And he was already laying on the bed when we came in here, right?" the first resident asks.

"Right."

"Did he move himself over?" the first resident asks.

From across the room, the circulator says, "No, we moved him over, he's a T4 paraplegic from the gunshot wound."

Both residents look up at the EKG as the complex develops peaked T-waves, widened QRS complexes, and degenerates into ventricular fibrillation.

"Calcium! Calcium! Get the paddles, God damn it, his potassium must be . . . !"

The door opens, "Don't bother with the calcium, Simulation's over."

Clinical lessons learned from scenario 15

Debriefing. The center of the debriefing table holds an open book—the Bible.

Resident 1 and resident 2 plunk themselves down in their seats, ticked off.

"Didn't you see the spinal cord thing?" the first one asks.

"What, who plucked your eyes out that you couldn't see it?" the second one snaps back.

The instructor flows into the room, hands facing palm down, at chest height.

Pushing his hands down in a placating motion, the instructor says, "Gentlemen, gentlemen, we are in the presence of Holy Writ, I would advise against rendering judgment against your fellow man. 'Judge not, lest ye be judged.'"

"Yeah," the first resident says, "and 'none so blind as those who will not see'!"

"Puh-leeze!" the instructor says, getting between the seething residents, "No holy wars in the Simulation Center!"

"All right," the instructor sits down, "how do you think it went?"

Neither resident talks, and they physically turn away from each other.

"OK, let me rephrase that," the instructor redirects, "what did you do right in there? Let's drop this 'You shoulda, I shoulda' stuff, and do a plus–delta debriefing. OK, the guy coded, you did some stuff wrong, we all know that, but let's be methodical about this."

"And cut yourselves, and each other, some slack," the instructor says. "Let me see here," he leafs through the Bible, "what's it say in here, oh yeah, 'The quality

| BOX 8–29 | Sux With Spinal Cord Injuries |

- **Increased end-plates in muscles**
- **Massive potassium release**
- **Hyperkalemic arrest**

of mercy is not strained, it droppeth as the gentle rain from heaven.' Think about that."

"That's not from the Bible," the second resident says, "that's from Shakespeare, *The Merchant of Venice*, when they're appealing to Shylock to not collect his pound of flesh."

Closing the Bible, the instructor says, "Well it *should* be in the Bible. Maybe it'll be in the second edition."

They lay out the plus side of the plus–delta debriefing.

<u>Plus</u>

1. Preoxygenated.
2. Noted the patient's somewhat rare condition, porphyria.
3. Paused to look up its major implication—avoiding certain drugs.
4. Breathed the patient down.
5. Diagnosed chest wall rigidity from the narcotic.
6. Diagnosing hyperkalemic arrest and moving toward treatment of same—calcium as the first step.

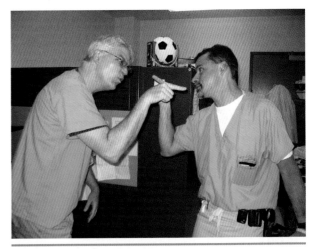

FIGURE 8–46 Once again, the fingers come out and the blame starts flying. Keep in mind, when you point *one* finger at another person, *three* are pointing right back at yourself.

Then they laid out the things they would change, the delta part of the debriefing.

Delta

1. Forgot to read the preop carefully.
2. Got blinded by the light—freaking out about porphyria and forgetting to check *all* the stuff on the history.
3. Syringe swap, forgetting to check the labels carefully and giving a very high dose of sufentanil.
4. High dose of sufentanil caused chest wall rigidity plus bradycardia.
5. Panicking and giving Sux, which led to hyperkalemic arrest.

"There's one last thing I'd put in that delta part," the instructor says. "You both were awfully quick to point the finger at the other guy. It takes two to tango when you were inducing this patient. You *both* had a chance to look at the preop, and you both had a chance to see about the T4 lesion."

"Another thing," the first resident admits, "I should have thought to ask the question. Any gunshot wound that does gut damage, even if it doesn't hit the spinal cord, can throw out a shock wave that can damage the spinal cord, so I should have at least considered that possibility."

"Here I stand, hat in hand." the second resident says, newly minted humility in his voice. "I was all going crazy about the whole cool porphyria, breathe-down-an-adult-for-the-first-time-thing, and I blanked on all the other stuff."

"Don't forget," the instructor intones, "at the heart of a *weird* case, is a *regular* case. You still have to do all the basic stuff—read the preop thoroughly, pay attention to labels, pay attention to the ABC." Tapping the Bible, "Don't be blinded by the burning bush and fall off the mountain. You still need to look where you're going, even when you're Moses and you're on a mission from God."

"Amen," the residents say, as one.

Summary. Success has many parents, but failure is always an orphan. These residents demonstrate the all-too-human failing of pointing a finger when something goes wrong. Better to keep that pointing finger stowed away.

Medically, this case points out several things.

Porphyria—the preferred method of induction is inhalation.

Read the labels! That much sufentanil causes chest wall rigidity and big time bradycardia.

Read the preop. You can miss big stuff, especially if you're all freaked out about an unexpected finding. Missing a spinal cord injury (which, yes, can happen), can lead to Sux, hyperkalemia, and an arrest.

When that happens, grab your Bible and start praying.

SCENARIO 16. **Rigid bronchoscopy can be a drag**
"OK," the instructor says, "time to hold hands again with Dr. Lang, your favorite surgeon."

The two anesthesia residents nod. Word's gotten out that Lang is the "killer surgeon" in the Simulation Center.

"Have to learn to deal with Lang here," the first anesthesia resident says. "There's sure to be 'Langs' out there once we're done with residency."

They look over the preop evaluation.

Patient is a 70-year-old man, drinker, smoker.

Scheduled procedure, rigid bronchoscopy, esophagoscopy, as part of a metastatic workup for laryngeal CA.

The anesthesia residents go into the Simulation OR, the patient is monitored, preoxygenating, and ready to go. Both residents go over the system, it looks good, and they induce. Lang tells them not to intubate, to induce anesthesia, give paralysis, and hand the airway over to him so he could place the rigid bronchoscope into the trachea for his examination.

"How long you going to be?" the first anesthesia resident asks Lang.

"Long as it takes," Lang says.

"Well, I'm just asking so I can dose my relaxant . . ." the resident goes on. If Lang is going to take a long time, the anesthesia resident might dose with vecuronium; if he's going to be quicker than quick, the resident may go with shorter-acting cisatracurium.

"Hey," Lang snaps, "as long as it takes, now get out of my way."

BOX 8-31 Chart

- **Read it**
- **Read it**
- **Read it**

BOX 8-30 Blinded By Weird Diseases

- **Step back**
- **Look at the entire patient**
- **Don't forget the basics**

Looking at each other, the anesthesia residents give the "Well, what do you expect from Lang?" look.

The saturation is 100%; the residents have 100% oxygen going and are anesthetizing with sevoflurane. The blood pressure and heart rate are normal.

Lang attempts to place the rigid bronchoscope and has a tough time getting it through the vocal cords.

"Can I help?" the first anesthesia resident asks, then tries to position the head a little more favorably.

"I've got it!" Lang says, "If I need a hand, I'll ask for it."

The saturation drops to 95%; still, the bronchoscope is not placed correctly.

"Um . . ." the second anesthesia resident says, "let us ventilate him for a second."

"Like hell!" Lang shouts, "I've got it."

The bronchoscope goes in, and the first anesthesia resident hooks up the circuit. He attempts to hand-

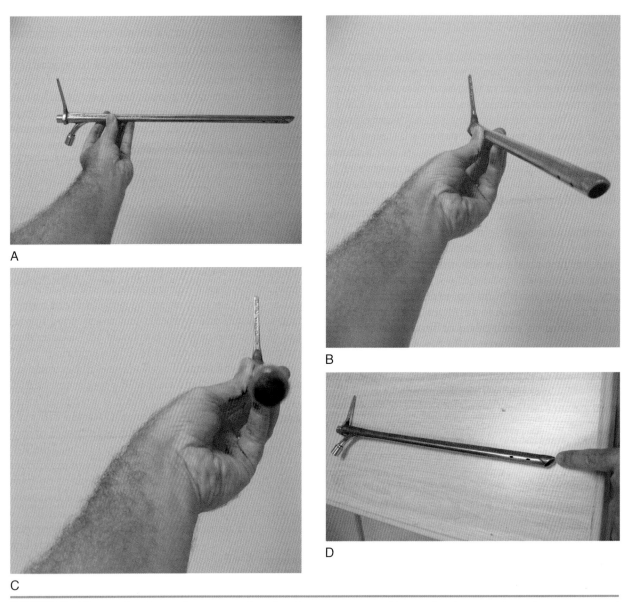

A

B

C

D

FIGURE 8–48   You don't have to be a surgeon, but when the surgeons are working on that airway you better have a pretty good idea of what they're using and how they use it. Here's a rigid bronchoscope—the "mother of all straight blades." This may save you if the patient has such enormous chunks of stuff in their trachea that you can't ventilate, even with the patient intubated. In goes the rigid scope, they pull out the chunks (*ick*, this is go gross), and the patient lives to fight another day.

ventilate. Inspiratory pressures go way up, no CO_2 appears on the end-tidal monitor. The pulse oximeter says 90% and proceeds downward.

"You're not in, you're not in," the second anesthesia resident says. "We can't ventilate!"

"I am too in, God damn it," Lang says, "here, look." He places the laryngoscope and lifts. Sure enough, the bronchoscope is, indeed, between the vocal cords.

"But . . ." the first anesthesia resident still can't move any air.

"It's in the right place, I'm telling you, it's in the right place, so shut up!" Lang says.

Saturation 80%.

"Oh," Lang says, then adjusts a switch in the bronchoscope. He had something turned the wrong way, not allowing ingress of oxygen into the lungs. "Try it now."

The anesthesia residents, nearly apoplectic by now, squeeze the bag like there is no tomorrow.

Saturation 75%, then it turns around, saturation 80%, 85%, 90%, and goes on up. Chest rise, end-tidal CO_2 appears, all's well.

Lang proceeds with the bronchoscope as if nothing happened.

"Done," the instructor says.

Clinical lessons learned from scenario 16

Debriefing. "Let's go back to the world of aviation before we look at our own scenario," the instructor says.

He passes out a handout, a 1995 article by Major Tony Kern of the United States Air Force, "Darker shades of blue: a case study of failed leadership."

On June 24, 1994, a B-52 takes off from a Washington state airbase to practice aerial maneuvers for an upcoming airshow. At only 250 feet above the ground, the enormous B-52 executes a tight turn, stalls, hits a power line, and crashes, killing its crew of four.

Tragic accident? Or a predictable inevitability?

Close review of one of the pilot's records reveals a systematic pattern of reckless flying. The pilot is a real "cowboy," ignoring warnings from fellow crew members after repeated close calls.

May 19, 1991: The pilot flies directly over an air show crowd, in violation of Federal Aviation Regulations.

July 12, 1991: The pilot flies too low during a ceremonial flight and executes banked turns that are too steep.

May 17, 1992: At another air show he again exceeds safety regulations, climbing too steeply and turning too sharply.

Comments from fellow flyers reveal concern, "I was amazed that they (the senior staff) let him keep doing that."

"[The pilot] broke the regulations or exceeded the limits . . . virtually every time he flew."

"I'm not going to fly with him, I think he's dangerous. He's going to kill somebody some day and it's not going to be me."

"And they let him keep going until he crashed, killing himself, three other people on board, and, just through luck, no one on the ground," the instructor says.

"Just like Lang" the second anesthesia resident says.

Lang, sitting at the table, says nothing.

"Well," the instructor says, "you tell me. Is it just like Lang?"

Lang raises his hand, palm outward, and looks down. He's handing carte blanche to the anesthesia residents.

"Well," the first anesthesia resident says, holding up the U.S. Air Force article, "you have a cowboy flying a B-52, and he 'pushes the envelope' right in front of entire air shows full of people, and all the other Air Force guys know he's out of control, and nobody does anything. Then he crashes.

"And here we have a guy who blow off our concerns, not trivial concerns, I mean, I can't move any air on the patient and everyone can hear that saturation going down. It's not like we're the only ones that know what that low-toned *boop—boop—boop* means. And Dr. Lang just doesn't get it."

The second anesthesia resident picks it up, "So let's say Dr. Lang is an attending, and here I am, lowly resident, and I'm freaking but my attending isn't in the room, so now what?"

"You tell me," Lang says. "Is it my bailiwick now? Since surgery started, and we've got surgery of the airway going, does that mean I'm in the driver's seat? You? Me because I 'rank' you? You because you 'rank' me in matters of airway concerns? What?"

Everyone at the table looks at everyone. No one says anything.

"OK," the instructor says, "impasse. Here's a rule to help you out. It's called the 'two-challenge' rule. It, too, comes from aviation experience.

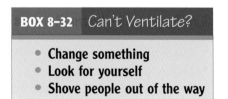

BOX 8-32 Can't Ventilate?

- **Change something**
- **Look for yourself**
- **Shove people out of the way**

"When danger is present, as it was here, then to protect the patient you challenge once," the instructor says.

"So," the second anesthesia resident says, "I say, 'We have an airway problem and I need to take over the airway', something like that?"

"Right," the instructor says, "then, if the culprit, if the source of danger doesn't respond, you challenge a second time."

The first anesthesia resident chimes in, "Dr. Lang, I am not kidding, we have a serious problem here, low sat and insufficient ventilation, something is wrong with this airway setup."

"Right," Lang says, "then, after the second challenge, you have the right, no, you have the obligation, to push me out of the way, pull out that bronchoscope, and intubate the patient."

Both anesthesia residents try to picture that actually happening.

"No," the instructor says, "this is it. This is the real thing, the 'two-challenge rule.' You cannot sit by when someone is doing something fatal. No matter what, you have to step in."

"That didn't happen in the Air Force with that cowboy pilot," Lang says. "Everyone commented on him, everyone talked about him, everyone judged him from the side. But no one in that cockpit challenged him when he was pushing the limits. And they paid for it."

"Don't let your patient pay for it," the instructor says.

"One more thing," the first anesthesia resident says, "should we know how to fix that bronchoscope? I mean, does that fall into our territory?"

"Yes and no," the instructor says. "I'd say the main thing is to know 'something's wrong, change something.' You don't want to just sit there, reinforcing failure, if you can't ventilate the patient. And the ultimate change is to pull the stupid thing out!"

Summary. Sharing the airway with the surgeons is enough to tighten any anesthesiologist's sphincter. You're right there, sort of, with control of the airway, sort of, but there's this surgeon there! And he or she may be managing the airway OK - or maybe not. Plus, the surgeon is focused on the *surgical* aspect of the airway (the lesion to excise or biopsy), and they're never quite as focused on the *air* part of the airway.

And therein lies the stress.

Lost ventilation means you have to strike quickly and decisively. In this case, a maladjusted bronchoscope didn't allow ventilation. Add to that the personality conflict of a surgeon who won't admit he's wrong and get out of the way, and you have a real dilemma.

Enter the "two-challenge rule." When danger strikes, give the "obstacle" two chances, then shove him or her out of the way and do what you have to do!

Good advice when flying a B-52, and good advice when flying an anesthesia machine.

SCENARIO 17. **Swan dive into the chest**

"Well," the instructor says, "you tell *me* what we should do."

A patient is on the table, intubated, a Swan-Ganz catheter in his right neck, all other monitors on including an arterial line.

On the view box is a chest X-ray. The entire right side of the chest is completely whited out, and the Swan-Ganz catheter is not in the heart. It's sort of looping around in the middle of the lung fields.

Inspiratory pressures are high, reaching $40\,cm$ of H_2O; and the saturation is 90% on 100% oxygen and $5\,cm$ of PEEP.

Both anesthesia residents look over the preop— the most important points are cardiac, vascular, and pulmonary.

> Cardiac: S/P CABG, now without symptoms and has a good EF on echo
> Vascular: $9\,cm$ aortic aneurysm, extending above the renal arteries
> Pulmonary: more than a pack-century of smoking, baseline ABGs show CO_2 retention and hypoxemia

On the monitor, the arterial line is fine, but the PA catheter doesn't show anything recognizable.

"Who put the Swan in?" the first anesthesia resident asks. "Can you aspirate on this thing?" She pulls on the distal port of the catheter, gets nothing, then pulls on the side port of the cordis, gets nothing. An IV bag is running in the side port.

The first anesthesia resident reaches up and shuts off the IV. "This thing isn't intravascular, it's going into the chest. That's normal saline in the right chest. We need a chest tube."

BOX 8-33 *Two-Challenge Rule*

- **Challenge**
- **Challenge again**
- **Punch his lights out and take over**

BOX 8-34 Central Line Placement

- Force it? Hmmm.
- Can't draw back? Hmmm.
- Get a CXR.

Nodding, the second anesthesia resident says, "Yeah, that's it. That thing . . . how did it go when it went in?" He looks around for the chart. Another anesthesiologist placed the line. That note says, "Wire required some force to place, negative aspiration once in, possibly kinked, floated Swan to wedge at 50."

"Wire required some force?" the second anesthesia resident says. "I thought that thing's supposed to slide in there like greased lightning. Not supposed to force it."

"Chest tube!" the first anesthesia resident says to no one in particular, then thinks better of it and says to the circulating nurse. "Excuse me, uh, what's your name?"

"Naomi."

"Naomi, yes, thanks. Naomi, could you please call the cardiothoracic surgeons and ask them to come here as soon as possible?" the first anesthesia resident asks. "We need a chest tube - and sooner rather than later."

"Got it," Naomi says.

From the overhead speakers, "Chest tube placed."

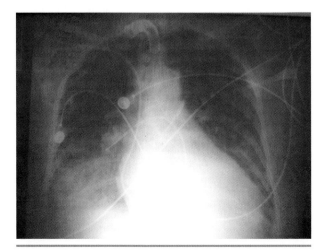

FIGURE 8–49 Something not as it should be? Get a chest X-ray. In this one, a central line is going straight into the chest, not even close to any vessel (don't ask). Chest X-rays are the "great revealers," showing us the lungs we dropped, the vessels we nicked, the tubes we misplaced. A lot of red faces and crumpled egos come from viewing a lot of chest X-rays.

The inspiratory pressures immediately drop, and the saturation rises to 96%.

"OK," the second anesthesia resident says, "now what? Do we go ahead or wake him up?"

Dr. Lang walks in the room. "I hear there's been a mishap?"

"Yes," the first anesthesia resident takes the helm. "During placement of a Swan-Ganz catheter, the line got into the pleural space and a liter of IV fluid entered the patient's right hemithorax. A chest tube has been placed, the fluid drained, and the patient is now stable. The question is, do we proceed with the operation?"

"What do you have for lines now?" the surgeon, Dr. Lang, asks.

"We'll have to pull this line, of course, then . . ." the second anesthesia resident starts.

"Then you're done, that's what," Lang says. "You're done, and we're not doing this damned case because you guys have gummed up the works. This guy's bad enough off, we don't need to get into this with one hand or, more accurately, one lung tied behind our back. Wake him up."

Unfazed, the first anesthesia resident says, "And if this thing ruptures, Dr. Lang? What's the game plan then?"

"Oh," Lang pauses.

"I mean, this is a hand grenade with the pin pulled, Dr. Lang, I just want to know what we do if all of a sudden he complains of sharp abdominal pain. God forbid, he complains of sharp pain stabbing through to his back up in his chest."

"Oh, OK," Lang says, "guess we do have to have plan B."

The second anesthesia resident turns off the anesthetic vapors and starts the process of waking the patient from anesthesia. Right away, the anesthesia resident draws up and gives 5 mg of labetalol. "I don't want this guy waking up, blowing apart his aneurysm, and forcing the issue."

"How about we stick him from the left subclavian?" Lang says. "I can do it, we do more subclavians than you do. We can float the Swan from there."

The first anesthesia resident looks over the left and right side of the patient's neck.

"No," she says, "no good. That Swan will float right past the rent, right past the hole. We could end up in the same place, the Swan poking through into the chest. This patient is just like a gunshot wound up high. We should go low. We should place a femoral line in this guy."

"Can you float the Swan from there?" the second anesthesia resident asks.

"Sure," the first resident says, "they do that in the cardiology lab all the time. It just looks a little funny on the CXR. It doesn't loop around like when it comes from the top, it just goes straight up and does a little jig to get in the PA."

Behind her, the patient's blood pressure rises to 170/90, and the heart rate climbs to 100. The second anesthesia resident is right on it, giving more labetalol and one squirt of 50 μg of nitroglycerin.

"An ounce of prevention is worth a pound of ruptured aneurysm," the second anesthesia resident quips. "By the by, do we need a Swan for this? How about a cordis in the femoral for volume and drips, and a TEE to monitor stuff up here. If all goes well, then at the end of the case, when all the volume shifts are done, we pull the TEE and just go with CVP?"

"Who's watching this guy in the ICU?" Lang asks. "We should talk to the ICU doc, that person may want the Swan in the unit."

BP 145/85, HR 75; the patient starts to blink.

"I think we're OK to extubate here," the second anesthesia resident says. Then he suctions, deflates the endotracheal tube, and extubates. Right after extubation, the patient makes a retching sound. The second anesthesia resident turns the patient's head to the side, puts the head down, and places a suction catheter in the mouth.

Door opens, instructor's head appears, "It's a wrap!"

Clinical lessons learned from scenario 17

Debriefing. "First things first," the instructor says at the start of the debriefing. "Let's work a little on documentation. What would you say in the chart if you were the one who doinked the Swan into the chest?"

"Wait!" the first anesthesia resident protests, "I didn't doink the Swan into the chest!"

The second anesthesia resident makes his fingers into a halo and holds it over his head, "I didn't do it, I swear. I didn't chop down the cherry tree with my little ax!"

Throwing down a few legal pads, the instructor says, "Enough! I'm deaf to your cries of innocence, write it down *as if* you were the culprit."

Just to set the mood, the instructor plays the theme music to *Perry Mason.* After a few minutes, "All right, all right, you're not writing the next Harry Potter book, let's see what you wrote."

Resident 1—Sterile P & D, R IJ approach, finder needle, Seldinger technique to place cordis for Swan. Some difficulty passing wire. Negative aspiration once line placed. CXR ordered. Fluid found in right chest. Chest tube placed.

Resident 2—Standard technique for placing right internal jugular line done. After placement, right chest found to be whited out. Chest tube placed.

After looking at the notes, the instructor says, pointing to the first resident, "Fine," and pointing to the second resident, "Bit skimpy. Flesh it out a little more. Tell everything that happened." Then the instructor sets down the legal pads, turns off the *Perry Mason* music, and asks, "Who are you writing these notes for?"

Both residents shrug.

"The lawyers?" they both guess.

The instructor moves his splayed out fingers back and forth in a teeter-totter motion. "Not quite. Close, but not quite. You guys familiar with Sun Tzu?"

Stares as blank as a newly opened package of computer paper.

"I'll take that as a 'no,'" the instructor says, deflated. "Sun Tzu was a Chinese philosopher from 3000 years ago or so. He wrote this book *The Art of War,* which is a real classic in military circles. We should have read it before going into Viet Nam. For that matter, we should have read it before going into Iraq. Anyway, Sun Tzu said 'Know your enemy and know yourself and you can fight a hundred battles without disaster.'

"So, you have to know your enemy when you're writing your notes too. And your enemy, believe it or not, is *not* the lawyer. It's the 12 people sitting in the jury box. Those are the enemy when it comes right down to something going to court. You have to know what a jury thinks, what they forgive, and what they don't forgive, when you write your notes."

Nary a flicker of recognition.

"OK, let me try another tack," the instructor says. "Write all your notes as if they are going to be splashed up on a courtroom wall years from now, long after you have forgotten all the details of the case. And picture your note in front of 12 jury members who are deciding your fate. Remember, it's not the *lawyer* who delivers the verdict, it's the *jury,* so you have to think— What are the *jurors* thinking?"

"So what are they thinking?" the first resident asks, "Doctors shouldn't make mistakes?"

"Believe it or not, they forgive mistakes," the instructor explains. "Think about our celebrity culture, the American public forgives anything— drugs, every sexual transgression, crime—but there are a couple things Americans won't forgive.

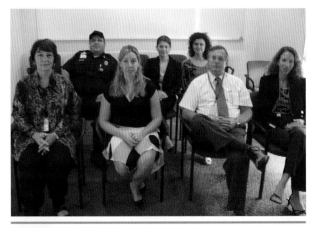

FIGURE 8–50 Every time you write a note ask yourself, "How will a jury view this?"

"Covering up and a cavalier attitude."

"Look at what brought Nixon down, if you can remember your ancient history. He does the Watergate thing—fine. But then he *covered up*. He *hid* it. That, no one forgives. So when you write your notes, you have to make sure you do not cover anything up. Just lay it all out. Say what happened. Don't think you can just jump over some unpleasant fact and hope no one notices. Let me tell you, the malpractice attorney *will* notice and will point it out to the jurors.

"In this note, for example, you have to say what happened—Swan-Ganz introduced into pleural space, one liter of crystalloid infused. That *is* what happened, and you *have to say it*. Don't get me wrong, you don't have to editorialize or draw attention to your screw-up.

"*Stupid me*, I stuck the Swan in the wrong place, *What a moron!*" the instructor says. "No need for that. Just a calm, 'Just the facts ma'am' description."

"And the second thing," the second resident says, "the cavalier attitude?"

"Right," the instructor pauses for a sip of Pellegrino, "right. Look, jurors have us pegged as rich bastard doctors driving drop-top BMWs and never drinking water from the tap, only expensive bottled water from Italy." The instructor slides the bottle of

BOX 8-35 Mistake Occurs?

- **Fix what needs fixing**
- **Document**
- **Follow up**

Pellegrino off the debriefing table and puts it underneath his chair. "So if you come across in your note as uncaring or indifferent, the jurors will kill you.

"'*Those rich sons-of-bitches, just last week I had to wait three hours in the doctor's office, and now this, the doctor hurts the patient and doesn't even care. Let's stick it to him!*'

"You don't need that. Your note should reflect everything you did to correct the mistake or make things better for the patient," the instructor explains. "That is, after all, what you actually *do*. You just have to make sure your note *says* it."

"If you don't write it," the second resident says, "you didn't do it, right?"

"Right."

"So" the first resident says, "let me give it a second shot here." She looks up at the ceiling and scratches her chin a little. "Swan placed in usual fashion, blah, blah, blah, up to the bad part. Then, um, OK, here goes.

"Swan noted to have negative aspiration and abnormal waveform. Fluids infused to this point 1000 cc crystalloid. Inspiratory pressures increased and saturation decreased. CXR ordered. Right, uh, crystalloid-o-thorax noted."

"Try 'fluid noted in right chest consistent with fluid infusion into pleura.'" the second resident says. "That's probably how Sun Tzu would say it."

"Yeah," the first resident agrees. "Immediately discontinued IV infusion, 100% oxygen, supportive care, and chest tube requested *stat*. Once fluid drained, will follow with serial CXRs, chest physiotherapy, and incentive spirometry."

"Any problem with chest physiotherapy in this patient?" the instructor asks.

"Oh yeah," the first resident says, "if they do that pounding on the chest with their cupped hands, I guess they could send a shock wave through his chest and pop his aneurysm.

"That would be not good," she says.

"Good," the instructor says. "That's the idea with the notes. Come across as honest, and come across as caring. Anything else with this case that merits our consideration, rumination, and obfuscation?"

Both residents roll their eyes. This is what comes of giving your attending a Word-a-Day calendar at Christmas.

"I liked how you woke him up," the first resident says. "Don't let him get all sympathetically juiced up as he emerges. Bad for the heart, and bad for the walls of that aneurysm."

The second resident takes a bow.

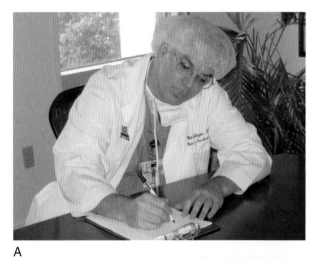

A

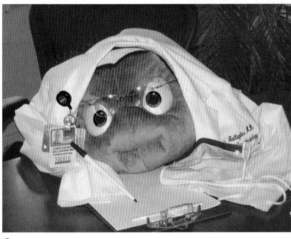

C

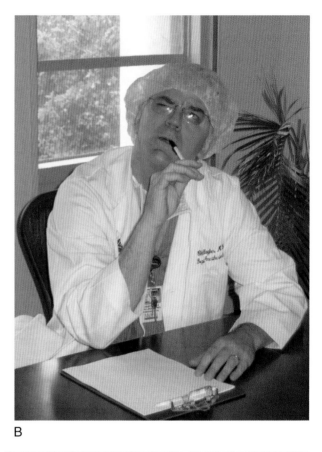

B

FIGURE 8–51 What will they think of me? Will they view me as a bastard, as a heartless doctor? Or will my note convey my inner beauty, my hidden wonderfulness? Will they see me as cute and adorable?

"What do you think about the lines in this case?" the second resident asks. "I mean, the thinking behind going femoral?"

"Well, think about it," the first resident says, "you've just poked a hole in something going into the chest, maybe the superior vena cava, maybe something feeding into it, anyway, it's something big. And the hole may have come from the dilator. That's a pretty big hole. So now if you stick again, you might hit that fresh hole, it might just have a little bitty platelet plug there. You could uncover that plug, push through it again, and end up in the caca again. You don't want that. Just go south, go femoral, you don't want to make the same mistake twice."

"Hard to argue with that," the instructor says. "Now how about a round of Pellegrino, you rich bastard doctors?"

Summary. We always beat the mantra into the residents, "Document, document, document!" but we

rarely look over their notes and give them a good critique. This exercise in the Simulator generated one of the more painful aspects of record keeping—recording a real-live complication in a complete professional manner. That record is your only friend if the complication comes to court, so it's worth making sure you come across in that note as:

Honest
Caring

Central lines have a host of complications, and entry into the pleura is one of them. If you recognize and treat the complication, good for you. Better yet, if you look for signs of trouble—a Swan tracing that looks abnormal, a line from which you can't aspirate—you may prevent trouble before it happens.

And once an area has been "violated" you have to look at all the options for big venous access or monitoring. You may have to avoid the "upper road"

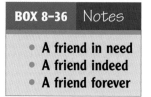

BOX 8-36 Notes

- A friend in need
- A friend indeed
- A friend forever

(because all roads from above lead to the SVC) and opt for the "lower road" (because all lower roads lead to the IVC). And keep in mind that you can get additional monitoring help from the TEE if floating a Swan presents hazards.

SCENARIO 18. **Pulling a fast one, epidural hematoma**

"The surgeon asked if you could see this patient, doctor," the step-down nurse explains. "She went ahead and pulled out your epidural catheter and said you might want to write something else for pain."

"The surgeon pulled the epidural?" the pain fellow asks. "She didn't want us to do it?"

"She said it had been in for 3 days, and it was time to come out," the step-down nurse explains. "She said she was doing you a favor. Could you write for a PCA or something?"

With the pain fellow are two medical students on the pain service.

"Let me take a look at this patient first," the pain fellow says, and they all go in the room.

Laying on the gurney, the patient is groaning. This is a standardized patient, not a mannequin.

"Hey, I'm Dr. Rodriguez," the pain fellow says, "how are you doing?"

"My back hurts," the patient says. "It hurts right back here." She points to her lower back.

"When did that start?" the first medical student asks.

"Since they pulled that thing out of my back, it's getting worse," the patient says.

The second medical student is looking over the chart. The patient has multiple sclerosis, had a hysterectomy 3 days before, and had the epidural placed for postop pain relief. She has a history of DVTs and was placed on low-molecular-weight heparin (enoxaparin 40 mg sub-q). At 10 a.m., she got her last dose of enoxaparin. The epidural was pulled at noon.

"Lift your leg," the pain fellow says. "Can you lift your leg?"

Going through the chart, the second medical student says, "Her neuro exam before was a little spotty. Her leg was a little weak before."

Up comes the leg, but it's weak, and the pain fellow can easily push it down.

"Does your leg feel funny or different?" the pain fellow asks.

"Yeah," the patient says, "it's tingly."

Again, the medical student speaks up, "her sensory exam before was spotty too according to this neurologist's note.

Examining the other leg, the pain fellow comes up with another spotty exam—a little weakness, a little tingling. Turning to the nurse in the room, he says, "Call MRI, we need a study *stat* to look for epidural hematoma."

Just then the surgical resident enters the room. "Hey, what's up?" she asks.

"Can we go out in the hallway a second, doctor?" the pain fellow says.

Out in the hallway, the pain fellow and the two medical students gather round the surgeon. "OK, here's the scoop," the pain fellow starts in, "we've got symptoms and physical signs of a possible epidural hematoma. Now, you pulled the epidural out, let's see, 2 hours after her last dose of low-molecular-weight-heparin, right?"

"But it's not like she's on Coumadin, it's not even regular heparin. It's just, you know, for DVTs," the surgeon explains. "Heparin's gone in 2 hours, right?"

"Well, actually, you're supposed to wait 12 hours after the last dose of low-molecular-weight heparin before you pull an epidural catheter. I mean, that's the recommendation of the Society of Regional Anesthesia."

"Are you sure she has an epidural hematoma?" the surgeon asks, now agitated. "She's got multiple sclerosis, you know. Her exam's always a little off the mark, you know, weak here, tingle there. That's what multiple sclerosis is! Shit, an epidural hematoma. Should we get a neuro consult first? Why don't we do that? This is probably just baseline, we don't have to go off our nut on this."

"No," the pain fellow says. "In case of doubt, get the study. If the study's negative, fine, no harm done. But if we wait, the damage will be permanent."

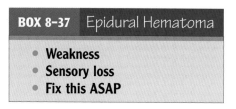

BOX 8-37 Epidural Hematoma

- Weakness
- Sensory loss
- Fix this ASAP

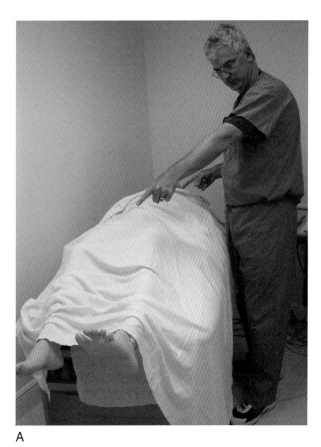

A

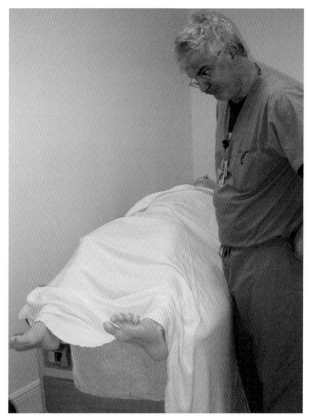

B

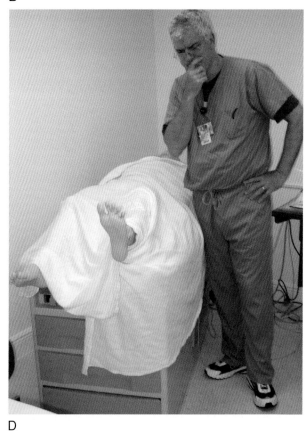

C

D

FIGURE 8–52 Epidural hematoma? Get to that bedside, do the exam yourself, and if there is any doubt get the neurosurgeons involved. This is a five-alarm fire, and time is of the essence. Get the imaging study and get that hematoma evacuated *now*!

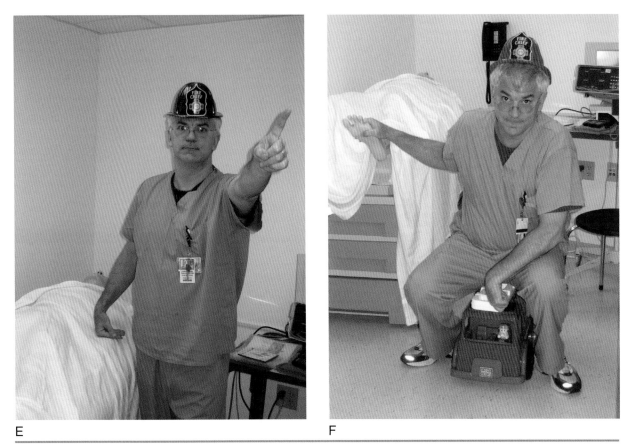

E   F

FIGURE 8–52 cont'd

They return to the room. "Are they ready for us in MRI?" the pain fellow asks. "We have to go right now."

Just as she hangs up the phone, the nurse says, "They're busy down there today, but they say they should be able to do her first thing on Thursday."

"*No!*" the pain fellow yells, "get me that number, we have to go now, now, now. And get neurosurgery on the phone too!"

"Chill!" the surgeon says, "he'll want to see the MRI before he does. . . ."

"No, wrongo," the pain fellow insists, "get neurosurgery in right away. They have to know about this too, they'll be pushing to go, go, go too."

At the patient's bedside, the medical students are examining the patient.

"Um," the first one says, "you might want to see this."

"Lift your leg," the second med student says.

Nothing. The patient can't move either leg at all.

Overhead speaker, "That's it, Simulation's done."

Clinical lessons learned from scenario 18

Debriefing. The surgeon, med students, and pain fellow sit at the debriefing table, a box of powdered sugar donuts in front of them—a *half-filled* box of donuts in front of them. Everyone has powdered sugar around their mouths.

Enter the debriefer and the miraculously cured patient.

"You guys ever get fed at home?" the patient asks.

"Don't reach in there, you'll lose a finger," the instructor warns.

After everyone reaches a comfortable glucose-rich cruising altitude, the conversation begins. "OK, there's a couple different flavors of lessons here. Let's do the medical stuff first."

A medical student produces some notes—"OK, the main thing is pulling the epidural catheter so soon after dosing the low-molecular-weight heparin. You put that catheter in, and maybe you ding a vessel or

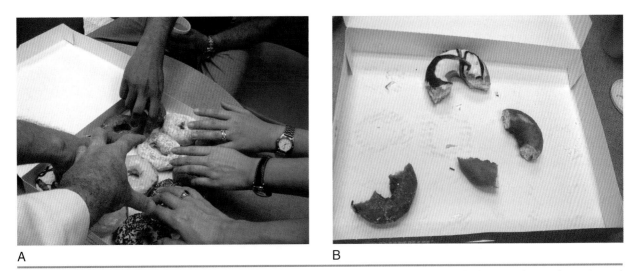

A   B

FIGURE 8–53   As health care professionals, we should take pride in setting a good example, both in our choice of nutrition and our conduct at the "donut box side."

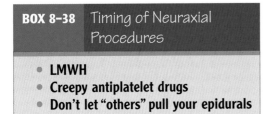

BOX 8–38   Timing of Neuraxial Procedures

- **LMWH**
- **Creepy antiplatelet drugs**
- **Don't let "others" pull your epidurals**

two. So if you are anticoagulated, you don't want to 'pull that plug' and let it bleed.

"It's got a half-life of 2 to 3 hours, has an antithrombotic effect for about 24 hours, doesn't get reversed by protamine, and, let me see, accumulates in renal failure patients."

The pain fellow's eyebrows go up. "Wow, med students *are* getting smarter."

"I got it off my Palm Pilot, I just did a search on Google, then went from there," the med student says. "Then I wrote it out by hand so you'd think I did all this in the library, the old-fashioned way."

Handing him another donut, the surgeon says, "Here, you earned it."

Then the other med student adds, "So you're supposed to wait 12 hours after the last dose before you place or remove a catheter."

"Right," the instructor says, picking through the donuts, "that's the medical schtick on this one. Anticoagulation is a real pain in the ass for us and our regional techniques. And everything now is antiplatelet. Why is that?" he asks the med students.

"The best current model for coronary thrombosis is rupture of a plaque, with aggregation of platelets at the site of the rupture," the first medical student says. "So more and more, they're zonking platelets with Plavix and all those other things."

"Yeah," the surgeon says, "and zonking those platelets may take the edge off heart attack land, but it makes stuff bad for us too."

"Right," the instructor moves on, "now let's go onto the next lesson—'the helpful person' who gets you in trouble. Let's put the clock on rewind and recreate the problem from the surgeon's point of view."

The surgeon lays it out, "You're following the patient, and you're happy but happy that the epidural is providing good pain relief. Remember, I see the patient every day, and I'm the reason they came to the hospital, so the patient and their family are relying on *me* to make things right."

"That's true," the patient (actually a CRNA working in the Simulator Center), says. "Things go wrong—get me my surgeon! The surgeon is the stopper, they're really the one you go to for answers."

"So, you know," the surgeon continues. "You see the epidural in, and you know it's been 3 days, and the last thing you want is an infection, so you decide to pull the catheter. You know, do the anesthesiologist a favor. They did you a favor by putting the epidural *in* in the first place, so now you just step in and pull it out."

"And you get the epidural hematoma," the pain fellow says.

"She *did* forget about the low-molecular-weight heparin," the instructor says. "So it's easy to blame her.

She pulled the catheter, she caused the hematoma. Vilify her, burn her at the malpractice stake. Then everyone feels better, right? Is that the best approach? The blame game?"

Shaking his head, the pain fellow says, "Well no. It's a system error, really. You should have a system set up where you *can't* pull it at the wrong time. Maybe tag it."

They all work together to devour the rest of the donuts and then design a *system* that would prevent this from happening again.

> Inform in-service nurses and medical staff on the new guidelines for removing catheters
>
> Tag the patient's chart with the last dose of LMWH given
>
> Tag the patient's bed
>
> Inform the patient so he/she can serve as the "final barrier" to catastrophe

"One last consideration," the instructor says, "before you all collapse upon yourselves in a reverie of self-congratulation. What do you do for the practitioner who has caused the screw-up? Say this had really happened, what do you say to the surgeon? 'Tough luck?' 'Too bad, couldn't have happened to a nicer person?'"

That stops everyone in their tracks.

"Think about it," the instructor continues. "This person has just made a mistake, a genuine mistake, and has made a patient paraplegic. Do you just hang this doctor out to dry?"

No one has a clue. Even a search on the all-knowing Google comes up a duster.

"Well, there is no magic bullet for this problem," the instructor says, "but you have to provide some kind of backup for these people in times of woe. Counseling, taking them off the schedule for a day or two, calling them and lending a sympathetic ear."

"Don't forget," the surgeon says, "today it's my mistake. Tomorrow it could be yours."

Summary. Know your coagulo-active medications. Wait 12 hours after the last dose of LMWH before placing a regional or pulling an epidural catheter.

For the antiplatelet meds ticlodipine and clopidogrel, the wait is much longer—7 days.

Epidural hematomas are five alarm fires—get neurosurgery and get the study *now*! This is not an "order and forget" kind of thing. This is something that you yourself shepherd every inch of the way. As this patient showed, you can go from vague symptoms (hard to tell

from her baseline multiple sclerosis) to flaccid paralysis in a short time.

Disasters are rarely isolated events—mistakes made by lone fools on desert islands. Disasters are more often a series of mistakes piled onto each other—the surgeon didn't stay up-to-date on LMWH; the anesthesiologist didn't make sure the surgeon knew; the nurse didn't stop the surgeon; the hospital didn't have a policy. When something like this occurs, the temptation is strong to blame one person with a resounding "Humph!" Patients are better served by a re-evaluation of all the events leading up to the problem and then re-designing the system to provide some checks and balances to prevent the error from recurring.

SCENARIO 19. **Juggling responsibilities, running two rooms with problems in each**

"Today," the instructor tells the anesthesia resident, "you get to be an attending."

Looking around, the anesthesia resident asks, "Where's my cup of coffee? Where are the keys to my Ferrari?"

"In room 1, a removal of a neck mass is going on under MAC. In room 2, which they're about to start, they're going to do a rigid bronchoscopy and tracheal dilatation on a guy with tracheal stenosis," the instructor explains.

The anesthesia resident looks over the preop on the patient in room 1—a small node on the back of the neck. A little more alarming is the preop for the patient in room 2. A morbidly obese (5'8", 285 pound) man with a history of poor compliance with his diabetes medications. A few years earlier, a bad bout of DKA landed him on a ventilator for 5 days, with resultant tracheal stenosis. Subsequently, the ENT service had dilated him three times and actually placed a metal mesh stent in the trachea. The patient never comes in for follow-up visits, just showing up in the ER with labored breathing and the need for another dilatation.

Plan—get the MAC going in room 1; then get room 2 going but shepherd this more difficult case all the way through. Damn, might not be enough time left for coffee drinking and Ferrari driving.

Into room 1 the resident goes. There is a medical student playing the part of the anesthesia provider in this room.

"How do you want me to do this?" the medical student asks.

"Give a little sedation, here, this stuff," the resident says, picking up a syringe of midazolam. "A milligram at a time, and keep talking to the patient. Remember, if they're talking, they're breathing. If they're not talking, they might not be breathing."

"What if I have to convert to a general anesthetic?" the med student asks.

The anesthesia resident mulls this over. This *is* the Simulator, and you don't want the medical student just sitting here. What the heck, give him a thrill.

"Tell you what," the resident explains, "induce with propofol and put this LMA in, then run the patient on vapors. Call me if you're in trouble."

"Any big deal if I do that?" the med student asks. "This is just a node, right, so no big deal if it's general or MAC, right?"

All the anesthesia resident can see is the morbidly obese airway problem in room 2, so his thoughts are anywhere but in room 1.

"Um, right. Asleep's fine," he says, then goes into room 2.

In room 2, an ENT surgeon (a fellow anesthesia resident plays the part), stands ready with a Dido laryngoscope. A medical student stands ready to function as anesthesia provider.

"OK to induce?" the med student asks. In her hands, she has propofol and succinylcholine ready to go, and she's chomping at the bit.

"Wait, just a minute, just wait," the anesthesia resident says, "we need a plan first. We have to talk to our ENT friends here.

"OK, so what's the plan?"

"Off to sleep," the ENT surgeon says, "then turn him over to me."

"You sure you can intubate him?" the anesthesia resident asks.

"Yep, I did his last two dilations. We know this guy from the inside out."

"Good," the anesthesia resident says. "Walk me through the sequence, what's first, when do we ventilate, what do you need to do?"

"I'll need him relaxed because I'll have this laryngoscope in the whole time," the ENT explains. "Then place the scope, look, place a small endotracheal tube, you breathe and get the sat up. Then out comes the endotracheal tube, I put in a dilator, inflate, hold it there as long as you say I can, then we pull out, put in a bigger endotracheal tube, you breathe, get the sat up, and we keep rolling like that."

"Endpoint?" the anesthesia resident asks.

"Once we can place an 8.0 ETT, we're done, probably take three, maybe four, dilatations."

The overhead speaker crackles, "Anesthesia to room 1, anesthesia to room 1." Somehow, the announcer manages to say it with the exact same intonation as Darth Vader.

"Just a sec," the anesthesia resident, a real Star Wars fan, says.

In room 1, the medical student says, "He was not liking it, said his shoulder really hurt, so I put him to sleep, OK?"

The simulator mannequin now has an LMA in and anesthetic vapors are on. Drapes cover the neck area, but all the vital signs are OK.

"Fine," the anesthesia resident hustles back to where all the action is in room 2.

Once in room 2, "OK, let's rock, we have a plan. But let's use Mivacron for relaxation. Sux won't last long enough."

The medical student knows her stuff, states the correct doses of both propofol and mivacurium, pre-oxygenates, then induces. After establishing a good airway, they turn the bed, and the ENT surgeon steps in, placing the Dido laryngoscope.

Saturation 96%, 94%, 92%.

"We better intubate," the medical student says.

The ENT surgeon places a 5.0 ETT. "Hook up!" he says.

Hooking up the breathing circuit, the student notices a large leak. "Um," she says, "I'm not seeing any CO_2 here, and I'm not getting much air in."

"Are you in?" the anesthesia resident asks, the tone heading upward in his voice.

Darth Vader on the speaker, "Anesthesia to room 1, the case is finished. Anesthesia to room 1, the case is finished."

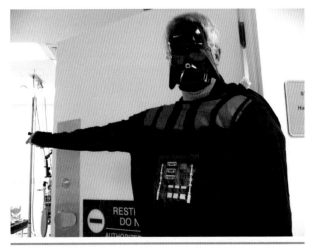

FIGURE 8–54 That person running the schedule may seem a little too powerful at times. But hey, they have to get the schedule done, so better go along with their requests. When they say, "Go ye and anesthetize," go do it.

"Just a second!" the anesthesia resident-turned attending shouts at the overhead speakers.

"Oh," the ENT surgeon says, "we forgot to inflate the cuff. Give me a syringe."

In go a few cc's of air, the seal is good, and ventilation proceeds OK.

Sat—89%, 91%, 95%.

"Right, OK," the anesthesia resident says, "don't pull the tube out until you get up to 99%, then you can do the next step, you know, the inflation thing. I'll be right back."

Hustling into room 1, the anesthesia resident sees the LMA getting pulled out. "We're done!" chirps the medical student. "Patient's awake and everything."

From the mannequin's speaker, the patient says, "My shoulder feels funny."

"OK," the anesthesia resident says, "probably that's just . . ."

"Anesthesia, room 2, anesthesia, room 2," Darth commands from overhead.

"My shoulder feels funny!" the patient says again. "I can't move it."

"Anesthesia, room 2, anesthesia room 2."

"Why does her shoulder feel funny, do you think," the med student asks.

"Anesthesia, room 2, anesthesia, room 2."

"My shoulder . . ."

"Why, tell me . . ."

"Anesthesia, room 2 . . ."

Spreading his legs to shoulder length, like an athlete preparing for anything, the anesthesia resident holds an arm up to the med student, "Hold that thought, I'll be right back!" then goes to room 2 and bursts in like a SWAT squad.

"Oh," the ENT says, "we just wanted to know. The sat's 98, is that good enough to go ahead and pull out and do the dilation?"

"Yeah," the anesthesia resident says.

Darth again, "Anesthesia, sign out in PACU."

"I'll be there in a sec!"

Darth rolls on, "Anesthesia, chill out, the Simulation is over."

Clinical lessons learned from scenario 19

Debriefing. Staggering into the debriefing room, the anesthesia resident plops down in a chair like a rag doll.

"No Ferrari for me!"

Everyone else sits down around the table. No black-caped, black-helmeted Darth Vader, though. More's the pity.

BOX 8-39 Nerve Injuries

- **Know anatomy**
- **Neck—watch for CN XI**
- **Under anesthesia, patient can't say "Ouch!"**

"Let's look at the rooms one at a time," the instructor says, "then once we have the individual things nailed, let's step back and look at the whole 'spread too thin' issue."

"What was the big deal about the patient's shoulder?" the anesthesia resident asks, finally un-rag-dolling himself. "Node biopsy, MAC, so she's a little sore at the site?"

Turning to the medical student in the first room, the instructor asks, "So, what was the little trap we laid there."

Instructor and medical student had colluded on this one. Having a confederate "in on something" is a little sneaky, somewhat unfair, and undoubtedly slimy. No wonder it's such a neat instructional tool!

"Node in the posterior neck," the medical student explains, "should always raise your hackles because cranial nerve XI runs back there, the spinal accessory nerve to the shoulder. If you do this under MAC, the patient can tell you if you're near the nerve. If you do this under general and you don't use a nerve stimulator, you can section the nerve and really weaken the patient's shoulder for life. That is a big no-no.

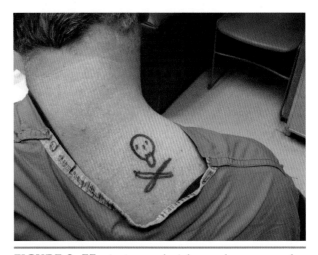

FIGURE 8-55 Again, you don't have to be a surgeon, but you have to know where they are going and what "landmines" await them. Here, a skull and crossbones indicates a danger area. A biopsy back here could snag the spinal accessory nerve and damage the shoulder.

"We knew you'd be focusing all your brain cells on the bad airway in the other room, so I just lightly threw in the suggestion that we go to general anesthesia."

"We baited you," the instructor says. "And you took the bait."

"Bastards, sneaky bastards," the anesthesia resident says.

Both instructor and medical student give appreciative nods. The instructor says, "I'll take that as compliment."

The ENT surgeon (to repeat, an actual anesthesia resident) goes on: "What about in our room? What's the lesson there?"

"Any trap? By the way, thanks for letting me use that Dido scope, it's clunky, but it's handy for shoving tissue out of the way. I can see how the ENT docs sometimes 'get it' with this when we can't 'get it' with our blades."

Picking up the Dido scope, the instructor looks it over and says, "Yeah, it is nice, we should use if every now and then. The fact that it's got a 'roof' on it keeps

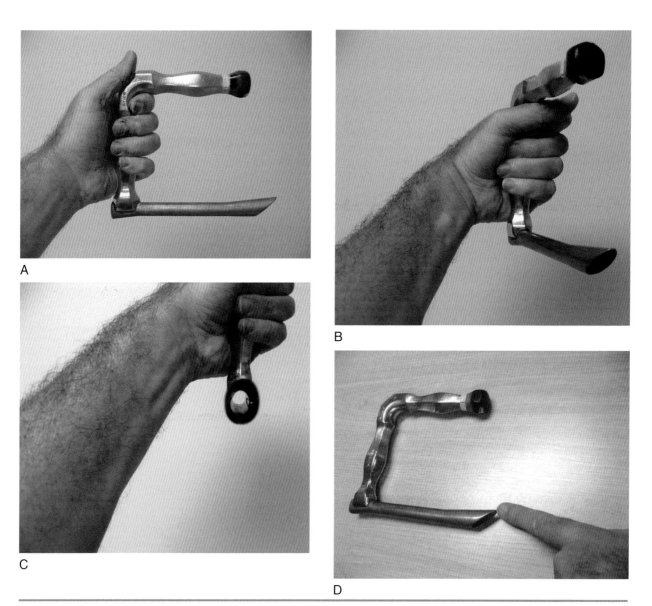

A

B

C

D

FIGURE 8–56 The Dido scope used by ENT. Big advantage of this honker: it has a "roof" on it, so soft tissue can't hang down and obscure the view. Many an ENT has bailed me out of trouble with this very scope.

tissue from hanging down and getting in your way. And yes, the ENT docs do save our butts from time to time. Learn to love your ENT, they are the ultimate 'airway getter.'"

The medical student from the second room, the anesthesia provider in that room, lays out the lesson, "The big thing was the airway and the 'what comes first, what comes second' plan. I thought the anesthesia resident did a good job. I mean, I knew just what we were going to do at each step, that's the main thing, right?"

"I did blow it when I forgot to inflate the endotracheal tube cuff, though," the anesthesia resident admits. "I got all jiggity about the complicated plan, then when it came down to a basic, 'Duh, inflate the cuff,' I kind of went into mind melt."

"Happens," the instructor says. "You're thinking of walking from point A to point B, and you get run over by a truck because you forgot to look both ways before you crossed the street on your way to point B."

Continuing, the instructor says, "OK, we forgot our anatomy in room 1, we came up with a good plan but got a little nervous in room 2, but still came out OK in there. What do we do about the bouncing back and forth? What do we do when we're getting overwhelmed by requests to be 'everywhere at once'? And believe you me, it happens."

Both medical students says, "Triage?"

Instructor and anesthesia residents raise their eyebrows and make the inverted smile facial expression that says, "Wow, that's surprisingly sharp."

"Yeah," the anesthesia resident says, "that's basically it. You have to pick the crisis and go to that. Hope they can tread water at the other one. I suppose you could call for help too. Have someone watch one room for you while you stay in the really bad room.

"It's tough when that overhead keeps going off because when they say they need you in a room, is it, 'They need me now, this is *stat*' or is it, 'Oh, we just have a little question for you'?"

"No magic answer for you there," the instructor says. "I guess that's why all the attendings drive Ferraris."

BOX 8–40 *Overwhelmed?*

- Slow down
- Get help
- Go back to ABC

Summary. The anesthesia resident discovers that life "at the top" has its own miseries. Watching more than one room can wear down the best of them.

You can never discount the smallest procedure. A MAC case for, what seems like a ditzel, can turn into a crippling injury if you forget your anatomy. Know where the surgeons are cutting and what landmines are in that area. For parotid tumors, everyone knows to watch out for the facial nerve. But you can forget that a node, even a seemingly superficial one, in the posterior area of the neck, can run right next to or on top of the XI cranial nerve.

Sharing the airway, as anesthesia and ENT were doing in room 2, always requires a pregame planning session. Who has the airway when? How and when do we ventilate? When will ENT be able to "get in there" and do their thing? And once the "battle is engaged," you have to still remember all your basics (like inflating the ETT cuff). Don't get blinded by the complexities and forget the humdrum stuff.

And finally, any anesthesia resident preparing for "release into the wild" should know how to handle multiple calls at once. Develop those triage skills that allow you to focus on the most pressing problem. Know what can go on the back burner for a while and what you need to take care of *now*. And don't forget the old mantra—"Call for help." That's not a sign of weakness, it's a sign of intelligence.

SCENARIO 20. **Pacing yourself, muscular dystrophy, and the need for a pacer**

"I'm supposed to know what Curschmann-Steinert syndrome is?" the anesthesia resident asks, his face utterly devoid of Curschmann-Steinert recognition.

His two fellow residents look just as clueless.

A 25-year-old patient with Curschmann-Steinert syndrome is scheduled for pacemaker placement.

The preop evaluator had mercy on them, "Myotonic dystrophy. PMH remarkable for diabetes mellitus, thyroid insufficiency, mild muscle weakness, and mild mental retardation."

Before the three residents go into the OR, they go into an examining room. They will interview a standardized patient (an actor who has a script and can act out the appropriate symptoms) before they go into the OR (where the action shifts to a mannequin).

"Hello Mr. Goodwin," the first resident says, extending a hand for a handshake.

Goodwin extends a hand, gives a handshake, and then keeps shaking the hand and shaking the hand, taking what seems like forever to release his grip.

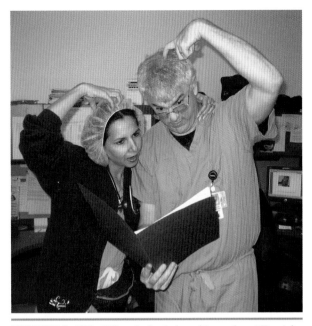

FIGURE 8–57   What the heck does this guy have? Don't let weird syndromes throw you off the track. Do a quick look in the textbooks or online. Then once the case gets going, pay attention to those good old basics—ABC.

The third anesthesia resident comes in the room a minute later, a printout on myotonic dystrophy hot from the laser printer. As the first anesthesia resident goes over the history and physical with Mr. Goodwin, the other two do a lightning review of this rare condition.

Acres of verbiage on nucleotide triplet mishaps, chromosome 19 aberrations—holy minestrone—they cut to the chase, anesthetic considerations.

The disease involves the muscle, and it affects anesthesia in a dozen ways.

- Muscles, once contracted, have a hard time un-contracting - hence the odd behavior of the patient. When he contracted his muscles to shake the first resident's hand, he had trouble releasing the "handshake muscles."
- Other muscles are involved, which can lead to bulbar weakness and recurrent aspiration, so you have to be careful with aspiration risk.
- They're sensitive to sedatives, so even small amounts of sedative hypnotics can lead to respiratory depression.
- Cardiac conduction is affected—hence the need for Mr. Goodwin to get a pacemaker.
- Pay attention to other endocrine systems, as diabetes, pancreatic, and thyroid dysfunction can occur.

Regional anesthesia is the way to go, if possible. Sux can cause a contraction that will "last and last the whole day long," so don't use it.

A host of other things can cause myotonia, shivering from cold, anticholinesterase drugs, and even surgical manipulation. Regional anesthesia, muscle relaxants, and inhalation agents (which cause good relaxation in normal patients) may not work in these patients. At times, infiltration of local anesthetic right into the muscle is the only thing that works.

All three residents get up to date on the anesthetic considerations of this rare disease, they wrap up the H&P and go into the OR.

Once into the operating room, they place the routine monitors, add supplemental oxygen, and then turn to the question of sedatives.

"Well," the second anesthesia resident says, "the surgeon can do this pacer under local, but we're going to have to give this guy something for sedation."

"Propofol?" the third one asks.

They all zip through the myotonic dystrophy handout. Who knows? Maybe the egg thing in propofol does something weird.

"Oops, here," the first anesthesia resident says, "pain from that injection can lead to contractions too."

"Damn," the second anesthesia resident says, "can't do *anything*!"

"Precedex, man, dexmedetomidine," the third resident says. "That'll sedate him. And it shouldn't stop him breathing."

All three heads shoot down to the paper.

"Precedex, Precedex, where the hell's the Precedex?"

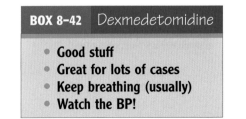

BOX 8-42	Dexmedetomidine

- **Good stuff**
- **Great for lots of cases**
- **Keep breathing (usually)**
- **Watch the BP!**

Across the room, the cardiologist says, "OK to start? Um, time is money, doctors. Time is money."

"Let's do it, let's do Precedex," the second anesthesia resident says.

The residents mix a mock concoction of dexmedetomidine, run it through an infusion pump, and start infusing it into the IV.

"If we have to intubate," the second anesthesia resident says. "If we do overdo it and have to take over respirations, we'll use mivacurium, and we'll have to intubate because he's an aspiration risk."

"Right," the others agree.

All the vital signs are fine, the surgeon starts working, then the EKG goes into third degree heart block. Blood pressure drops to 70/40, the pulse oximeter stops picking up, the patient starts making nauseated sounds.

"Do you have the pads on?" the cardiologist asks. "Do you have the external pads on? The Zoll pads for external pacing if we need it?"

"Oh!"

"Oh!"

"Oh!"

"Get 'em on!" the cardiologist yells. "I'm not in yet, I can't pace from here!"

The residents look around, there is a defibrillator, they roll it over to the patient and start opening drawers like mad. "There aren't any pads in here!"

"Get some!"

"Forget the stick, start CPR!"

The door opens, "Forget CPR, the Simulation's over."

Clinical lessons learned from scenario 20

Debriefing. Three ticked-off residents sulk in the debriefing room.

"Anyone know how to work this cappuccino machine?" the instructor asks, pointing into the lounge. Like lounges everywhere, the Simulator lounge has a regular coffee machine that everyone knows how to work and a multiarmed, European-looking cappuccino thingie that no one knows how to work.

All three residents shake their head.

"All right," the cardiologist (a medical student working on a Simulator project) says. "Here's the defibrillator and here are the paddles you use for pacing."

In the middle of the debriefing table is a mannequin. The residents place the pads, adjust the buttons on the pacer, and set the pacer at 80.

"I see and I forget, I do and I remember," the instructor says.

"OK, you guys went over the myotonic dystrophy stuff pretty well, and all the considerations you talked about," the instructor says. "And you definitely did the right thing, getting a quick Google search and getting the latest greatest anesthetic considerations on this rare disease. No one can remember all this stuff, but you can always look it up.

"Tell me, what went into your decision to use the dexmedetomidine?" the instructor asks. "Take me through the thinking."

"All right," the first resident says, "you have to figure, this is a rare disease, and let's face it, dexmedetomidine is a pretty new drug. How likely is it that anyone has done a study, safety of sedating with dexmedetomidine in myotonic dystrophy?"

The second anesthesia resident goes ahead, "So we don't have *perfect science*, but we can go with *best guess* and have the appropriate backup in case we get it wrong. So we had the right muscle relaxant, Mivacron —you know, no need to reverse that—in case we *do* oversedate and cause a respiratory arrest."

"Right," the third resident is no shrinking violet. "So you figure, dex provides sedation, which this patient will probably need, he is mildly impaired and may not hold still, but we want to stay with regional if at all possible. So dex it is."

Then attention turns to the question of the pacer.

"OK, now let's address the question of 'blinded by the light,'" the instructor says.

All eyes go down onto the table top, looking for a convenient crack that they might crawl into and disappear.

"What do you do when you *might* need pacing or *might* need defibrillation in a case?" the instructor asks.

"You put on the pads," the resident chorus says.

"And when someone has a bizarre-o disease that you've never heard of but that has a million implications for anesthesia, does that change anything?" the instructor is enjoying this too much.

"I'll bet you pulled wings off flies when you were a little kid, didn't you?" the second anesthesia resident asks.

With a smile, the instructor says, "Yes, now that you mention it. Don't avoid the subject."

BOX 8-43 External Pacer Pads

- **Think of them**
- **Put on early**
- **Do a dry run with the controls**

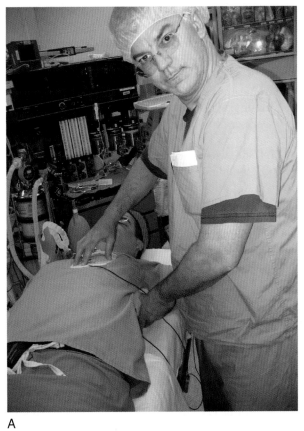

A

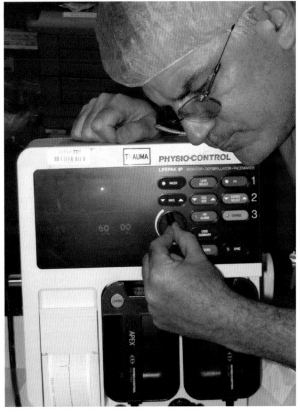

B

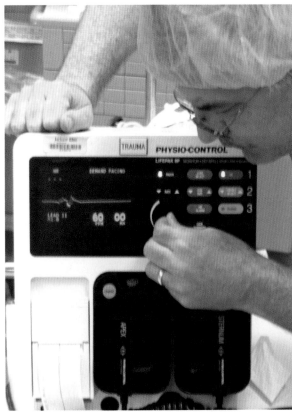

C

FIGURE 8–58 Just as you need to "fiddle" with the defibrillator to make sure you know how the buttons work, you need to fiddle with the external pacer buttons.

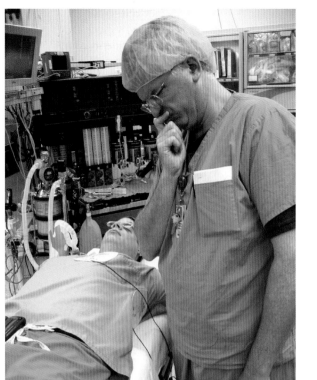

A

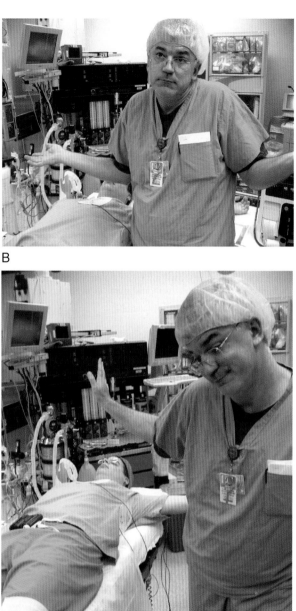

B

C

FIGURE 8–59 **A.** If it's an emergency and you can't figure it out, the patient may suffer. Do this in the simulator first so you'll have it down when the big day comes. **B.** Of note, here, the hapless practitioner forgot that the pads have to be on *skin*, not just on the patient's *shirt*. Oh well. **C.** Sorry.

"No," the first resident says, "you're right. It's a lesson worth learning—you *do* get all freaked out. And sure enough, what bites you in the ass? The weird thing? The one in 10,000 thing?"

"No," the second resident says, "it's always the basics, always the basics, always the basics."

After the debriefing the residents try to work the cappuccino machine. One scalds his middle finger on the steam apparatus, and after 25 minutes they give up and drink the regular coffee.

Summary. Oh, if only anesthesia were "plug and play"—the same for everyone. But alas, it isn't. And specific diseases have specific prohibitions.

Spinal cord injury? Burn? MH? Can't give sux. Everyone knows that.

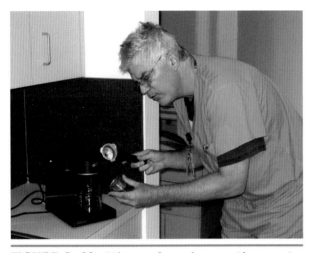

FIGURE 8–60 Who can figure those stupid cappuccino machines anyway? Just give me the regular coffee pot. If I toss enough heavy whipping cream and sugar in there, it's just about the same thing.

But what happens when you hit a real oddball, a disease you've never seen before and may have not even heard of, except in passing during some dim and distant lecture hall?

Look it up! With today's technology, you should never have to stumble blind into the land of "Gee Whiz, can I give *this* drug in the face of *this* disease?" And the residents did their due diligence on this patient with myotonic dystrophy.

But they hit a snag forgetting the basics. We talk forever about "multitasking," but our brains are not that good at it. With all the concentration focusing on this disease, its many prohibitions and restrictions and the danger of oversedation in this patient population, the residents forgot a fundamental point.

The operation itself—not just the rare disease—requires some preparation. This patient has a conduction problem in his heart. If the conduction system fails, the patient may go into third degree heart block, a potentially fatal rhythm. So you must be ready for that. Until the wire is in and the pacemaker is functioning, that means external pacing, and *that* means having the external equipment ready to go.

They didn't.

Oh well. As the saying goes in the Simulation Center, "Kill them *here*, so you don't kill them *out there*."

SCENARIO 21. **TEE time, TEE in an unstable patient**

"Thanks for the donuts," the instructor says. "This demonstrates excellent insight into what affects your evaluation."

Looking down at his feet and scuffing the floor, the senior anesthesia resident says, "Shucks."

A pair of junior anesthesia residents come out of the OR and approach the donut bearer. "We've got a case in here that we can't figure out."

They bring the senior up to date as they go in the room. "This guy was selling Bibles in a bar last night at 2 a.m. when some kind of ecclesiastical difference arose."

The other junior resident continues, "So in a pitch of religious fervor, one of the theological disputants beat the hell—pardon the appropriateness of the analogy—out of this guy. We're fixing facial fractures right now, and we've already done a negative lap to see if he's bleeding in his belly."

"The assailants didn't limit their fury to his face, then?" the senior resident asks.

"No," junior resident #1 says. "It was a somewhat generalized dishing out of disgruntlement."

"Pneumo? Hemothorax? Anything in the chest?" the senior asks.

"We thought of that, CXR is negative," junior resident #2 says.

In the operating room, the patient is all draped out, and a CXR is on the view box. On the monitors, the sat is 100%; they are on 100% oxygen, on no inhalation agents, and the arterial line trace is reading 85/55.

"Little low," the senior says. "What's going on?"

"Good question!" the juniors say. "We've gone through everything and can't peg what's going on. This is a young guy, and it shouldn't be so low!"

"OK, let's see what you have so far," the senior says.

"Hey!" the surgeon says, "He's movin'!"

"Got it!" the senior resident says, giving some muscle relaxant. "Did you guys use cisatracurium before?"

"Yes."

"OK if I give rocuronium now, then?" the senior asks.

"No," junior #1 says, "don't mix muscle relaxant families, you might get a synergistic response."

(The surgeon in the field does a low-tech simulation of the patient moving; he grabs the simulator and shakes it around a little.)

"We went ahead and started an epi drip," junior #2 says, "and that helped a little."

"But you still don't really know what's going on, right?" the senior asks.

Nods of agreement.

"Did you get an arterial blood gas?" the senior asks. "Don't forget, it's always a good time for a blood gas;

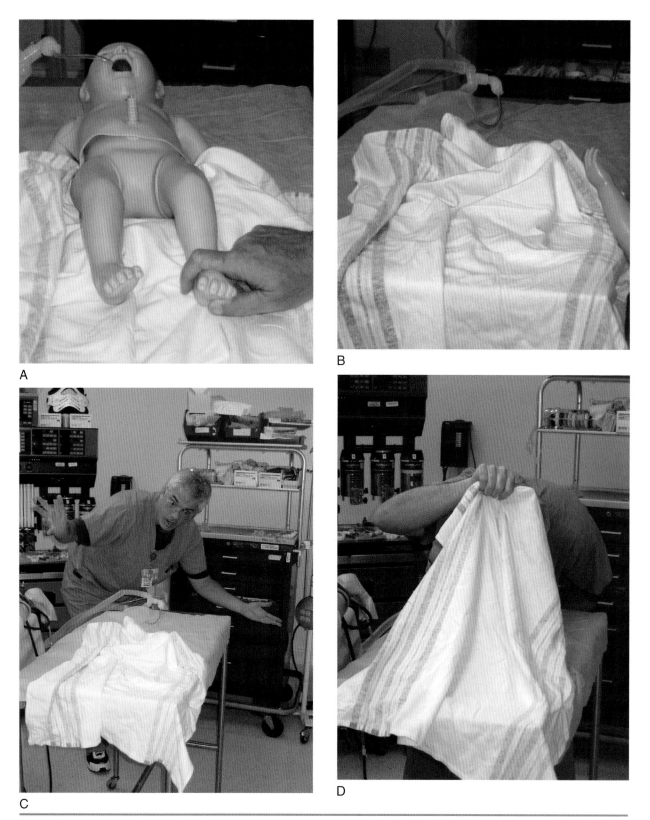

FIGURE 8–61 To create "surgical movement" the surgeon in the field can give the patient a little tug. This is low technology, but effective. In the case illustrated above, it's quite effective! Not to mention amusing.

and when things aren't going right, it's *really* a good time for an arterial blood gas."

They'd gotten one, and things looked OK on it. Normal acid-base, normal glucose, good oxygenation and good carbon dioxide elimination. Hematocrit a little low, 31, but not so low as to explain the instability.

"So how do we figure out what's going on?" the senior asks. "What's our next best move when we have unexplained hemodynamic instability?"

"Swan?" junior #2 asks. "Should we float a Swan?"

"All right, where you going to put it?"

"Um," the juniors look at the field, drapes all over the face and neck. "Antecubital? Can you do that?"

"Can, but not done much."

"Femoral? I guess the surgeons would have to do that, huh?" junior #1 says.

"They would."

They ask the surgeon, who grumbles a little, but puts in the femoral sheath; and then, under guidance from the anesthesia residents, floats the Swan. (On the monitor screen, the waveforms of CVP, then RV, then PA, then wedge appear in succession, creating the feel of a Swan being placed.)

PA 30/18, CVP 12, wedge 10, cardiac output 4.0.

They puzzle over the numbers.

"Well, he could be full, I guess, or. . . ." junior #2 says.

"Or he could be, well, depending on his baseline, he could be . . . he could need more fluid . . . um," junior #1 says.

"So, in summary, we kind of still don't really know what's going on, is that what you're telling me? We have a bunch of numbers, but we're still in the dark about whether he's full or empty, whether the heart is good or bad, or whether there might be something else going on, right?" the senior resident asks.

Both juniors agree.

"So now what do we do, magically take a picture of the heart and instantaneously clear away the fog?

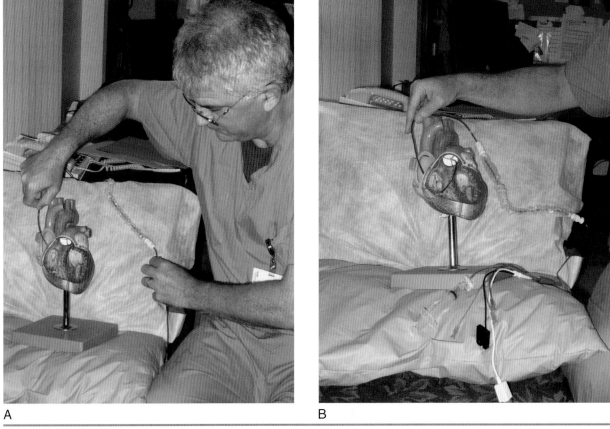

A B

FIGURE 8–62 Want to demonstrate how a Swan meanders through the heart? Grab a Swan and a little model and show the students how it goes through the various chambers.

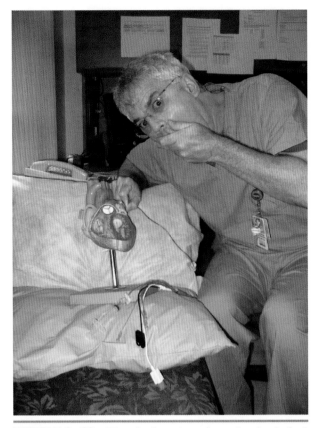

FIGURE 8–63 Here the Swan is on the, wait, what is that? The Swan on the left? Oops.

senior continues, "don't force it. You don't want an esophageal tear. If it gets stuck at all, place your laryngoscope, lift up, and take a look. Always better to do that than to force it."

Junior resident #1 does the placement; then they pull the probe out, and junior #2 places it again.

"What's the number one complication of placing these things?" the senior asks.

"Esophageal tear?"

"Blood pressure going up?"

"Nope," the senior says, "distraction. You fall in love with this TEE image, and you forget about the patient. They wake up, they move, their blood pressure plummets, you disconnect the ventilator—all that stuff can happen, but here you are - glued to the damned TEE - and you forget about the patient. So don't forget to look up and make sure the patient is doing OK before you go ga-ga over the TEE view."

On the TV screen, a video of the TEE shows a dilated and barely moving right ventricle. The left ventricle appears OK.

"What's the diagnosis?" the senior asks.

"Doesn't look like that right heart is doing too much," junior #1 says.

"Maybe an infarct, contusion maybe, on the right?" junior #2 ventures.

"Where's the right heart sit?" the senior asks. "Right under the sternum, right? And when this guy's buddies were beating the daylight out of him, some of those shots must have hit him in the chest. This guy probably has a cardiac contusion with right heart failure—that's why his blood pressure's low.

"Bingo, now you have a diagnosis!"

Overhead, "Bingo, now we can have the rest of the donuts. Simulation's over."

They file out of the room with more *Hallelujah Chorus* playing.

Clinical lessons learned from scenario 21

Debriefing. "How does anyone ever get skinny in this department?" junior #2 ask, helping himself to a cream-filled.

Wouldn't that miracle maneuver be handy right about now?" the senior resident says.

"Um," junior #2 says, "echo?"

Over the speakers, the *Hallelujah Chorus* blasts out, loud enough to make everyone's sternum function like a woofer in a stereo speaker. Just as quickly, it cuts off.

"Good idea," the senior resident says.

(To keep from damaging the upper airway of the expensive mannequin, an intubating dummy is rolled in the room along with an old TEE probe. This way, the resident can practice placing the probe without risk of damaging pricey equipment. A TV is also brought in to play a video of a TEE. In effect, then, the resident "places the TEE" and then "sees what the TEE shows.")

The senior resident instructs on placing the TEE probe, "First, make sure the probe is unlocked. You want this thing wiggling its way down the esophagus, not ramming down like a sword in a sword-swallowing carnival sideshow.

"Now, a little anterior flexion, so it will follow the curve of the pharynx and head for the esophagus," the

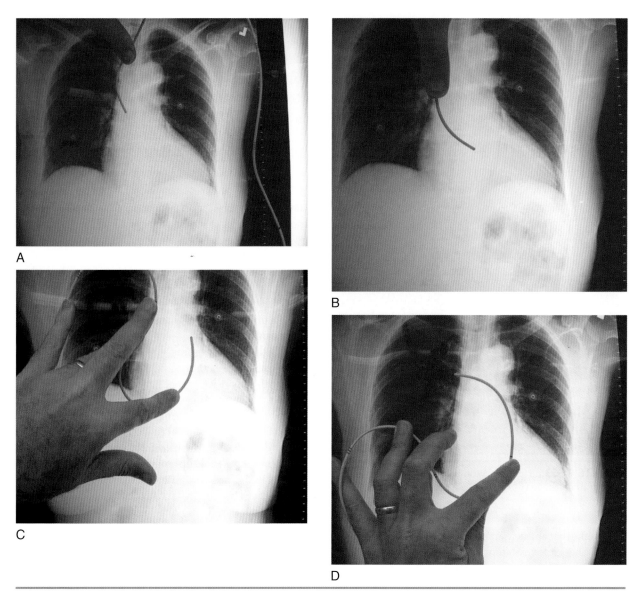

A

B

C

D

FIGURE 8-64   Back to our old friend the CXR to show the "Swan trek."

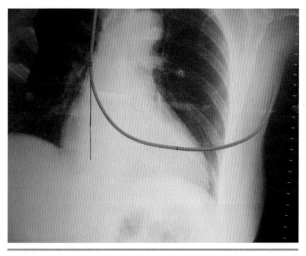

FIGURE 8-65   Here, a Paceport Swan with the wire extended. This helps you visualize just exactly what is going on.

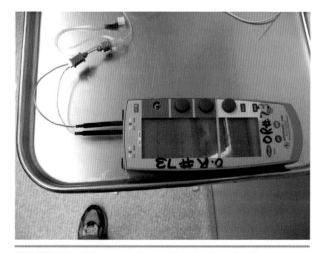

FIGURE 8-66   Don't forget the niggling details. Hook up to the pacer (remember the broken one with the missing knob?) and make sure you know how to set that puppy.

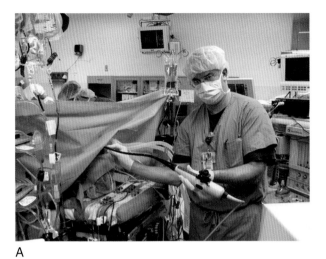

A

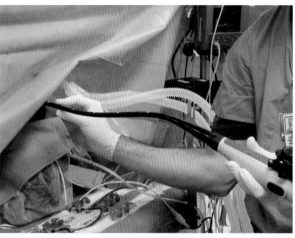

B

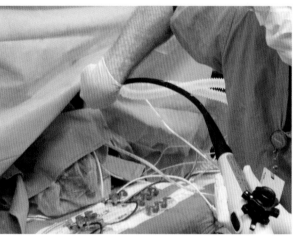

C

FIGURE 8-67 Gentle, gentle with the TEE, don't force it!

"My belly used to jiggle when I walked," junior #1 says. "Now it jiggles when I brush my teeth. It's discouraging. Hey, hand me that last glazed, would you?"

"Let's number everything here on the board, every last thing that you think we did in this one," the instructor says. "But we'll save the whole TEE thing 'til last 'cause that's obviously the biggie."

They come up with:

Assessed the all-important "something is wrong here"

Called for help (a lesson worth learning over and over again)

Rounded up the usual suspects by looking for bleeding in the abdomen and chest and then sending off a blood gas

Buying time with an epi drip and keeping the patient still with muscle relaxants—imperfect solutions but things you have to do in such a case. All agreed a BIS would be handy (not yet available on this Simulator mannequin, though you can always get around it by having the instructor state a given BIS value)

Looking at hemodynamics with a PA catheter

So overall, the junior residents acquitted themselves well. The instructor gives a quick refresher on hemodynamic instability by going back to basics.

"Always think 'ABC,' and you guys did," the instructor starts. "And when you come to the 'C' part of 'ABC,' then think of three more things, rate, rhythm, contractility. So once you've done that, and there was nothing in the rate or rhythm part of the equation to account for this hypotension, you have to think about contractility."

"Enter the TEE?" junior #2 asks.

"Well, yes," the instructor says, "but give me a second.

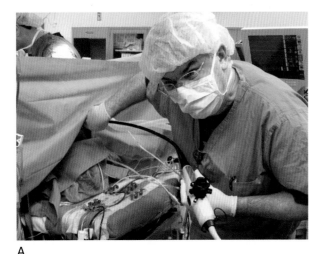

A

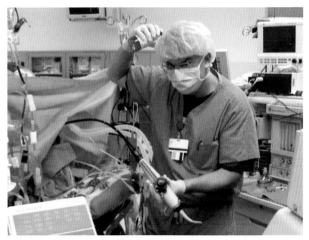

B

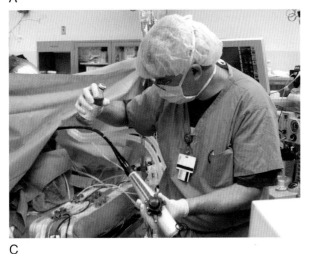

C

FIGURE 8–68 Slip it in with your fingers or else use the laryngoscope. Don't shove and shove, and especially don't pound it in with a glass albumin bottle. That is *way* not the right way to do it!

"Go back to the history, this guy got pounded. And pounding gives you the visible injuries—the facial injuries they're repairing—and the invisible stuff. Fractured spleen, epidural hematoma, fractured kidney, fractured liver—that's a good time, trust me—pulmonary contusion and the case here, cardiac contusion. So review the history to help you assess where to hunt."

"And TEE is the way to go," junior #2 won't let go of this bone.

"You got it," the senior resident says. "You don't have to be a wizard or take that perioperative TEE exam to be able to tell the biggies—heart empty or full, ventricle good or bad, tamponade yes or no. I mean, just like that you can peg those things. And that can usually bail you out of most hemodynamic jams."

"It's your window to the world," the instructor finishes.

Summary. Nothing tightens your sphincter like a patient who is not responding to "the usual stuff we do." And when you are barely anesthetizing a patient, or not anesthetizing him *at all*, and his blood pressure is still in the basement, you have some figuring out to do and fast.

ABC, ABC, ABC—check all the usual stuff, looking for the common causes of hemodynamic trouble. Face it, after trauma, it's usually hypovolemia of some sort (actual blood loss or "virtual blood loss" from tamponade or pneumothorax impeding venous return).

But sometimes you're still stuck. That's the time to call for help, review what you've done so far, and get another brain going over the differential diagnosis. Pride has no place with an unstable patient! If the help comes and saves the day, good for them, and good for you for *asking* for them!

Think TEE.

Easy to place, pretty easy to interpret, and the quickest "turnaround time" you could ask for. In the blink of an eye, you can usually peg what's wrong. In this case, right heart failure from a contusion. Not that this was any miracle cure—right heart failure is difficult to treat, involving judicious inotropic support and fluid management. But you're a lot better off *with* a diagnosis that *without* one.

SCENARIO 22. Sailing with rear admirals, colonoscopy

"You're working with the rear admirals today," the instructor tells the two anesthesia residents.

"Rear admirals?" the first anesthesia resident asks.

"Rear admirals. The colonoscopists."

"Oh," the residents say.

In the operating room, there is a mannequin on its side. A GI fellow is positioned with a colonoscope. Replacing the bottom part of the anesthesia mannequin is a GI simulator that can admit a colonoscope and provides a simulated colonoscopy for the GI fellow to work with while the anesthesia residents work on the "anesthetic half" of the patient. Standard monitors are hooked up, and the patient has nasal oxygen on.

Sat 99%, BP 160/100, HR 95, sinus rhythm.

"I'm kind of nervous," the patient (mannequin) says.

Lightning review of the preop—everything is in order, patient is NPO, had a bowel prep with low-residue diet for 48 hours, has a history of hypertension and a family history of polyps, so this 47-year-old author is coming in for a "preemptive strike" on any colon polyps.

"Any contraindications to proceed?" the GI fellow asks.

"Contraindications?" the first anesthesia resident asks, then turns to the second resident and hisses, "Shit, are we supposed to know the contraindications to colonoscopy?"

"No contraindications!" the second anesthesia resident chirps. "No toxic megacolon, no fulminant colitis, and no evidence of perforated viscus. As soon as we get a little sedation on board, we'll be ready to go. Just give us a second here."

"How'd you know that stuff?" the first anesthesia resident says in a toxic megawhisper.

"The instructor sends us some reading material in an e-mail before we come to the Simulator," the second anesthesia resident says, "if you check your e-mail and do the reading assignment, you'd know this stuff too."

BOX 8-45 | *Colonoscopy Considerations*

- **Patient on side**
- **Watch for oversedation**
- **Vagal responses**

"Remind me to kill you later," the first anesthesia resident says.

"Let's go with just a skosh of Versed," the second anesthesia resident says, "then intermittent propofol."

The saturation drops to 92%, the first anesthesia resident lifts the chin and encourages the patient to take a deep breath. "At least I know that, even if I don't check my e-mail. How much propofol, you figure?"

"A 2003 study showed that, on average, a colonoscopy could be performed with propofol with an average dose of just under 300 mg, so figure 15 cc is about as far as we should have to go," the second anesthesia resident says. "Alternatively, we could do the traditional Versed/fentanyl route, with doses around 7 mg of Versed and about 2 cc (about 100 µg) of fentanyl."

"Well aren't you just a font of gastroenterologic pharmacologic wizardry today," the first anesthesia resident says. "I suppose that was in the...."

"No," the second anesthesia resident interrupts, "I looked that up myself."

"Remind me to kill you slowly and horribly later," the first anesthesia resident says. "I want to hear you scream and watch you struggle."

"Everything OK up there?" the GI fellow asks.

"Couldn't be better!" the first anesthesia resident says, "Patient's doing fine, and we're just like two peas in a pod up here!"

The pulse oximeter suddenly slows, hitting a rate of 29, the blood pressure cycles, but isn't saying anything yet.

"Oh," the patient groans, "I'm feeling sick. I don't feel so good."

The first resident grabs a syringe of atropine, "Symptomatic bradycardia, let's go with atropine 0.4 mg."

Atropine goes in, heart rate returns to normal.

"How you doing, sir?" the first anesthesia resident asks.

"Better, better," the patient says.

Finishing up the GI study, the fellow says, "All done here," then he pulls the scope out.

"That's all folks!" the overhead intercom says.

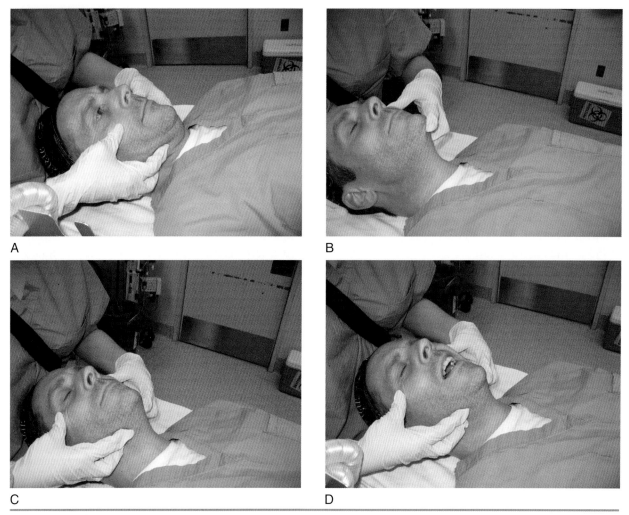

A   B

C   D

FIGURE 8–69   Chin lift, chin lift, chin lift. Simple technique but a real life saver. Use two hands if you have to. Note that doing this on a fully awake person can be a tad uncomfortable. When a patient is in laryngospasm, pulling up on that jaw may not really "break" the laryngospasm, but it may cause so much pain that the patient catapults himself right out of stage II (sort of asleep) to stage 0 (a level that does not even exist, but it means you're really awake).

Clinical lessons learned from scenario 22

Debriefing. Rain pounds the windows of the debriefing room.

"Fool, this cold night will turn us all to fools and madmen," the GI fellow says.

"Who said that?" the first anesthesia resident asks.

"I just did."

"No, who said it . . . you know. . . ."

"Oh, Shakespeare, in *King Lear*."

The instructor comes into the room and tosses down an article on sedation for colonoscopy.

"Uh," turning to the first anesthesia resident, "did you check your e-mail and do the assigned reading?"

"Um, the short answer to that would be, well, no," the first anesthesia resident admits.

"Might I go on record as saying that *reading stuff* has been the basis of education since the invention of writing, some 5000 years ago?" the instructor states.

"It's hard to disagree with that," the first anesthesia resident says. "In the Simulator, isn't the patient supposed to die or something? We saw a vagal response, we sedated him some, but we, you know, I thought the Simulator always went to a code and a disaster and the end of life as we know it."

"Good question," the instructor says. "It's good to know you are still capable of *thinking*, even if you seem to have lost the art of *reading*."

The resident shrivels into his chair.

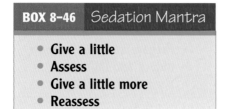

BOX 8-46 Sedation Mantra

- **Give a little**
- **Assess**
- **Give a little more**
- **Reassess**

"No, the Simulator is not just *the death machine*. The Simulator is a place to learn something, pure and simple," the instructor explains. "And a lot of you are going to go out into the world and do MAC cases, sedation in colonoscopy suites and such. And you have to know how to do these cases just like you have to do the big "mondo" killer thoracic cases. And one place to learn safely is here in the Simulator.

"Let's play the DVD."

The DVD rolls until the hissing exchange between the anesthesia residents.

"What were you thinking when goody-two-shoes here could quote chapter and verse on the doses of sedation," the instructor asks.

"Truth to tell," the first anesthesia resident says, "I wish I had that stuff down too. I mean, you're going into this blind and kind of thinking, 'Well, I'll give a little sedation and see what happens'—that's what you usually do. But it does make sense to have a little science behind your decision making."

"So in this era of 'evidence-based medicine' it really does make sense to look at the, well, the 'evidence,' right?" the instructor asks.

"True," the second anesthesia resident says, "but still the mantra of sedation is the same. Give some, assess, give some, assess, then react to changes. My learned confrere may not have checked his e-mail and may not have jumped into the literature, but he lifted the chin when the saturation went down, kept talking to the patient to make sure he was still breathing, and reacted quickly when the patient developed symptomatic bradycardia."

"He did good medicine," the instructor says.

"Yep," the second anesthesia resident says.

"That's all I'd want from the anesthesiologist in my colonoscopy suite," the GI fellow adds.

"Well then," the instructor says as he walks to the rain-battered windows, "I guess we'll just have to let the resident live."

Summary. As the instructor said, every scenario in the Simulator does not have to be a 100 megaton nuclear warhead explosion. The Simulator is a great place for

any lesson, even a review of MAC procedures. When combined with a partial task trainer—here, the colonoscopy Simulator—you can even get in some interdisciplinary training and communication.

Evidence-based medicine is out there for a reason, and no practitioner should get lax about "keeping up." If you're going to be doing a lot of work in a GI suite, then read the latest. Propofol works fine for sedation, as do Versed and fentanyl. As with any other sedation technique, vigilance is the key, so keep assessing the patient's breathing! Remember, the symbol for the American Society of Anesthesiologists is the lighthouse, always sweeping its light around, ever vigilant.

Complications of colonoscopy are rare, but hemodynamic derangements, particularly vagal responses to all the bowel inflation, are a threat. Keep your eyes peeled for bowel perforation (incidence 0.1% to 0.3%).

And keep eating your shredded wheat and bran muffins!

SCENARIO 23. **Shortcuts and shortfalls with the anesthesia machine**

It's medical student day in the Simulator. The instructor can spot them as they come in. The students look as if their mothers had just scrubbed their faces with a hot wash rag. Red, flushed, beaming, curious. Not yet jaded by a cruel and uncaring world.

Hate to maim the little monsters at such a tender age, the instructor thinks to herself.

"Cool!"

"Wow, this is great!"

"Is this where we do the simulations? Look at this stuff!"

Med students are easy to impress. The instructor thinks back to the time she bought pizza for the

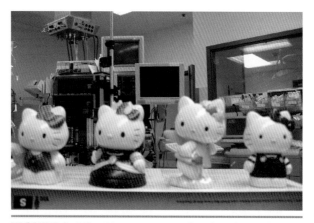

FIGURE 8-70 Oh yippee, it's med student day in the Simulator! Ah, the first blush of youth.

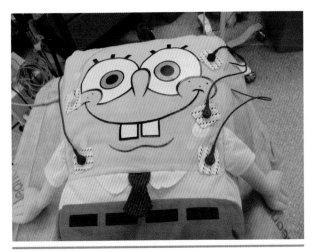

FIGURE 8–71 Tailor the lesson to the students. Here, Sponge Bob is happy to show the students where to put the EKG electrodes. "Green and white, on the right, Christmas colors down."

medical students who were with her on a call night. Near deity status—and all for the price of one large sausage and pepperoni, thick crust.

If only everyone were so easy to charm!

"OK, what we're going to do today is the most basic, basic, basic induction," the instructor explains. "We'll set up the room and go through what we do to make a person go from the land of the awake to the land of the anesthetized, OK?"

"Cool!"

"Yeah, do we get to give the drugs ourselves? Great!"

"Oh man, we should do this every day!"

God Almighty, the instructor thinks, life should be this good *all* the time. I better not buy them lunch, they'll erect a statue in my honor in front of the med school.

They go through a machine check, detailing how to ventilate the patient using the bag and mask. Using the mnemonic MSMADE, they get ready to go.

Machine, suction, monitors, anesthetics, drugs, emergency meds.

"Let's do an induction," the instructor says, "and each of you will get to do it."

It takes a little while to get the sequence down, but after a half hour the students catch on.

Greet the patient, check the consent, make sure you're doing the right thing to the right person.

Apply monitors—EKG, blood pressure cuff, pulse oximeter.

Secure the patient's arms with arm straps.

Preoxygenate
Sedate.
Double check that everything is ready.
Give induction agent.
Take over breathing for the patient.
Once you can adequately ventilate, give a paralytic agent.
Intubate.
Check tube position.
Hook up to the ventilator.
Check vital signs, then start anesthetics.

"Hey," the instructor says, "you guys are great. Way smarter than when I went to med school a thousand years ago."

The students nearly bust their buttons.

This love fest is getting a little treacly for the instructor—time to shake it up a bit. But how to do this without crushing their budding egos?

"I'm going to bring you all into the control room," the instructor explains, "all except one, and we're going to see what happens when we take shortcuts."

Good, that's the way to go, the instructor thinks. I'll enlist them to make one mistake on purpose. That'll make the point but won't snap their egos during these delicate formative years. They'll have plenty of opportunity for failure, humiliation, and degradation during their residency years.

Shortcut #1: Failure to check the machine.

The medical student goes into the room, hooks the patient up to the monitors, induces, and tries to mask-ventilate the patient. No go! A plastic wrapper is still around one of the Baralyme (CO_2 absorber) containers, making it impossible to move air through the system. Now the patient is apneic, but there is no way to move air.

"Call a code!" the medical student yells. She figures that a code will get a team there that can find a way to breathe for the patient. Good thinking! A code team will bring an Ambu-bag, and that is just what you need.

Shortcut #2: Failure to make sure suction is ready to go.

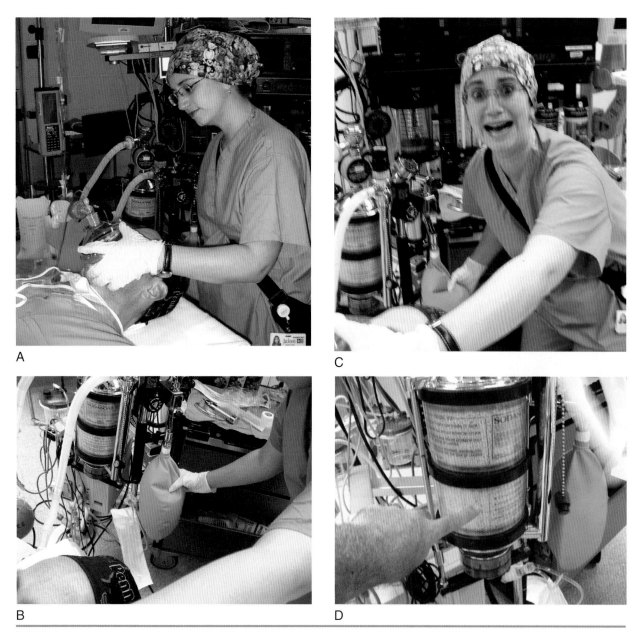

FIGURE 8-72 A snappy little scenario. The resident attempts to mask and can't ventilate. What happened? The plastic wrapper is still around the Baralyme, and the circuit is thus "plugged." As always, in the Simulator you can sabotage the equipment and put the "patient at risk" without actually putting anybody at risk.

This medical student checks the machine, but at induction the patient vomits. (You *can* make a mannequin vomit, but it's messy, takes a long time to set up and clean up, and you worry that the liquid might seep down into the delicate electronic workings around the neck, so most Simulator people just make retching noises through the mannequin speakers and tell the participants to 'act like emesis is there'.)

Reaching for the suction, the medical student discovers that although the suction works the tubing is wound around a Bovie. When he tries to put the Yankaur into the patient's mouth, it won't reach.

"Hey, free up that suction tubing!" the medical student shouts at the circulating nurse (a secretary at the Simulation Center who functions as "anyone and everyone" in the scenarios). Another good move.

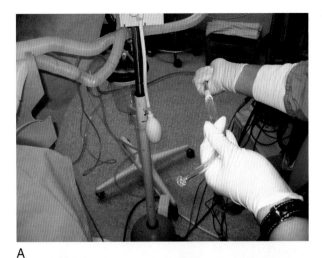

A

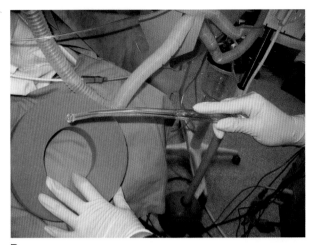

B

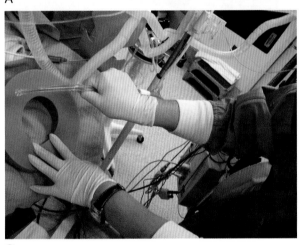

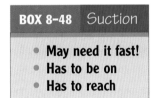

C

FIGURE 8–73 Damn, the suction is too short, or wrapped around something, or who knows what. Bottom line—*the damned thing can't reach*. Even this *simplest* of problems can lead to the most *complex* of disasters.

BOX 8-48 Suction
• **May need it fast!**
• **Has to be on**
• **Has to reach**

BOX 8-49 Preoxygenate
• **Don't skip this, ever**
• **Each induction is a "plunge into the unknown"**
• **Never know when difficulty may arise**

Damn, these med students *are* clever. Maybe there is hope for the future.

Shortcut #3: Failure to preoxygenate.

Into the room, monitors on, off to sleep. Lo and behold, the patient, who did not look difficult to intubate, now turns out to be unexpectedly difficult to intubate. Saturation drops rapidly to the 80% range.

Abandoning the intubation, the med student reverts to mask ventilation, and the saturation rises to the mid 90s.

"Um," the medical student says, "get a tracheostomy kit!"

Instead, the instructor rolls in with a fiberoptic cart. "No need to cut quite yet, let's see if we can get it with this."

The session ends with each of the med students looking through the scope as they intubate with the fiberoptic. When the instructor wraps things up, the students are beside themselves with separation anxiety and grief. They never want to stop.

"Don't worry," the instructor assuages them, "we have to do a debriefing session before you go."

Like happy Golden Retriever puppies the med students tumble into the debriefing room.

Clinical lessons learned from scenario 23

Debriefing. "Cool!"

"Wow!"

"Nice conference room!"

Rolling her eyes, the instructor thinks, "Was I *ever* this way? Will I ever *get back to being this way*, or is the Age of Innocence lost forever in my world-weary soul?"

On the screen, the instructor puts up a slide, a flight path drawing of a plane attempting to land in Dubrovnik, Croatia on April 3, 1996.

"Let's talk about the shortcuts we did in the OR," the instructor says. "And then we'll talk about how shortcuts affected this flight."

"What was that thing with the machine?" the first medical student asks. "How come I couldn't ventilate the guy?"

"The soda lime absorber needs to be changed out periodically," the instructor explains. "Techs may come in the room, after you've checked the machine, and they'll change out that absorber. If they don't take the plastic covering off the absorber, it's just like having a plug in the middle of your system, and you can't move air."

"The techs shouldn't do that, though, should they?" the med student asks.

"No" the instructor says, "they shouldn't, but the fact is they sometimes do. That's why you have to always check that machine again—at least make sure you can move air through the system each time you are about to take over a patient's breathing. Let's say you do forget, and something is wrong with the machine, your best bet is to take the machine out of the equation entirely. Just get an Ambu-bag and an oxygen cylinder."

"How about that suction thing?" the second medical student asks.

"You tell me," the instructor bounces the question back.

"Well, I knew the suction was on, but I didn't do a 'test run'. I didn't reach it over and make sure I could actually stick it in the patient's mouth. I guess it's better to practice it beforehand, before you need it, rather than when badness happens, huh?"

"You got it!" the instructor encourages. (God, rein it in, she thinks, I'm sounding like a cheerleader.)

"Now let's look at the preoxygenation shortcut, what's the big mistake there?"

"In case you get in trouble, you want your reserve tanks filled up," the third medical student states. "Just like scuba diving. Fill the tanks all the way because you never know when you might need extra time under water."

"That's it," the instructor explains. "Full preoxygenation gives you about an extra minute and a half of time before you desaturate if you get in trouble. So, for example, a crummy 'Take a few breaths' preoxygenation *will* help you. But a full 3 minutes of complete lung denitrogenation will help you *more*. And because trouble doesn't ring a bell, you want to always be prepared for unexpected trouble.

"Let's look to aviation—we do that a lot in the Simulator—to see about this whole shortcut business," the instructor explains. She then details the flight that killed Commerce Secretary Ronald Brown and 34 other people in 1996. Shortcuts in the safety realm pile up in the retelling.

> Neither pilot had ever flown into Dubrovnik before. Dubrovnik sits on a narrow strip of flat land with mountains to the north and northwest. Even a casual glance by a nonaviator would reveal the danger of such an airport. But that's OK, let's just go ahead.
>
> The former Yugoslavia was now split into warring factions, with certain air corridors "off limits" and dangerous. This might not have been the country to fly into. But that's OK, let's just go ahead.
>
> During this whirlwind political and economic tour, Ronald Brown was making many stops, placing a lot of pressure on the crew to keep to a tight schedule. But that's OK, let's just go ahead.
>
> Visibility was poor that day, with rain and fog shrouding the mountains. But that's OK. . . .
>
> The nondirectional navigation beacon at Dubrovnik airport did not meet guidelines from the International Civil Aviation Organization. But no one bothered to check that.
>
> The crew needed two directional devices (called ADFs) on board to make an accurate instrument approach to the airport. They only had one on board. But that's OK. . . .

"Don't kid yourself," the instructor says, "when you go into anesthesia, you will be under a lot of pressure to do shortcuts yourself. Anything to get the cases going, right? 'Come on, don't check the machine again, let's go!'"

Back to the 1996 plane flight.

Shortcut, shortcut, shortcut. Maybe we could plan this trip better, but let's just do a shortcut and go ahead. Maybe we should consider the weather or the pressure on the crew—nah, let's just skip those considerations and go ahead. Maybe we should check out what kind of equipment the airport has, for that matter, what kind of equipment the *airplane* has. No, forget it, let's just get going.

So with all these shortcuts "on board," so to speak, Air Force CT-43A (a Boeing 737) plane flew just a *few degrees off the correct bearing*. No big deal, right? Heading 119 degrees instead of 110 degrees.

The airport runway was at 110 degrees.

A 2200 foot mountain was at 119 degrees.

The plane did the ultimate shortcut, landing earlier than expected. Only this landing was nose first at 133 knots right into the side of the mountain.

Summary. Discipline in anesthesia means going over the basics and checking all your stuff each and every time. This "beginner's Simulation" with medical students merits attention, even from experienced anesthesia people.

Check that machine, you never know when it will malfunction. You don't want to "find out something's wrong" when the patient is under anesthesia and apneic.

Check the suction, do a test run. Patients can vomit and aspirate in a split second, and you will need to get that suction there just as fast. Make sure the darned thing reaches!

Drugs lined up and labeled, patient well preoxygenated—each time, every time. The siren song of "shortcut" is tempting, but it can lead you to disaster—so plug your ears and don't listen to it!

The aviation examples are out there for us to study—that's why they fit so well into simulation education. Cockiness and pushing ahead without adequate planning or adequate equipment drives planes into mountainsides. Cockiness and pushing ahead without planning or adequate equipment drives anesthesiologists into "mountainsides" as well.

BOX 8–50	Short Cuts

- **Bad habit**
- **One fine day this will bite your head off**

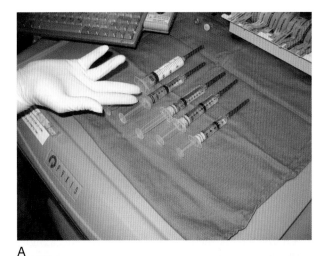

A

B

FIGURE 8–74   Neat, neat, neat. Keep the drugs all nice and neat (**A**). If you have a mess (**B**), you won't be able to find the drug you need in a hurry.

SCENARIO 24. **Heartbreak during a heart transplant**

"The donor's in Baltimore," the instructor says, "but they want you to take the recipient in the room now, flying time is about an hour and a half."

The two cardiac anesthesia fellows ask the obvious question, "What are we transplanting?"

"A heart," the instructor says. "First you'll be talking to the patient in the standardized patient room, then we'll go to the OR.

In the standardized patient room, a patient (medical student coached in what to say) is sitting bolt upright on a gurney, nasal oxygen in place, and an infusion pump on an IV stand beside the patient. The pump is infusing into his arm. There are all kinds of decorations hanging off the IV pump—Mardi Gras beads and such.

Brightening visibly when the doctors enter the room, the patient says, "Is it good? Have they looked at the heart yet?"

The two fellows look at each other, "Don't think they've seen it yet."

"Three times I've gotten the call, twice I go to the OR," the patient says, "and, you know, no good. You guys want some beads?" She reaches for the IV pole and hands them each a Mardi Gras necklace.

"Let's party!" she says.

After their anesthetic history and physical, the fellows explain the procedure, go over the risks, round up the usual suspects.

Fellow #1 says, "We're on your side here. This should be the start of a new life for you."

"Man, you guys just don't know," the patient says. "You know, you have a baby, happiest day of your life, then you just feel so run down afterward, you figure, you know, you figure you're supposed to be run down after you have a baby, right?

"I can still remember when the echo tech put that thing on me and he says, 'Oh shit.' And I'm going, 'What?' and he says, 'I'm not supposed to tell you this, but you got it, lady, you got a cardiomyopathy.' And here I am. Got my little friend here," she points to the infusion pump—milrinone. "My sister's watching the baby. I see him every now and then, but I'm just too tired, I mean, I get short of breath just looking at him."

"Hope that heart's good," she says, and shakes their hands.

Over to the operating room.

The mannequin's speakers relay the same voice as from the standardized patient room.

"Can you guys pray with me before we go to sleep?" she asks.

She has all her monitors on, including a line and Swan-Ganz catheter.

The fellows look at each other, "Sure."

"Jesus, it is into thy hands that I hand myself, please guide the hands of these good doctors, as they are the instruments of thy will, amen," she prays.

"Amen," the fellows say.

On the monitor, the numbers tell the story of a bad heart—blood pressure 90/60, PA 70/45. Systemic and pulmonary pressures are almost the same.

"Keep the milrinone going?" fellow #2 asks.

"Yeah," fellow #1 says, "you induce, I'll take the airway."

Induction—the fellow gives ketamine and Sux, keeps a syringe of epinephrine, $8\,\mu g/cc$ in his hand in case she crashes.

Blood pressure dips a little, then goes back to baseline. The heart rate goes from its baseline 115 to 125.

"You want to slow that heart rate down?" fellow #2 asks.

"No way, not on your life," fellow #1 says. "That heart must be awful, if we slow it down at all, kaboom, she'll crash and burn."

The surgeons drape and start going.

"We ready to cross clamp?" the surgeon asks. (Surgery in the Simulator can go in fast motion, moving right ahead to the next "decision point.")

The first cardiac fellow says, "Wait, we have to get word from the donor team. Where's the heart?"

"Haven't heard yet, better wait," the second cardiac fellow says. "Wait a minute, we better pull that Swan back."

The fellow pulls the Swan-Ganz catheter back to the CVP. If they wouldn't, then there'd be a nasty surprise when the surgeons cut the heart out. There would be a severed Swan-Ganz catheter in the middle of it!

"We better start some nitric oxide," the first cardiac fellow says, "We have some nasty PA hypertension here."

A "dummy" nitric oxide container is brought in the room. Nitric oxide costs thousands of dollars to use, so actually using it in the Simulator is prohibitive. But the fellows set up the complicated gadgetry to deliver this potent inhaled pulmonary vasodilator.

BOX 8–51	*Special and Unexpected Patient Requests*

- **Within reason, honor them**
- **Look at things from the patient's point of view**
- **You'd be scared too**

BOX 8–52	*Inducing in a Transplant*

- **Don't wait too long—increase organ's ischemic time**
- **Don't go too soon—make sure the organ is good**

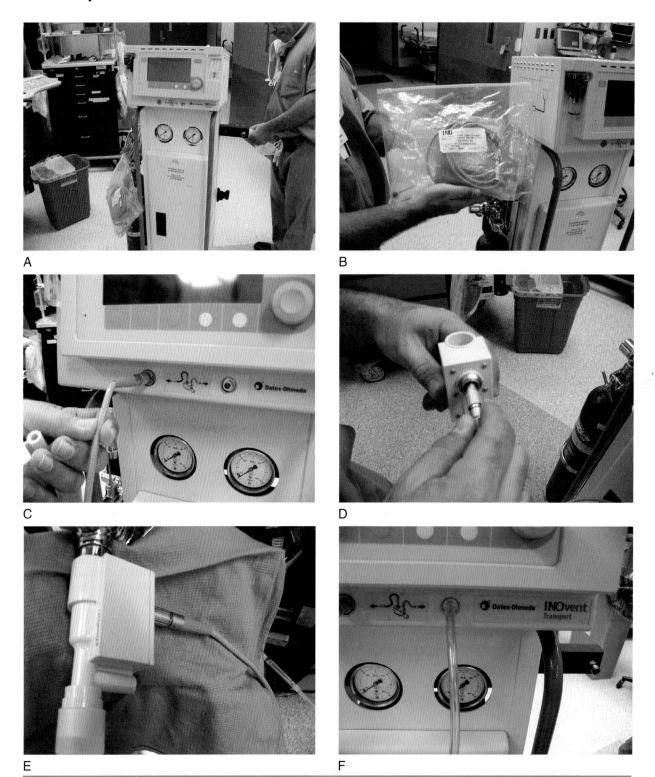

FIGURE 8-75 This shows the complete setup of the NO machine. Be sure and do this before you have to. The connections are complex, and you don't want to be figuring this out in the middle of the night during a lung transplant with the patient dying of pulmonary hypertension right in front of your eyes.

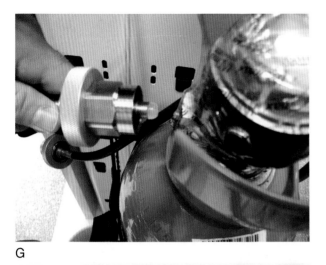

G

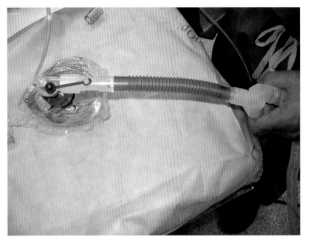

H

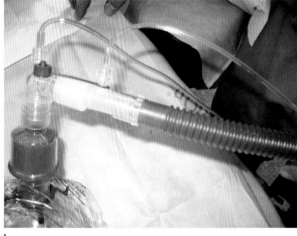

I

FIGURE 8-75 cont'd

The surgeons (two Simulator Center secretaries) are waiting.

Just then, the telephone rings. Picking it up, the second cardiac fellow says, "Hello."

A voice on the phone says, "Wake her up, there'll be no transplant tonight."

"What?" the cardiac fellow doesn't believe it.

"The plane from Baltimore went down."

Overhead, "Simulation's over."

Clinical lessons learned from scenario 24

Debriefing. Both cardiac fellows are visibly shaken in the debriefing room.

"Man, that is unfair," the first one says. "I mean no way. That just does not happen."

"How could, I mean, would they let you get that far, well, I guess you would," the second fellow says, "but still."

The patient rolls into the debriefing room, still pushing the merrily decorated IV pole, and sits at the debriefing table.

"What would you say to her right now?" the instructor asks.

Looking down at the table, neither fellow says a thing.

"Is this so far-fetched?" the instructor asks.

Turning sideways, so he doesn't have to face the patient, the first fellow says, "You're stuck between a rock and a hard place here. You want to keep ischemic time for the donated heart to a minimum. So you have to get the recipient in the room and get going early, especially if it's not a virgin chest. I mean, if this woman has had earlier heart operations, the surgeons will have to take down all the scarring and such and that takes a while. If we wait until the new heart has actually arrived and *then* start opening, the donated heart sits there, ischemic. So we can't do that."

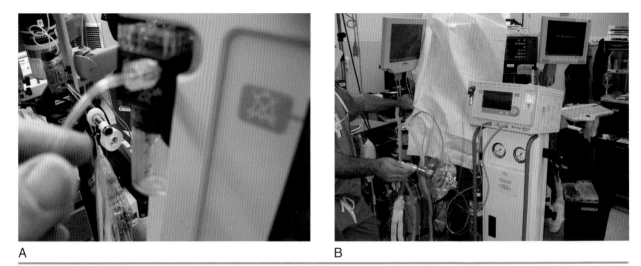

A   B

FIGURE 8–76   This stuff is *expensive*! Does it work? Well, not all the time. It is an attempt at that magic bullet that drops pulmonary pressures but doesn't touch systemic pressures. If only it did always work. If you find yourself "going to nitric oxide," you're in for a long night.

"And planes do go down," the instructor says. "Ambulances carrying organs get into wrecks just like regular cars get into wrecks, right?"

"I guess," the second fellow says.

"So then, this could happen, right?" the instructor asks.

Neither fellow can deny that.

"So then, here she is, here's the patient, what do you say to her?" the instructor asks.

"Wouldn't the surgeon have to . . . you know . . . do the talking?" the first fellow asks.

"She prayed with you," the instructor says, "and she asked to talk to you."

"God," the fellows say.

"Funny you should mention that," the instructor says.

The patient breaks the ice, "I heard I didn't get the heart."

Both fellows nod with the pursed lips that say, "Yep."

"What happened?"

Taking a clinical tack, the first fellow lays it out in sequence, "From our standpoint, we got all ready, then had you go off to sleep. We gave you special medications that don't depress your heart much, what with it being so weak and all. And we kept your milrinone going."

She taps the infusion pump, "My little friend here."

"Right, your little friend there. And we started an inhaled drug, called nitric oxide, to try to make the pressures in your lungs go down."

"Can't I breathe that now? Like an asthma inhaler or something?" she asks.

"Well, no," the second fellow picks up. "That only works if you breathe it in all the time, like when you're on a ventilator and have a breathing tube in."

"OK," she says, "then what happened."

"Well," fellow #2 keeps going, "we had to get you off to sleep so the surgeons would have enough time to . . . to get where they're going and so the donated heart would have the least time, um, the least time before it would go into you."

"Who gave me their heart?" the patient asks. "That's quite a gift you know."

"Oh," the fellows look at each other, "that we don't know."

There's a bit of an awkward silence as the whole table tries to rearrange their thoughts.

"Well," the first fellow starts again, "we had you as good as we could get you, and the whole system was working, when we found out the plane from . . . from the where the donor was didn't make it. It went down. So the heart was on board."

"A lot of hearts were on board," the patient says. "There were a whole lot of hearts on board that plane."

"Yeah," the first fellow says, "yeah, I guess there were."

Summary. Transplants are emotional events, often lost as we grumble in the middle of the night. "Another transplant at 2 a.m., damnation!"

We, face it, view the patients as a set of variables that we try to manage just right. And that is all well and good. Heart transplant patients have poor cardiac function, requiring delicate induction, maintenance of hemodynamics, and exotic maneuvers such as nitric oxide. The fellows did all that and did it well.

Transplants require timing and coordination, thank God for cell phones with a national reach! And you have to balance a short ischemic time ("Get the recipient in the room!") with practical considerations ("You can't have the recipient under anesthesia for 5 hours just waiting for the organ to arrive.").

Then look at things from the patient's point of view. This is a life-saving and life-changing event for them. This isn't just a "2 a.m. pain in the ass." This is a new life! Transplant recipients tend to know the score, know their disease, and know the numbers. A heart transplant candidate knows that death is sitting in the corner, marking time and tapping his watch. When that beeper goes off or the call comes, their hopes go through the roof. And rightfully so. You would feel the same!

They've often ended up on constant infusions of inotropes—the patient's "little friend." And you'll see them making the best of their situation—decorating the IV pole they're chained to, getting to know all the staff, reading up on all the medications. It's a whole world, this "waiting for the transplant" world.

No surprise, then, that patients take a proprietary interest in you, more so than in other cases. Their strong religious feelings may sustain them, and they may want to share those with you, in the way of a prayer.

So this scenario encompassed all this—the physiologic challenges of the heart transplant, plus the heavy emotional overlay of this procedure. And now this twist, the patient goes under anesthesia expecting to wake up with a new heart and wakes up with the old one in place, the infusion pump still attached, and the tragic story of the donor procurement team to deal with.

How do you manage this near-impossible scenario? Is there a way to "do this right"?

Say a prayer.

SCENARIO 25. **Don't delay! Burns and airways**
Two anesthesia interns are in the Simulator. They sniff the air.

"Why does it smell like barbeque in here?" the first anesthesia intern asks.

The instructor had brought in barbeque for two reasons, for lunch and to make a point.

"There's a patient in the emergency room," the instructor says, "He was trying to open a barrel of flammable liquid and he couldn't pry it off."

"What did he do?" the second intern asks.

"He couldn't find a crowbar, so he opened it with a blow torch."

"Bad move," the first intern says.

"You could say that," the instructor answers.

The two interns go into the emergency room. A Laerdal Sim man is on the gurney, black powder is around his face. From his speakers, the patient says, "Listen, I know that wasn't the brightest maneuver, but I'm feeling fine. How about some salve or something, then I'm out of here. I don't got any insurance and I can't pay for none of this."

The monitor shows sinus tachycardia with a rate of 120. Oxygen saturation 95%. Blood pressure 150/90.

"Let's put him on oxygen," the first intern tells the ER nurse. "Five liters mask."

"Any chart on this guy?" the second intern asks. The ER nurse hands him a chart. Both look it over.

"Says here you're on some medications sir?" the first intern says, "What do you take again?"

The patient says, his voice a little higher now, "I take some water pill for blood pressure."

"OK, OK," the interns keep looking over the chart. "You had a knee scope?"

His voice continues to creep upward in tone, "Yeah, I twisted it playing softball."

Saturation is now 99%.

"Hey, he's got smoke all around his nose, shouldn't we intubate him?" the second intern says.

"His sat's 99%," the first one says. "Feeling OK sir?"

No response.

"Sir?"

Nothing.

"Get me the Ambu-bag," the first intern tells the ER nurse. "And get me the intubation kit. You're right, we should intubate him."

With Ambu-bag in hand, the first intern attempts to mask—no air moves. Saturation drops to 90% and keeps going down.

In goes the laryngoscope, everything is swollen and intubation is impossible. Saturation is unobtainable, and multifocal ectopy starts.

"Gimme an LMA," the second intern says, "and call for help."

Overhead, the call goes out, "Any anesthesiologist to the ER *stat*."

LMA goes in, nothing.

"Get me a 14 gauge angiocath, we have to do a cric!" the first intern says. "Jet ventilation, we gotta do it."

The first intern places the angiocath through the cricothyroid membrane. "OK, let's hook up!"

"Hook up what?"

"The jet ventilator!"

"What jet ventilator?"

Everyone looks around. Oh yeah, there is nothing to hook up to.

"You have a cric kit?" the first intern asks the ER nurse.

"No."

"Gimme a Swan introducer kit, it'll have to do," the first intern shouts.

He tears open the kit, puts the wire through the 14 gauge, pulls out the angiocath, cuts a hole, then slides a 4.0 uncuffed into the trachea (the first thing someone hands him) and hooks up oxygen.

The sat rises and the ectopy goes away.

"All over but the screaming," the instructor says over the intercom.

Clinical lessons learned from scenario 25

Debriefing. The interns look wind-blown, as if they just finished a long interstate drive with a convertible.

"OK guys," the instructor starts, "tell me how you think it went."

"Look," the first one says, "just go ahead and call the unemployment office. Tell them to save two places in line."

"We blew it," the second intern says. "We forgot the prime rule of burns, secure the airway right away, don't wait until you lose it because then you're screwed every which way but loose."

"That barbeque should have been a tip," the first intern says. "As soon as we smelled that charred flesh, we should have known. You even had the smoke around his nose."

"Right, well," the instructor says, "there's a reason all this stuff is written down. Now tell me, tell me so I know *you* know, what are the indications for securing an airway right away when you have a burn victim."

"Burnt nose hair, ash around the mouth, or a history of fire in a closed space like a mobile home," the first intern said.

"Steam too," the second intern said. "steam can sneak through the cords and zap the lungs."

"Let me simplify it," the instructor says, "if there's a burn, a chemical burn even, and you *think* of intu-

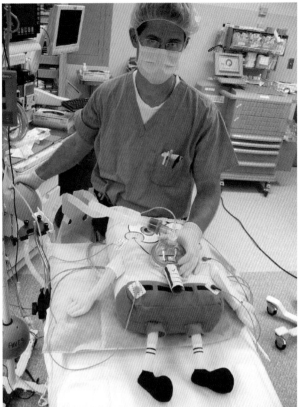

A

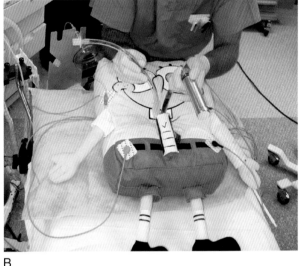

B

FIGURE 8–77 The lost airway is no joke, but we rarely practice it. Here, a resident goes through a dry run of losing an airway and then using a Swan introducer kit to secure the airway surgically. He should have been tipped off by Sponge Bob's prominent incisors that this could be a difficult airway.

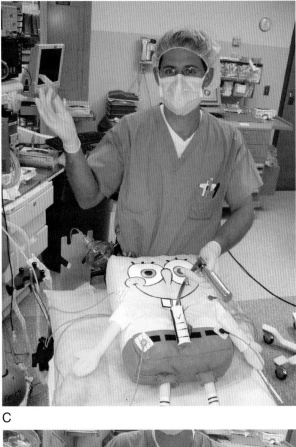

C

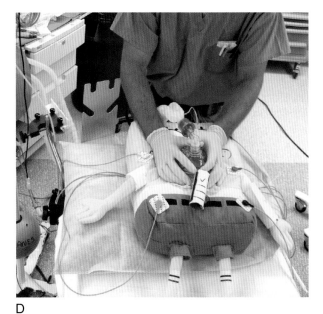

D

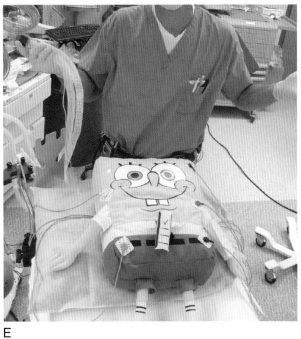

E

F

FIGURE 8-77 cont'd

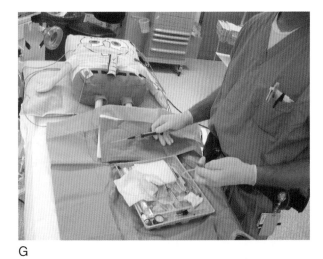

G

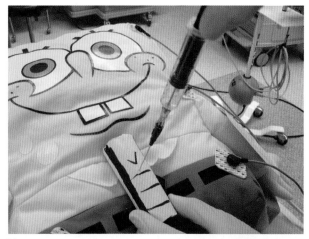

H

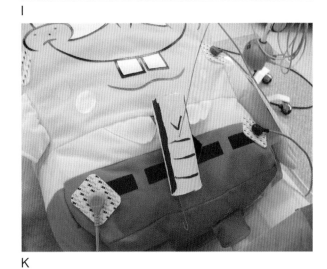

I

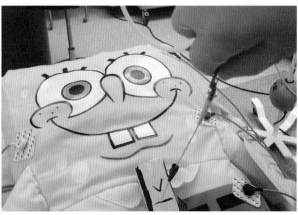

J

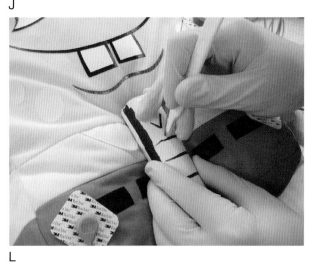

K

L

FIGURE 8–77   cont'd

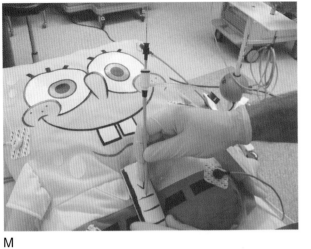

M

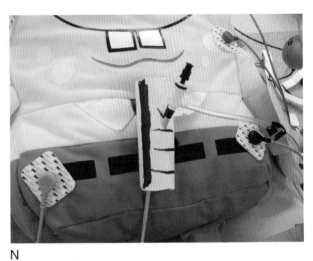

N

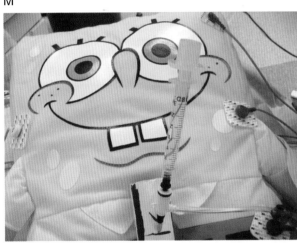

O

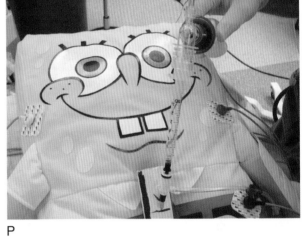

P

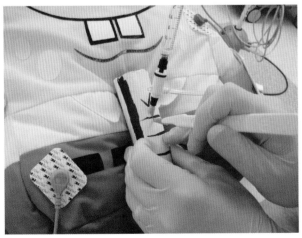

Q

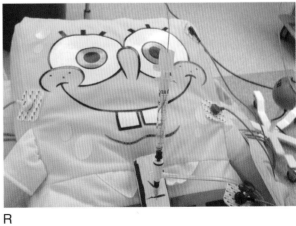

R

FIGURE 8–77 cont'd

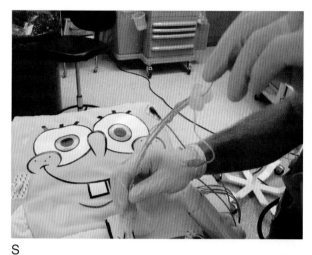

S

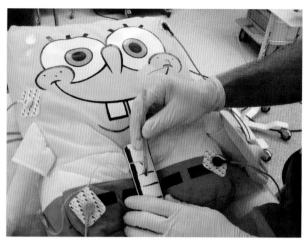

T

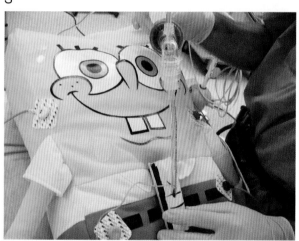

U

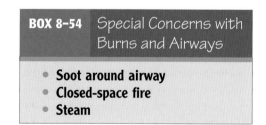

FIGURE 8–77   cont'd

BOX 8-53	Fires and Airways

- **In case of doubt, intubate**
- **Airway swells shut fast**
- **Once lost, that airway slams shut and stays shut!**

BOX 8-54	Special Concerns with Burns and Airways

- **Soot around airway**
- **Closed-space fire**
- **Steam**

bating, do it. If later on it turns out that you didn't need to, well then, the guy sits on a ventilator for a while. That's not the end of the world. But if you wait, and that airway closes off, well, that *is* the end of the world. I mean, that airway swells shut, and you have nothing, but nothing. Plus, this edematous, swollen shut airway is real friable and any instrumentation will stir up bleeding."

"What clues was he giving you?" the instructor asks.

They review the DVD. What completely escaped the residents during the scenario becomes glaringly apparent during the video replay.

"His voice keeps getting higher," the first intern says. "His voice keeps getting higher and higher and higher. His airway is closing off."

"One thing about the Simulator," the instructor says, "we can't recreate the rocking motions of the obstructed airway. We should have a way of having the abdomen stick out and the chest cave in, the classic sign of obstruction. But they just don't have that yet."

They review the cric sequence.

"Pretty good," the second intern says. "But that thing about 'what to hook to'. I guess that's a real problem."

"Yeah," the first intern says, "we're always talking about doing jet ventilation, but what am I supposed to do, carry a jet ventilator around with me?"

"Good point," the instructor says, "the actual mechanism might not be there when you need it. But you did the next best thing."

"Just think of the trachea as a big vein that has air in it instead of blood," the first intern says. "You're just putting a giant IV in a big, rigid, crunchy vein. That's the way to look at a surgical airway."

"How about doing a real trach?" the instructor asks.

"Takes too long, too bloody," the second intern says. "When you have no time, you have to go high and shallow, you have to go for the cricothyroid membrane."

Paper plates all around, and the gang starts in on the sloppy Joe barbeque sandwiches.

"Or better yet," the first intern wipes barbeque juice off his chin, "we intubate the guy right away and avoid this whole mess. God, how did we miss that?"

"Hey," the instructor forgives, "if you knew everything, you wouldn't have to do a residency. And if you knew everything, there'd be no need to pay me my fantastic academic salary."

Summary. Burns and airways—scary business. No matter how good the patient looks initially, that airway may swell shut in no time, leaving you with a surgical airway and a coding patient.

Saturation OK? Doesn't matter, that will change fast.

Patient says he/she is OK? Doesn't matter, they won't feel OK when that airway slams shut.

Always err on the side of caution when an airway is threatened. And swelling from a fire is always a threat to the airway.

Think about all the surgical airway options before you need to employ them. Here, the residents were caught short with "half a jet ventilation" setup. The catheter was in, but what to hook it up to? Fortunately, the intern kept his cool, cut an opening, and got something in there. Imperfect, yes, but capable of delivering *some* oxygen.

SCENARIO 26. **Dangerous hallways, hallway hypertension**

"OK," the instructor tells the two residents in the hallway, "you're going into a heart case, and guess what, the case is over. All you have to do is transport this guy to the ICU. What we're going to do is have you move him over to a bed and just go across the room. With all the connections to the mannequin, it's too hard to go down the hall. We'll do a 'pretend transfer' but you'll still have all the hoops to jump through for a transfer, OK?"

Done and done. The residents go into the OR and take over the case from another "resident" (a medical student who then goes into the control room and observes).

"We just finished an aortic valve replacement on this 45-year-old guy," the medical student explains.

"That's pretty young for an aortic valve," the first resident says.

"He had a bicuspid aortic valve," the student explains. "They get stenotic pretty early."

He goes on, "My wife's having triplets, so I have to go right now. This guy has a good ventricle, thick walls, and no other medical problems. No allergies. I'm aiming at fast-tracking him so haven't given much in the way of narcotics. He was easy to intubate, but he's still bleeding a little. Plan to keep him intubated for just another couple of hours to see if this bleeding keeps up. If he dries up, you can extubate him in the unit. Got it?"

"What are you on?" the second resident asks.

"I just turned the Forane off. I have some nitroglycerin hanging in case you need it," the student says. Getting the thumbs up from the residents, he leaves.

"Triplets—oy, better him than me," the first resident says.

"Does that happen when you have sex three times in a row?" the second resident asks.

Shrugging, the first resident says, "How could I possibly know?"

On the monitors—SaO$_2$ 99%, arterial trace BP 140/85, P 80. The ventilator is on. A transport bed is brought in. IV bags, the NTG pump, a carrier bag—a whole tangle of lines is hanging on the IV poles.

Both residents start moving stuff over.

"Do we have a transport monitor?" the first resident asks. One is brought in (by the medical student, who functions in whatever role is needed, then goes back to the control room).

Tangling with the transport cables, the first resident cannot get the art line to zero. For three full minutes, no blood pressure is visible. The surgeon (med student

> **BOX 8-55** Hallway Hypertension
>
> - **Anesthetic wears off**
> - **You're stuck in hallway**
> - **Pressure goes through the roof**

who put on a different gown and cap and looks, amazingly, like a different person) comes in.

"Guys," he bellows, "you're killing me here. I've got a fresh aortic valve in, a fresh gash in this guy's aorta, and I want to know what the blood pressure's doing!"

"We, uh," the first resident says, "can't get this, uh. . . ."

"The hell with it," the second resident says, then reconnects to the original arterial line. BP 280/130.

"You are going to tear that aorta apart, get that blood pressure down now!" The surgeon is apoplectic.

"Whoa," the first resident says, then reaches back to the cart. There must be a syringe of something there.

The second resident turns the Forane back on.

Nitroglycerin, aha, the first resident picks up a syringe of nitroglycerin 200 μg/cc, and gives 0.5 cc.

BP 290/140.

"Get ready to open—this aorta will tear!"

Forane 5%, another 0.5 cc of nitroglycerin, then 1 cc, then another.

BP 150/60.

"Better," the surgeon says, "Don't let that blood pressure get away from you."

"Turn that Forane down," the first resident says, "we don't want to overshoot."

Forane back to 2% and then off as the blood pressure goes to 80/40.

"Oh," the second resident says. "The transducer is on the floor."

"What?" the first resident asks, then looks and sees the transducer on the floor.

"Oh God," he says, "if the transducer's on the floor, then that pressure's falsely elevated. His real pressure must be. . . ."

He lifts the transducer up to the patient's level.

BP 50/20.

"Oh man, now *I'm* going to have triplets," the first resident says, "give me some Neo!"

Fluids, neosynephrine 200 μg, and a calcium bolus, and the blood pressure normalizes.

"It's a boy!" the overhead speaker says, "and a girl, and another girl! Simulation's over!"

Clinical lessons learned from scenario 26

Debriefing. Dark clouds are rolling into the afternoon sky through the windows. Distant rumbles.

Three Beanie Babies sit in the center of the debriefing room, a blue ribbon around one, and pink ribbons around the other two.

"I trust mother and babies are doing well," the first resident asks. That gets a nod from the proud papa.

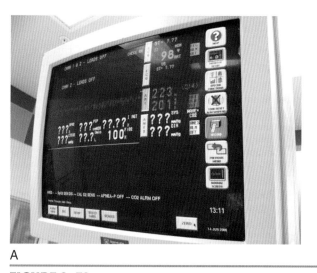

A

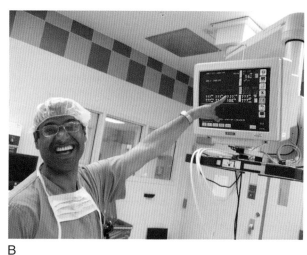

B

FIGURE 8–78 "Hey, get that pressure down, what the hell is going on here!" In the simulator, re-create reality with the screaming, abusive, throat-slashing behavior that our beloved surgery brethren sometimes display.

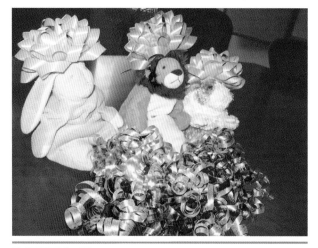

FIGURE 8–79 Hey, this explains where those triplets came from!

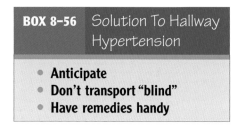

BOX 8-56	Solution To Hallway Hypertension

- **Anticipate**
- **Don't transport "blind"**
- **Have remedies handy**

"OK," the instructor opens, "let's talk about the transport monster. Let's talk about that God-awful twilight zone where disaster awaits around every corner. Tell me first, what can go wrong during *any* transport?"

The two residents come up with a list.

1. Extubation.
2. Line pulls out.
3. Transducer falls, disconnects, or the stopcock gets bumped.
4. Oxygen failure (empty tank or hose to Ambu-bag disconnects).
5. Hemodynamic instability.
6. Monitor failure (battery dies).
7. Getting stuck somewhere (waiting for elevator, hallway cluttered).

"You forgot my favorite one," the instructor says. After a while, the residents get it.

"Distraction," they say.

"Boy howdy, distraction," the instructor says. "During a case, you're glued to those monitors, and you're 'riding the pony' very carefully. You keep up with the volume, you titrate the medications just so,

BOX 8-57	Transport Monster

- **Tubes come out**
- **Monitors die**
- **Instability**

you respond to the slightest changes in vital signs. You are totally focused.

"Then transport comes along, and all your priorities change—don't tangle the lines, move the pump over, is the transport monitor charged, does this bed have a pole? There're a million and one things—all of them important—that pull and yank at your attention. Plus, you're pulling and yanking on things that have been in one place during the case."

"And boom, down goes the transducer," the medical student says, perhaps a little *too* helpfully. Both residents pick up Beanie Babies and throw them at the medical student.

"Hey, that's child abuse!" the med student yells.

"Let me show you a little med student abuse," the second resident says.

"Children, children," the instructor says, picking up the third Beanie Baby and hugging it, "don't make me chain you under the staircase again!"

"The transducer is a problem," the instructor brings her unruly charges under control, "and that's a thing that's easy to miss when you're looking at a hundred things. What could you have done when you first saw that sky-high pressure?"

"Feel a pulse," the first resident says. "Go back to basics and see if you really do feel a pounding pulse, telling you that, yeah, the pressure is nearly 300."

"Ding!" the instructor says. "Remember in all this high-tech jumble that the best monitor is still *you*. There's no electricity, no battery failure, no misplaced transducer between you and your fingertips, or you and your eyes. A 'monitor' is something that 'looks at' something. That's the original meaning of the word. So use *yourself*, your powers of observation, as the first line of defense for your patient."

BOX 8-58	Monitors

- **Battery operated? They will fail**
- **Eyes? Never fail**
- **Best monitor? Eyes**

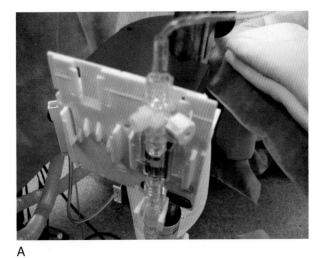

A

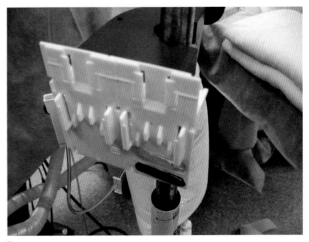

B

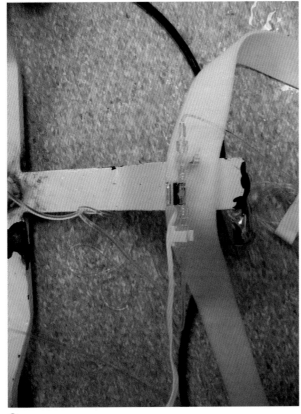

C

FIGURE 8-80 Aha, the old transducer on the floor trick. This creates a falsely high pressure reading—which ties in with the general principle: Don't accept any reading at face value. Realize that any electronic signal is just that, an electronic signal, at one step removed from reality. So double check things—electrodes come loose, transducers fall, oximetric Swans need to be re-zeroed.

"Chest rise, color, pulse," the first resident says. "If you've got that, you've got something."

A lightning strike hits just outside the building, and the lights flicker in the debriefing room.

Everyone stops for a second; then the resident lifts the Beanie Baby and looks at it. He flips over the name tag.

"Thunder baby?" the medical student asks. "Thor baby?"

The instructor redirects traffic, "What is the special concern here, at the end of an aortic valve replacement?"

"If this guy had aortic stenosis," the second resident says, "his ventricular walls are thick. So when the aortic obstruction is taken away, the stenotic valve is taken out of the way, the patient can generate tremendous pressures—high blood pressures that hit right at the surgical site, the aortotomy, the cut in the aorta. That surgeon was right, that aorta *was* going to blow if the blood pressure stayed that high."

"So what do you do about that?" the instructor asks.

"Well," the first resident says, "you have to make more preparations for preventing 'hallway hypertension'. If you just keep the anesthetic vapor going to right until the end of the case, when you leave the room you're going to get in trouble. The vapor comes off as the patient is transported, and the blood pressure rises, rises, rises. By the time you get to the ICU, the blood pressure is through the roof."

"Options?" the instructor asks. Another list appears on the white board.

1. Turn down vapors; replace with narcotics.
2. Start dexmedetomidine drip; get to a steady state.
3. Start propofol drip and use that as a "hallway TIVA."
4. Have an effective antihypertensive on board, such as Cardene or Nipride.
5. Keep a few syringes handy (propofol, NTG, Cardene) in case the blood pressure gets out of control and you need bolus help.

"And don't be afraid to get an extra hand in there to help you out," the first resident says. "One person watches the monitors only while the other moves over the lines and pumps and stuff."

"Yeah," the second resident says, picking up a Beanie Baby, "get Transport Beanie here to help you out." Then he turns to the toy and shakes it, "And don't let the stupid transducer fall on the floor!"

"Hey," the instructor says, taking away Transport Beanie, "don't do that. You'll give it 'shaken Beanie syndrome.'"

Summary. Picture transport as a multiheaded dog, with each head ready to bite you. We tend to plan our lines, our induction, our airway management; but you rarely hear someone discussing 'transport plans' for a patient. Transport is viewed as a 'given,' but this case illustrates how wrong that assumption can be.

During the case your attention is on the patient. During transport your attention is pulled in a dozen directions.

Moving something puts that 'something' at risk—endotracheal tube, central line, IV, transducer, NG tube, Foley, surgical drain. What the hand of mankind placed *into* the patient, the hand of transportkind can pull *out of* the patient.

Don't let yourself fly blind if the transport monitor is giving you trouble. Go back to the "old reliables" until the better monitor can be brought into the room. In a case with real hemodynamic "swing potential," this is doubly true.

Plan ahead to prevent "hallway hypertension." When vapors come off, the pressure rises. Do you have something to replace the vapors? Sedative? Antihypertensive? If not, then you are in for an unpleasant surprise as you wind down the hallway.

Keep an eye on transducer levels. Lift a transducer, and the apparent blood pressure drops. Drop a transducer, and the apparent blood pressure rises. Don't treat these "phantom blood pressures"—make sure you have the accurate number before you act.

When all else fails (and it will), go with your own senses and get your hand on that pulse.

And never shake a Beanie Baby.

SCENARIO 27. | Presto-chango with the syringes

"Mix and match today," the instructor says. "We'll have a partial-task trainer, an arterial line practice device, to the left of the METI simulator mannequin. Put the art line in, and then we'll start the case, all right?"

Three anesthesia residents are in the scenario. Two will do the scenario in the OR while the third sits in the control room. The control room resident "sees things from the instructor's viewpoint" and gets a different take on the lesson.

The first resident asks, "So I sort of pretend this art line device is the actual patient?"

"Right," the instructor clarifies, "then once it's in, proceed with the case."

This combination of partial-task trainer plus Simulator mannequin gives residents both a hands-on task scenario (the art line) and an anesthesia scenario (the mannequin). Plus, it mimics real life because you often put in an arterial line before you start a case.

"I drew up the meds," the instructor says. "Go ahead and sedate this patient as you would a regular patient before the case starts."

Instructor and control-room resident leave the OR and go to the control room. They watch things through the one-way mirror.

A senior resident and a junior resident are left in the operating room. "Go ahead and do the art line," the senior says.

"I've only done a couple," the junior says. "Any tips?"

"Yeah, here," the senior says. "First make a good wrist roll and make sure the hand is bent back. You want as straight a shot as possible. Think of a plane flying into the Holland Tunnel. If you come in at a sharp angle, you won't go very far in the tunnel. If you come in at a flat, flat angle, and you don't have to hop up an over anything, then you should be able to slide pretty far in the tunnel. That's the key to getting both the needle in and the catheter. If you don't flatten the wrist, and the thenar eminence sticks up and in your way, you'll never get that shallow angle into the artery."

Over the loudspeaker, "Don't you want to review the case before you stick this guy?"

The residents look up, "Oh yeah."

The patient is a 55-year-old man with known CAD and a long smoking history; he's now here for a carotid endarterectomy for 90% stenosis of the right carotid with symptoms of TIA. Psychiatric history: anxiety disorder.

"We better sedate him," the junior says. "He'll be awfully anxious for this arterial stick."

As if on cue, the patient speaks, "What are you guys doing? Is this going to hurt?"

He has a blood pressure cuff on—BP 160/85. EKG shows sinus rhythm of 80, and his saturation is 97%.

"Right, sir," the senior resident starts, "we need this special IV here in your wrist to watch your blood pressure real close. We'll give you a little something to help you relax and some local numbing medicine here in your wrist."

"I don't know," the patient says, "can't you put it in after I'm asleep?"

"We really need this to watch your blood pressure closely as you go off to sleep," the junior says, "here, we'll give you some medicine to help you relax."

A syringe labeled Versed sits on the anesthesia cart, the junior gives 2 mg. Then he stands by the side of the patient and gets ready to start the art line.

"No," the senior says, "try sitting down. Makes it a lot easier to do the art line. If you're standing and bending over, you end up with a sore back. If you sit, then all you're thinking about are the little muscles in your hand. Makes it a lot easier to concentrate on the line."

Sitting down, the junior says, "Got it."

"Ouch! That hurts!" the patient says.

"OK," the senior resident says. "I'll give a little pain reliever here."

He picks up a syringe labeled fentanyl and gives 0.5 cc.

In the control room, the third resident is watching the action. "Is that the syringe you told me about?" she asks. "Is that the mislabeled syringe?"

"Yep," the instructor says.

"The one with undiluted norepinephrine?"

"Yep."

"You're a real bastard, you know that?" the resident says.

"I'll take that as a compliment."

"I feel funny," the patient says. "My heart feels like it's going fast."

Both residents are hunched over the arterial line.

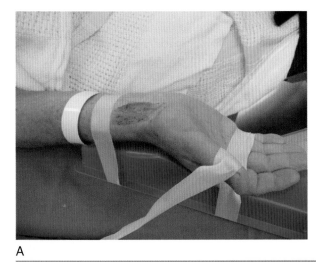
A

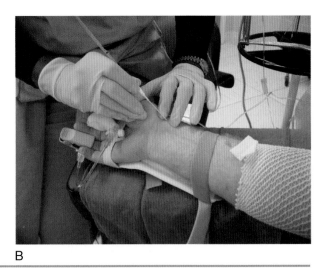
B

FIGURE 8–81 A few pictures from a real live patient showing art line placement. Come in at a shallow angle, get the flash, advance a little, then slide it up, and there you are. When do you need an art line? Beat-to-beat blood pressure measurements and for taking blood gas samples. You are rarely unhappy to have an art line in.

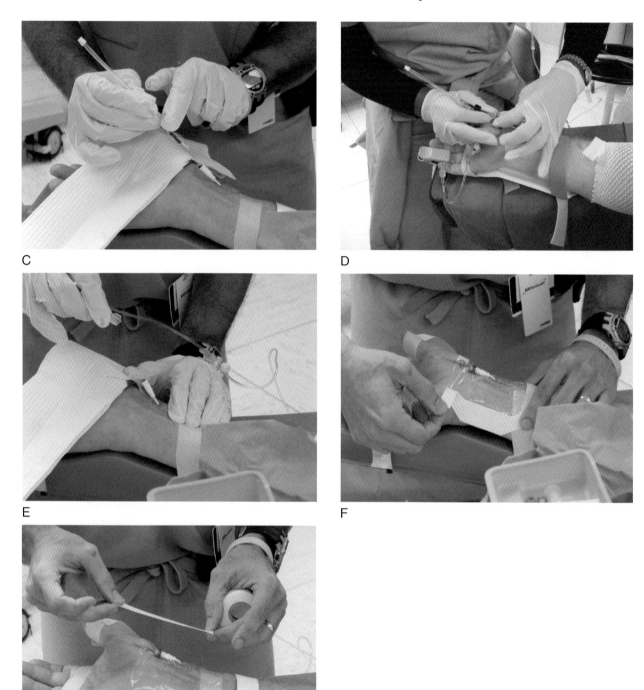

C

D

E

F

G

FIGURE 8–81 cont'd

"That's probably his anxiety," the junior resident says. "Maybe he's hurting from this. Give him a little more fentanyl."

On the monitor, the heart rate is 110.

The senior gives a full 1 cc of "fentanyl."

"I'm not kidding, my heart feels really funny, it's going really really fast," the patient says, alarm in his voice.

EKG shows sinus tachycardia with a rate of 140.

"My chest hurts, I'm not kidding," the patient says.

The junior resident gets the arterial line in and hooks it up. As soon as it's hooked up, the art line trace appears on the monitors.

BP 330/160.

"What the. . . .?" both residents say.

"Holy shit, get that blood pressure down," the junior resident says. "Wait, are we zeroed OK, did the transducer fall down?" The transducer is level.

"Oh God!" the patient says, then falls silent.

"OK," the senior resident says. "No way he's got a pressure that high. What did we give him? What did we give him again?"

"Little Versed, little fent, that's it," the junior says. "We better intubate this guy, he'll be in pulmonary edema and cardiac failure in no time with this pressure."

The senior picks up the syringes, looks at the labels. "Who drew these up?"

"I didn't," the junior resident is applying the face mask and preoxygenating the patient in anticipation of intubation.

"Me neither," the senior says, hurried. "To hell with it, throw out all the old syringes, I'm drawing up all new ones. That must have been straight epi or something. This is a syringe swap! God damn it, something we gave was undiluted something."

"I'd better intubate," the junior resident says. "ABC, man. Let's get the A and B part at least."

"Stand down," the instructor says over the intercom, "Simulation's over."

Clinical lessons learned from scenario 27

Debriefing. "Do you know why they told me to stand up when my teacher walked into the room?" the instructor asks.

The three residents around the table shake their heads.

"Because when your teacher walks into the room, God has just sent you a messenger," the instructor says. "What message is God trying to send to you today?"

BOX 8-59	Syringe Swap

- **Happens**
- **Keep suspicion up**
- **Draw up all new stuff**

"Don't give undiluted epinephrine," the senior resident says.

"It was undiluted norepinephrine," the control room resident corrects.

"Think about it," the instructor says, "if that were epinephrine, what would have happened?"

"A lot more beta effect," the junior resident says. "More tachycardia, probably way up to 200 or so, probably V tach or V fib."

"Correct," the instructor says. "there is a little beta effect with norepinephrine, it's not all alpha, although that predominates. What would have happened if you had given, say, undiluted phenylephrine. Any tachycardia?"

The control room resident sees her chance, as she won't be able to answer much from the OR scene (when you're in the safe confines of the control room, you generally sit out the discussion of what happened in the OR unless a general question like this comes up). "You'd see the big blood pressure jump but no tachycardia. You'd probably see a big reflex *bradycardia*, as a matter of fact."

"Yes," the instructor explains. "Now why am I even asking you this? I mean, you're not expected to give undiluted epinephrine or undiluted norepinephrine, are you?"

That's true. No one has an answer to that.

"Because it can happen," the instructor says, pulling out a bottle of fentanyl and a bottle of norepinephrine. They look almost identical. He shows two other bottles that almost look identical—dexamethasone and norepinephrine. "Do you see how similar these bottles look? I'm surprised these switches don't happen more often."

Around the table, the residents look over the bottles. Man, they *would* be easy to mix up!

"A syringe swap is about as bad a thing as you will see," the instructor says. "And it is easy to panic when it happens. But you are to be consultants, and a consultant is like an actor."

That draws blank stares.

"An actor must know his lines, correct?" the instructor says. "He, or she, must know the lines down cold. And the good actor knows the lines of *everyone else* too. That way, if another actor forgets a line or skips ahead, the good actor knows what to do. The good actor can respond to any emergency.

"And the good doctor knows how to respond to any emergency too. Even as catastrophic a problem as a syringe swap."

Now the lights go on.

"So I should be able to tell what has been given, even in a syringe swap, even if I didn't do the swap," the senior resident says.

"Yes."

"That's not easy," the junior resident says.

"Nothing worth your while is easy," the instructor says. "That is why you must study hard and pay attention to your lessons. It's the easiest thing in the world to skip your studies and become a bad doctor. But that is not what you have chosen to do, is it?"

"How do you prevent a syringe swap?" the junior resident asks.

"You tell me," the instructor bounces the question back.

"Well, draw up your own stuff, look at the drug before you draw it up, look at it after you draw it up, and make sure you're not distracted while you're doing it," the junior says.

"How do you prevent this from happening on a more systematic level?" the instructor asks.

"Oh," the control room resident jumps in, "I read this, somewhere." She searches her memory banks. Where was that? On the Internet somewhere? Anyway, "The best thing for big time vasoactive drugs is to make it really hard to draw them up by mistake. So, instead of having a bunch of norepinephrine bottles sitting in a drawer, there should only be one, and it should be shrink wrapped to a 100 cc bag of saline. So, to just grab it and draw it up, you'd have this 100 cc bag to contend with, and you'd be reminded, 'Oh yeah, I've got to dilute this stuff first.'"

"Why would you need a drawer with 20 vials of norepinephrine anyway?" the junior resident asks. "At most, you'd just need one."

"Right again," the instructor says, "when they lay out drugs, there should be some rationale to it, not just throwing all the drugs in a drawer and saying, 'Fine, we have all the bases covered.' There should be some real forethought into, 'What could go wrong here?'"

"So we diagnosed the trouble, now what?" the instructor asks.

"After we gave all that norepi?" the senior asks. "Well, once you know what happened, then you could either ride it out, let the drug wear off, or try to treat."

"With what?"

"The one thing you *don't* want to give is esmolol," the senior says. "You have this heart in big trouble, pushing against unbelievable afterload. If you then weaken the heart with esmolol, you'll probably cause a cardiac arrest."

"Better to give something to unload like nitroglycerin or Nipride?" the junior asks.

"That is right," the instructor says. "Afterload is what's getting you, so unload the afterload. As these syringe swaps unfold, most of the time it takes a while to figure out what's going on, and by the time you do, the drug has worn off."

"Would you proceed with the case?" the control room resident asks.

Both junior and senior look down at the table for a few seconds, then the senior responds, "This guy could very well have had an MI here. That or a stroke. I'd let the dust settle first. Maybe get some enzymes."

"I don't know," the junior says, "if this guy is having bad TIA symptoms, and he's really at risk for a stroke, you can't just sit on him forever."

"So you'd have to talk with your colleague about this," the instructor says. "What do you tell him happened?"

All the residents picture the horribleness of that conversation.

"Well," the junior says, "I guess you'd have to tell the surgeon exactly what happened. No other way."

"Speak the truth," the instructor says. "You are a doctor and a professional. Nothing less than the truth will do."

Summary. First the technical stuff. Arterial lines require placing a catheter in a tiny, tiny vessel. (The next time you see an operation on the wrist, take a look at the radial artery, you'll be amazed how small it is.) Do everything in your power to make the stick easy.

> Line up the artery so you can enter it at a good angle.
> Sit down to take the pressure off your lower back. It also allows you to concentrate on your little hand muscles.

Now, the big lesson—syringe swap.

Always be aware of the *possibility* of a drug swap. We are human, and the people we work with are human. Sometime, somewhere the wrong thing will be in that syringe. (Do everything in your power to avoid this, obviously.) When the swap happens, keep your cool, try to peg the most likely mistake, redraw new drugs yourself, and stick with ABC.

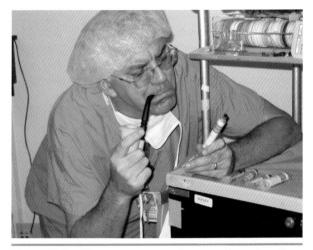

FIGURE 8–82 Syringe swap. It happens. Always be a Sherlock Holmes when something really whacko occurs. It may very well be that the wrong syringe is the culprit. Elementary, my dear Watson.

On a legal note, don't throw those syringes away. *Quarantine* them. Keep them separate from the patient but keep them around so you can analyze them later and see what happened. And when you document this and report it—honesty is the *best* policy—the *only* policy.

And keep your eyes open for messengers. They are sent to you every day.

SCENARIO 28. **Prone position potpourri**

"Hey, that's a department store mannequin," the CA-2 says.

"Good pick up," the CA-3 says. "Your powers of observation shine as brightly as ever."

A pair of senior medical students, interested in anesthesiology, join the anesthesia residents in the operating room at the Simulation lab. The instructor enters the room to clear up the mystery.

"Why the extra dummy, you ask?" the instructor explains, "Today we're going to do a prone case. You can roll the METI human simulator prone, but, from an owner's perspective, that's just scary as hell. All those hoses and connections, coming out the back— no thank you.

"So here's what we're going to do. You'll induce on the METI, and all vital signs you'll follow with the monitors on the METI. Then when we move prone, you're going to actually move the department store mannequin prone. Got it? We want to do the drill of moving prone, pay attention to positioning and stuff. Then once we're prone, you'll have to sort of 'imagine' the METI as being prone. Got it?"

After one quick demonstration of the plan, the students and residents "have it." This combination pack of Simulator-for-vital-signs and additional-prop-for-additional-lessons works well. It's just a greater extension of our request that students in the Simulator "suspend their disbelief" during the scenarios.

The medical students put on the monitors, and under the direction of the residents induce the patient. He is a 49-year-old man who was lifting weights when he suffered a slipped L3-4 disc, developed a foot drop, and is now here for urgent laminectomy.

"Going to use Sux for muscle relaxation?" the CA-3 asks.

"Is the foot drop one of those neuromuscular contraindications for Sux?" the first medical student asks. "Like a spinal cord injury? This is sort of like a spinal cord injury, isn't it?"

"Not really," the CA-2 says, warming to the task of "teacher" for the med students. "There hasn't been enough time to develop additional end-plates on the muscle to present a risk for hyperkalemia. So as far as that goes, you don't have a contraindication to Sux. There might be another reason though, a surgical reason."

Picking it up, the second med student says, "The surgeon may not want the person paralyzed. He may want to see the leg jump if he's too close to a nerve."

Turning to his fellow resident, the CA-3 says, "They're smarter than we were when we were in medical school."

"They're smarter than *you* are now," the CA-2 replies.

Induction goes smoothly, but the med students flounder with the intubation.

"Here," the CA-3 demonstrates, "you're not putting the laryngoscope all the way in. You're just putting it in a little and hoping the vocal cords are there. I got news for you, the vocal cords are not visible 1 inch inside the mouth. Maybe if you're intubating a gerbil, but in a human adult they're deeper. Put the blade all the way in, all the way to the right, then lift along the direction of the handle. Don't crank back, you'll generate dental work. Lift along the direction of the handle, then pull back, back, back, until you see the epiglottis plop down. There, you see it?"

The med students stick their heads nearly into the dummy's mouth to see. Their heads clunk with a sickening thud.

"Uh, one at a time," the CA-3 says, then turns to his fellow resident, "Maybe they're *not* so smart as we give them credit for."

"Once that epiglottis plunks into view, don't lift right away, you have to put the laryngoscope just a little bitty bit, so you engage the tip of the blade into the vallecula," the CA-3 explains. "Then you lift, and the epiglottis should pop up and give you a good view."

With meticulous planning and some "After 'you's,'" the medical students manage to see without further cranial collisions.

Between intubation attempts (each student requires two more tries), the CA-2 tells them an important point, "Between intubation attempts, be sure to pull out and mask-ventilate. Don't kill the patient trying to intubate. Remember, you don't *have* to intubate, but you *do* have to ventilate."

Once both students have intubated, the team turns to moving the patient prone, and they go to the department store dummy. To add realism, they tape a sawed-off endotracheal tube to its mouth and put monitors on it.

Overhead on the intercom, "We'll tread water on the vital signs. Just go through the drill of moving prone."

"Do you know how many people it takes to move a patient prone?" the CA-3 asks the med students. They shake their heads, "One more than whoever's in the room. No matter how you divvy it up, there's always one arm or one leg that flops around and scares the hell out of you. So get as many people as you can."

"Here's the real deal, up here at the head," the CA-2 demonstrates. "Start with your arms crossed when you hold the head, and plan it out so once you've flipped the patient over and he goes prone, your arms won't be crossed. Because that's when you're going to need to be holding the head steady and firm." He shows them.

"Take a good look at the monitors one last time before you move, then disconnect as much stuff as you can, pulse oximeter the last monitor, and oxygen the last thing," the CA-3 says. "Then once you've flipped, go in reverse order, hook up oxygen first, then pulse oximeter, then the rest of the monitors. Listen for breath sounds because that tube can move around.

Very easy, if the head is flexed, for that tube to go into the right mainstem."

"Anything else before we go?" the second med student asks.

"Protect the eyes," the CA-2 says. "Once you flip, it's a pain to worm underneath there and put goop in the eyes or tape them. So do that ahead of time."

They do the flip, and, sure enough, the mannequins left arm flops out at a crazy angle.

"Catch it!" the first med student shouts.

"Broken arm, brachial plexus stretch, yuck," the CA-3 says. "Moving is not for sissies. You gotta watch everything."

Stepping back, the residents let the med students hook everything up. Once that's all done, they then reconnect all the monitors and the ventilator to the METI. To add to the realism, a sheet completely covers the METI so everyone can now imagine it being prone.

The high inspiratory pressure alarm goes off. Vital signs are high normal, with a blood pressure 155/90, HR 95, SaO₂ 99%.

Switching to hand ventilation, the CA-2 starts trying to figure out the cause of the high inspiratory pressure. Hand ventilation is difficult.

"What do you think's going on?" the CA-3 asks the med students.

"Kink in the tube?" the first one asks.

"Asthma?" the second one tries.

Turning up the sevoflurane, the CA-2 says, "Maybe he's just light. Remember, he's not paralyzed, we used Sux and it wore off. We just did a stimulating thing with the move prone. His endotracheal tube was getting jiggled all around. Could be deep and be hitting the carina." He pulls the endotracheal tube back a little after checking breath sounds.

The inspiratory pressures go down, and the case smooths out.

"Cookie time!" the overhead speaker announces. "Time for all the good girls and boys to have cookies and milk. The scenario is over."

Clinical lessons learned from scenario 28

Debriefing. A plate of chocolate chip cookies and a half gallon of skim milk preside over the debriefing table.

"Cookies at 10 in the morning," the CA-3 says, "I could learn to like the Simulation Center."

"Cookies and skim milk," the CA-2 adds, "that's kind of like, 'I'll have two slices of key lime pie and a Diet Coke,' right?"

BOX 8-60	*Going Prone*

- **Keep arms untangled**
- **Get lots of help, then get one more helper**
- **Watch the neck, watch the neck, watch the neck**

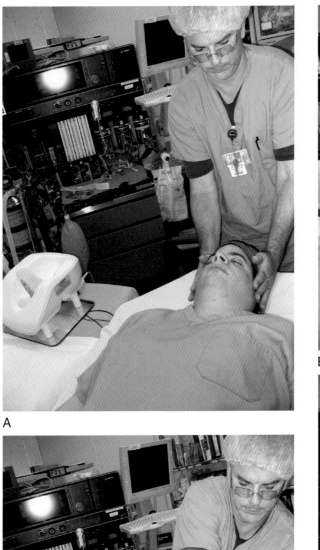

A

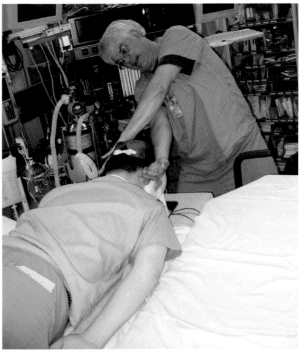

B

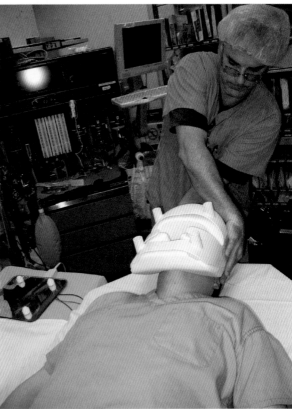

C

D

FIGURE 8–83 **A, B.** When you move someone to a prone position and you start out with your own arms straight, by the time the patient is prone your arms are all tangled and you can't control anything. **C, D.** If you start out with your arms crossed and your facemask in place, by the time the patient is prone your arms are nice and untangled.

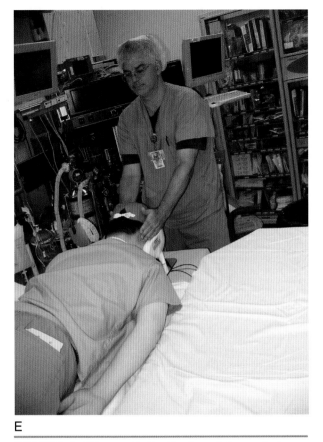

E

FIGURE 8–83 cont'd **E**. Caption—Aah, much better. Much easier to control the head and neck with your arms like this.

Further ironic observations take a back seat while everyone divvies up the cookies.

"Milk, it does a body good," the instructor says. "Take it from a native cheesehead."

"What were the biggies in today's scenarios?"

"Can you use Sux when someone has a, well, a 'little' neurologic problem?" the first med student asks.

The instructor lists it on the white board, some chocolate smearing off his writing hand on to the board. An attempt to erase the chocolate just smears it further, convulsing the room with laughter.

"Glad to see you're so easily amused," the instructor says. "What else, quick, before you wet your pants laughing."

"Can you use Sux when the surgeon wants to 'see a nerve jump'?" the second med student offers.

"Tricky aspects of moving," the ·CA-2 says. "Oh, and differential of high inspiratory pressures."

"That all? What did you guys spend a lot of time doing with the medical students?" the instructor asks.

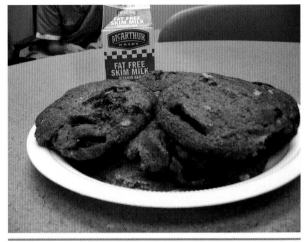

FIGURE 8–84 Chocolate chip cookies and skim milk. That is living.

"Intubation."

"Right, intubation," the instructor says. "Worth a review."

"Let's go over intubation first," the instructor says. "The tongue has two parts, a wiggly part at the end, and a fixed root at its base. When you are first learning to intubate, your biggest problem is the wiggly end of the tongue. You tend to put the laryngoscope just a little ways into the mouth because you're hesitant. Then, when you try to look, the slippery eel of a tongue slides and slithers across the laryngoscope, you can't see anything, and you end up with the scope on the *left* side of the mouth, instead of the *right* side where it belongs.

"The cure? Put the laryngoscope all the way in. I'm forever batting med students on the back of their 'laryngoscope hand' saying 'deeper, deeper.'"

"When you put the laryngoscope all the way in, you'll be hooking the base, the immobile part of the tongue," the pornographically gifted instructor continues. "Then, when you lift and look, you won't have that tongue sliding over the blade and obscuring your view."

With an intubating dummy, just down the table from the rapidly emptying cookie plate, the instructor demonstrates.

BOX 8-61 Intubation

- Get mouth open
- Scope all the way in
- Lift along the direction of the handle

"Now, let's look at the questions about succinylcholine," the instructor says. "What's the big concern?"

The first med student has done her homework, "Because Sux causes a depolarization, you are concerned if the muscle has abnormal end-plates. If, because of spinal cord injury, prolonged immobilization, burns, or abnormal muscle development such as Duchenne's muscular dystrophy you have too many end plates, you'll get a kind of 'super-depolarization.' Instead of a small rise in potassium, which everyone gets, you'll see a huge rise in potassium. High enough to arrest the heart."

"And in this case?" the instructor asks.

"Well, this is a little fuzzy," the med student says, "he does have some loss, I mean his foot is weak. But I don't know if that's 'enough' to give you the big bad depolarization. How much is too much?"

"Truth to tell, I don't know," the instructor says. "In case of doubt, probably better to go with the nondepolarizer."

"But if the surgeon wants to see the nerve jump?" the CA-2 asks.

"If you use a short-acting drug such as mivacurium, or cisatracurium, it should wear off by the time you secure the tube, move him prone, reconnect, and then they prep. There's usually enough time so it's not a problem," the CA-3 explains.

"Let's go over the move again," the instructor says, then actually leads them back into the OR to physically reenact the move.

"Let me show you the thing with the head again," the instructor says, "this is important. Think through the hand movements ahead of time, to make sure that your hands won't be all catty-wampus once you've moved prone. You really want to be able to control the head once you move him over. Figure that everyone you move *may* have cervical disc troubles, so you don't want to wrench their neck around.

"The arms are the forgotten element. People watch the tube, watch the head, but you've gotta make sure someone is watching each arm or else one of 'em will get away from you, as happened this time. Now once you've moved them prone, go over every spot—neck, eyes, breasts, genitalia, pressure spots on the knees, everything. An old trick is to put yourself in the position the patient is in. If *you* feel uncomfortable, the *patient* is feeling uncomfortable too. Don't trust the nurses to pad and position, don't trust the surgeons to pad and position. *You* go over every last inch of the patient and make sure *you* are satisfied. There is no more sickening feeling than taking down those drapes and seeing something awful and wondering, 'How

long has that arm been twisted like that?' or 'I hope the leg hasn't been off the table long.'"

"OK," the instructor says, "last point, we're almost out of cookies."

"When the ventilator alarm goes off," the first medical student offers.

"Right, when the ventilator alarm goes off," the instructor repeats. "Let's walk through that."

The CA-2 takes this ball and runs with it, "The differential is long, everything from kinked, clogged, misplaced, or displaced tube, all the way to problems inside the chest, such as pneumothorax or even a tumor squashing the bronchi. The lung tissue itself can be a problem, with asthma topping the list. So you have a lot of stuff to choose from, but you want to go with common stuff first."

"You hear hoofbeats, think horses," the instructor helps out. "Don't immediately think of unicorns."

"Right," the CA-2 says. "This guy has no history of asthma, nor have we done anything to invade his chest, like a central line or anything. So you turn to the more common things. We just moved him, we intubated with Sux, which has probably worn off because the med students took forever to intubate."

"Hey!" they both protest through cookie-filled mouths.

"So most likely, the patient is fighting us, resisting the ventilator's inspiratory efforts with his expiratory efforts, making the high pressure alarm go off. So I deepened the anesthetic. Plus, I did a check of breath sounds and pulled the tube back a little, just in case we were hitting the carina."

"Hey," the CA-2 says, "there aren't any more cookies."

"Well then," the instructor says, "this is like a party that ran out of beer. Time to close up shop."

Summary. When first starting simulations, it's tempting to try to teach everything under the sun. But a more productive tact is to just pick a few important take-home lessons and make sure they stick. With mixed batches (residents and med students), you can also give the residents a chance to do a little teaching of their own.

Intubation is not a "given," and even senior residents can do with a review of the anatomy. Understanding the two parts of the tongue—mobile and fixed—helps guide the beginning laryngoscopists around this slippery obstacle. Put the blade all the way in, then pull back. You'll get to the cords much faster that way than tip-toeing down the tongue, a micron at a time.

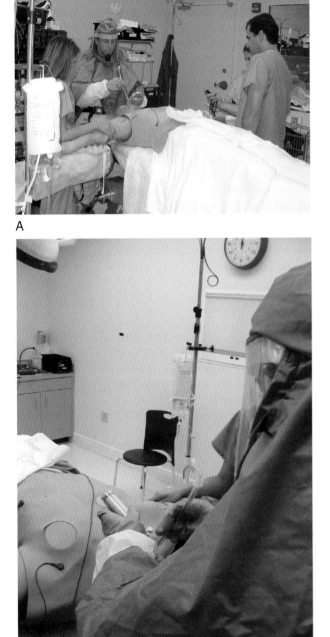

A

B

FIGURE 8–85 Intubation is not a given. God forbid a chemical or biologic attack occurs someday—we'll be intubating in these clunky Haz Mat suits. (I did it myself; and, believe it or not, you actually *can* do it.)

Sux is one of the few drugs we use that can "kill instantly." That hyperkalemic thunderbolt as always looking for a chance to strike—spinal cord injury, crush injury, immobilization (in some cases after just

a few days!), intra-abdominal abscess, burn, muscle abnormalities. And in gray zones, where you're just not sure, you would sure hate to be "the next case report of hyperkalemic arrest with succinylcholine use."

Moving a patient prone is another minefield, with potential injury at every turn—lose control and twist the neck, arm, or leg, put pressure on the eyes, hyper-flex or extend the neck, forget to pad a pressure point, forget to secure something, which then slips out while the patient is under the drapes. So practicing this maneuver with a dummy makes sense. You can demonstrate all the wrong things and rehearse all the right things with no harm to the patient.

Finally, managing routine problems is a great Simulator exercise. Bucking and high pressures, the endotracheal tube slipping down into the right mainstem—these are bread-and-butter problems. But common problems need fixing too! And a quick fix. With the patient fighting the tube, it's only a matter of seconds before the surgeon is fighting you, so you need to identify the problem, rule out more serious dilemmas (pneumothorax, for example), and keep the case going smoothly.

Smooth, mmmmm, just like those smooth creamy chocolate chips, melting in the middle of a still-warm batch of cookies, right out of the oven.

SCENARIO 29. **Plane crashes and AICDs**

"Is she in the OR?" the first anesthesia resident asks.

"No, in the holding area," the instructor explains. One area of the Simulation Center has a full operating room setup, with a mannequin in there. Another area of the simulation center has a mannequin in a more generic setting. The latter area can function as a holding area, PACU, ICU, or ER. "She's in there while we wait for the AICD rep to show up."

The two anesthesia residents, both CA-1s, go into the holding area. In there, a CA-3 is looking over the chart next to the patient. Next to him, the patient is moaning, has oxygen on, an IV, and an arterial line. On the monitors, the BP is 100/60, P 120, sat 94%.

"What's the scoop?" the first CA-1 asks.

The CA-3 fills in. "This 73-year-old woman, just had an AICD put in 2 months ago, looks like she's got an acute belly. Probably blew out a diverticulum. Now they've got to explore her."

All this time the patient continues to moan.

"Abdomen's tight as a drum, we're just waiting for the AICD rep to come here and turn the AICD off before we go back," the CA-3 says.

"You have to turn those things off?" the second CA-1 asks.

"Yeah," the CA-3 explains. "The AICD might see a Bovie signal, think it's V tach, and fire."

The first CA-1 says, "That's right. You can't put a magnet on it, can you? Doesn't a magnet screw it up?"

"Correct," the CA-3 says. "These babies cost 25 to 30 thou. Something like that. A magnet could reprogram it and screw the whole thing up."

"When's the AICD rep coming?" the first CA-1 asks.

"She said something about traffic," the CA-3 says, "maybe 45 minutes. Let me go out and give her a call and see if she can come a little sooner." The CA-3 walks out of the room.

Left in the holding area, the two CA-1s confer.

"She must be dry as hell, let's put in a central line, she'll need one for sure if she's got a bowel process going on," the second one says. "Plus, we don't want to just sit here!"

Over the intercom, "Go ahead. There's a partial task trainer in the corner where you can practice putting in central lines."

The instructor comes in the room and guides them through the central line placement.

"More suspension of disbelief here, doctors, just pretend this is the patient you're putting the line in," the instructor says. Once the trainer is draped, the instructor gives some instructions on placing a central line.

"Forget all the stuff about triangles, high approach, low approach, and all that bologna. The only landmark that means anything is the carotid. Fact is, the internal jugular vein lays close up next to the carotid and that's all there is to it. Feel the carotid, go next to it. That's it.

"Now once you've felt the carotid pulse, don't keep pressing down hard. That would flatten the easily compressible internal jugular vein. If you ever do this with a Site-Rite echo system, and I suggest you do, you'll see just how flat you can make the vein if you press down hard."

First one, then the other, CA-1 place the central line. Then they return to the simulator mannequin. Now there is a CVP trace as well as an arterial trace.

BP 90/50, P 130, CVP 0, SaO$_2$ 92%. She continues to groan.

"All right, we need to tank her up some here, let's send a blood gas, see where we are with the hematocrit, then we fix her up," the first CA-1 says.

Intercom—"Blood gas shows metabolic acidosis and a hematocrit of 46."

"OK, she's volume contracted for sure," the second CA-1 says. "Let's start with some albumin, tank her up until we get the acidosis turned around, urine output good, and that CVP at least up to the middle range, say 6."

The CA-3 comes back in the room. "Some truck turned over on the interstate, the AICD rep is still held up, so we can't go in the room."

"All right, well, we've got a plan here," the first CA-1 says. "We've got it under control."

After a few minutes, they've given fluids, but the CVP stays low, no urine comes out of the Foley, and the blood pressure goes to 85/45 with a heart rate of 140.

"Guess we're getting septic, let's start a norepinephrine drip," the first CA-1 says. "We better switch the CVP over to a Swan if we're ever going to get a handle on these hemodynamics."

"Is there another AICD rep?" the second CA-1 asks. "Maybe someone in house, from the cath lab or the EP study lab who can help us with this AICD?"

"Good idea," the CA-3 says, "but there's an EP conference this week. I think they're all out of town. We have to wait for that AICD rep out there in traffic."

"OK," the first CA-1 says. "Let's switch over to a Swan."

A PA pressure trace now appears on the monitor. PA 45/28, CVP 3, wedge 3.

"Looks dry, but, well. . . ." the first CA-1 says. "Pressure's only 80/40 now. Maybe it's time for epi. What do you think?"

"I think the Simulation's over," the instructor says over the intercom.

Clinical lessons learned from scenario 29

Debriefing. Expecting to see an article on Swans or sepsis, the CA-1s are surprised to see a newspaper article waiting for them on the debriefing table.

"Navy outlines errors preceding fatal submarine crash," *New York Times,* May 8, 2005, Section YT, page 23.

"What's this?" the first CA-1 asks.

"Read it," the CA-3 says. "It has everything to do with this case."

Both CA-1s raise their eyebrows and give each other a "Where are they going with this?" look.

January 8, 2005, depth 500 feet, location 360 miles southeast of Guam, aboard the nuclear submarine San Francisco. The submarine is proceeding at top speed, 33 knots. Everything on board the ship is, well, ship-

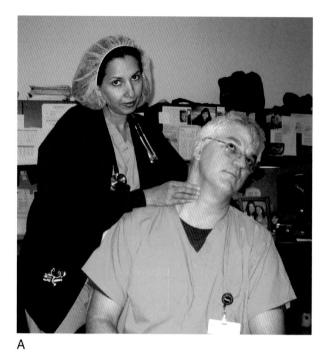

A

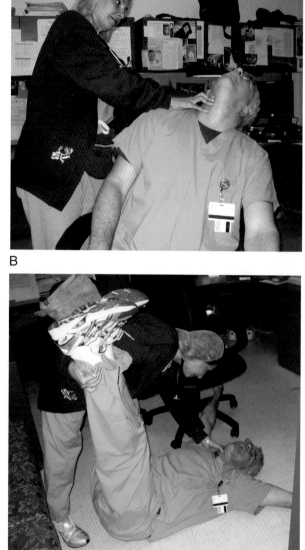

B

C

FIGURE 8–86 Now the carotid is a damned good landmark, but don't press on it too hard. You could throw off a plaque or you could elicit a vagal response. See how this skilled clinician continues to feel the carotid while resuscitating the patient! This is the stuff of reality shows.

shape. Modern equipment, well trained crew, double-hulled construction for safety. Only two problems—they do not have accurate charts of the area. They are not taking frequent depth soundings.

The submarine is sailing blind.

The San Francisco smashes into an undersea mountain. One sailor is thrown into a metal casing and killed. 20 others are injured, and $88 million in damage occurs. Thanks to the double-hulled construction, the ship is able to surface and get back to port.

"What does this story have to do with how you handled this case?" the instructor asks.

No clue of recognition from the CA-1s. Nary a flicker of cerebral activity. For a moment, the instructor fears brain death in his junior residents. Maybe a quick cold-caloric study?

"OK, let me lay it out for you," the instructor prays it's not too late for these CA-1s, "What did that submarine *really need*?"

"A map," the first CA-1 says.

"Right," the instructor agrees, "a map. That submarine needed a chart, to see where to go. Without a good chart, this submarine smashed into an underwater mountain. The most important thing to underwater sailing is *knowing what's down there*. You know, reef, mountain, rock, depth, whatever. If you don't have the most important thing, you crash!"

"They might have done everything else right, you know, had the bow planes adjusted, had the depth gauge set right, had the periscope tucked, whatever it is you do on a submarine. But they didn't do the most important thing!"

"What did this patient need? What was wrong with her?" the CA-3 asks.

"She needed her AICD turned off," the first CA-1 says.

"*Wrong!*" the CA-3 shouts and slams his fist on the table. "*Wrong, wrong, a thousand times wrong!*"

BOX 8–62	*Basics*

- Don't get lost in the trivia
- What's the MAIN thing wrong?
- Fix the MAIN thing

Even the instructor flinches a little at this outburst. This is what happens when you enlist senior residents to teach. Sometimes they fall prey to "irrational exuberance."

"What your learned confrere is trying to emphasize is, think about what this patient's pathology is," the instructor says, mollification in her voice.

"Oh," the second CA-1 says. "She needed an exploratory laparotomy for a ruptured diverticulum."

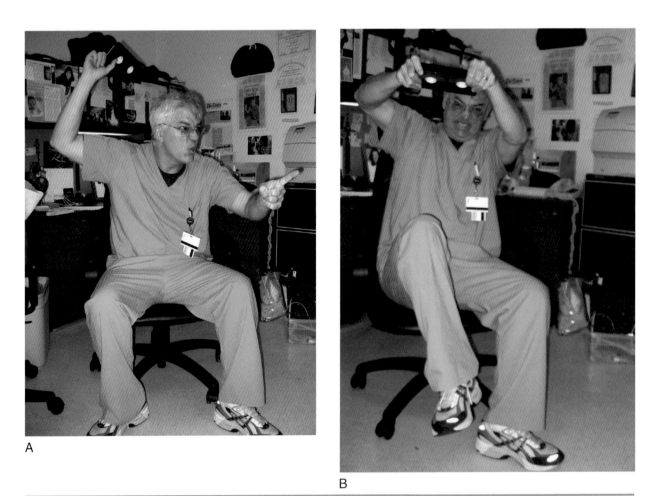

A

B

FIGURE 8–87 Of course you want to wax enthusiastic and put some emotion into your teaching methods. But don't let yourself fall prey to irrational exuberance in your ardor to instruct.

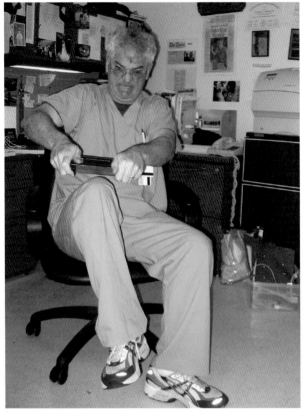

C

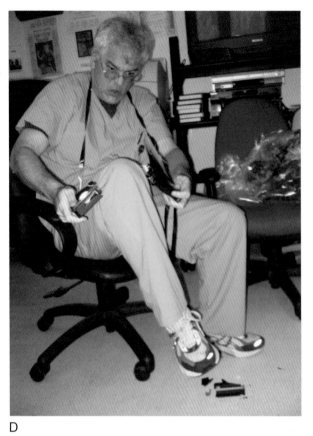

D

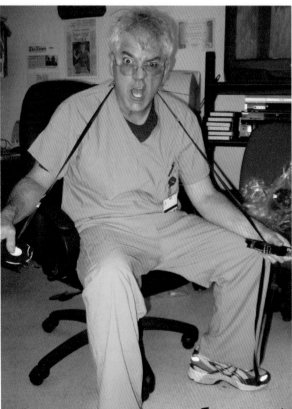

E

FIGURE 8-87 cont'd

"Exactly!" the CA-3 is back in the arena. "She had a hole in her intestinal tract. She was spilling stool into her abdomen, that's what happens when you blow a diverticulum. She needed to get explored, opened, and cleaned out. Nothing else can cure her."

"What about the AICD?" the first CA-1 says.

"That's a side track," the CA-3 says. "Yes, in a routine case, you need to turn it off. But this is not a routine case! This woman is dying, dying, dying. You're doing all the other stuff right—placing a central line, correctly analyzing the blood gases, resuscitating with volume—but all of that is secondary. The killing lesion is the hole in the intestine, and you can be the world's greatest resuscitator, but she'll still die of peritonitis.

"You can do a case with the AICD in and on. It might be a pain, it might fire. You might have to go with a bipolar in the field. Hell, you might even need to have the surgeons skip the Bovie altogether and *tie off* the bleeders. God, imagine that.

"But the bottom line is this, if you don't open this woman and clean out her belly, she's a goner. Better to proceed in a less-than-perfect way than to sit around and let her die. That rep may be stuck in traffic until you bury this patient. That is not doing the patient any favors!"

"But you told us. . . ." the second CA-1 says. "You said we needed to wait."

Smiling and looking at the instructor, the CA-3 says, "Well, you can't believe everything you hear, can you?"

"Your senior colleague was what we call an *agent provocateur*," the instructor explains, "a plant, by yours truly. I wanted her to lead you down the garden path, to implant the premise—*We have to wait for the AICD rep*—and see if you guys would just accept that. You fell for it."

"And once we got involved in the details of fluid resuscitation and CVP and Swan and stuff, we never came back and challenged that premise," the first CA-1 says.

"Exactamundo," the instructor says.

On the white board, the CA-3 writes "crisis resource management."

"One of the big rules in crisis resource management is the idea of global reassessment," the CA-3 says, then writes that down too. Continuing, she says, "You're consultants, you can't get too drawn into the details. You have to step back every now and then and look over the entire situation. Do you need to retool your thinking? Do you need to take an entirely different approach? In this case, I strait-jacketed you into one

---

> **BOX 8-63** Submarine Safety
>
> - Avoid mountains
> - Don't open any windows

---

mind set—*We have to wait for the AICD rep, we have to wait for the AICD rep, we have to wait for the AICD rep.* You would have kept that up right until she died of sepsis."

The CA-1s nod. "You got us," the first one says.

"Once you start thinking that way, you just don't shake it," the second one says. "And I never thought to question the CA-3."

"Lesson learned," the instructor summarizes. "Question everything. Your patient's life depends on it."

Summary. Crash! Every patient has crash potential, just as every submarine has crash potential. If you forget the most important thing—the underwater chart (submarine) or the diagnosis (patient)—you increase your crash potential!

First, some clinical points the CA-1s got right.

Central line—with a big belly case and lots of fluid shifts anticipated, a CVP is a good idea. The instructor's review of the landmarks hits a major point—find that carotid. That pulse tells you where big red is, go lateral to that, and you're there. Good idea to learn how to use that Site-Rite as well!

The CA-1s pegged the blood gas right. High hematocrit? Not a sign of good health, this is a sign of hemoconcentration. Acidosis? Cells are crying out for help, that's the simplest way to analyze metabolic acidosis. So fix what you can fix. In this case, the residents focused on fluid resuscitation.

But the junior residents got led astray by the initial mind set. They got all wrapped up in the need to turn off the AICD and forgot that a stool-infected peritoneum presented the real problem.

Step back, reassess, re-examine the initial premise. Make sure you have the right "mental map." That's what makes a good submarine captain. And that's what makes a good doctor.

SCENARIO 30. Far from home, sedation in the CT scanner

"You're in the dungeon today," the instructor says. "Radiology."

"Far from home and far from help," the CA-1 resident says.

The CA-2 and CA-3, also assigned to the Simulator that day, agree.

"Here's your case," the instructor hands them a sheet. "Your case will take place in the CT scanner. We'll be in the operating room Simulation room. Pretend that the anesthesia machine is far enough away to not interfere with the CT scanner. Imagine too, that the patient is slid head first into a CT scanner."

The three residents look over the preop. A 38-year-old man fell off a ladder and hit his head. He is now going for CT to look for an intracranial bleed. No other medical history. Airway OK, C-spine cleared. Last ate 2 hours ago.

"Like some other cases, we'll have one of you in the control room with me," the instructor says.

The residents play "rock, paper, scissors" to determine who goes in the control room. After four rounds (everyone kept putting down "rock" at the same time), the CA-3 emerges victorious.

In the control room, the group settles in, puts up a routine set of vital signs, and looks through the one-way mirror.

"I've just got to know," the CA-3 says, "what are you going to do?"

"Stay tuned," the instructor says. "Watch along and see what you would do if you were in there. No freebies just because you're in here."

In the operating room, the CA-2 and CA-1 interview the patient.

"How are you doing, Mr. Cooper?" the CA-2 asks.

"Unnnnnh," Mr. Cooper says.

"No, really," the CA-2 insists, "I need you to tell me. I need to hear you tell me."

"Fine," Cooper snaps. "I'm fine, just, my head hurts, you know, I don't want to talk so much."

In the control room, the CA-3 says, "That's good. Assessing level of consciousness. Don't want Mr. Cooper slipping down below Glasgow Coma Scale 8—you'd then have to intubate him."

"How are we going to sedate him?" the CA-1 asks. "I'm trying to think of something that won't cloud him up too much or raise his CO_2 much."

"Good question," the CA-2 says. "Propofol, no. Versed, maybe, but he might get a little disinhibited and squirm. Narcotics? No, that'll raise his CO_2, no good for his brain. Dex? Yeah, that's good. Might slow your breathing some. OK, here's the deal, nothing is an absolutely free ride. But let's go with Dex."

"Let's cross one bridge right now," the CA-1 says. "What is our threshold for saying, 'To hell with it, let's intubate him'?"

"Good, good, grasshopper," the CA-3 says in the control room, putting on his best Kung Fu accent.

"I hate it when they're smart," the instructor says, "it makes it so hard to humiliate them later."

"Let's set that bar really low," the CA-2 says. "Worst thing we can do for this guy is oversedate him, let his CO_2 rise, increase blood flow to his brain, and screw this whole deal up. In case of doubt, off to sleep and secure everything."

They hang a pump of dexmedetomidine, push the patient "into the CT scanner" (to achieve a feel for this, the anesthesia machine is at the patient's feet; at his head, two IV poles with a drape across the top of them creates an ersatz CT scanner).

Once the patient is in the scanner, all monitors are go, and there is a good CO_2 pattern.

"Well blow me down," the CA-3 says. "They keep doing everything right. What can we do to these fine fellows?"

The instructor tells the technician, "Now."

In the OR, the lights go out. All electricity is gone, the monitors go dark.

"Hey!" the CA-2 and CA-1 yell.

"Is the CT scanner still working?" the CA-2 asks.

"Must not be," the CA-1 says.

Bang, bang, bang! Drawers fly open and shut, "Where's a flashlight!" "Here's one!"

The CA-1 turns one on, the light comes on, flickers, and dies.

"Go get one!" the CA-2 says. The door opens and shuts as the CA-1 runs out.

"How you doing, Mr. Cooper!" the CA-2 shouts. "Mr. Cooper!" Though dark in the OR, there's enough light creeping under the door so the CA-2 can grope up to the head of the bed. He reaches in the "CT scanner" and puts his hand over Mr. Cooper's chest and mouth.

"I'm feeling his chest going up and down," the CA-2 shouts to the control room. "My hand is over his mouth to see if I can feel wind moving. My hand is on the pulse, and it feels OK."

"Mr. Cooper," the CA-2 shouts, "I really need you to tell me how you're doing."

Without waiting, he pulls Cooper out of the CT scanner, grabs an Ambu-bag, and opens a cylinder of oxygen.

"Hey!" Cooper yells, "Take that thing off my face!"

The CA-2 reaches over to the cart, pulls out a little plastic stick, bends it, something goes "Crack!" and an eerie yellow light appears. He's just pulled out a phosphorescent stick that sends out a chemical light.

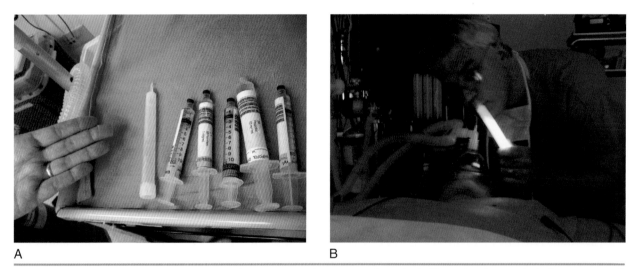

A   B

FIGURE 8–88 What do you do when the lights go out? If you're too clever by half, you break out a little fluorescent stick that you just happened to have on hand. In the Simulator, you can do little tricks like this to see if the resident really is "ready for anything."

"The ultimate light source," the CA-2 says, "don't leave home without it."

The lights come back on, just as the CA-1 bursts back into the room with a flashlight.

"Wait! Turn the lights back off!" the CA-1 shouts, "I've got the flashlight!"

"That's rich," the CA-3 says in the control room.

Leaning into the microphone, the instructor says, "No need, we're done. Head to the conference room."

Clinical lessons learned from scenario 30

Debriefing. Everyone crowds around the CA-2 with his cool, hip glowing device.

"Man, it really works!"

"This is too much!"

"What's the 800 number to get this thing?"

"Break it up, break it up!" the instructor says, pushing aside the crowd. "Take your seats, you rabid consumers."

Everyone sits down.

"Now gimme that thing," the instructor says, looking the thing over. "What's the 800 number to get this thing?"

After a flurry of scribbling down the 800 number, the residents turn their attention to the debriefing.

"How do you think it went?" the instructor asks.

Both CA-2 and CA-1 have a chagrined look, saying without words, "We should have made sure where the flashlight was."

Reading their minds, the instructor says, "Forget the power outage for a second, we'll get to that. How

BOX 8-64	Other Equipment

- **Flashlights**
- **Fire extinguishers**
- **O₂ shut off**

do you feel your assessment was in this case? Remember, what we're most interested in here is your *thinking*, your *decision making*."

"I thought we did OK," the CA-1 says. "Sedation in radiology land is always something you approach with a lot of caution."

"Why is that?" the CA-3 says.

"You have to be like a turtle in these 'off-site' anesthetizing locales," the CA-2 explains. "You have to carry your house on your back, like a turtle does. Anything special, like equipment or drugs, and you better have it with you because tech help is far away. And the techs might not even know where you are."

"Plus," the CA-1 (wise beyond her years) says, "help from another anesthesiologist may be far away too. When the call goes out, 'Anyone to room 3, *stat!*' everyone piles into room 3 in 10 seconds. When the call goes out, 'Anyone to PET scanner, *stat!*' everyone says, 'Where the hell is the PET scanner?'"

"And," the CA-2 says, "we've got an additional consideration here. Possible intracranial bleed. So for that reason we kept talking to this guy. If his sensorium gets clouded, and he can't respond appropriately, we have to assume the worst. He's bleeding, his ICP is climbing, he may not be able to protect his airway, plus he's got a full stomach.

"And sedating in someone with increased ICP is a real tough balancing act. Just the teeniest amount of sedation could increase that ICP past the point of no return. And you can mix or match pathology here too. You give a little sedation, he bleeds a little more. A patient who was fine a minute ago can be moribund now. And you can muddy the waters yourself—you give a lot of sedation, now the guy is slurring his words. Is that because of your sedation, or because he's about to herniate?"

Turning to the CA-3, the instructor says, "See what I mean when you have a bunch of really good residents? How do I justify my grossly inflated paycheck when the damn residents know more than I do?"

The CA-3 shrugs.

"Now, to the power outage, talk to me," the instructor says.

"Mea culpa," the CA-2 says. "Part of check out should always include making sure there is a working flashlight nearby. 'Trouble doesn't ring a bell,' as they say. As the senior resident in the room, I should have taken it upon myself to make sure there was a flashlight nearby."

"Any other 'weird' stuff you should always know about?" the instructor asks.

Eyes go around the table, no one tumbles to it.

"How about the fire extinguisher?" the instructor asks.

All three residents say, "Oh!" and lift their hands up, the universal sign for "I should have thought of that."

"Oxygen shut off? Fire alarm?" the instructor hammers on them. "Shouldn't you always know where they are too? Doesn't JACHO tell us that we all need to know where this stuff is?"

"JACHO not enough for you?" the instructor says. "Let me pull an ACGME core clinical competency on you. As part of the 'systems-based medicine' area, residents should know about things such as fire alarms, extinguishers, and the like. It's not part of our *regular* equipment checkout, but it *is* stuff we need to know."

Heads are hanging all over the table. We were rolling on the ICP stuff, and now we're getting roasted alive on fire extinguishers. How appropriate an analogy!

"But who are we kidding?" the instructor says, holding up the glowing stick. "Anyone who has a flashlight ready to go like that. Man. That is just too good.

I was going to throw all of you out the window. But now, I just might let you live.

"Go forth and sin no more."

Summary. Off-site anesthesia can be a real stressor. The key to surviving this is to think ahead, "What might I need?" and then make sure you bring it along. Better yet, bring two of them along in case one doesn't work. Think of yourself as going up in a space ship—if you don't have it, you won't be able to get it.

Sedation in the CT scanner can also lay a lot of stress on your own cardiovascular system, let alone the patient's. Any question about the neuro status? Better to play it safe and secure the airway. If you do sedate, use the light touch and stay in constant communication with the patient. If they're talking and making sense, you're golden. If they're not talking and not making sense, something might be amiss!

Anesthesia equipment deserves a good going over. We need to know our laryngoscopes, ventilator, and vaporizers. But in a larger context, we need to know about other facets of equipment too—flashlights, fire

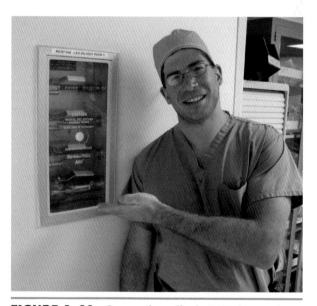

FIGURE 8-89 Oxygen shut-off valve? We have to know about that too. You probably walk past one every day without noticing it!

extinguishers, oxygen shut off, alarms. After all, lights do go out, electricity fails, fires happen. And as consultants, we need to be ready for, not just the routine, but everything.

So the next time you watch late-night TV, and you see one of those glowing stick thingamabobs, get it. And since you get two of them (for the low, low price of $19.99), send one to me!

SCENARIO 31. **ICU dilemmas: to extubate or not to extubate, that is the question**

"Welcome to the cardiac ICU," the instructor says. "Today, you'll be taking care of fresh hearts. Right now, there are two of them, eagerly awaiting your tender ministrations."

In the ICU portion of the simulator, there are two Laerdal simulators. Two anesthesia residents are assigned to go into the ICU. As with other simulations, a third resident will be in the control room, getting a different angle on the action.

Patient #1 is in the first bed, extubated, nasal cannula on, with his monitors showing a sat of 88%, BP 100/60, HR 75.

Patient #2 is in the second bed, is on a ventilator, with his monitors showing a sat of 99%, BP 150/85, HR 80. The ventilator is functioning and has a rate of 10.

The residents glance around then go over to patient #1. An ICU nurse (one of the Simulation Center's secretary) is at the bedside.

The first resident asks, "What's the story here?"

"This patient just came from the OR," the ICU nurse says. "Fast track after an off-pump bypass. They extubated on the table. Jehovah's Witness."

A chart at bedside has the rest of the information— Good EF to start the case, starting hematocrit 39, patient absolutely refuses blood bank blood but will take cell saver blood. The surgeon's note says a CABG × 3 was done without problems.

"Why did they extubate on the table?" the second resident asks. "What's the rush?"

"What's the patient's temperature?" the first resident asks.

The ICU nurse shrugs. (When nonmedical people "fill in" during scenarios, they are generally good at scripted responses but not at making up answers to unscripted questions. In its own way, that's fine, because a lot of time you can't get information in the real world either.) On the monitor, though, the temperature is shown: 34.3°C.

"Let's put him on a 100% rebreather mask," the first resident says. "See if we can get that sat up a little,

and let's get a Bair Hugger warming blanket on him. Do we have a blood gas?"

"Here you go," the ICU nurse hands over a slip of paper. 7.32 pH, 40 P_{CO_2}, 58 P_{O_2}, 88 oxygen saturation, −6 base excess, 42 hematocrit.

"Houston," the first resident says, "we have a problem."

"Yeah, no kidding we have a problem," the second resident says. "Think we should reintubate the guy?"

Over the intercom, a voice says, "Rebreather mask on the way, Bair Hugger on the way."

On the 100% rebreather mask, the patient's saturation creeps up to 90%.

"Mmmm, not quite yet. What do you make of the hematocrit?" the second resident says.

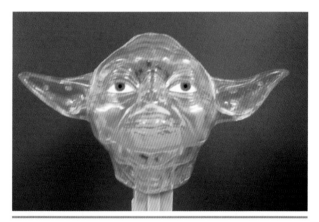

FIGURE 8–90 Feel the force.

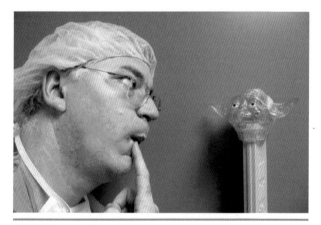

FIGURE 8–91 If something in your "inner force" feels uncomfortable, then probably something is wrong. Trust your feelings, Luke, trust those feelings, then make sure the patient is OK. Classic example? A nagging tachycardia that isn't responding to the "usual stuff." You just can't shake the feeling that "something is not right about that." You send a gas, whoa! Hematocrit 17! That explains it!

"Started out at 39, now he's at 42. And he's a Jehovah's Witness who won't take blood," the first resident says. "I'd say one of two things. We're either seeing a miracle of spontaneous hemato-generation, or else this guy is major league volume-depleted. This is hemoconcentration. That would go along with the base deficit of 6 as well. He's acidotic because he needs volume."

"Why'd they extubate him so cold, I wonder," the second resident asks. "Guy's a heart patient, last thing you need is an extubation at 34.3°. I'll bet the surgeon said, 'Extubate him on the table.' I'll bet you a million dollars that's what happened."

"Let's give him fluid, warm fluid," the first resident tells the ICU nurse. "Give him a liter of LR, then repeat the blood gas. OK? We better take a look next door, just make sure we don't get too wrapped up here and miss something fatal over here."

In the control room, the third resident is throwing himself at the controls. "Come on, let me kill this guy. Let's rock and roll and zap him! Isn't that what we're here for? Which one of these buttons will make him go into V fib?"

The technician holds the resident back, "Slow down, Killer."

"Believe it or not," the instructor tries to throw cold water on the murderous rage of the resident, "that isn't actually the be-all, end-all of simulation. We're not just a 'practice running a code place.' We're more of a 'can you think this stuff through' kind of a place."

A sulky pout from the resident, "OK, if you say so."

Technician and instructor look at each other. (Does this guy have ex-girlfriends buried in his back yard?)

The two residents in the ICU walk over to the second patient, the one on the ventilator.

Without getting asked, the ICU nurse gives them a report. "This man also had an off-pump CABG, but as you can see he's not intubated. The plan is to get him extubated over the next 2 hours or so."

"Is he bleeding?", the first resident asks.

"No."

"Any problems intraop?"

"No."

"Hard to intubate?"

"Um, I don't know."

The residents check the chart, sure enough, the intubation note catches their eyes, "Attempts × 3, MAC 3, no view, change to Miller 2, barely saw posterior arytenoids, passed blind. Decadron given for anticipated airway edema."

"Aha," the second resident says, "the game's afoot!"

"OK," the first resident says, "let's put his head up, try to get the swelling down. Easy on the fluids, if everything else is dandy, and let's start weaning him down. Let's make sure we're around when it's time to extubate, and let's do the whole 'what-happens-if-we-have-to-reintubate-him' thing happens."

They return to the first patient. A repeat blood gas shows the base excess is down to −3 after 2 liters of fluids. His Po_2 is up to 75.

"On the right track here," the first resident says.

"We're ready to extubate over here," the ICU nurse says. (In the "Simulator time zone" time always fast-forwards to the next event. You don't sit around for 6 hours while they wean the patient down.)

The residents go over the checklist of extubation.

"Muscle relaxants reversed?"

"Check."

"Warm, stable, not bleeding, nothing arguing against extubating? Neuro status good? He can protect his airway?"

"Roger."

"Blood gases OK, mechanics OK?"

"Roger wilco."

"What's with all this pilot talk? Are you some kind of ex-top gun F-15 jockey?"

"No," the first resident says, "but I liked Kelly McGillis in that movie."

"God all fishhooks," the second resident says, rolling his eyes. "All right, how about the fancy stuff for his airway? And just say OK, OK?"

"Roger that."

"Kill me now."

They have a fiberoptic brought in, let the cuff down and make sure the patient can breathe around the tube, and place a tube changer down the endotracheal tube to serve as a guide in case they need to slide the tube back in. They are ready, but ready.

The first resident asks, "In the real world, do they actually tolerate that tube changer sitting in their trachea? I would think they would gag and splutter like crazy."

"At this point, just before you extubate, they are kind of 'used to' the endotracheal tube sitting in their trachea. The tube changer is actually smaller. So, yeah, they do actually tolerate it. I've seen it with my own two eyes. It does look kind of odd, though."

In the control room, the third resident continues to stalk around, trying to find a way to code the patient.

"Come on, let's fibrillate him!"

"Why? They did everything right?"

"Oh, don't you guys ever have any fun in here!"

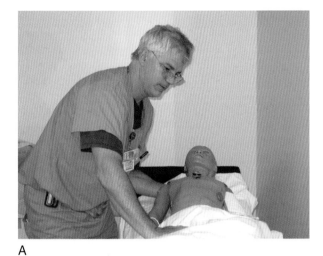

A

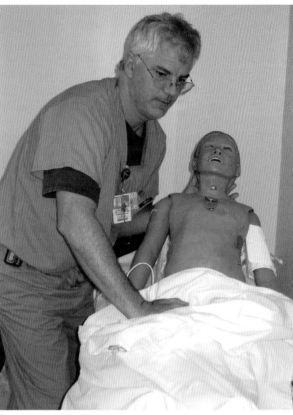

B

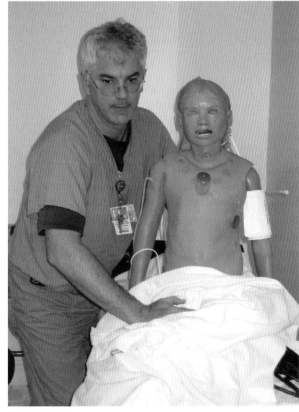

C

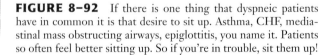

FIGURE 8–92   If there is one thing that dyspneic patients have in common it is that desire to sit up. Asthma, CHF, mediastinal mass obstructing airways, epiglottitis, you name it. Patients so often feel better sitting up. So if you're in trouble, sit them up!

The instructor leans into the intercom microphone, "Thus ends another chapter in the never-ending saga, Days of our Simulator. Head to the conference room."

"10-4," the first resident says.

The second resident grabs him by the throat and starts choking him, "10–4 this, good buddy!"

Clinical lessons learned from scenario 31

Debriefing. In the debriefing room, the first resident rubs his neck, "I think you subluxed something. Hope you have a good lawyer."

"Let's talk about fast tracking, early extubation, and the push to move faster," the instructor says. "I'll

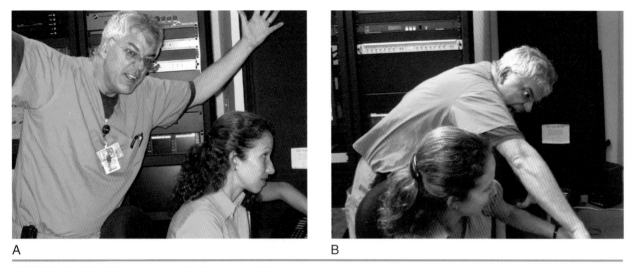

A   B

FIGURE 8–93 "Come on, let's fibrillate him!" When you first start teaching in the simulator, there is a temptation to always "go to the nth degree," make everyone die, turn every scenario into a code. No need! There are a hundred lessons, a thousand lessons that you can teach without going the "way of the code."

address this to our murderous friend who joined us in the control room." She fills them in on how their fellow resident kept wanting to fibrillate the patients.

"That first patient shows what can go wrong when you get all wrapped up in this 'Extubate on the table' business," the control room resident says. "I think whoever extubated was hot-dogging. Trying to impress the surgeon, impress the nurses, impress somebody.

"The patient's cold, the patient's not maintaining adequate oxygenation, the patient's in a bad metabolic state—look at the acidosis. This patient had a lot of reasons *not* to get extubated. So what did they do? 'Ooh, let's be really slick. Let's do a heart and extubate on the table!' Then look what happens. The guy slides into the ICU with one engine on fire, the landing gear shot away, and smoke in the cockpit."

"Not more pilot talk!" the second resident shouts.

"What?"

"Forget it."

The instructor jumps in, "Let's play the Talmudic scholar. Argue for me the opposite. Why *is* it a good idea to try to extubate soon?"

"You get your thoracic pump working for you, instead of the ventilator working against venous return," the first resident says. "The sooner he's extubated, the sooner he can cough, expand his lungs, prevent iatrogenic pneumonia. The patient breathing on his/her own is normal physiology. A ventilator breathing for the patient is abnormal physiology, now matter how you slice it or dice it."

"So there's good reason to stay away from the 'Give them 100 cc of fentanyl and let them sleep overnight' anesthesia of 20 years ago," the control room resident says. "But you still need to use your common sense. Don't go nuts trying to extubate early just so you can say you did it. Better to keep that airway protected during transport, let everything settle down in the ICU, then extubate once you get the 'all clear.'"

"All right," the instructor says, "let's go over the second patient, the difficult intubation. Take me along on your thinking there."

"You should have let me fibrillate that guy," the control room resident says.

"Back, back!" the instructor holds up an imaginary chair and cracks an imaginary whip.

"Caution's the byword here," the second resident says. "Don't burn any bridges. Always be ready to go back one step. That's why we made sure to have all the good stuff in the room in case we needed to reintubate—tube changer, fiberoptic."

"Give me a really imaginative way you could be 'ready to go' with that fiberoptic," the instructor says. "I mean, this will be a little over-the-top, but tell me how you could be ready, but ready."

A little time passes as the residents mull this over.

"Well," the control room resident says, "I guess you could vasoconstrict the nose, topicalize it, load an endotracheal tube into the nose, make sure that you can actually see the cords, and then extubate. If you get in trouble, you can slide that baby right in."

BOX 8-66	Extubating in the Unit

- Don't be a hero
- Have backup plan
- Tube exchanger?

"Even with all that, should you have the tube exchanger sitting in there?" the instructor asks.

"Yep," the second resident says. "Have a belt *and* suspenders. That way your pants never fall down."

"More important than all the reintubation stuff though," the first resident says, "is making sure that all the other stuff is OK before you do the extubation. Look over the metabolic picture, make sure the patient's neuro status is OK. Give them the good once-over before you go for broke."

"Time well spent," the instructor affirms.

"Still," the control room resident hovers around his favorite subject, "would have been fun to code the guy."

Summary. Fast tracking is hot right now. Economic pressures push us to do cases faster, faster, faster. This mind set can get in the way of common sense—if someone shouldn't be extubated, they shouldn't be extubated no matter what the 'economic climate.'

Extubation is a question of common sense—Does this patient need the tube to oxygenate, to get rid of carbon dioxide, or to keep the airway patent or protected? Is there anything *else* going on that would stress this patient out—metabolic problems, bleeding, hemodynamic instability, need for reoperation? If the answer to any of these questions is yes, don't take the tube out.

Extubation is not rocket science!

One way of looking at the endotracheal tube is this—Stand at the end of the bed. If the endotracheal tube looks like an "incidental finding," like a cigarette hanging out of the patient's mouth, you can take it out. If, in contrast, the endotracheal tube looks like a spike, holding the patient onto earth, preventing him from floating up to heaven, by all means keep the tube in.

The "tube changer in the endotracheal tube" is a great way to keep your options open. As counterintuitive as it may seem, patients do actually tolerate this maneuver. And remember some of the old chestnuts when it comes to extubating a patient with a difficult airway.

Extubate during the day, when there are people around.

Have stuff ready, just in case.

Go over everything else (blood gases, neuro check, mechanics) with a fine toothcomb to make sure all the "stuff other than the airway" is optimal.

SCENARIO 32: **In a high state of dudgeon over high blood pressure**

"It's up to you whether to go ahead on this guy," the instructor says. "He's in the holding area. His surgeon is in there too."

The two anesthesia residents go into the holding area. A surgeon (another anesthesia resident, coached to play the part) is pacing back and forth next to the patient (the Simulator).

"This is elective, this is elective, I know, I know," the surgeon says, hands up in a defensive posture. "This doesn't absolutely, positively have to go, I know. But I just want you guys to look this over and think about it, OK. Just think about it."

The holding area chart tells the story. The patient is a 58-year-old man with known CAD and S/P stent placement a year ago with no subsequent symptoms and no subsequent EKG changes. On arrival in the holding area for his outpatient lap cholecystectomy, his blood pressure was 160/110. He was given some clonidine PO, and now his blood pressure is 130/85.

A note at the bottom of the chart says, "Anesthesiologist refuses to do case. Blood pressure not optimized on arrival."

Looking at each other, the residents wonder what to do.

"Will one of you guys sleep this guy?" the surgeon asks. "Huh? Or do I send this guy home? What, what, or maybe do a spinal, if that's safer, I don't know." The surgeon stalks out of the room.

"Como esta senor?" the first resident asks. (The preop says the patient speaks Spanish only. The rest of the conversation is translated into English, however.)

"Fine," the patient says.

"And lately, been doing OK, getting around all right?" the second resident asks.

"When I don't have the pain under my ribs here," the patient says, "You know, after I eat."

"That's not like when you had the heart trouble, is it?" the second resident asks. "Like when you had the heart stent?"

"No, no. No trouble with that at all. Fine since they did that thing, you know, the Roto-rooter (using the same term in Spanish, of note) in my heart."

"Do any exercise?" the first resident asks.

"Yeah, some," the patient says. "Walk around the block a few times. Don't really jog or anything like that. Suppose I should."

"OK, give us a minute," the residents go to a corner of the room.

"Big deal," the first resident says, "his pressure's a little high, gets a little medication, and now he's fine. I say we go ahead."

"What about the note from the other anesthesiologist?" the second resident says. "Doesn't that paint us into a corner? Legally, I mean?"

"Well," the first resident thinks about it a little. "Medically, the thing to do is to proceed. We'll document like crazy and just do the right thing. That's what we should do."

They discuss this with the surgeon and then go into the OR. Everyone goes over to the OR simulation room, where the mannequin is monitored and ready to go.

"How we going to do this induction?" the first resident says. "Think we need an A-line?"

"Yeah. CAD, blood pressure required some treatment already. Our induction stuff might combine with that antihypertensive agent and, boom, pressure's in the basement and we've got ischemia on our hands," the second resident says. "Low risk procedure, high payoff."

"Art line's in," the intercom says, and an art trace appears on the monitor.

The residents induce, and the blood pressure goes through a few swings before it settles down. Up go the drapes, and the surgeon proceeds.

"Hey!" the surgeon says, "His stomach is full of air. Did you decompress his stomach?"

"No problem," the first resident says, then attempts to place an OG in the patient.

(Before the scenario, the instructor placed an IV cap in the esophagus, making it impossible to pass a gastric tube.)

No go, the tube won't pass for the first resident, then the second resident tries. No luck.

"Hey!" the surgeon shouts again. "I can't do this case with the stomach in my way. What's going on up there?"

Lift the chin, still no go. Turn the head to the side. The residents try every trick in the book but they cannot get that damned OG to go in. They try going nasally, but still no.

"Do I need to come up there and put the stupid tube in? What's the matter with you guys?" the surgeon's tone is rising.

"Time out," the first resident says, then looks over at the monitor. "Don't let's get all wound up about this OG tube and forget to take care of the patient."

Sure enough, the blood pressure has drifted up to 180/100, the heart rate to 100 and the first hint of maybe ST depression! They deepen the anesthetic, get the vital signs under better control, and get back to the problem of the OG tube.

"OK," the first resident says, "here's what we're going to do. Here's the ultimate when the gastric tube just won't go."

He cuts an endotracheal tube longitudinally, then places the laryngoscope and deliberately intubates the esophagus with this sliced endotracheal tube.

"Usually the gastric tube gets hung up high, coiling in the hypopharynx," the first resident says. "When we put the gastric tube through this endotracheal tube, that gets us most of the way there, at least through the hypopharynx and on into the esophagus. If that doesn't do it, then to hell with it, we need someone to take a look with a scope, because he might have some weird outpouching or something, some constriction, and we don't want to force it."

Once he places the endotracheal tube and puts the gastric tube inside, the intercom crackles, "No need for further heroics. We're done."

The instructor comes in the room and pulls out the IV cap.

"Sneaky son-of-a-bitch," the first resident says.

"I'll take that as a compliment."

Clinical lessons learned from scenario 32

Debriefing. "No Christmas ham for you!" the first resident says.

"I don't eat ham," the instructor says.

"All right then, no Christmas matzoh for you then," the first resident says.

"But . . . forget it," the instructor says. "I'm glad you know more about hypertension than about comparative religions. Tell me what your thinking was on the decision to proceed."

In a surprise move, the surgeon speaks first, "We talk a lot about elective cases, but something you want to keep in mind is that these aren't totally elective. I mean this guy is hurting! He's symptomatic from his gallbladder disease, that's why he came to see me. If we put him off and put him off and put him off, that's a lot of misery this guy is going through.

"Plus he's arranged time off from work, his brother came in town to watch the kids, his whole extended family is on tenterhooks. He got onto the OR schedule. There's a lot of stuff that gets put in place before an 'elective' case rolls into the operating room. I mean, if he's got something that's *really going to kill him*, then, no, that's not the time to operate. I'm not cavalier. If he gets a stroke or an MI, this doesn't just hang on your necks, it hangs on mine too. The family comes to me and says, 'What happened?' and I can't just say 'It's anesthesia's fault.' They don't care about anesthesia, they came to see me."

"Such eloquence from a surgeon," the first resident says. "And to think, you're actually one of *us*, not even a surgeon. You sound more like a surgeon than a *real* surgeon."

"Thanks," the surgeon says, "I did a little acting in college. You should see me do *A Streetcar Named Desire*. 'Stella!'"

Appreciative nods and smiles all around the debriefing table.

He holds up one hand, "Please, please, I'd like to take this moment to thank the Academy."

"What about the legal question," the instructor interrupts the thespian reverie. "One anesthesiologist has already weighed in against proceeding."

"Here's my take," the second resident says, "This is very much like Dr. McCoy on Star Trek, but, I'm a doctor, not a lawyer. This guy has easily controllable blood pressure. He is symptom-free, EKG change-free, and gives a good history of doing walks around the block. He's good to go, and we should proceed. If you send him off, hoping that he'll be 'optimized,' I got news for you. He won't come back optimized, he'll probably come back worse, as a matter of fact. So document and go."

"Good enough," the instructor says. "Now, the NG, or OG."

"Thanks for putting that obstruction there," the first resident says.

"It is through pain that we grow," the instructor explains.

"You have to know what the surgeon needs," the first resident says. "It's not just a luxury that the stomach get decompressed, There's a lot of stuff in there when they do a lap choly, and a big air balloon of a stomach will get in his way."

The surgeon speaks up, "I like that trick of the sliced endotracheal tube."

"Very handy," the first resident says. "It really does get you past the easy-to-coil-in upper pharynx. And once past that, unless some heartless bastard has placed an obstruction in your way, it should go."

"But when you're doing funky stuff like that, it is easy to take your 'eyes off the road,' isn't it?" the instructor says.

"Oh yes," the second resident says. "Very easy. You have to step back every now and then and remind yourself—Take care of the patient, don't kill the patient while you're placing a gastric tube."

Turning to the surgeon, the instructor asks, "Did you ever do any stand-up comedy in addition to your acting?"

"So the soda lime absorber traveling salesman goes into a bar. . . ."

Summary. To proceed or not to proceed, that is the question. That is *the* question that faces anesthesiologists every day. In some cases, it's easy.

> Emergency: life, limb or sight at risk, you have to go
> Elective: patient just ate? No way.

Then there are the multiple gray zones.

> Asthma: is it under "good control" or the "best possible" control?
> Diabetes: how high is too high on the glucose?
> Hypertension: how high do you dare go before you say "no"?

Absolutely rigid guidelines are tough to come by and tougher to enforce in the real world, especially when, with our short-acting medications, we can fix most things. So you're left with the vague directive, "Evaluate each case on its own merits."

Here, the residents decided that, with good blood pressure control and a good exercise history, proceeding was the best thing to do.

The gastric tube, probably the last thing on the residents' mind, presented the next dilemma. As with all other procedures (TEE, central line, art line), the key idea here is to *take care of the patient*, not *do the procedure*. The procedure is always secondary. It doesn't do any good to place an NG tube perfectly and then discover you have an NG sitting in the stomach of a recently deceased patient!

And when it comes to acting, remember the advice of Spencer Tracy, "Learn your lines and don't trip over the furniture."

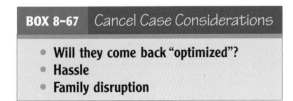

BOX 8–67 *Cancel Case Considerations*

- **Will they come back "optimized"?**
- **Hassle**
- **Family disruption**

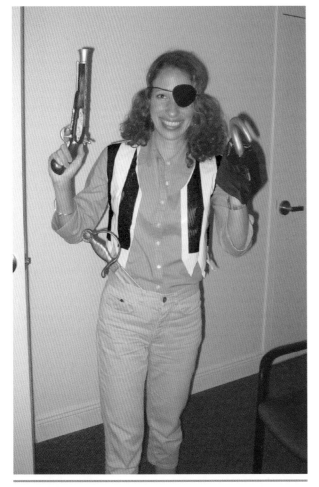

FIGURE 8–94 Ahoy matie! This scenario of "creating an anesthetic from scratch" is based on an actual case. One of the attendings here at Jackson had to call a cruise ship (or was it a pirate ship?) and "talk them through" a Sux drip, ketamine drip anesthetic. And the patient survived.

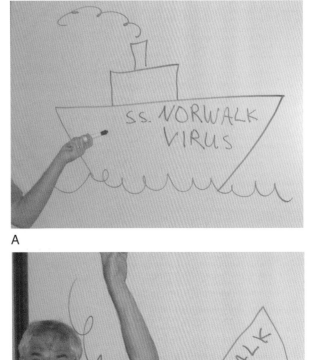

FIGURE 8–95 Don't go down with the ship. Pay attention to the basics, back to ABC, and you can even give an anesthetic under the most basic circumstances. So long as you have the airway—some way to provide pain relief and amnesia—you should be able to keep the ship afloat.

| SCENARIO 33. | **Cobbling together an anesthetic on the high seas**

"What's with the pirate getup?" the first resident asks of the instructor.

Standing with the complete pirate "do," the instructor pulls out a whistle and blows it. "Now here this, now here this. You are on board the newest cruise ship, the SS Norwalk Virus, ship's flag Liberia. You will proceed to the ship's sick bay for a consult. A surgeon is waiting for you there along with a patient."

The two residents go into the "sick bay" where a patient (Simulator) waits as does a surgeon (another anesthesia resident, primed to play the part of the surgeon). The patient (female, as indicated by a wig) is moaning like anything.

On the monitor, the blood pressure is 85/50, pulse is 140, Sao_2 is 98% on 3 L nasal cannula. There is a small portable ventilator by the side of the bed and an IV bag hanging.

"This woman's last period was 3 months ago, she is having sharp pains in her abdomen," the surgeon says. "It is my feeling she has a ruptured ectopic pregnancy, and we need to operate."

"OK," the first resident says, then looks around. "Let's go into the operating room. No time to wait. Is she typed and crossed?"

"Perhaps you do not understand our situation, doctors," the surgeon says. "We are on board the SS Norwalk Virus, 8 hours out of Aruba. We have no blood bank. We have normal saline and that is it."

"Then we'd better evacuate her," the second resident says. "Get a Coast Guard helicopter out here."

"Aruba has no Coast Guard, and the American Coast Guard can't reach this far out," the surgeon says. "Gentlemen, we are on our own."

Looking for the usual stockpile of labeled syringes, the residents get a puzzled expression on their faces.

"All you have here is midazolam, Sux, and ketamine," the first resident says. "Do you have an anesthesia machine?"

"No."

"Narcotics?"

"Vicodin pills."

"Muscle relaxants other than Sux?"

"No."

"God Almighty," the first resident says.

The two residents keep looking around, hoping somehow, by looking, more drugs will magically appear on the SS Norwalk Virus. No luck.

"OK," the second resident says, taking charge. "Let's get at least a couple liters of fluid in her, then we go. Sux and ketamine. Not the worlds' greatest combo, but that's what we got. We'll give a little Versed up front and hope we don't get any recall."

"I don't suppose you have a BIS monitor on board," the first resident says, then laughs.

"We do have airway stuff, right?" the first resident says. "I mean, you have to have a code cart."

They do, and the residents make sure the light works in the laryngoscope. They also hook up an Ambu-bag to the portable ventilator, make sure it works, check suction, and check the oxygen source.

"How we going to keep her relaxed?" the first resident asks.

"Sux drip," the second resident says.

"What the hell do we know from a Sux drip?"

"Let's go to the Internet while we load her up with fluids."

Fortunately, the ship has Internet access, and the residents get a plan ready.

Sux—Intubate with the usual dose, then mix 500 mg in 500 cc NS and run at 15 drops/min (1 cc/min, about 60 mg/hr) and titrate up as needed. The patient could need as much as 10 cc/min to keep relaxed.

Ketamine—induce with 2 mg/kg, then mix up an infusion of 500 mg in 500 cc and run this at 15 drops/min (1 cc/min, about 60 mg/hr) and titrate up, looking for signs of light anesthesia (tearing, movement, tachycardia—which, admittedly, would be hard to diagnose against this backdrop of severe anemia).

Versed—4 mg at induction, then 2 mg every half hour to keep amnesia on board.

"Given the amount of bleeding, the plan would be to keep her intubated and sedated until port is reached. In the meantime, full steam ahead for Aruba! Make sure the captain knows," the first resident says.

"Let's do one more thing," the second resident says, "let's prep and drape her at the start, like a C-section. I don't think this makeshift pseudoanesthetic will be any great shakes, so the sooner out, the better."

They induce, intubate, and the case gets going. After induction, the heart rate goes to 160, and the blood pressure stays in the 85 to 90 systolic range.

"Slow her down?" the first resident asks.

"No way, she's young, this is all compensatory," the second resident says.

After a few minutes: "She's moving!" the surgeon yells.

They increase the Sux drip, then give a bolus of 25 mg of ketamine.

"Land ho!" the instructor shouts over the intercom and follows it with a shrill blast of the whistle. "All hands to the debriefing room!"

Clinical lessons learned from scenario 33

Debriefing. Merry sea shanties are belting out over a boombox in the debriefing room.

"What do you do with a drunken sailor,
"What do you do with a drunken sailor,
"What do you do with a drunken sailor, ear-ligh in the mor-ning?"

"You're enjoying this way too much," the surgeon tells the instructor.

"Hey," the instructor defends herself, "if you can't have fun at work, don't go to work!"

"OK, talk my arm off."

The first resident takes the lead, "Well here we are, sort of stranded on Gilligan's Island, with someone about to die if we don't do something. A ruptured ectopic might as well be a firehose of blood emptying into the abdomen. Nothing will tamponade it, and the belly will 'accept' most of your blood volume. You can die in just a few hours, and this woman is already showing signs of severe hypovolemia."

"So," the second resident picks up, "we have to cobble an anesthetic together. This is, really, kind of like in the ICU when they have to do a procedure. Once you have the airway secured, it's just a question of giving enough IV agent to keep the patient relaxed, amnestic, and asleep."

"Did you worry about a phase II block from the succinylcholine?" the instructor asks.

> **BOX 8-68** *Jury-Rigged Anesthetic*
>
> - **If you have to, you have to**
> - **Support ABC**
> - **Secure airway, if at all possible**
> - **You'll be amazed, it can be done**

"Not really," the first resident says. "I was figuring, even if it happened, I was going to keep her intubated at the end of this case. This is such unfamiliar turf here that I just said to myself—'So what if she's into phase II, just protect that airway and keep some sedative on board until we get to Aruba and can get her into a real ICU.' That was it. Keep it simple, stupid."

"Tachycardia bother you? I mean, isn't everything in anesthesia now about preventing tachycardia with beta blockers?"

"Different patient population there," the second anesthesia resident says. "That's the CAD crowd you're talking about. This is a young woman, and she is trying to keep everything perfused with Kool-Aid blood. Who knows how low her hematocrit is going? Any attempt to slow her down would just pull the rug out from underneath her compensatory mechanisms. Probably kill her."

"If it helps," the first resident says, "this ship probably doesn't even have any beta blockers."

"We have Dramamine for sea sickness," the surgeon says. "Plenty of that!"

Summary. As an anesthesiologist, you may get "called upon" to provide anesthesia in some "less than optimal" places—medical missionary work, out in the wilds on a safari, on a cruise ship. Strange stories abound of anesthesiologists getting "pressed into service" in odd places under odd circumstances.

Doctors first! Specialists second! When the call comes, you have to help out!

These residents quickly grasped the situation, and converted their OR/ICU skills into a shipboard kind-of-OR, kind-of-ICU anesthetic. Stick to the basics—get that airway, resuscitate with what you can, head for safe harbor (literally), and use what you have.

Young patients can take a lot of punishment and still come back for more, as this young woman did.

ABC, ABC, ABC.

SCENARIO 34. **Say this 10 times fast: papilloma in the pregnant patient**

"You better take a look at this woman, she doesn't sound too good," the instructor says, and leads the anesthesia residents into the examining room. A standardized patient is sitting there. Stridor, inspiratory and expiratory, is audible across the room.

She can talk, but with some effort, "Papillomas, I've got . . . papillomas."

Her chart lists a diagnosis of recurrent respiratory papillomatosis. She is a 28-year-old scheduled for excision of these subglottic lesions today. Also noted on her chart, she has a positive pregnancy test.

"How far along are you?" the first resident asks.

"14 weeks."

The chart also notes that the surgeons do not want the patient intubated. Because the lesions are subglottic, an endotracheal tube may "scrape off" the lesions, making them tumble farther down the trachea, seeding little respiratory papillomas all the way, creating a real nightmare later. A forest of respiratory papillomas all throughout the respiratory tree.

The anesthesia residents confer among themselves.

"Jet ventilation?" the second resident asks.

"No," the first resident answers, "the puff from that jet ventilator could break off the papilloma too and blow that little monster 10 miles down the respiratory tree."

"OK, so we can't intubate, we can't jet ventilate, and we probably don't even want to do positive-pressure ventilation, period," the second resident says. "So she'll have to breathe spontaneously, I guess, the whole time. Will they be able to put in their, what's that thing called? The ENT-o-scope. The laryngoscope with the covered bridge thing?"

"The Dido laryngoscope," the first resident says. "I think it was named after the famous ENT doctor named Dr. Laryngoscope."

"God help us."

In the hallway, on the way to the operating room, the anesthesia residents go over a few more plans.

"She's pregnant, 14 weeks," the first resident says, "should we delay this?"

"No way, her airway's gonna get more and more narrow as she swells with pregnancy, and she's stridorous already, we better go ahead."

"Aspiration prophylaxis?" the first resident asks. "She *is* pregnant, and we're not going to have her airway secured, you know."

"Right. We'll do the whole nine yards, metoclopramide, ranitidine, nonparticulate oral antacid. Then, Prop drip, breathe her deep but deep, then see if they can put the scope in. We won't be able to use relaxant, or else we'd have to do assist her breathing, and we don't want to do that unless we have to."

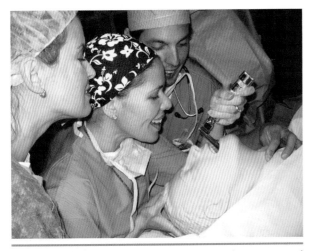

FIGURE 8–96 Sharing the airway can become a real bummer. Pretty soon it seems like the whole Mormon Tabernacle Choir is hovering around the airway. Don't be afraid to push some people back so you can get a "clear shot." One constant danger with a lot of people is disconnection as someone bumps the hoses. Keep in mind the old adage, "When there are seven nursemaids, the baby drowns."

"Wait," the first resident says, "she's sure to have questions about the baby. We better go back in there and talk to her."

In the examining room, the residents reintroduce themselves to the patient.

"How will my . . . baby do?" the patient asks. "Is the . . . is the anes . . . anesthesia OK for a . . . baby?"

The first resident takes the lead, "Bottom line, anesthesia has been proven safe over many years and many cases. Lots of pregnant women have had operations, and the test of time has shown us that this is safe. You are at 14 weeks, so a lot of the initial formation of major organs and such is done, and anesthetics haven't been linked with malformations.

"Now, in general, we put off entirely elective cases if you're pregnant, just along the lines of—don't expose a baby to unnecessary medications unless you have to. But this case is not really something we can put off. You're working a little at your breathing now, and this will get worse as time goes on. So to take good care of you, we need to take these things out.

"One rule always holds true, 'To take good care of baby, take good care of Mommy.' And that's just what we'll do today."

As they walk out of the room, the second resident says, "You're good. One day, if you keep this up, you might, just *might*, be as good as I am."

"I can only hope."

In the operating room, the residents get everything ready. They have a 6.0 endotracheal tube there, just in case, but will do everything in their power to avoid using it.

Monitors, preoxygenation, all vital signs are OK.

They start a propofol drip (a dummy drip with saline in it, but they program the pump as if it were the real thing) at 150 µg/kg/min. With the mask on, they dial the sevoflurane up, performing an inhalation induction. No muscle relaxants are given.

After 3 minutes, the ENT surgeon (the second anesthesia resident does this, playing the part of the surgeon), places the Dido scope, reaches in, and pretends to scrape the lesions clean.

Pulling out, he says, "OK, we would basically repeat this as often as necessary. Breathe down, stop, place the scope, scrape the lesions, and go until done."

"Truth to tell," the first anesthesia resident says, "to keep her down, we'd probably have to trickle in some narcotics, but I'm talking 10 µg, maybe 25 µg of fentanyl at a time. Never want to give so much that she'd stop breathing."

"Good enough," the overhead loudspeaker says, "done!"

Clinical lessons learned from scenario 34

Debriefing. "Lot going on here," the instructor says. "Just lay it out for me again."

The second resident says, "Pregnant, aspiration risk, can't instrument the airway, patient already symptomatic, will need to put a laryngoscope in without muscle relaxant. You're right, a lot's going on here."

"And you're committed to spontaneously ventilating," the first resident says. "Mask intubating an adult too, not the usual thing. You're heading into some different turf here."

"What about placing the laryngoscope?" the instructor asks. "How can you instrument an airway without paralyzing the patient first?"

You don't absolutely have to. You just have to get them good and deep. Breathe them deep and have some propofol going."

The second resident continues, "Best thing is, ENT is cool. You work with them, they know about

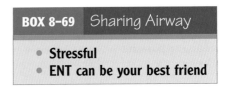

BOX 8-69 Sharing Airway

- **Stressful**
- **ENT can be your best friend**

the airway, they know you can't paralyze. Hell, they appreciate that you're not just ramming the tube in and screwing it all up. They'll be cool if they have to wait a minute while you deepen the patient."

"Talk to me about narcotics," the instructor asks.

"Tread lightly," the first resident says, "tread real lightly. Just trickle it in, because you don't want apnea. And a slug of fentanyl will give you apnea. Give a little bit at a time, dilute it down, even, and just give $10\,\mu g$ at a time. The narcotic helps blunt the sympathetic response all right. And the narcotic reduces the MAC, but you just have to tiptoe with it."

"And let's play out the 'Delay this until she's not pregnant anymore' scene," the instructor says.

"We covered that in the hallway," the first resident says. "Her airway was sure to get edematous as she progressed. That, plus the possibility that the papillomas would extend, would really get her in trouble."

"And the longer you wait the 'more of a full stomach' she is," the second resident says. "Imagine taking this on 3 months from now, when she is physically and hormonally even more of an aspiration risk."

"No, thank you," the first resident says. "Damn, I just thought of something. We should have put on those special masks, shouldn't we? Those masks that filter out the viruses and stuff when you're doing papillomas in the genital region."

The instructor raises his eyes, "You're right! By Jiminy you are right. I hadn't thought of that myself! Glad I thought of it now, though."

Summary. Sharing the airway with ENT places a strain on any anesthesia situation. And some cases are more difficult than others. Here, the lesions are subglottic and the endotracheal tube itself could knock the lesions deeper into the respiratory tree.

When does a pregnant patient "become" a full stomach? At 14 weeks, she has probably "turned the corner" and represents an aspiration risk. But you have to weigh that aspiration risk against the other danger—spreading the papillomas further.

Thank goodness for sevoflurane—a quick-onset, nonpungent inhalation anesthetic agent. Perfect for inhalation induction in a child, and—surprise, surprise—perfect for inhalation induction in an adult as well.

We are creatures of habit, and we tend to think along similar lines all the time—to place a laryngoscope, we need muscle relaxant. Not true! Get a patient deep enough, and you can indeed place a laryngoscope. Might not be perfect, might not be optimal, but it should be good enough to get the case done.

So with a little clever maneuvering, planning, and discussing with the surgeon, you can accomplish this little "miracle of miracles," cleaning out the trachea of papillomas.

SCENARIO 35. **Love is a many-splendored thing, clotted aortic valve in a parturient**

"Love must be in the air," the instructor says, "because your next patient is also pregnant."

"Cupid's arrows fly thick around here," the first anesthesia resident says. "Maybe one will strike me."

"Um," the second anesthesia resident says, "you've been married twice already, Romeo. Cupid's found the range on you."

The residents look over the patient's history.

She is a 32-year-old woman, 4 years S/P aortic valve replacement. She had a congenital bicuspid aortic valve, developed symptomatic aortic stenosis, and had the replacement. As she would require lifelong anticoagulation, she was strongly advised against becoming pregnant. But pregnancy arrived one day. Her Coumadin was discontinued, and her obstetrician placed her on enoxaparin. She was now in the emergency room and very short of breath. She is about 24 weeks pregnant. The ER doc says her chest sounds odd, that he can't hear a mechanical click, and he suspects something is wrong with the valve. He's called for an echo, but wants someone from anesthesia to see her because she looks so bad she might need to be intubated soon.

"Then without further ado," the residents go in the standardized patient room. A pregnant woman is sitting in there, bolt upright, with an oxygen mask on, and she is gasping.

"What's going on?" the first anesthesia resident asks.

She looks at him but can't say anything, she just continues to sit there and puff.

The pulse oximeter cannot pick up anything.

"Get the cart," the first resident says. "Whatever the valve problem, we are just about to have a respiratory arrest. She can't even say a full sentence."

"Ma'am, we're going to have to put a breathing tube in your mouth to help you breath."

She just continues to look forward.

The instructor comes in the room, "OK, the cart is sent for, now we'll go to the OR. Transthoracic echo shows this." He holds up an echo that shows a clot causing almost complete occlusion of the artificial aortic valve. Distension is present in the left ventricle, and the EF is almost nil.

In the operating room, the patient (METI simulator) is propped upright. A fetal heart tone monitor is in the corner, with an obstetrician (a secretary from the center) there. "Can we get a fetal heart tone before she goes to sleep? We have to do a section before you replace the aortic valve."

Gasping sounds escape from the patient, and an arterial trace shows a blood pressure of 60/40. The EKG shows sinus tachycardia with a rate of 150, and the pulse oximeter still can't pick it up."

"No time for that," the first resident says, putting the laryngoscope in her mouth.

"No meds?" the second resident says.

"Sux and some scopolamine, nothing else," the first resident says. Intubation proceeds OK, and the blood pressure holds at 60/40. "Get CT surgery in here, we need to go, she won't make it through a C-section, we've got to get her on bypass."

"Left uterine displacement? Head down?" the second resident asks.

"OK," the first resident says, "we can do that now, since we got the airway."

They put the patient flat, slide a pillow under her right hip, and the blood pressure goes to 40/20.

"Start CPR!" the first resident says, "Get the surgeon in here, splash and slash, come on, we have to go, I'm giving heparin."

The obstetrician steps out of the room, puts on a different gown, and comes back in, "CT surgery, what's up?" (One person can play different characters. Just changing one little thing is sufficient to convey the message—new person.)

"We have to go on bypass now," the second resident says. "This pregnant woman occluded her prosthetic aortic valve and has essentially put a cork in her left ventricle. Heparin's in and CPR is in progress."

"OK," the CT surgeon says, "let's do it."

Over the intercom, "OK, the valve has been replaced, and now it's time to come off bypass, got it?"

The residents nod.

"For the record," the first resident says, "I'll go over the stuff we'd check before coming off bypass.

A—airway: Turn on the ventilator and make sure the lungs go up and go down.

B—bureaucracy: Make sure "everything metabolic" is OK—hematocrit, potassium, oxygen, glucose, pH, temperature.

C—circulation: Get the best rhythm and rate, then focus on the contractility of the heart.

They turn the ventilator on. The arterial trace reaches 75/47 but just won't climb. An epinephrine drip starts (saline run through a real pump, programmed just like in the operating room to make sure the residents know how to work the pump).

BP 95/60.

Looking in the field, the surgeon says, "Looks good." Then, "Hey, what's going on with my suture line!"

BP 240/130.

"What's going on, the blood pressure is too high, my suture line is going to tear!" the surgeon yells.

The first resident looks at the pump. Epinephrine is infusing at $2\,\mu g/kg/min$, that is, a rate of 150 $\mu g/min$—a full 70 times the normal dose.

"No!" he shouts, "It's supposed to be $2\,\mu g/min$, that's it. Not $2\,\mu g/kg/min$! That's way too much!" He disconnects the pump, let's the blood pressure come down, then restarts the pump at $2\,\mu g/min$.

"Oh God, that's right," the second anesthesia resident says. "I was thinking of dobutamine or dopamine, those things are $\mu g/kg/min$. Sorry."

"You gotta watch that," the first resident says.

"Guess we can put the fetal heart rate monitor on now," the surgeon says, "That OK with you guys?"

"Sure."

The fetal heart rate shows a rate of 130, but there is very little variability.

"Do we need to section?" the surgeon asks.

"No variability can be a bad one," the second resident says. "Call OB."

"Wait, hold that call," the first resident says. "This kid's only at 24 weeks, this would be too early, I mean, this kid would be so premature I don't think many make it at this age.

"Wait, no, wait a minute, I just thought of something too. Loss of variability, wait, that's a regular reaction to general anesthesia in a baby. That's right. Now that Mom's stable, we have her on some Forane, so that's a normal response to anesthesia. We don't need to cut here."

"Oh yeah," the second resident says.

"Oh yeah is right," the intercom says. "And 'oh we're done' is right too."

BOX 8-70 *Crashing?*
• **ABC**
• **Forget "routine," get going**
• **Delay = death**

Clinical lessons learned from scenario 35

Debriefing. "No chocolates?" the first resident asks.

"What?" the instructor answers back.

"Well, you know, all this talk about Cupid before. I figure we rated some chocolates, that's all."

"Here," the instructor throws down some Oreos. "'A kid'll eat the middle of an Oreo first, and save the chocolate cookie outsides for last.' Isn't that sort of how the Oreo jingle goes?"

"There, now that you're all sugared up, tell me a little about this case you just did," the instructor asks. She eats the cookies straight, none of this eat the middle part first business.

"The patient's in extremis," the first resident starts, "that's for sure. You've just slammed the door shut on a valve sitting at the exit point of the left ventricle. No flow out the ventricle, and you are a dead man."

"Or a dead Mom, in this case," the second resident says.

"Right. And you have the additional problem that CPR is not effective with a gravid uterus sitting there, so you could argue to do the C-section right away to make CPR effective. Toss in this extra cookie, though, CPR in the face of an occluded artificial valve is *also* ineffective. Let's face it, CPR gives you, maybe, on a good day, an EF of 10%. And 10% EF pounding against an occluded valve, well, forget it."

"What's your thinking on the age of the baby," the instructor asks.

"Those neonatologists are miracle workers, and they're forever getting 1 pound peanuts through the neonatal ICU," the second resident says. "But if we can at all deliver them a baby a little farther along, we're avoiding lots of lung trouble and necrotizing enterocolitis and retrolental fibroplasias. So, hey, get Mom through the troubles, and you may be able to get baby through, too."

"What are the numbers?" the first resident asks.

"Fetal survival after cardiopulmonary bypass is about 50%, but it's hard to say—is it bypass or the stress of surgery. You're not exactly doing elective, minor surgery in these cases."

"What's your goal on bypass as far as pressure goes?" the instructor asks.

Neither resident can answer that one.

"That's admittedly a pretty specialized question," the instructor says. "Our best guess physiologically is to keep the blood pressure about 80 during bypass because the placental villi are pressure-dependent. No one knows if pulsatile or not makes a difference."

"That would be a hard study to design," the first resident says.

"Amen."

"Why do you think she crashed when you laid her back and put the hip roll underneath her," the instructor says. As she asks the question, she rolls the DVD from the scenario. Sure enough, they have to start CPR when the patient is put flat and then put in left uterine displacement.

"I'd point a finger at the clot in the aortic valve," the first resident says. "Who knows what configuration that clot has? Maybe just moving it around a little converted a partial block into a complete block."

"Any drug going to help you at that point?"

"You could always blast her with epinephrine," the second resident says. "That usually rallies just about anyone for a minute or two. But the die was cast here. She needed her chest opened and needed to get on bypass. That's pretty much it."

They look over the rest of the recorded session.

"I like that, when you come off—the ABC thing," the instructor says. "It keeps you from forgetting stuff."

"Airway. Bureaucracy. Cardiac. I might have to steal that."

Blushing, the second resident relives his mistake on the infusion pump as he sees it on the DVD.

"Man, I gotta remember that," he says. "I blew it with that μg/kg/min instead of the μg/min."

"Here's another one," the first resident says. "Mix any inotrope or vasoactive drug in 250 cc. Start the drip at 15 cc/hr. Go up or down based on response. Using that formula, you are never far off. You might be a *little* but never a *lot*. And because everything is based on response anyway, who cares about the exact dose?"

"Another good trick. Here," the instructor throws him another Oreo, "a reward for your fancy tricks."

The second resident gives the first a sidelong glance, "Here," he throws another Oreo, "see if you can roll over and play dead now."

Summary. This case is a killer, with a rapidly decompensating patient and a lot of confounding variables. An immature baby on board, a heart with a stopper in it, and no time. So the residents needed to make their choice—fix the valve first—and get a move on.

This woman's problem, incidentally, was preventable. A pregnant woman cannot take warfarin during early pregnancy for fear of birth defects. But a pregnant woman with an artificial valve must remain anticoagulated or the valve clots off (as happened here). What to do? Recommendations are heparin throughout pregnancy or else heparin during the first trimester, warfarin during the second trimester (after organogenesis is complete), then heparin during the last trimester. A pretty exhausting regimen!

Is enoxaparin approved for anticoagulation for pregnant patients with artificial valves? No.

Once the patient made it through the initial "excitement," the residents faced two additional dilemmas.

First, what to do in the face of the alarming "loss of variability" on the FHR monitor? Luckily, someone had done his reading and remembered that this is a normal response to anesthesia. What do you know? Reading your anesthesia book can prevent an unnecessary C-section and premature baby!

Second, the error programming the epinephrine infusion pump. It's easy to get mixed up with which drug is mcg/min, which is mcg/kg/min. The best defense against a gross error is to use common sense. The "mix whatever you want, start at 15 cc/hr and go

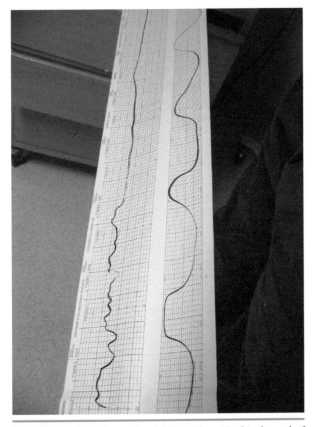

FIGURE 8–97 Loss of variability. Oh no! Is this the end of the world? No, the baby is just responding to general anesthesia. Back to "Know your strips." If you don't read them right, you could end up jumping into an unnecessary and premature C-section.

up or down based on effect" rule is a good one. You can always get more precise later. But initially, start your drug at a reasonable starting dose (and 15 cc/hr is a reasonable starting dose), you can always fine-tune later. Remember, it's the patient's *response* that counts, not the exact dosage of the drug.

SCENARIO 36. **Talkative patient from Chernobyl with ankylosing spondylitis**

"Hope you're good at regional," the instructor says.

"Why?" the anesthesia residents ask.

"This guy could sure use one."

The preop evaluation lays out a pretty grim story. A 62-year-old Russian man with ankylosing spondylitis, non-insulin-dependent diabetes mellitus, COPD, hepatitis, peripheral vascular disease, S/P right BKA 2 years ago, S/P left BKA 10 days ago, now with a gangrenous stump requiring revision. His most recent operation was done under a spinal, but the note says, "Took more than a dozen attempts, and the patient states he'd rather die than go through that again."

Physical exam is remarkable for a pronounced C shape of his entire back, with his "chin resting on his chest and fixed there."

The instructor leads them to the examining room, where the patient (a coached medical student) is sitting in a wheelchair, a blanket over his (what would have been amputated in real life) legs. His chin rests squarely on his chest, and the patient looks up at the anesthesia residents by lifting his eyes and tilting back his entire body.

Before the residents can ask a question, the patient speaks in a Russian accent, "You know where I am from?"

The residents know he's from Russia. Where, exactly, doesn't really matter, the issue here is that C-shaped neck and the airway problems attendant.

"Little village, north of Kiev," the patient goes on, "you knowing where that near?"

Neither resident could point out Kiev if their lives depended on it.

"That where Chernobyl plant is, atom plant, that why I this way," the patient says. "Never bent like this, then big fire in Chernobyl and say can't walk in woods. Too much dirty in woods from air from plant. Can't eat mushrooms, can't drink water. Where I am supposed to drink? You eat without mushrooms. Mushrooms I like, they out there in woods. Why I not eat? Now I bent, and no one believe me."

The two anesthesia residents look at each other, sort of wanting to move along, but sort of not wanting to cut the patient off.

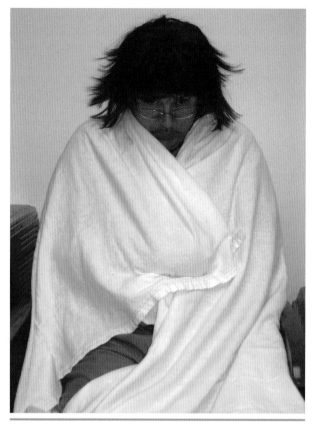

FIGURE 8–98 Ankylosing spondylitis with fixed flexion in the neck. A real airway nightmare. The chin is stuck on the chest, you can't extend anything, and the "old reliable" (a trach in case all else fails) is not even an option. Yikes!

"OK," the first resident says. "I see you don't want us to put that numbing medicine in your back, to numb you up for this leg operation?"

"You say numbing, I say numbing medicine not so good," the patient says. "Must be come from Russia. Ha! That joke. Get it, come from Russia. Mafia probably take all numbing medicine out, send you vodka instead, that why I am hurting so much. Ha! Why you doctors always so serious?"

Nervous titters from the resident. "Hey, that's a good one," the second resident tosses out an anemic response. "We were thinking of giving you some numbing medicine—good stuff this time. Numbing medicine we won't put in your back but in your leg, it's called a fem-sciatic block, that should make you numb enough for the operation. OK?"

"Fine," the patient says, "long as not Russian. Long as, maybe, Japanese. Make good cars, maybe make good numbing medicine too. Ha ha! Come on, doctors, little smile. Not always so serious. Look at

me. Legs gone, bent like, what you say, bent like, you know that thing you eat with salt."

"Pretzel."

"Pretzel, that right, pretzel," the patient says. "I am having sugar disease, bad heart. I not bother you long, pretty soon I gone, you know that. Just we have a little fun before I go, OK? You think they have bent coffin for me? Maybe make special pretzel coffin, just for me? That funny to see. Get one more joke. Even dead, make people laugh."

The first anesthesia resident wants to steer back to the anesthetic plan and is waffling a little on how just to do this.

"Go ahead," the patient says, "you want more doctor talk, go ahead."

"Right," the first resident says. "This numbing medicine in your leg, this special block. You know, with the Japanese numbing medicine . . ."

"Good," the patient says, "Doctor is making joke now too. Very good. I don't even care you kill me now, at least I die laughing."

A wan smile on his face, the first anesthesia resident plows on, "In case this numbing stuff doesn't work—and sometimes it doesn't—we'll have to put a breathing tube in you while you're still awake. A little sleepy, and we'll numb you up, but you'll still be awake so you can keep breathing OK for us. And once the tube's in, then you'll go to sleep. But because your head is curved around, we can't put the tube in after you're asleep, that would be too dangerous. Is that OK with you?"

"Fine, any doctor tell joke can doing anything with me," the patient says.

In the operating room, the residents hook up the monitors to the mannequin. (It's too hard to bend the mannequin into a C, so the residents are told to imagine this is the same patient.)

With erasable magic marker, they draw the landmarks for a femoral block, then demonstrate how they would place the block. Although they can't stick the mannequin, they go through the motions of drawing up the local anesthetic, show how they'd use the nerve stimulator, aspiration before injection, and frequent checking of vital signs and symptoms to guard against intravascular injection. On the department store mannequin (more easily turned prone), they do the same for the sciatic portion of the block.

Over the intercom, the instructor says, "The block fails."

"OK, on to plan B," the second resident says. "Awake fiberoptic."

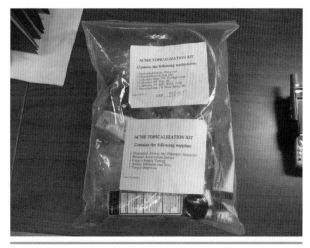

FIGURE 8–99   If you have all your "airway prep" things in one bag, life is much easier. You don't have to spend all day running around getting stuff. You spend your time doing what you should be doing—topicalizing the airway.

BOX 8-71   Awake Intubation Logistics

- **Know where the stuff is**
- **Have your own "tricks" handy**
- **Look slick, be slick**

Pulling out a plastic bag, the first resident says, "Behold, the Acme Topicalization Kit."

"What's this?" the second resident asks.

"An ingenious device of my own invention. Because the hardest thing about doing an awake intubation is 'getting all the stuff,' I put all the stuff I could possibly need in this handy traveling case."

The bag holds:

1 Diphenhydramine 50 mg vial
2 Glycopyrrolate 0.2 mg vials
1 Lidocaine ointment 5%, 35.44 g tube
1 Lidocaine 4% topical liquid bottle
1 Lidocaine 2% jelly 30 ml tube
1 Phenylephrine 1% nose spray bottle
1 Ovassapian airway
1 Mucosal atomization device
1 Oxygen supply tubing (female-female connections)
1 Miller airway
1 Tongue depressor

"Wow," the second resident says. "Nice."

"Hey," the patient says through the mannequin's speakers, "my leg, can still feel it. Must have used Russian numbing medicine again!"

Placing all that local in the mannequin would be a mess, so the residents again go through a kind of "mock topicalization" showing how they would topicalize.

First one, then another resident actually do place the endotracheal tube, going nasally.

Half way through the intubation, the blood pressure rises to 180/110 and the heart rate goes to 120.

The residents keep charging ahead and intubate.

Once intubated, they give propofol and the blood pressure drops back to normal.

The intercom crackles, "OK folks, all done."

Clinical lessons learned from scenario 36

Debriefing. The patient sits at the debriefing table but is now able to lift his neck out of the extreme C position, but he stays "in character" for the purpose of the debriefing.

"Today we're going to focus on one core clinical competency—professionalism, and then we'll take on the medical aspects, which are tough, let's face it."

"What's our best approach with a talkative patient like this?" the first resident asks. "It's good to bond with the patient, I know, and you don't want to come across as all officious and business-like, but how do you keep the conversation on the straight and narrow?"

"You tell me," the instructor says. More than just shelling out pat answers, the instructor tries to let the residents hunt around a little and come up with their own answers. For that reason, Simulator sessions aren't scheduled to a razor-thin edge. There's always some extra time thrown in for "resident discovery."

"Well," the second resident says, "let the patient have their say. Not forever, but let them speak up a little. This is *their* day, after all. This is 'just another case' to us, just another 'airway to conquer.' But this is an operation for them. Hell, it's an operation *on* them. So we should cut them a little slack. It's not like *every* patient talks this way. If one patient goes on and on a little bit, I guess you can look at it the same as when it takes you a long time to get an IV in."

"There's another thing," the first resident says. "This may sound a little corny, but I hear some of the best stories this way. Some old vet with something to say, some story about way back when. You hear the coolest stuff."

The patient loses the accent but keeps the character. "I know the doctors want to keep things moving along, like a factory. And the way you talk to me makes a difference. If you convey the idea that I'm just a slab

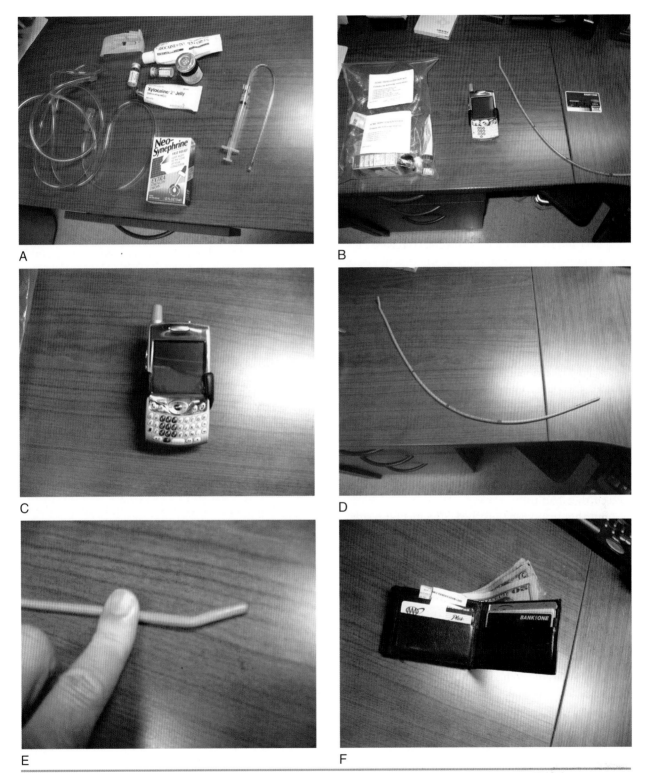

FIGURE 8-100 **A.** Local, a mucosal atomization device, neo in case you go through the nose, airways. It's all here. **B.** Keep some other stuff around too. **C.** A phone to call for help. **D.** An intubating stylet. **E.** Note the end of the Eschmann intubating stylet: It curves up just a little bitty bit to give you that anterior-heading millimeter or two. This can save your butt. **F.** And plenty of money to keep your malpractice premiums up to date in case, well, you know.

of meat, ready for the conveyor belt so you can lop another hunk of my leg off, well, that just doesn't sit well with me.

"Where I come from, neighbors take time to talk to each other. Doctors take time to talk to their patients. Hell, in Russia, they don't *have* anything else they can offer the patients, so they *better* talk to them.

"Then you come here and zoom, zoom, zoom. Everything is fast. And the hospital might as well be a drive-through window at McDonald's. So yeah, I want you to talk to me, I'm sorry if I don't fit in your Palm Pilot schedule."

No response to that, but the looks at the debriefing table say that the lesson struck home.

"Can't improve on that," the instructor says. "Um, this is kind of from the sublime to the ridiculous, but let's shift gears and look at the medical angles at work here."

"Typical capitalist, imperialist pig," the patient says. After the earlier discussion, everyone was pretty wound up. So this served as the perfect release, and the whole gang cracks up.

"Placing a regional in a patient with a bad airway, take me through your thinking," the instructor says.

"OK," the first resident says, "you always have to have plan B ready, because no regional is a guarantee, no way. Plus you have to have 'situational awareness' regarding the surgical site. Can the surgeons help you out, can the surgeons stop if the block doesn't work. This case, they're out on a limb, they could give some local if they had to."

"But this airway isn't just bad," the second resident says, "this is the worst possible bad in the universe bad. Even the ultimate fall-back, the surgeon-bail-us-out trach, is not an option here. Look at the neck, the chin is sitting on top of the place where you'd put the trach. There's no way to cut into this guy's airway. You'd have to, I don't know, cut into the chest or something."

"Hence," the first resident says, as he pulls out his Acme Airway Kit, "the need for the Acme Airway Kit. Always ready to prep someone in a New York minute."

Everyone in the room looks over the kit. Appreciative oohs and aahs.

"Yeah, I guess you are ready, aren't you?" the instructor says. "One thing you missed, though."

The first resident looks shocked, shocked by the news, "What?"

"Should have given him the glycopyrrolate earlier, given it time to work. His mouth wouldn't have had time to get dry before you did the topical."

Snapping his fingers, the resident says, "You're right, you got me there."

"One more thing," the instructor says.

"I thought you only had one thing!"

"I lied, I had *two* one things," the instructor says, then plays the DVD. "See here, halfway into the intubation, where the blood pressure and heart rate are heading too high?"

The residents nod agreement.

"Take a time out, stop for a second, give a little more labetalol or something to get the vital signs under control. That's the beauty of the awake intubation. Because they're still breathing, there's no rush, so you can stop. Get a handle on the vitals, then start again. Got it?"

"Got it."

Summary. A French saying speaks volumes in a single phrase, "There is no such thing as sickness, there are only sick people." In our madness to pigeonhole patients' diagnoses, categorize the problems, and deal with said problems efficiently, we can lose sight of "the patient who is living and breathing underneath the problem list." This patient demonstrated this very idea.

A Russian immigrant, coming from a blighted landscape in the shadow of Chernobyl, this man had a lot on his mind. Yes, he suffered from multisystem disease, he presented the ultimate airway nightmare to an anesthesiologist, and he needed an operation sooner rather than later. But beneath all that "interesting and challenging pathology" beat the heart of a human being. A human being who wanted to talk with his doctors a little, crack a few jokes, take a step back (even if he had no legs to do so) and just breathe in the crisp air of companionship for a few minutes before he had to submit to the knife again.

Give the man his moment in the sun. Do all the right stuff, yes. Plan your regional block carefully, aspirate to avoid an intravascular injection, have plan B ready, and put together a useful airway kit so you can prep and secure the airway in an efficient and comfortable fashion. All good. And listen to your instructor when she reminds you to address the hypertension and tachycardia in midintubation. Good advice. But keep your human being cap on too.

For just a second, before you go completely "clinical," take a step back. The world won't end if you take a few minutes to listen to a story, hear a joke, and tell one yourself. Patients appreciate it. Patients deserve that much.

SCENARIO 37.   **Who'd a thunk it? An arm block that gets weird**

"Tennis elbow, you say?" the first resident asks. "Did he get it playing, um, tennis?"

"This is the funniest thing, and this has nothing to do with this Simulation," the instructor explains, "but most of the people with *tennis elbow*, get it from doing something *other than tennis*. Golf, racquetball, squash, even baseball. Isn't that the weirdest thing. Some orthopod guy told me that once."

That earns an appreciative nod from the anesthesia residents.

"We're going to cobble a lot of stuff together today," the instructor continues, "give you a funny kind of regional workout for this case. We always ask you to suspend disbelief here in the Simulation Center. Today we're really asking you to suspend disbelief. You game?"

"Sure," the second resident says. "Tennis, anyone."

The two residents go into the OR room. There is a skeleton there, some block needles, a couple skin markers, and the METI simulator.

"Let's start out with you talking to the patient," the instructor says, then walks out of the room.

Going through a routine preop checklist, the residents uncover a 20-something ASA 1 patient. When given the option of a regional block versus general anesthesia, the patient (through the mannequin speakers) asks, "Tell me about that, doc."

Starting in, the first resident says, "Because we're going to be operating on the elbow, our best bet would be an interscalene block. That's up here in the neck region (she points on herself). We give you a little sedation, then numb you up, and then use a little needle connected to a little electrical stimulator to find just the right spot to place the local anesthetic."

"When we inject the local anesthetic," the second resident says, "we'll be asking you a few questions."

"Why is that?" the patient asks. "Can't you just do that when I'm asleep?"

"Actually, we need you awake and talking to us to make sure the needle is in the right place and hasn't slipped to the wrong place."

"OK."

The residents hook up monitors, check all their airway equipment, suction, all the stuff you'd need for a general anesthetic, then start sedating the patient. After 2 mg of midazolam, the patient is still easily arousable but has slight slurring of speech.

"We'll put the medicine in now," the first resident says.

"Time out!" over the intercom.

To go through the interscalene block, each resident serves as the other's model. In turn, they lie down on a gurney, turn their head, and let the other draw the landmarks and put a little X where they would place the needle. Then they both get up, go over to the model of the skeleton, and indicate with a block needle where they would go.

"Now fish around in here a little," the instructor says, pointing to the skeleton. "Show me what you would hit if 'the best-laid plans o' mice an' men gang aft agley' during your interscalene block."

One resident goes straight down, "You could drop a lung."

Going too medially, the other resident says, "You can go intrathecal, or hit a blood vessel. If you go intra-arterial, you will have the world's fastest onset seizure. You could also go epidurally."

"And then there's the good old, 'you just plain miss' and the block doesn't work," the first resident says. "I myself, not to brag here too much, have perfected that block myself."

With a saline syringe, extension tubing, a block needle, and a nerve stimulator, they go through the motions of the block.

Now, having gotten the landmarks on a human (each other) and shown where to go (on the skeleton), they go back to the Simulator.

"How does the arm feel? Heavy? Numb?" the second resident asks.

"Yeah," the patient says, "feels funny all right."

The surgeon (Simulation Center secretary) starts the operation, "Hey, he's moving."

"That feels a little sharp!" the patient says.

"OK, probably just taking a little while to set up," the first resident says, then gives 1 cc of fentanyl. In the meantime, the second resident sets up a propofol infusion.

"He's still moving," the surgeon says. "I don't think he's liking this much."

"Hey, doctors," the patient says, "no kidding, I don't think I'm as numb as I should be. I can feel him working down there. *Ow!*"

"Want to get this propofol drip going?" the second resident asks.

"No," the first resident says. "Time out, everybody! Sir," she addresses the patient, "we're going to give you some medicine to go to sleep now."

"Feel free!" the patient says.

The residents give 150 mg of propofol, place a #4 LMA, and turn on vapors.

"OK, go to the recovery room," the instructor says over the intercom.

Trooping over to the other Simulation room, the residents come upon the patient (the surgeon, now turned into the patient) lying on a gurney.

"How are you doing?" the first resident asks.

"I don't know what you guys gave me, but my right elbow doesn't hurt too much now at all."

"I told you we just needed to let it set up a little longer," the second resident hisses.

But before she can gloat, the patient adds, "Funniest thing, though. You didn't put any of that stuff in my left arm, did you?"

Looking at each other, then at the patient, "No, why?"

"Because part of my left arm and forearm feel numb now too, why would that be?"

The residents look at him. Neither says anything.

"OK, we're done!" the instructor says.

The patient gives the residents a wave, a weak wave, goodbye.

Clinical lessons learned from scenario 37

Debriefing. "Wait a minute, wait a minute," the first resident says. "I want to do an exam on that patient. I want to see just what the hell was going on with that other arm."

The Simulation Center secretary has to beg off. His daughter is in a softball tournament, and he has to bail out early. But the instructor (all-knowing, all-seeing, all-conniving) helps out.

"Go ahead, examine me."

The residents go through a sensory and motor exam on the instructor, who gives a perfect rendition of a cervical epidural block. Sensory and motor loss from C4 to C6.

"Where was your needle?" the instructor asks.

"Too lateral, no, wait," the first resident says. "No it wouldn't be lateral. We must have been too medial."

They dredge out an anatomy book from the Simulation Center library and take a good look at the neck.

"Crowded place," the second resident says. "No wonder you hear so many spooky stories about neck sticks."

BOX 8–72 *Neck Stick Misadventures*

- **Intravascular**
- **Intrathecal**
- **Epidural**
- **Intra-nothingness**

"We must have gone too medial," the first resident says. "We went too medial, and the local anesthetic creeped up a dural sleeve, went across and into the epidural space."

"Well bend me over an Adirondack chair and give me 50 lashes with a crushed velvet whip," the second resident says. "I couldn't do that stick if I tried on a hundred patients for a thousand years."

Instructor and first resident are trying to do a visual on the Adirondack chair and the crushed velvet whip.

Gathering what professionalism is possible under the circumstances, the instructor says, "Well, hit it you did. And that explains the block not exactly working, and that explains the contralateral symptoms."

"Crushed velvet?" the first resident asks.

"It's an acquired taste," the second resident says. "What about the rest of the case. I mean, other than this phantasmogoric needle malplacement, what do you think about the other stuff we did."

They go to the DVD.

"Good explanation to the patient of how you'll do the block," the instructor says. "Do you think you're soft-pedaling the risks and benefits a little?"

"That's a toughie," the Adirondack chair/crushed velvet whip aficionado says. "If you want to get all legal-eagle about it, I suppose you have to read every patient the riot act, go through every single possible complication in the world, including death. But these people know the score. They sign the consent. I don't think you're doing them any favors with this big 'scare the hell out of them' bit."

"I don't know about that," the first resident says. "If something *does* go wrong, and you *didn't* tell them, that could be trouble too."

"I got news for you, cowboy," the second resident says, "if something goes wrong, your having said something won't make any difference anyway. Just tell them the main things, then take good care of the guy.

"What say you?"

A shrug of the shoulders from the instructor, "You can argue it either way, I've gotta tell you."

"That's nice and clear," the first resident says.

"How about the 'going to sleep' part?" They review that part of the DVD.

"You tell me," the instructor asks.

"Once the regional has bitten the dust," the second resident says, "better to just bag it and go with a general. Otherwise you end up sedating and sedating, and pretty soon you end up with a RAG."

"What's a RAG?" the first resident asks.

"A room air general," the second resident explains. "A half-assed general anesthetic where they're sedated too much, no way are they really induced, their airway is pseudo-protected at best, and you are inviting disaster."

Looking at the DVD, the instructor says, "Which it looks like you were getting ready to do here, weren't you? I mean look, there's some midazolam on board, you gave some fentanyl, and here you are brewing up a propofol cocktail."

The second resident frowns as she sees that she was, indeed, doing just that.

"I was younger then," she says. "More foolish. Now that I've got a few more minutes under my belt, I see the error of my ways."

Summary. Necks should have a warning tattooed on them, "Abandon all hope, ye who enter here." Well maybe it's not actually that bad, but depositing local anesthetic in the neck always merits a good deal of caution. There's a lot of stuff in there! There is the brachial sheath, amen, and that is just the place to put local anesthetic if you're looking to block the elbow and upper arm. But there's a lot of other stuff too— blood vessels, CSF, epidural space, nerves, lungs— lions and tigers and bears, oh my!

That needle can go in the wrong place, and that local anesthetic can go in the wrong place—both of which you need to avoid if possible but react to the incorrect placement when it does happen.

Sedation in the regional patient also requires a deft hand. You want the patient comfortable and relaxed— Isn't that what *you* would want?—But you need good cooperation too. No less an authority than the Society of Regional Anesthesia reminds us that nerve injury in the oversedated patient is a real risk.

And this simulation, even with its focus on landmarks both external and skeletal, still draws attention to our other important duty—talking to the patient. As the instructor points out in his waffling answer during the debriefing, detailing risks to our patients is a debatable topic. You can argue that we should tell the patients every possible thing that can go wrong. And you can argue that we should strike a more reassuring tone, with less detail about the risks. Why didn't the instructor give an authoritative, definitive answer to this question?

Because there is none.

SCENARIO 38. Medical students take over the place, a routine induction

"Hysterectomy, huh?" the senior anesthesia resident says. "Anything special here?" She looks over the preop. "Heart murmur as a child, but none lately, no

heart symptoms." She looks up at the instructor, "So, what exactly do you want me to do here?"

A couple of medical students are with the senior anesthesia resident today in the Simulator. The instructor says, "Just show them how you get going in an efficient fashion, that's the main thing. Give a blow-by-blow of how you do this routine case, so they can get a feel for how giving an anesthetic goes."

The medical students are early in their third year, still displaying the "Gee whiz, this is so much more fun than sitting in the lecture hall" look. They don't yet have the "Yeah, I already saw that, yawn" look of the fourth year medical students.

In the operating room of the Simulation Center, the senior anesthesia resident takes the students on a guided tour. The students have the bounding energy of wire terriers chasing after blown soap bubbles.

"One of you want to put in an arterial line? These cases can get a little bloody?"

If two people were capable of trampling each other to death, it would have happened as the med students push forward to do the art line. The resident points to the art line partial task Simulator by the wall. "You, you go ahead and put it in; then after it's in, we'll look at the waveform up here on the monitor."

Once again, the combination of partial task trainers next to the mannequin allows some "task work"; then with a little leap of faith, you just incorporate that task into the simulation.

"And you," the resident points to the second student (who might have imploded without getting something to do), "help me put on the monitors."

In order, the resident and student:

Put the oxygen mask on, held in place by a black strap.
Go to the right side of the patient, put on the two right-sided EKG leads, strap down the arm, and put on the blood pressure cuff.
Go to the left side and place the three left-sided EKG pads, the pulse oximeter, and the arm strap; then rig the left wrist as if the art line were there.
Come to the head of the bed.
Double check that the suction and airway equipment are ready to go.

"There, see, one trip around the patient," the resident says, "and the whole time the patient is preoxygenating, so we're ready to go right when we get up here. Got it? Boom. No wasted time. When you go out in the real world, keep this in mind. The sooner you go, the sooner you go home. Know what I mean?

If you can shave a few minutes off the start of your case, and you do five cases a day, then you go home a half hour earlier."

"I got it!" the med student shouts in triumph over at the art line simulator. Even though he has a surgical mask on, you can tell he's smiling by the fattened cheeks under the lateral aspects of his eyes and the crinkliness around his eyes. His happiness seems so absolute, he could die right now and feel his life had been complete.

The resident goes around the patient and undoes all the monitors.

"OK, you guys each do it."

Both medical students go around, putting on the monitors a few times.

"Green and white, on the right, Christmas colors down," the resident says, citing one of the many mnemonics for placing EKG electrodes on.

"Watch the tubing to the blood pressure cuff," the resident instructs. If it folds back or kinks on itself, you won't get a reading."

An arterial line setup is in the room. "Let's look this over," the resident says, "what can go wrong here."

The students stare at this new apparatus like kindergarteners staring at the Rosetta Stone.

"OK," the resident sighs, drawing on Job-like reserves of patience, "let's go over this. This is all high-pressure tubing, and the key is just 'following the pressure.' So if you turn the stopcock off to the artery, you lose the pressure. If you turn it on to the artery, the pressure comes to here, the transducer. And if you turn it this way, opening it up, the arterial line does what?"

Now the eyes above the masks are furrowed. "Wouldn't the blood just come back?" the first furrowed student says.

"Yes," the resident explains, "that is called a 'linoleum transfusion.'"

The students scan and rescan their memory banks for mention of a "linoleum transfusion." Could that have been the lecture on hematology they missed? One of them pulls out a Palm Pilot that has several textbooks encoded in a handy-dandy, accessible, cross-

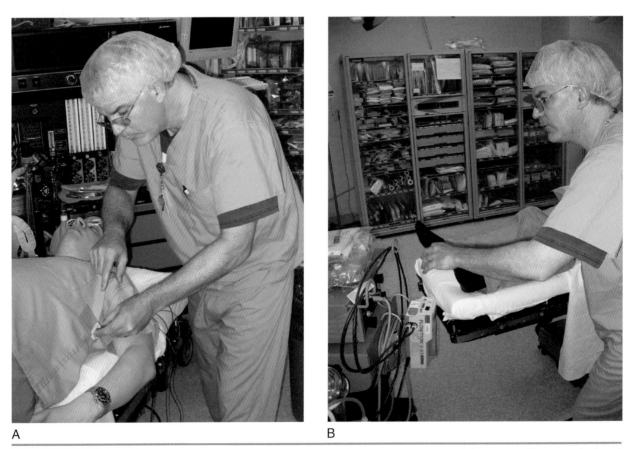

A   B

FIGURE 8–101   Learning "room logistics." Try to do all your work in "one sweep" around the patient. If you run back and forth, tripping all over stuff, you waste time and look like a moron. Rather than learn this under the prying (and judgmental) eyes of an actual OR staff, practice this efficiency in the simulator.

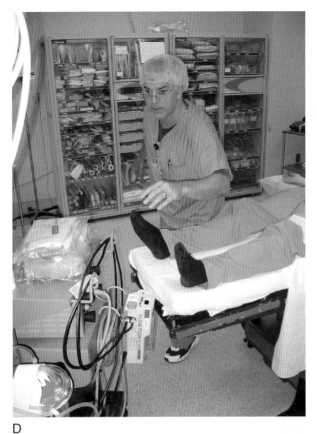

C

D

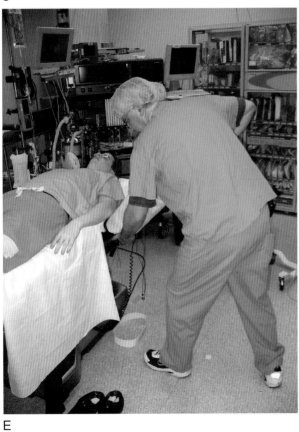

E

F

FIGURE 8–101 cont'd

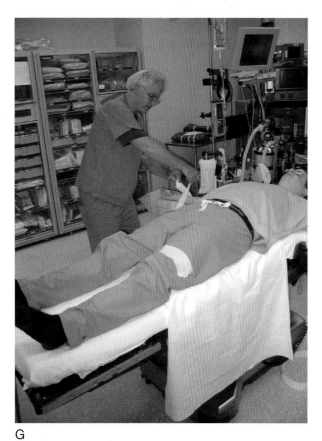

G

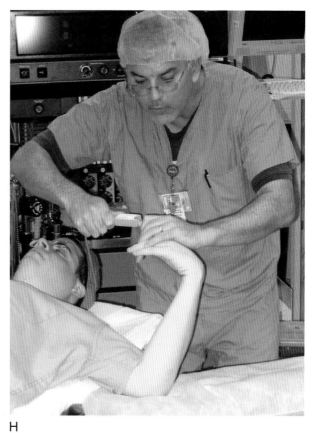

H

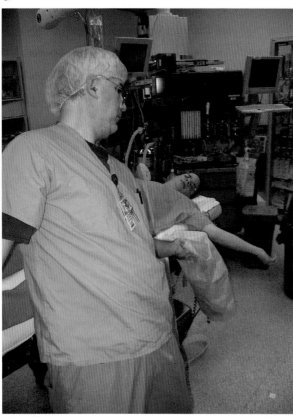

I

J

FIGURE 8–101 cont'd

BOX 8-73	Arterial Lines

- **Sit down**
- **Get good position**
- **Check all the tubings and connections**

referenced format. He dutifully enters "linoleum transfusion."

From the control room, through the two-way mirror, gales of laughter escape through the "soundproof" wall.

"Uh," the resident says, "that is, actually, a joke. You won't find 'linoleum transfusion' in there anywhere. I just meant the blood would drip out onto the floor."

"Oh, I get it!" the second med student says.

Putting away the Palm Pilot, the first med student doesn't seem very amused.

"Right, so long as we're having fun with the art line, let me show you a few other things."

She shows them how all the connections of the art line need to be double-checked, as every one can come loose and result in the infamous "linoleum transfusion." Then attention turns to the pressure bag, and the resident shows how you have to inflate it, make sure it stays inflated, and check it periodically during the case.

"If you don't," she explains, "the blood pressure appears damped." She draws a picture of a damped line, "and you might think the pressure is lower than it actually is."

Once "all things arterial line" are explained, they proceed to induction.

"So," the resident says, "take me through the drugs you would give for a generic, regular old induction."

"First, sedate the patient," the first med student says. "Give Versed, right?"

"Good. Then what?"

"Intubate?" the first med student asks.

"Uh, no, with Versed, you're just sedated. You need to be *induced*, you need to be *unconscious*, first."

"Oh yeah, oh yeah. I'm so stupid, right, right, what was I thinking?" the first med student trips over himself. "Right, you give propofol, until they are asleep."

"Induced," the resident corrects, "induced is what you want to say. Asleep is at night at home with your teddy bear and Minnie Mouse night light."

"Induced," the first med student says.

"Let me!" the second med student wants in on the action. "Then once they're induced, you paralyze them, right?"

"Well," the resident tries to check the students' irrational exuberance, "first you make sure you can breathe for them. And then you give the paralytic."

"Like succinylcholine, right?" the second medical student asks.

"Yes, if there is no contraindication to Sux, you can use that."

"Then we intubate?" the first med student is back in the fray.

"Well, even Sux takes a little while to work, you have to keep breathing for them, hand-ventilating until the Sux kicks in; then we intubate," the resident says. "Got it? Let's do it again a few times together."

Each med student does his own induction.

Sedate
Induction
Breathe
Muscle relaxant
Breathe
Intubate
Make sure tube is in the right place
Turn on ventilator
Turn on anesthetic agent

In military drill-type fashion, they go over this a few times until the sequence becomes clear and the med students understand the "why" of each step.

Once they have the drill down, they ramp it up a little and pay close attention to the vital signs as they induce. And once they induce:

Sedate, blood pressure goes down a little.
Induce, blood pressure goes down more.
Breathe.
Give paralytic.
Intubate, blood pressure goes up.
Make sure tube is in the right place.
Turn on ventilator, blood pressure goes down a little.
Turn on anesthetic agent, blood pressure goes down a little.

BOX 8-74	Give What, When, in a Routine Induction?

- **Sedate**
- **Induce**
- **Mask**
- **Paralyze**
- **Mask**
- **Intubate**

The intercom speaks, "This is the voice of the linoleum transfusion monster. You are done with today's lesson, pack it up."

Clinical lessons learned from scenario 38

Debriefing. In the debriefing room, the "wire terriers" are bouncing all over the place.

"Oh, man, did you see me get that art line?"

"What was I thinking, intubating after Versed. I'm so dumb!"

"Did you see the cords?"

"That dummy's mouth is hard to open!"

"They never let me do anything on the Medicine rotation, here we got to do everything!"

Instructor and resident are sitting at the table, sipping bad coffee made palatable by type II diabetes-inducing levels of processed white sugar.

"Make sure the med students only get decaf, OK?" the instructor says.

"Check," the resident responds.

"OK, kiddos," the instructor tries to rein in the youthful exuberance. "Let's give it a once over, what we did just now."

On the DVD replay, they look over the residents' setup and preparation.

"No doubling back, no retracing her steps," the instructor points out. "She plans ahead what she'll need to do on each side of the bed, so she won't have to come back. Doing this efficiently ties in with a core clinical competency we call 'systems based practice.' We work in a medical system, not just a vacuum. Time and resources are valuable commodities, and you have to use them well. So note how the resident doesn't waste any time in the operating room. Even preoxygenating *first* means you'll get going just that much quicker."

"And you want to look slick," the resident says. "This is not just a hot-dog maneuver, this matters. Face it, you are judged every day by how you do in the OR. Nurses are watching, techs are watching, surgeons are watching. If you bumble around and flounder like a fish out of water, people notice. If you *look* disorganized, guess what, you *are* disorganized."

"But does it really matter what people think?" the first med student asks.

"Yes, it does, don't kid yourself," the instructor says. "You need the confidence and support of the people around you. If you don't enjoy their confidence, if they don't believe in you, then pretty soon work becomes very unpleasant. This is not just kow-towing to peer pressure in junior high. This is the way the world is. Prepare well, work well, look good, be good, take good care of the patients. That is the essence of working in a system. And that is the essence of 'systems based practice.'"

They look over the sequence of induction again, drilling the points a few more times.

First, induce unconsciousness.
Ensure adequate ventilation.
Give muscle relaxant.
Continue ventilation.
Intubate, make sure you *did* intubate.
Ventilate.
Check vital signs, then start the volatile anesthetic.

"At this stage," the instructor says, "this is the main stuff for you to know. There are a hundred variations on this theme—rapid sequence induction is a little different, inducing an unstable patient requires some fiddling, a difficult airway requires a different approach—but for now, this is the gist of most anesthetics."

In the debriefing room, they handle the tubing, transducer and cable of the arterial line and review the mishaps that can befall this monitor.

"Biggest thing is the connections, check the connections," the instructor explains. "One loose connection anywhere along this line of things, and you'll lose your trace and maybe lose some blood. There are horror stories of a stopcock bumped in a tucked arm and the patient exsanguinates all over the floor. Gotta be careful with these things!"

Summary. In talks with Simulator instructors across the land, one major use of Simulators becomes clear—showing beginners how to do anesthesia. Whether medical students or beginning residents, the Simulator is the place to "do it first."

It's easy to forget, once you've done anesthesia for a while, what a baffling place the OR can be. Lines and tubing everywhere. A hundred things to do. You might have read a little about anesthesia and know some of the theory, but simple things (where do the leads go again? How do I make sure the blood pressure cuff works?) can throw you off.

And the medical student thinking you intubate after giving Versed? His confusion is understandable. The sequence of drugs and sequence of patient responses is not a given, when you are beginning.

So the Simulator is just the place. Beginning residents or medical students can flounder around, ask questions galore (without a nervous patient hearing and wondering, "Do these clowns know what they are doing?"), and learn the ropes in safety.

And for the more advanced resident? Efficiency and "looking slick" are important aspects of your practice, especially once residency is over and you are "released into the wild." In the Simulator, a resident can go over his/her motions, under scrutiny, and find weak spots and inefficiencies. Better to find them out early and correct them than to carry these bad habits out into private practice.

And finally, the Simulator is a great place for an instructor to touch on some of the "softer, fuzzier" facets of the ACGME core clinical competencies. Here, the instructor specifically mentioned and taught about "systems-based medicine." The residents need to learn this. And the residencies need to teach it, or else the big bad ACGME dragon will come and eat you up!

SCENARIO 39. **Blood bath during a hysterectomy**
"I thought we already did a hysterectomy," the senior resident says. "Last week with those yappy med students."

This time, the senior resident is with one of the ICU fellows.

"Who knows?" the instructor says. "Maybe last year's birds don't live in this year's nests."

"Same patient?" the resident asks. "She has a recurrent uterus?"

"Alright," the instructor yields, "it's her identical twin sister."

Looking over the preop, the fellow says, "Good enough, let's do it."

Same history, a murmur during childhood but no symptoms, now in for a hysterectomy. This time in the operating room the ICU fellow does the room setup and does his best to demonstrate time-and-motion efficiency.

"Little rusty," the resident observes. "Too much time in the intensive care unit. It's good you're back here for a little brush-up."

The fellow insists on a central line as well as an art line for this hysterectomy, "These OBs, they can lose a lot of blood with these things."

"During a hysterectomy?"

"You'd be surprised."

The fellow induces, intubates, and the patient is draped. Surgery begins. The surgeon (a medical student taking on Simulation as a special research project) says, "This is a pretty big uterus, I'm losing a lot of blood."

On the monitors, the CVP drops from 8 to 3, the heart rate rises to 120, and the blood pressure drops

---

BOX 8-75 | *Lose Volume?*

- **Give volume**
- **Need more, give more**
- **This is not rocket science either**

---

from 140/80 to 100/50. All this is consistent with a blood loss of 1000 cc.

"Let's get some blood in here," the resident says.

A nurse comes in with two bags of blood.

"Wait a minute," the fellow says, "these don't match. That medical record number is different than this patient's."

"It may be another 20 minutes before we can get some more blood up here," the resident says. "Let's buy time with some albumin."

Albumin would be too expensive to use in the Simulator, so they hang two bags *labeled* albumin.

"Let's put her head down," the fellow says, "and get this fluid in a little faster." He puts the volume under pressure.

"Hey, look at the STs," the resident says.

On the EKG, the ST segments go up.

On the intercom, the instructor says, "The BIS monitor has just gone from 55 to 12." (The simulator doesn't have a BIS built in, so "ad hoc" reports like this bring the BIS into the scenario.)

"Why should her STs go up, she's only 40. Her pressure's not that low," the resident says.

Multifocal ectopy starts on the screen.

"Something is weird here, this doesn't make sense," the fellow says. "Let's send a gas."

"I'm having a lot of trouble in here," the surgeon says. Audible from the field is the sound of lots of clicking and unclicking as the surgeon keeps readjusting clamps.

"Get the echo, get the echo!" the fellow says.

"What?" the resident asks.

The blood pressure is now 60/40, the ST segments are tombstone-shaped, and the patient is having runs of V tach.

"Echo on the way," the intercom says. "Echo image on the TV." (In a shortcut right to the TEE image, the instructor plays an image on a TV in the OR.)

Bright echoes fill the left and right ventricles, a snowstorm, a blizzard of white inside the heart. Panning up, when the interatrial septum comes into view, bubbles are clearly crossing from right to left.

"V fib!" the resident shouts. "Get the cart, we gotta shock!"

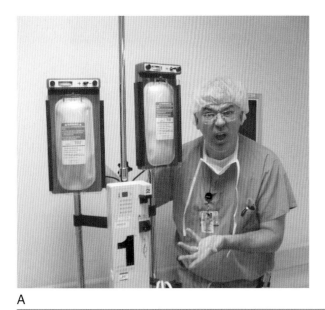

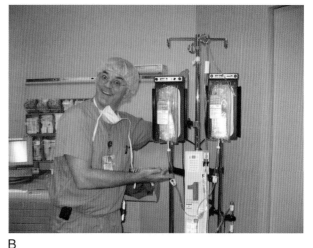

B

A

FIGURE 8–102   Rapid infuser for a major Kahuna blood loss procedure? Just the ticket. But, to sound like a broken record, don't learn to set this up *when you are in trouble*. Learn to do this *ahead* of time, in the calm cool setting of the nonemergency. And you can also make mistakes with this in the practice run. See the problems when it *doesn't* count to prevent mistakes when it *does* count.

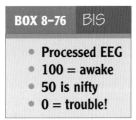

BOX 8-76   BIS

- **Processed EEG**
- **100 = awake**
- **50 is nifty**
- **0 = trouble!**

"Get a chest cutter, get a thoracic surgeon!" the fellow shouts.

Overhead, "The BIS is 0. Cardiac surgery on the way."

The instructor (in surgical garb) bursts into the room, "What did you do now? Do you need a trach or what?"

"I don't know, the patient coded . . . ," the resident starts.

"I'm giving heparin right now," the fellow says. "We need to get her on bypass, right now!"

"Heparin?" the OB shouts. "We're already bleeding like stink down here!"

"Cut the chest, now," the ICU fellow says, evenly, "this is this woman's only chance. Start CPR right now. And down in the field, flood everything with saline, clamp everything you see. This is an air embolus from the field and we've got paradoxical transit of the air. We don't get on bypass and empty this heart out, she's dead."

"OK," the chest surgeon says, "get me a saw. I'll start CPR."

"And we're done," the chest surgeon-turned instructor says."

Clinical lessons learned from scenario 39

Debriefing. "Man," the resident says in the debriefing room, "things were indeed a little more eventful this time."

"What, now in retrospect, do you make of that heart murmur as a kid," the instructor asks.

"Had to be a PFO, patent foramen ovale," the resident says. "Must have closed off and there goes the murmur, but then the foramen ovale must have stayed probe-patent."

"Just sitting around, waiting for the right chance to screw us up," the fellow says.

They play the DVD of the scenario.

"Damn, I am rusty," the fellow admits. "Just a few months out of the OR, and I look like a CA-1 blundering around. I better get in here more often."

The fellow keeps retracing his steps, forgets to put the straps on the patient's arms, then drops syringes, a real Keystone Kops operation. Later, when things start to go to pieces, they slow down the DVD and replay a few parts.

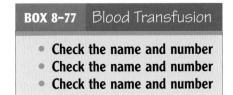

BOX 8-77 *Blood Transfusion*

- Check the name and number
- Check the name and number
- Check the name and number

"Where do you think the air embolus came from?" the instructor asks.

On the DVD, the surgeon keeps opening and closing the clamps. With the blood pressure dropping, the resident and fellow drop the head of the bed. The nurse comes in with the wrong blood supply.

"Hey, at least I caught that," the fellow says. "Don't I get a free weekend in Vegas or something for doing that right?"

"Wow, you did something right," the instructor says. "Catch me, I'm fainting. Now look at what happens next."

"We've got all the stuff in place," the resident says, "the heart is lower than the surgical field, and so air can entrain. And every time the OB opens and repositions a clamp, a big vein might take a gulp of air."

The STs go up, the BIS goes down, and the patient becomes unstable.

"So, my mind's eye sees the air getting in the right ventricle, bad enough. You get enough air and you get an air lock," the fellow says. "But air is now also jumping across the probe patent foramen ovale, maybe from us pushing fluid in so fast through the central line, and now air is on the left side."

"Air in the coronaries," the resident says, "that makes the heart ischemic. Air up top, in the carotids, and now you're BIS is getting zapped because cerebral blood flow is impaired."

"That, or, with the blood pressure dropping, that could also be giving your BIS a drop," the fellow says. "Either way, that processed EEG signal is getting weaker, and the patient is in trouble."

"Air in the ventricle, actually, air in both ventricles," the fellow says, as the TEE image is shown.

"What makes the air so bright?" the medical student asks.

"Ultrasound doesn't conduct well in air," the fellow explains. "Air might as well be opaque so far as the ultrasound beam is concerned. So each bubble, even the tiniest one, throws this big shadow. If you have a lot of air, a lot of bubbles, it opacifies the ventricle, all you see is this sheet of white."

"OK," the instructor says, "you have this mondo air embolus, what do you do?"

"Stop the source of entrainment," the resident says, "so you have the surgeon flood the field. And if things are bad enough, like here, you have to go all the way with hemodynamic support, all the way to CPR."

"Could you have tried to aspirate air out of your central line?" the medical student asks. "Could that have maybe helped a little?"

Both resident and fellow smack their respective foreheads with the heel of their hands.

"Yeah."

"We should have thought of that."

"Tell you what, though," the instructor says. "With that big of a problem, you were probably right doing what you did. You would need to crack the chest, get that air out directly, and maybe even suck air out of the coronaries with a little 25 gauge needle."

"What about the air in the head?" the fellow asks. "Hyperbaric chamber?"

"That's what I was thinking," the resident says. "I don't know if she would survive this big of an insult, but if she did you might make a beeline for a hyperbaric chamber to see if you can shrink those air bubbles in the cerebral circulation. Try to get back some brain function."

"Is this where the expression 'air head' came from?" the med student asks.

Fellow, instructor, and resident stop in their tracks and look at the med student.

"This student is a keeper," the fellow says. "Do not throw this one into the trash compactor like you did the last one. Will you promise me that?"

"Agreed and done," the instructor says.

Summary. One initial premise for a scenario can serve different functions. In the previous scenario, a "simple hysterectomy" served as a platform for an introductory lesson. Medical students learned the mechanics of doing a generic case. No complexities, no subtleties, no complications. This same premise, a "simple hysterectomy," took a turn down Catastrophe Lane for a senior resident and ICU fellow.

At the start of the case, the simulation arena served as a much-needed review for someone "too long from the OR." And this is the perfect place to "scrape the rust off" and get back into the OR groove if you've been away for a while. Better to look clumsy and oafish in the Simulator than to do the same in front of a rapt audience in a real operating room.

Blood transfusion? Remember, always remember the number one cause of transfusion reactions is a clerical error, sending the wrong blood to the wrong place. In the hubbub of an unstable patient losing lots of

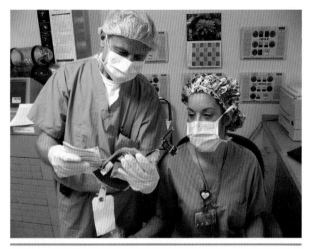

FIGURE 8–104 Name and number, blood type. Check that blood before you give it! Still, even with all our computers and tracking systems, the most common cause of transfusion reaction is clerical error. Hammer that point into your head!

blood, it's easy to short-circuit the paperwork. Fight that temptation—you have to make sure that *this* patient is matched with *this* unit.

Funny, or to be more accurate, *not* funny, how the littlest things can come back to haunt you. The only thing of any note whatsoever in this woman's history was her "childhood heart murmur," which went away and had never come back to haunt her. Well, it came back to haunt her today. With unexpectedly high blood loss, a head-down position, and frequently opened and closed clamps in a vascular area, air got into her circulation. And not just on the right. Her probe-patent foramen ovale (recall, 25% of people have such a creature!) allowed her air embolus to cross over to the left side of her heart, creating havoc in the coronary and cerebral (and no doubt other vascular beds) circulation.

TEE to the rescue again? Yes! Once again, when hemodynamic things are just not adding up, and the patient is going downhill, downhill, downhill, a TEE is a good idea. Without the TEE nailing the diagnosis of massive air on the right and the left, you would have been left with an "I don't know what went wrong, she just crashed" explanation. Pretty limp stuff, that.

Open your eyes so you may see. And while you're at it, put in the TEE so you can see even better.

SCENARIO 40. **Taking a lesson from the railways, correct site surgery**

"Why did you ask me to bring in a Thomas the Train train set?" the senior anesthesia resident asks.

"Trust me," the instructor says, "I'm a doctor, I don't just play one on TV. Put the train set in the debriefing room, then come to the operating room."

In the operating room, there is another combo pack—mannequin Simulator by an anesthesia machine and partial task trainer.

"Today we're going to do a transarterial technique for an arm block," the instructor says. "We've jury-rigged some IV tubing so you can practice the aspiration technique."

The IV tubing has some red-dyed water in it. The tubing itself lies in some Styrofoam packing to give the idea of the artery embedded in the tissue. As usual, the plan is to do the technique, then move to the Simulator to "play out" the rest of the scenario.

The two residents look over the "axillary block trainer." "Did Rube Goldberg invent this thing?" the first resident asks.

"Do you have a patent on it?" the junior resident asks.

"How sharper than a serpent's tooth is the ingratitude of whining residents, if I may misquote Holy Scripture," the instructor says, then leaves the room.

The anesthesia preop describes a construction worker, hurt in a fall, now in for débridement of his left forearm. He agrees to a regional block, so the residents go to the partial task trainer.

"I've never done one of these," the junior resident says. "How about I watch you do it, then I do it."

"See one, do one, serve as an expert witness for the plaintiff on one," the senior resident says.

"First let me show you the mistake most people make," the senior resident says. "You go through the artery, come back until you can aspirate, then go forward so you're on the far side of the artery, but you go too far."

As he leans over the fake arm, the senior resident bumps a little paper onto the floor. The paper lands, writing side up.

RIGHT ARM.

The senior resident continues, "The way this works is to just go past the artery, I mean just, just past the artery." Demonstrating, he shows the right technique.

Artery, you can aspirate.

Through, you can't aspirate.

Back, just until you can aspirate.

Through, but just barely, just barely, to make sure you are just deep to the artery.

Then he shows the wrong way.

Artery, you can aspirate.

Through, you can't aspirate.

Back, until you can aspirate.

Through, way through, a few centimeters, which puts you through the axillary sheath and too deep.

"When you go too deep like this," the senior resident says, "you get what's called a Z-79 block."

"What's that?"

"Z-79 is some annotation they used to show that endotracheal tubes are hypoallergenic or something. Endotracheal tubes used to have 'Z-79' written on them. I don't think they do anymore. Anyway, a 'Z-79' block means you supplement with an endotracheal tube; in other words, the block doesn't work."

The junior resident sets up and does the block. He goes through, back, and just through again a few times to get the feel of the "just through."

"Purists say you put half the local on the far side of the artery, half on the near side; let me show you," the senior resident explains. After the needle is just through the far side, he injects half the local. "Break it up, the injection, because you never know when you might be going intravascular. Give a few cc's, aspirate, ask the patient if they feel anything funny."

"Sir," the senior resident asks the patient (the Simulator next to the partial-task trainer arm block gizmo), "let me know if you feel any ringing in your ears, or a funny taste in your mouth, or if you feel lightheaded or your heart is racing, OK?"

"OK," the patient says, "none of that. You guys doing OK?"

"Sure, we're fine."

"Now, you put about two-thirds of the local on the far side," the senior resident continues, "because you're pretty sure you're in the right place there. When you pull back, and come back through the artery, you can sort of pucker the artery back with you. The needle 'hangs on' to the artery until you're way back; and by the time you're finally free of the artery, the artery may spring back. Guess what, you're out of the sheath. I mean, I've been pulling back through the artery and aspirating, and it seems like I'm about to come out of the skin with the needle, and I'm still aspirating blood. So you can imagine you could be out."

"Whoa."

"Yeah," the senior resident affirms. "But usually the two-thirds on the other side will do it. That'll usually give you the block you need.

The junior resident does the procedure until he's satisfied he has it down.

"Why do the transarterial approach?" the junior asks. "Isn't the nerve stimulator more, um, scientific?"

"Yes," the senior says, "but out in the real world, the nerve stimulator is gone, it's lost, it's broken, no one has a 9 volt battery. It's good to know how to do a jungle block, just using the artery.

"When you're done, put the arm up on the patient's chest. If you're in there, he won't be able to straighten out his arm in just a few minutes. But when you ask him to lift it, don't let him do it alone—his arm will fall on his face and you'll be doing a repair of a nasal fracture too."

Once both residents have done the block to their satisfaction, the patient speaks up, "How come my left arm still hurts."

"What?"

"My left arm, how come my left arm still hurts?" the patient asks. "My right arm feels all numb, but that's not where I got hurt. You guys numbed up the arm they're not operating on."

The junior resident looks down on the floor and picks up the piece of paper.

RIGHT ARM.

"Um," the junior says as he shows it to the senior, "we have a little problem here."

Over the intercom, "Please go to examining room 1, the patient's wife is in there and wants to hear what happened."

The residents look at each other, then at the RIGHT ARM paper, then back at each other.

In the examining room, a woman (Simulation Center secretary) sits in a chair. "How's my baby doing? I heard there's some delay starting the case? Something about the wrong arm?"

The residents enter the room.

"First, he's doing fine, that's the main thing," the senior resident says. "Let me explain what happened. For this operation, we can have the patient go to sleep, or put just the arm to sleep with numbing medicine. Now, after we had your husband in the room and were ready to go, we put the numbing medicine in and put the arm to sleep. There was no bad reaction or anything, but as it turned out we placed the numbing medicine in the right arm, not the left."

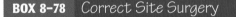

BOX 8–78 *Correct Site Surgery*

- *You* make sure
- Have patient confirm
- *You* make sure (did I already say that?)

"How could that happen?" the wife asks.

"Well, it was a mistake, that is all there is to it. It was a mistake, and it was our mistake, and we're sorry. Now, your husband still needs an operation, but we can't put the numbing medicine in the other arm right now. That would be too much numbing medicine in the system all at once. So he will go to sleep for this operation."

"How do I know you won't do something else wrong!" the woman shouts. "I want another doctor to take care of my husband, someone a little more careful!"

"That's perfectly understandable," the junior resident says. "And we will be happy to arrange that."

"All done!" the instructor says.

Clinical lessons learned from scenario 40

Debriefing. "I don't know," the senior resident says, a little miffed, "I think this whole wrong side thing was a setup and smells not entirely unlike bullshit, if you pardon my French."

Shrugging, the instructor holds up the RIGHT ARM paper. "OK, so it was a little contrived, so shoot me."

"I liked the fake arterial arm block thing," the junior resident says.

"Good," the instructor says. "That's the kind of ass-kissing I like to hear. Now we're going to do a little exercise in note-writing here. I want both of you to write a procedure note on what just happened. While you work on that, I'm going out to do important 'attending-like' things." He hands them each a yellow legal pad.

"What are important 'attending-like' things?" the senior resident asks.

"Read e-mails I don't want to read and send e-mails no one else wants to read. That's what you do when you're at the top," the attending answers.

The residents document the block, noting all the details. Then they lay out the mistake made (wrong side) and detail the discussion with the wife.

After his crucial e-mail foray, the instructor returns and looks over the notes.

"Good, good," he says, then lays down the legal pads. "Who are you writing these notes for?"

"The jury!" the residents sing in unison.

"Very good!" says the instructor. "And what won't they forgive?"

"Mistakes?" guesses the resident.

"No, surprisingly," the wife of the patient says. "People know that mistakes happen. As we discussed before (remember?) the two things a jury won't forgive are dishonesty and a callous attitude. Those are the two things *I* would be most ticked off about. And that same attitude goes through juries. When you guys met with me, told me what happened straight up, and were willing to listen to my complaints, that made a big impression. And when I said I wanted someone else to take care of him, and you agreed, well that told me you weren't hard-headed jerks who would just blow off my concerns. You seemed to care."

"What's with the train?" the senior resident asks.

Pushing the train off the tracks and onto the floor, the instructor recreates a crash. Thomas the Tank Engine does a header onto the debriefing room carpet.

"Amagasaki, Japan, April 25, 2005. A West Japan Railway train takes a corner too fast, derails, and kills 107 people—the worst train wreck in Japan in 40 years. That would qualify as a mistake, I would say."

Looking down on the floor, the junior resident says, "Thomas the Tank Engine thinks so."

"What's the response of the company? Severalfold:

2 Drivers on the train call on their cell phones to report the disaster, the company tells them to leave the scene immediately, even as injured and trapped passengers are screaming in the background.

43 Company executives hear about the crash and go bowling.

19 Employees hear about the catastrophe on the golf course. They keep playing.

"That's pretty cold," the senior resident says.

"West Japan Railway is the poster child for the wrong response to a mistake," the instructor says. "No matter what you do, no matter how egregious the error, at least show concern after the fact. You can't undo the crash, but you can sure tell go to the site and try to pry people free once it has happened. Admittedly, this is a pretty extreme example, but it makes the point. When you make a mistake, in medicine or in railroads, make sure you are honest, and make sure that you are concerned in the aftermath. The callous, cavalier response to a disaster sets you up for the next disaster."

"The legal disaster," the junior resident says.

"Right you are."

"Let's get back on track here," the senior resident says, putting Thomas the Tank Engine back on the wooden track. He pauses for effect, everyone tumbles to it, then groans out loud.

"Thank you," the senior resident says, "it's good to know my genius is appreciated."

BOX 8-79 Notes

- **Complete**
- **Honest**
- **Caring**

"Let's go over the whole 'wrong side' issue," the instructor says. "I'll admit this was a little bit of a setup here, but it's still worth going over."

"Time out, that's the thing to do," the junior resident says. "Before you lay a finger on the patient, do a time out and make sure the consent, the schedule, the patient, everybody agrees on the side of the operation. It takes about 30 seconds and it can spare you a real headache."

"Correct," the senior resident says. "Make sure the patient marks the side, and ask them which side before you give any sedation."

"Make sure you have the right side—make that the correct side," the instructor says, "then 'All Aboard!'"

Summary. Once again, a cobbled-together simulator/partial task trainer delivers a combined clinical/behavioral lesson. The senior resident gives his junior colleague a few tips on transarterial blocks. Then both residents learn about the sticky and diffi-

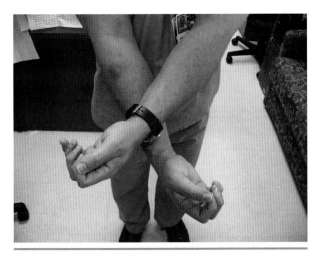

FIGURE 8-105 How on earth could we ever mix up the right and the left? How on earth could we ever do "wrong-sided surgery"? You'd be amazed. Make sure you do a "time out" before you start surgery, making sure that you are doing the correct side. Talk to the patient ahead of time, have him/her mark the spot. As this patient demonstrates, you can mix them up and make it tricky. Quick, which arm is the left one? No fair, you noticed the watch.

cult terrain of "what do you do after you make a mistake."

Of all the regional blocks, the axillary block is the one that every anesthesiologist should know how to do. You may never do a fem-sciatic block after residency, but any resident worth his/her salt should be able to numb up an arm. "No blood, no block" is the watchword for the low-tech (and remarkably reliable) transarterial block. Key to the block is not going too deep on the far side. That sheath is thin, so just go a skosh past the artery.

Unless you're working on the nose, umbilicus, or some other midline structure, you always run the risk of operating on the wrong side of the patient. Double check, triple check to make sure you are doing the procedure on the correct side. Pitfalls can happen when the patient can't help you (unconscious or pediatric patient, ICU patient on a ventilator) or when, for example, both arms are bandaged, or both legs appear ischemic. Don't shrug off or laugh at the possibility of wrong-side surgery. It happens every day!

And one day it will happen to you. A mistake. We're all human, and mistakes happen. Your best bet when you make a mistake—be honest and forthcoming, don't be afraid to apologize, and come across as caring. The callous, the unfeeling, the dishonest doctor is setting him/herself up for big trouble. Use the example of the West Japan Railway of what *not* to do. When your train crashes, roll up your emotional sleeves and start prying apart the wreckage to search for survivors.

SCENARIO 41. **Situational awareness during an amniotic fluid embolus**

"The resident in the delivery room is coming up on 80 hours for these last 2 weeks," the instructor says, "He *has* to go, or the entire program will get dinged. So can you go in there and relieve him. He's babysitting a twin delivery. Good epidural, I think both babies are out, they're just working on the placenta. Anyway, get him out, finish that up for me, would you?"

"Your slightest whim is my most ardent command," the CA-2 says.

A CA-1, less prone to purple prose, is also there. "Yeah, like he says."

The two go in the room and relieve another anesthesia resident (secretary from the Simulation Center). Stirrups are on the bed and an OB (medical student) is at work. "Just got one more placenta to go here, she's not hurting, so we should be fine."

"Twins OK?" the CA-1 asks.

"Off to the nursery," the OB says. "A little early, they might need some O₂ for a little while. Maybe a little time under the French fry lights."

"How are you doing, ma'am," the CA-2 asks the patient (the METI simulator).

"Fine," she says. "Two at once, I don't know if I'm going to get any sl. . . ."

All at once, she stops talking and starts coughing, a dry, barking, nonproductive cough.

"I can't . . . it's hard to . . . ," the patient stops talking. Her saturation drops to 80% then becomes unobtainable. The blood pressure cuff starts cycling but can't come up with any numbers right away. Ectopy appears on the EKG.

"Oxygen! Get the mask on her!" the CA-2 says.

"High spinal?" the CA-1 asks.

"I'm not sure, but let's secure the airway, she's about to code."

The CA-2 opens up the fluids.

"Just give Sux, no agents," the CA-2 says.

After giving 100 of Sux, the CA-1 reaches up and gives cricoid pressure, "Oops, I should have done that first."

"Forget it," the CA-2 says, then intubates. "Do we have a pulse?"

The CA-1 reaches up and feels a faint brachial pulse, "Got one here."

"Then she must be at least around 80," the CA-2 says. "This could be an amniotic fluid embolus or could be a plain old pulmonary embolus; either way, we're going to need some lines. You put an art line in, I'll do the central line."

"Want me to turn on the ventilator?" the CA-1 asks.

"Oh shit, right, God, what was I thinking?" the CA-2 says. "Get the code cart in here."

"What's going on?" the OB asks.

"Big dive in vital signs, all of a sudden. I'm going with some kind of embolus."

"Did you bolus the epidural lately, could that be it?" the OB offers.

Both residents look up at the epidural infusion pump, nothing awry there. "No, no boluses here. Are you about done there? I'm afraid if you reach around any more, you might introduce more amniotic fluid into her circulation."

"Done here! What can I do?" the OB asks.

"We'll need an ICU bed, and talk to her husband or whoever's around. She's sure to be on a vent for a while, and who knows how this will turn out."

"Got it."

On the monitors, an art line trace and a CVP trace appear. The BP is 70/40 and the CVP is 22.

"Damn, man, we're flying blind, we better go with a Swan here," the CA-2 says.

A PA trace appears a few minutes later. PA 34/22 with a wedge of 6.

"All right, this does look like an embolus, we got a plug on the right side and not much is getting to the left side. And we're getting some pulmonary hypertension, probably from all that stuff in the lungs," the CA-2 says.

From the foot of the bed, "We've got some serious bleeding down here."

"OK, here's what we're going to do," the CA-2 says, "you're going to give blood and just keep sending blood gases and lab work. Got that? Blood gases, lab work, give blood. I'm going to do the hemodynamic support. OK? I'll mix the epi, milrinone and norepinephrine, and steer the hemodynamics. Got it?"

"Got it," the CA-1 starts hanging blood. Every minute, the instructor sends in a blood gas or other lab value.

"'Crit's low, only 20, I'm hanging more blood."

"PT's 16, hanging FFP, and sending a TEG."

"TEG's back, looks like the platelets aren't working, hanging platelets."

In the meantime, the CA-2 keeps everyone abreast of the hemodynamic plans.

"Gave a milrinone bolus, 3 mg, starting norepinephrine drip, we're sure to lose our SVR, and I'm cranking up the epinephrine."

"Isn't that what you do in a heart case?" the CA-1 asks.

"I got news for you pal," the CA-2 answers, "this *is* a heart case."

Over the next 10 minutes, the blood pressure rises to 90/60, the heart rate goes to 130 (high inotropic support is going), and the saturation rises to 90% but stays there, despite PEEP, suctioning, and inhaled beta agonists.

"OK gang, we're done with this scenario, wrap it up," the instructor writes on a blood gas form.

The CA-1, cranked up to respond to each blood gas, reads the note and doesn't get it at first.

"Oh, hey," the CA-1 says, "we're done."

The CA-2, also wound up and completely "into" the scenario, has a hard time coming down too.

"What?"

"We're done."

"Oh."

Clinical lessons learned from scenario 41

Debriefing. "We're going back to the aviation industry for this one, OK?" the instructor says. "We're going

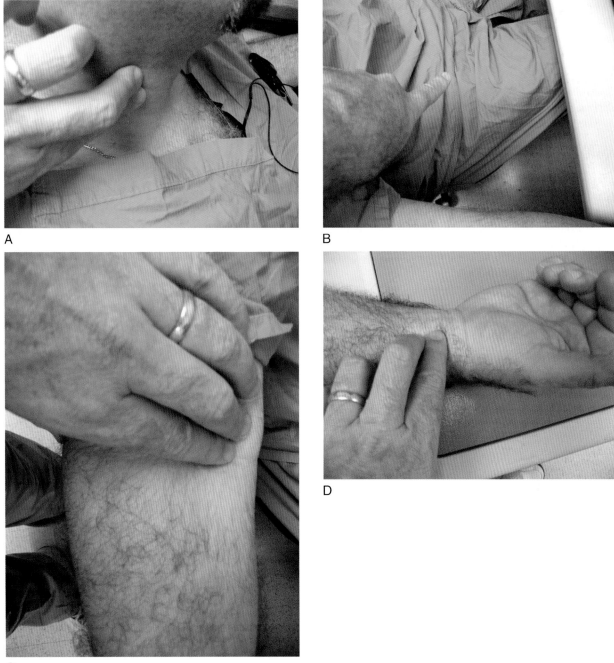

A

B

C

D

FIGURE 8–106 **A.** Don't forget the low tech. When all else fails (battery dies on the monitor, for example), feel for a pulse. If you can feel the carotid, you have about 60 systolic. **B.** Feel the femoral? About 70 systolic. (I didn't get permission to go groping around in this person's femoral area. He told me I should go get a life.) **C.** Brachial, about 80. **D.** Radial, about 90. Never lose track of the "old way of diagnosing trouble"—breath sounds, pulses, color. In this heavily computerized age, we can become too dependent on "stuff" and forget that direct physical observation and examination can give us lots of information when "the power goes out."

to look at everything that happened from the angle of 'situational awareness.'"

"Shoot," the CA-1 says.

Up on the white board, the instructor writes three things.

1. Ambiguity
2. Fixation on a task
3. Gut feeling.

"When the aviation industry did a big study on airplane crashes, especially perfectly good planes hitting perfectly hard earth, they uncovered some patterns that indicated the pilots had lost 'situational awareness.' They weren't tuned in to what was going on.

"Ambiguity is the inability to resolve discrepancies logically. In planes it can be that the instruments say you're straight and level, but the seat of your pants feel like the plane is turning.

"Fixation on a task means you have lost your priorities. In planes, the pilot may fixate on something nonessential (an alarm indicating the windshield wiper fluid is low) while the plane flies into a mountain.

"Gut feeling is important! Even in this era of super-high-tech gadgetry. Voice recorders from crashed planes have ominous comments like 'This isn't right.' 'Let's just climb and go to another airport.' 'I don't like this, something's wrong here.' That little tiny voice inside of you that cries out to be heard *deserves* to be heard. So listen to it."

The team reviews the entire DVD of the scenario, first all the way through, then going back and looking at individual items, trying to link the situational awareness lesson to their experience in the operating room.

"There, pause the DVD," the CA-2 says when the patient first does something odd—when she starts to cough. "Right there, I'm hearing this woman cough and I'm thinking, what the hell does this mean? Ambiguity, right there. She's perfectly healthy, no history of asthma, it's not like she could have aspirated, I mean, she was just talking to me. Then this cough, and right afterward" (they advance the DVD) "her sat drops. That's a pretty tough thing to figure out right there."

"It was an amniotic fluid embolus, wasn't it?"

"You think so?" the instructor asks.

"I do," the CA-1 says. "More common with multiple births. Sudden onset of hypoxemia and hemodynamic instability in an otherwise healthy patient. You could, I guess, invoke a regular pulmonary embolus. That can happen, too, with the hypercoagulable state of pregnancy. Kind of hard to tell them apart."

"So we're back to ambiguity," the CA-2 says. "But it's not like we were frozen, we didn't do the 'deer in

BOX 8–80	Amniotic Fluid Embolus

- **Often fatal**
- **Major support**
- **ABC**

the headlights' thing just because we weren't absolutely sure of the diagnosis."

The DVD bears him out. They did move fast.

"Let's see if we can smoke out some fixation on a task," the instructor asks.

"Bingo," the CA-2 says, "right there, after I intubated. I was so fixed on getting the airway secured that I forgot to turn on the stupid ventilator after I intubated. Duh!"

"Lucky I was there to save your sorry ass," the CA-1 snipes.

"Take it easy, I might be chief resident next year, making the call schedule," the CA-2 says. "Then we'll see whose ass is in what kind of shape."

"Enough!" the instructor says. "Jump on that last idea, gut feeling."

On the DVD, they stop when the CA-2 says *"Big dive in vital signs, all of a sudden. I'm going with some kind of embolus."*

"That's good, right there," the instructor says. "Your gut says this is something awful, and you proceed to follow your gut instinct, lines, ICU arrangements, inotropes."

"Looks like you guys had real situational awareness here."

"Let's get back to where you divvied up the responsibilities," the instructor says, "take me through your thinking."

"A CA-1 has handled some trauma, so he can handle blood gases, hanging blood and products," the CA-2 explains. "But I'm a little more familiar with inotropes and Swan numbers. So I figured I'll have the CA-1 do CA-1 things, and I'll do the CA-2 things."

"You flew it straight and level," the CA-1 says. "Can we get any in-flight drinks now?"

Summary. Amniotic fluid embolus is a diagnosis of exclusion, but you had better get excluding and diagnosing fast! This disastrous obstetric complication still has high mortality. Worst of all, you can't predict or prevent an amniotic fluid embolus. It can be a true "bolt from the blue." Your only hope is to always have that diagnosis "ready to go" and to start aggressive resuscitative care right away.

In this scenario, the residents took over a routine case that turned real bad real fast. By keeping "situational awareness," they were able to move in the right direction, and with one glitch (forgetting to turn on the ventilator, but the junior resident caught it), they brought the patient back.

When assigning tasks, it's important to have the right people doing the right things. A flat-out emergency is not the time to in-service a junior resident on the complicated machinations of unfamiliar inotropes. Let the senior handle the inotropes, let the junior hang the blood.

When did the "obstetric case" turn into a "heart case"? When things got bad. That is the good thing about knowing cardiac medications, inotropes, and resuscitation—you never know when *any* case will turn into a *heart* case. Then it's lines, epi, milrinone, levo, and you're off to the races.

SCENARIO 42. Morbid obesity

"What, exactly, is *heavy biscuit poisoning*?" the first medical student asks.

"Poor choice of words," the instructor says. "Let me see that preop."

A 45-year-old, 5′7″, 480-pound victim of heavy biscuit poisoning.

"God, I'm going to have to kill someone," the instructor says, tearing up the preop. "Try this."

A 45-year-old, 5′7″, 480-pound patient suffering from morbid obesity is in for bariatric surgery.

Fortunately, the med students keep a grim face on as the instructor loses his cool.

"That's half the fricking problem! Us, us, and our stupid, snippy comments about obesity! God Almighty, if we made fun of diabetics or epileptics or paraplegics like this, they'd burn us at the stake in Times Square! They'd feed our fingers into a paper shredder!"

"Point well taken," the second medical student says.

"Quit agreeing with me!"

"Sorry."

"No," the steam stops hissing out of the instructor's ears, "no. Sorry, OK, lost it there for a second. But the point is still worth making, even if I went 'coo coo for Cocoa Puffs' there for a minute. Today we're going to take care of a morbidly obese patient in the operating room, and we're going to see how this multisystem disease—and it is a disease, not an excuse for jokes—affects different organ systems. Got it?"

The three medical students are standing rigid as tent poles, afraid of doing anything but nodding.

"Relax," the instructor assures, "I promise I won't go postal on you again, OK?"

They all troop into the operating room. To convey morbid obesity, the Simulator has pillows wrapped by sheets around the abdomen and chest, and extra padding around the head and upper arms.

"How you doing Mr. Vickery?" the instructor asks.

"Ready to get going!" the patient (mannequin's speakers) says. "Going to turn things around, and today's the day we start!"

"OK if I talk about you a little bit, Mr. Vickery, as we get you ready to go to sleep? We have some medical students and they're eager to learn about this procedure."

"Go ahead, talk away," Mr. Vickery says.

"You go ahead and put the monitors on while I talk," the instructor says. The med students start putting on leads, blood pressure cuff, and pulse oximeter. "The bariatric surgery situation is getting to be more and more commonplace. This used to be the exclusive domain of a few specialty centers, but as word of the procedure's success spread more and more surgeons learned how to do it. Most places now do it by laparoscopic technique, and the really experienced hands can do it in about 2 hours, which is pretty amazing if you think about it."

"I can't get this blood pressure cuff on," the third med student says. "Even with the thigh cuff, I just can't get it around here."

The instructor tries, "Cuffs are cylindrical, if you look at them, built perfectly if your patient has a stovepipe-shaped arm. But the bariatric population often has a triangular upper arm, with an extremely wide area up near the shoulder. It's almost impossible to get a good fit sometimes."

"Can you use the forearm?" the med student asks.

"Yes," the instructor says, "but let's put in an arterial line, make sure we get a good accurate reading the whole time. Mr. Vickery, we're going to have to put an arterial line in your left hand here, a kind of special IV that let's us look at your blood pressure."

"Fine."

All the med students go over to the art line partial task trainer, so they can each "put in" an art line.

While they're working there, the instructor continues, "In this population, art lines are generally easier to put in than venous lines. The wrist doesn't have as much adipose deposition, and the artery is fixed in place. Veins tend to be a little tougher. If you have to go with a central line in these people, it's a good idea to use the Site Rite echo system. That allows you to see the vessel with an echo image, rather than just sticking blindly. And these patients have difficult landmarks, so the Site Rite is just the thing.

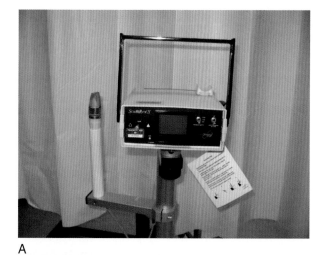

A

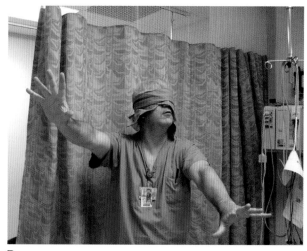

B

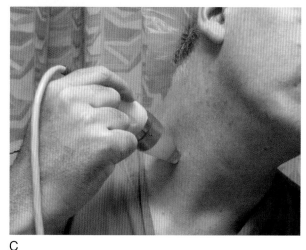

C

FIGURE 8–107 Why go blind with a neck stick when you can use the Site Rite or other echo location devices. Sure, with an easy central line, you don't need it. But when the going gets tough (multiple sticks, scars, obesity), the tough get echoing.

The med students, done with the art line, look over the Site Rite. To show its use, the instructor lies down on a gurney, has the students get an image of his neck vessels, then goes through a few maneuvers to show how the internal jugular vein can vary in size.

"Watch as I do a Valsalva maneuver," the instructor says. As he does this, the internal jugular vein gets gigantic.

"Whoa, that's amazing," the second med student says.

"That vessel is very stretchy, and can really change in size a lot. Now, press down real hard and see what happens."

As the med students push on his neck, the internal jugular gets as flat as a sheet of paper.

"That's what happens if you press real hard, you almost obliterate the lumen, making it nearly impossible to stick."

Now they all return to the patient. The monitors are all on, the oxygen is on, and they are ready to induce.

"Go ahead," the instructor says. "Each of you will induce and intubate."

The first med student jumps in. As soon as the propofol and Sux are in, the saturation starts to drop: 98, 95, 92, 89.

He tries to mask-ventilate, but there is a lot of squeaking and flatulence noises, the sat continues to drop.

"I better intubate," the first med student says. He places the laryngoscope, gets a view, and places the tube. Hooking up to 100% oxygen, he starts ventilating. There is a continued dip, then the sat turns around.

85, 82, 79, 83, 85, 89, 93, 98.

"Next!" the instructor says, and pulls out the endotracheal tube. "You saw what happened, what do you think you can do differently this time?"

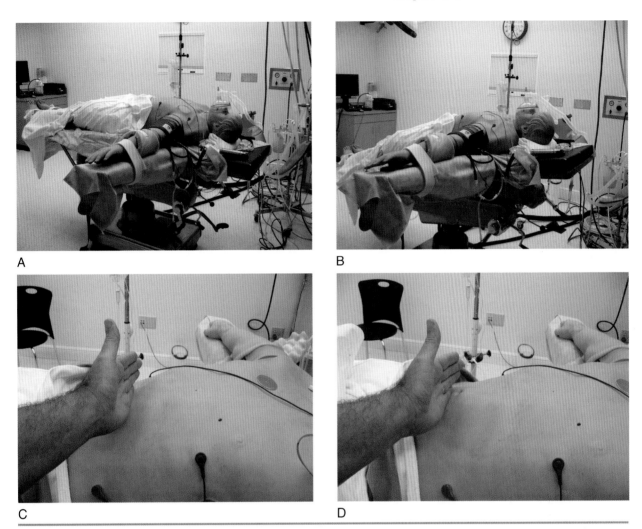

FIGURE 8–109 **A, B.** Roll that table into a little reverse T-burg and it makes the patient less likely to desaturate and easier to ventilate. **C, D.** Why? The diaphragm moves down just a touch, opening up the lungs, giving you more FRC and improving the whole respiratory situation. This head-up trick is especially useful in the obese patient. Lying flat, these patients can desaturate in no time.

The second med student, a little pale after seeing the sat drop so low just now, shrugs her shoulders.

"Try this," the instructor says, and puts the patient in a little reverse Trendelenburg.

She preoxygenates the patient, gives propofol and Sux, and starts mask-ventilating. There are fewer embarrassing flatulence sounds. The sat drops but not as bad this time.

98, 95, 94, 93.

She places the laryngoscope, intubates, and a shallower "swoop down, then swing up" occurs.

93, 90, 88, 90, 93, 96, 99.

"Third time's a charm," the instructor says. "Any ideas on how to do even better?"

"Um, cancel the case?" the third med student offers.

"Comedy Central is still hiring, I hear," the instructor says, "any other ideas, though, before you become the next Eddie Murphy?"

"Awake?"

"Good," the instructor says. "Awake intubation is a good option when you are really concerned about someone desaturating fast. Even if the airway's good, a person of this habitus can desaturate, even if you do everything right!"

All three med students intubate fiberoptically. The saturation doesn't budge.

"See?"

"I see and I believe!" the first med student says.

"That's it, lunch time!"

"But wait," the second med student says, "we were just getting started, this is too much fun!"

Clinical lessons learned from scenario 42

Debriefing. "Pizza!"

"Isn't this kind of fattening?" the third med student says. "I mean, in light of the case we just did, um. . . ."

"What, because we're discussing morbid obesity, we should eat bean sprouts and spring water for lunch?" the instructor asks. "Come on, dig in."

All three med students look at each other, give each other a "What the hell" shrug, and start grabbing slices.

"Who here saw *Supersize Me*?" the instructor asks.

All three raise their hands.

"The systemic review at the end of the movie should be required viewing for all medical students. The guy goes over his entire body and describes the effect of obesity and, really, malnutrition on every organ system. But which systems interest us most?"

"Heart."

"Lungs."

"Airway."

"Well what do you know, the Three Musketeers hit the three major ones," the instructor congratulates them. "Tell me about the airway."

The third med student says, "Lot of floppy, redundant tissue in the upper airway, and the head and neck can be so thick that you can't really extend them well to get a good view of the cords. What else? The tongue can be real big too. That would be a problem."

"You," the instructor says, pointing to the first med student, "you mentioned the lungs."

"Yeah, the abdomen pushes up on the lungs, squishing them, giving them a restrictive defect. Less FRC, quicker to desaturate. Well, we sure saw that here. That guy desaturated in a heartbeat."

"Speaking of heartbeats," the instructor now points to the second med student, "tell me about the heart and obesity."

"If you want to look at it from a left side/right side point of view," the third med student says, "the left

heart has to work extra hard to provide blood flow to all this extra tissue. And the left heart's blood supply could be impaired from high cholesterol leading to coronary artery disease. Then on the right side, these patients can have sleep apnea, chronic hypoxemia, and develop cor pulmonale. So both right and left are at risk."

"Good. One thing I liked about this whole discussion, did you notice we kept things professional and physiologic? There are organ systems at risk, and there are strategies to reduce that risk. This is not, 'Make fun of the patient day.' You got that?"

Each med student gets it, then gives a long look to that last piece of pizza.

It stays in the box.

Summary. Nothing challenges our professionalism more than the obese population. The temptation to take cheap shots, make fun of the patients, or blame them for their condition is there, no doubt. But the facts are that obesity is here to stay, it is a serious disease with multiple, poorly understood causes, and it presents us with serious challenges. Whether society needs to change, personal responsibility needs to change, economic factors need to change—all that is beyond our scope and is essentially irrelevant when we are faced with a morbidly obese patient on our OR table right now.

We can't "wish them to be thin," no matter how much we would like to.

In this scenario, the instructor made the point that obesity is not a laughing matter. Then, by demonstration, the instructor gave some practical points about care of the morbidly obese:

Blood pressure cuffs may not fit.

Arterial lines are easier than IVs.

Tilting the patient head up helps keep the saturation up.

An awake intubation keeps the saturation up too.

By doing three different induction sequences, the instructor showed, first hand, the various options and how each resulted in different "oxygen saturation flight paths." These head-to-head comparisons brand the lesson into the students' brains.

Are students usually disappointed when the session is over? You bet they are. The only complaint we ever get is, "Why can't we come here more often?"

BOX 8–81 *Obesity*

- **Reverse T-burg**
- **Quick desaturation**
- **Consider awake**
- **Art line better than poorly functioning cuff**

SCENARIO 43. **Tracheostomy, what could possibly go wrong?**

"Ever done a trach before?" the instructor asks.

"Yeah," the first resident says.

"Me too," the second resident says.

"OK," the instructor says, "here's your patient."

Patient is a 65-year-old, vent-dependent COPD patient requiring 15 of PEEP and 70% F_{IO_2}, now for trach.

"Got it," the residents say.

In the operating room, the patient is already intubated, and monitors are on. He is on 100% oxygen, 10 of PEEP, and has a saturation of 94%. Blood pressure 160/86, HR 95. The patient is draped, and the surgeon (med student) is ready to begin.

"OK to start?" the surgeon asks.

"Fire away," the first resident says. "Guess we could give some relaxant and a little narcotic." She looks over the vital signs. "Should be able to tolerate some vapors." On goes the Forane.

"OK, I'm getting down to the trachea now. You may get a leak in your cuff soon," the surgeon says. (The medical student has a script in the field and is reading off this script.)

"All right," the second resident says. "Wonder what they want us to do for this?"

"I don't know, stand here, look interested?" the first resident says.

"*Fire!*" the surgeon yells, and runs out of the room.

Over the intercom a deafening shout, "Fire, room 1; fire room 1!"

To create the notion of a fire, the surgeon laid a bright red napkin right on the trachea before he ran out of the room.

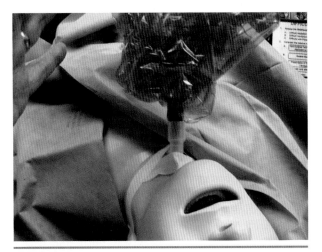

FIGURE 8–110 Airway fire, a nightmare you never want to see. Any time you have a source of ignition (Bovey, for example), and high ambient oxygen, you could trigger a fire. Even in as mundane a case as a trach, there is a real danger of a spark causing a fire if that Bovey hits a trachea filled with 100% oxygen. If there should be a fire, pull out the tube, turn off the oxygen, then once the fire is out, resecure the airway.

The intercom continues, "There is fire coming out of your endotracheal tube!"

Both residents step back, then look at each other. There isn't, of course, actual fire coming out of the endotracheal tube, but the intercom re-emphasizes the point. "Fire is coming out of your endotracheal tube!"

The first resident reaches over, grabs the tube, and pulls it out. The second resident goes around to the field, sees the red napkin (the fire), and pulls all the drapes off, puts them on the floor.

"Any water in here, give me a bottle of water!" the first resident shouts.

"Use the fire extinguisher!" the second resident yells, just as he reaches for another endotracheal tube. "I'm assuming the fire is out, and I'm going to reintubate."

Per intercom, "Fire's out."

The second resident reintubates. As he does this, the first resident grabs a (dummy) fire extinguisher, pulls the pin, and sweeps it over the area of the drapes, then aims it on the patient.

After the intubation, the second resident looks back at the monitors. "Any CO_2?"

The intercom crackles again, "The fire melted the sampling tubing, you don't have access to end-tidal CO_2."

Stethescopes on the chest, "Sounds good. Good chest rise. Get me a code tray, they'll have an end-tidal CO_2 confirmation device."

"Where the hell's the surgeon?" the first resident asks.

"Took off," the intercom says. "OK, wrap it up. Brush the charcoal off and let's go to the debriefing room."

Clinical lessons learned from scenario 43

Debriefing. The instructor is sitting at the debriefing table wearing a red fireman's hat.

"Very funny," the first resident says. "Hilarious."

"That was too much," the second resident says. "Major freakazoid, that was."

"We're all going to jump in a time machine, and go backward in time," the instructor-cum-firehat says. "Back to the original preop. And let's put on," she points to the fireman's hat, "not our fireman's hats. Let's put on our thinking hats this time."

A 65-year-old, vent-dependent COPD patient requiring 15 of PEEP and 70% F_{IO_2}—now in for a trach

"When is a trach an emergency?" the instructor asks.

"When that's the only way of securing an airway," the first resident says. "Say you can't intubate, can't ventilate. Or if someone has a really wrecked airway, tumor, trauma, burn, and you can't go from 'up top.' Then it's an emergency."

"Is this an emergency?"

"No, this is more housekeeping," the second resident says. "Doesn't have to be done today. Guy's probably been intubated for a month of Sundays already."

"Let me rephrase the question then," the instructor says, "*should* he be done today?"

"Oh, I get it," the first resident says, a light bulb going off above her head. "Yeah, I get it. No, this patient should *not* get done today. Look at those settings: 70% oxygen, 15 of PEEP. That's a hell of a lot of ventilatory support—15 of PEEP, come on, that's a lot. And even with all that PEEP, we're still above 50% oxygen, we're still giving toxic levels of oxygen. If you disconnect this guy for just a little bit, just for a second, such as when you switch over the endotracheal tube for the tracheostomy tube, you lose all that PEEP and the saturation drops like a stone."

"And how about the fire?" the instructor asks. "Before we get into how you handled the fire itself, think about how 15 of PEEP and 70% oxygen set you up for a fire."

The second resident picks up the discussion, "We blew it there, too. If the surgeon brings the Bovie near the opened trachea, you have a fire source near a column of oxygen. Kaboomo. In a trach, we should lower the F_{IO_2} when the surgeon gets ready to open the trachea to prevent a fire. And with this patient, requiring such high F_{IO_2} and so much PEEP, we just wouldn't be able to do that. We were painted into a corner."

"Did you even think to lower the F_{IO_2}?" the instructor asks.

"No."

"I guess when you think of fires, you always think of laser beams in the airway," the first resident says.

"Right," the instructor says, "you get in that pattern of thinking. You have to think like a consultant each

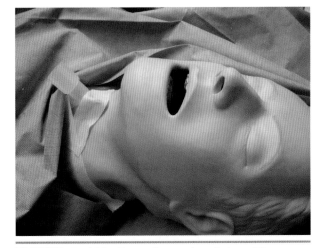

FIGURE 8-111 Don't forget the obvious. If someone comes down with a fully functional tracheostomy, well, guess what? You have your airway. This "overlooking the obvious" is not limited to trachs. You may struggle forever to place an IV line when the patient tells you, "I have a line here in my neck, doctor." Oh boy.

time. Is there a fire source, is there an oxygen source? If those two exist, you can have a fire."

Everyone now sits through the DVD replay.

"Damned clever how you made that fire," the first resident says.

"We asked about doing an actual fire, but the sprinkler system would probably go off, and a few residents would probably find a way to burn themselves to death, so we had to give it up."

"The fatalities among the residents I could handle. But I would hate to mop up after the sprinkler system went off."

"OK," the first resident says, "fire in the tube. Do I turn off the oxygen first or pull the tube out first."

"Pull out the tube," the instructor says. "Once the tube's out, the oxygen isn't being delivered right to the field anymore."

"And the drapes?" the second resident asks.

"No, what you guys did was right, take them down. Take away another fuel source. Then douse them or use the extinguisher."

"Then reintubate, right?"

"Right. You now have an airway burn, and what's the first thing you do in a burned airway? Secure the airway before it swells shut."

They look at the sequence again.

"Did I actually say that?" the first resident asks. At the very beginning of the OR scenario, she is talking to the surgeon and says, "*Fire away.*"

BOX 8-82 Airway Fire

- **Tube out**
- **O_2 off**
- **Reintubate**

Summary. Airway fires are rare but devastating. The reaction of the surgeon in this scenario is not uncommon—panic and bailing out. People have been knocked over as people flee, literally, from the flames on an operating room table. So if there is ever a test of "coolness under fire," this is it (pardon the pun).

As with every other clinical venture, a little planning and forethought can prevent a catastrophe and obviate the need for "OR heroics."

Don't trach someone who needs monster vent support. That will just lay the groundwork for a big desat intraop and possible crash.

Plan out your oxygen delivery during a trach. Here's one approach.

Get the F_{IO_2} as low as the patient can tolerate during early dissection, when there's sure to be a lot of Bovie work.

Once the surgeons are right on top of the trachea and about to enter it, ask them if they are really and truly done with the Bovie.

If they are, increase the F_{IO_2} and give the lungs a little "reserve oxygen for the switchover."

Remind the surgeons that "Bovie time is over."

Now, with some reserve oxygen on board, you are set for that period of apnea and nervousness as you pull the ETT and place the trach.

Heaven forbid a fire does occur, but if it does you have to move quickly. Get the endotracheal tube out of there, turn the oxygen off, resecure the airway. Douse flames with liquid or an extinguisher.

Better yet, pray this never happens to you.

SCENARIO 44. **Quadraplegic patient and an untoward reaction**

The residents are standing by the OR table. From the patient, a curious whistling and clicking sound is coming. A trach tube is taped to his neck (indicating the patient has an indwelling tracheostomy). The patient is blinking.

"Let's step out in the hall while they prep the patient," the instructor says.

Out in the hallway, the anesthesia residents gather around the instructor.

"What's up with the whistling and stuff?" the CA-1 asks.

"Here's your preop."

Case: A 34-year-old policeman, shot in the line of duty, now with C5 quadriplegia. Vent-dependent through tracheostomy. S/P several diverting procedures; now in for a urethral dilatation. Labs normal.

"I still don't get it," the CA-2 says. "What's going on with the whistling and, what would you call it, knickering sounds?"

"What do you think he was trying to say?" the instructor asks.

"Got me," the CA-1 says.

"Seemed like he was just trying to get our attention," the CA-2 says.

"Well think about it for a second," the instructor says. "You're quadriplegic, trached, and can't really talk to anyone. What's the only way you can get heard? What's the only way you can reach out in any way to anyone? You can't talk. But you can, if you work it just right, put together a kind of a whistle, and a kind of a, right, that's the name of it, a kind of knickering sound."

"So that's what a quadriplegic patient does?" the CA-2 asks.

"Yeah," the instructor says. "That is what they do sometimes. It's hard to figure out exactly what they might want, but sometimes you can read their lips or something, maybe they have an itch on their face and they want it scratched. That might sound trivial, but that is real torture to quadriplegics. And a little scratch from you might just make their day."

"So this patient has no feeling from C5 down?" the CA-1 asks.

"Correct."

"And they're doing a urethral stent?"

"Correct, what kind of anesthesia do you want to give him?"

The CA-2 is ready to jump all over that, but the instructor waves him off, letting the CA-1 walk right into the trap.

"I don't think he really needs any anesthesia, does he?" the CA-1 says.

Behind the CA-1, the CA-2 is ready to raise his voice in protest, but again the instructor shakes his head. "Let's play this out," the instructor is saying.

The residents return to the operating room, put the monitors on the patient, and the CA-1 tells the surgeon to proceed.

Taking a back seat, the CA-2 just waits in the wings.

"I'm starting!" the surgeon (the instructor in a surgical gown) says.

At first, the vital signs are all normal, and you hear nothing from the patient. The CA-1 has a trach collar around the trach site for supplemental oxygen.

After a minute, the patient starts to whistle and knicker, again and again. The heart rate slows noticeably, going from a resting heart rate of 100 down to the 40s.

"What the hell's going on?" the CA-1 says. The CA-2 presses the blood pressure cuff, which takes its time cycling before it comes to rest at 260/130.

More whistling, more knickering.

Over the intercom, the instructor says, "The patient's face is all red and flushed."

(Just as there is no BIS built into the Simulator, there is no way to make a face look different, so the intercom and a little imagination have to do.)

"Holy shit," the CA-1 says, "I need a hand here, get my attending, wait . . ." turning to the CA-2, "I think I need a hand here."

"OK," the CA-2 says, "you've got a case of autonomic hyperreflexia." Raising his voice, "Hold off on the instrumentation down there a minute, OK, we have to get a handle on things here."

"OK," the surgeon says.

"He's flushed because there's compensatory vasodilation above the spinal cord lesion, below the lesion there's tremendous vasoconstriction," the CA-2 explains. Then he draws up some nitroglycerin, gives a few little boluses, 50 μg at a time, to get the blood pressure down. "Not too much. Don't want to overshoot."

"What now?" the CA-1 says.

"Now that we have things under control, we have to induce anesthesia before the surgeon can proceed. This reaction is preventable with anesthesia, either spinal or a general. How do you think we should do this?"

The CA-1 is still rattled. "He has a cervical fracture, do we need to do an awake fiberoptic?"

"Uh, you have the easiest airway in the world," the CA-2 says. "Don't forget this." He points to the trach.

"Oh yeah," the CA-1 says with a nervous giggle.

They hook up the circuit, turn on the anesthetic vapors, and turn on the ventilator.

The surgeon looks up above the drapes.

"OK, done."

Clinical lessons learned from scenario 44

Debriefing. "Why did you let me do that?" the CA-1 asks. "You guys let me step right onto that landmine."

BOX 8-83　Autonomic Hyperreflexia

- **Reflexes interrupted**
- **Constrict below injury**
- **Try to compensate (vasodilate, slow heart rate) above**

The CA-2 and the instructor both raise their hands.

"Guilty as charged," the CA-2 says. "I knew the guy would have autonomic hyperreflexia if we let the surgeon proceed. But they waved me off."

"That's one thing that really sets us apart here in the Simulator versus in the real world," the instructor says. "In the operating room, with a real patient, I would never in a million years let you make that mistake. I would catch you, explain the whole thing, then make sure you did the right thing. And that is all well and good.

"But here we do have a rare luxury. We can let you wander down the garden path. Now, instead of just getting a lecture on autonomic hyperreflexia, or seeing some PowerPoint presentation. You got to trigger it, see it happen, and see how to treat it. All in the 'holy shit' setting of it really happening right in front of you. That makes a lesson you'll never forget. That's one thing we do here. Not just a lesson, a lesson with a real emotional tag.

"If you think about it, most of what you learn is in this low-level, emotionally flat-as-Nebraska state where people are talking to you, 'Blah, blah, blah.' Or else you're curled up in a chair at home, reading a book, skipping over paragraphs hear and there, and absorbing about 0.01% of what you read. But then you do this case, you see the pressure through the roof, you see, well, you imagine seeing, the red face, and all of a sudden, autonomic hyperreflexia has earned a real nesting spot in your brain stem."

"It sure does," the CA-1 says.

They look at the DVD.

"How could I forget about the trach?" the CA-1 says.

"Well, think about it," the instructor says. "You were pretty much in a panic when things went haywire, right?"

"Right."

"And what's the first thing that malfunctions in an emergency?"

"Your brain."

"Right," the instructor says, "your brain. That's why the *best* thing you did was call for help. You got that all-important second pair of eyes and second brain in the room to look things over and help you out.

"When you were decompensating, you were getting all wrapped up in your ego, you know, 'Oh no, this is *my* case and *I* screwed it up,' you lost touch with reality. You forgot your own name, probably."

"I did."

"So you call for help, your helper pegs the diagnosis, makes a good recommendation, points to the trach. . . ."

"Please, don't rub it in."

"And you're golden. What could be better?" the instructor wraps it all up with a nice ribbon.

Summary. We need to understand the needs of quadriplegic patients, just as we understand the needs of all our other patients. The high quadriplegic, on a ventilator, unable to move, may seem so disconnected from us that we can almost ignore them. Wrong move! Have a heart. Remember the golden rule, is that how *you* would want medical people to treat you? Even if you can't clearly communicate with them, make an effort. You might not get through very well, but you are doing the right thing.

This simulator scenario was a little cruel, because the beginning resident was allowed to impale himself. OK, no one said we *always* give them a break in the Simulator. Every now and then, for learning purposes, it's worth letting the dangerous or deadly thing happen. That's the beauty and wonder of the Simulator—no one gets hurt!

When the spinal cord is sectioned, the normal autonomic feedback loops are interrupted. Although the patient's pain fibers are interrupted, their spinal reflex arc (which doesn't have to go up to the brain to work) is still intact. With painful stimulation or visceral manipulation, a signal goes to the spinal cord. In a reflex, the body below the level of spinal cord injury goes into intense vasoconstriction, driving the blood pressure sky high. The heart responds to this (recall: the vagal innervation of the heart comes from a cranial nerve, well above this patient's C5 lesion) hypertension with reflex bradycardia. This is the heart's normal reponse to hypertension.

Another reflex response is the body's desperate attempt to lower the blood pressure. In the intact area (above the spinal cord lesion), the body does its level best to lower the blood pressure by vasodilating. Hence, the patient's flushed appearance. As well, his face probably felt hot, which made him uncomfortable, so he started trying to get everyone's attention again, whistling and knickering."

Treatment? First, get things under control. Stop the stimulation that's causing all the trouble, get a handle on the hemodynamics, then induce anesthesia so they can proceed with the case.

Oh, and don't forget if they already have a trach in.

SCENARIO 45. | **Coils in the neuroradiology suite**

"We're coiling today, in the radiology suite," the instructor says. "You know what that's all about?"

"Yes," the CA-3 says.

"No," the CA-2 says.

"Fill her in."

The CA-3 lays it out, "Way back a hundred years ago, when our instructor was training, all cerebral vascular malformations had to get clipped surgically."

"Hey, wait a minute," the instructor protests, "that was only 95 years ago that I was training."

"Yeah, well, whatever," the CA-3 goes on. "In the 1980s, some smart people developed the Guglielmi detachable coil. It's kind of like stenting the heart, except instead of trying to keep a vessel open, you're trying to make a portion of the vessel close. They go in through the femoral artery, and guide the wire up to the base of the aneurysm. Then they feed this little bitty coil—it looks like a little Slinky—into the aneurysm. They put a little current through the wire, which cuts the coil free. The neuroradiologists do this with progressively smaller and smaller coils until the aneurysm is all packed up with the coils. This effectively obliterates the aneurysm from the circulation, and that's it."

"That pretty much sums it up," the instructor says.

"Wait, wait, wait," the CA-2 says. "What about the other stuff?"

"What other stuff?"

"You know, what other stuff can go wrong?" the CA-1 asks. "I heard about you guys last week and letting the CA-1 trigger autonomic hyperreflexia. You're not going to sit back and let me go supernova. At least give me a hint or two."

On his face, the look of an angel, "Us, let you get in trouble? Who on earth would ever make you think that? Some bad, bad person must be making up stories about us here."

The CA-3, well versed in all matters of the coil, tells about possible complications, "You are poking a little thing into a thin-walled aneurysm. So you can rupture the aneurysm."

"Then you basically shift into intracranial bleed mode, right?" the CA-2 asks.

"That's it. Ready to rock?" the CA-3 asks.

They read the anesthetic preop together.

Case: A 49-year-old woman with hypertension, diabetes, and smoking history. Presents with blurred vision and found to have an anterior cerebral artery aneurysm. Physical exam—airway OK.

The patient is on the OR table, with routine monitors on.

"I think we're going to need an art line," the CA-2 says. "We have an aneurysm here and don't want wide blood pressure swings."

(Both residents are facile with art line placement so they skip the art line partial-task trainer.) An art line trace appears on the screen.

Induction proceeds with propofol, rocuronium, and fentanyl. Intubation goes well, but after the tube is in the blood pressure rises from a baseline 140 to 180.

"Yeeee, no good," the CA-2 says and gives another 40 mg of propofol. "Not too high, not too low, ju-u-u-u-st right."

The vital signs straighten out.

Before the CA-3 can say anything, the CA-2 says, "I'll send a gas. This woman has diabetes, and we're doing something that might threaten cerebral cells. We don't want hyperglycemia."

"Or *hypoglycemia*," the CA-3 warns. "Remember, hyperglycemia can be a problem, and there is some theory about getting glucose too high and injuring cells. But you go wild with that insulin and drive that glucose down to 5, and I'll tell you, you're going to have some neuronal injury to write home about."

The neuroradiologist (Simulation Center secretary) says, "OK, we're half an hour into this, I have femoral access, and I'm going to advance the wire."

"Heparin," the CA-3 says. "We better give heparin. All those wires in the cerebral circulation can get thrombi on them. And you just don't want that in your cerebral circulation. Giving heparin!"

Over the intercom, "Noted. An ACT was sent off and is 300."

"That's in the right range," the neuroradiologist says. (Actors in the Simulation Center are coached on the kinds of things that surgeons and radiologists would normally know.)

"Hey, she's moving!" the neuroradiologist grabs the Simulator and shakes it around, imitating a patient

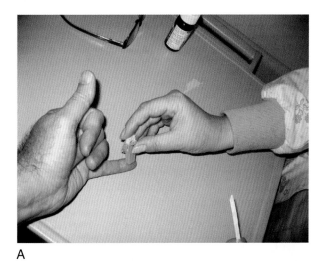

A

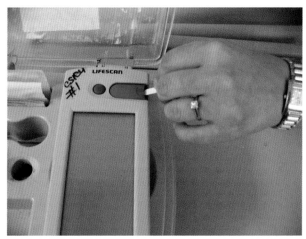

B

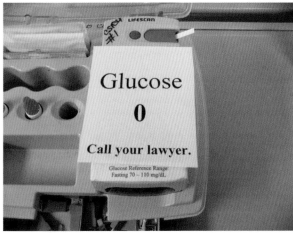

C

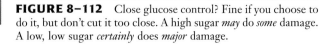

FIGURE 8–112   Close glucose control? Fine if you choose to do it, but don't cut it too close. A high sugar *may* do *some* damage. A low, low sugar *certainly* does *major* damage.

bucking. "This is bad, real bad. I'm deploying the coil right now!"

The CA-2 switches to hand ventilation, turns up the anesthetic vapors, gives 50 mg of propofol and 20 mg more of rocuronium.

"Damn, where's the twitch monitor?" the CA-2 asks.

"You were doing so good, I thought you'd have it on. I thought you thought of everything," the CA-3 says.

"Let me know when she stops moving, this is just not acceptable, do you hear me?" the neuroradiologist is hopping mad.

"Got it, got it," the CA-3 reassures, "she's holding still now."

"I cannot interpret these last images," the neuroradiologist says. "I'm trying to do some digital subtraction images here, and that movement just ruins the shot. I sure as hell hope I didn't puncture anything. Can't you people keep this patient still? Isn't that what you're paid to do?"

"Got it, we got you covered," the CA-2 says.

"We're 3 hours into this now," the neuroradiologist says, about another half hour to go." (In the Simulator, time can go on "fast forward.")

The two residents look over the screen, everything looks OK.

"What's that in the corner, is that the temperature?" the CA-3 asks.

"That is, yeah, that is the temperature," the CA-2 says.

32.3°C.

"What the hell?" the CA-2 asks.

"OK, we're done," the neuroradiologist says. "I'm going to need to do a neuro exam as soon as possible to make sure we didn't occlude anything. Could you wake her up right away please?"

"Uh. . . ." the CA-2 stammers. "This may take a little while. Could I get a Bair Hugger please?"

The instructor sticks his head in the door, "We're done."

Clinical lessons learned from scenario 45

Debriefing. The neuroradiologist pops into the debriefing room, "Listen, I got news for you. If you can't keep the patient still and warm, there are plenty of people out there who can. You got that? Plenty of other people can sleep my patients and not give me half the hassle you did. Keep that in mind before you buy yourself that next yacht." She slams the door on her way out.

A pall hangs over the room and no one says anything for a while.

"In case any of you think that is an unlikely exchange, then you're in for an icy cold wake-up shower when you go out into private practice," the instructor says. "Here, you automatically get cases. Here, you always have operations landing in your lap. Out there, you tick someone off? Guess what. They snap their fingers and get someone else, just like that."

"You are kidding, aren't you?" the CA-2 asks.

"I speak not with fork-ed tongue," the instructor says. "Don't believe me, just ask your CA-3 friend."

"That's right," the CA-3 confirms, "last year's class is out there, and a couple of them have already pissed people off. Now they're not getting as many cases. It happens."

"Damn."

"OK, let's go over the case. How do you think it went? Anything you'd change?"

"Blew it on two accounts," the CA-2 critiques, "forgot the importance of keeping the patient relaxed, and forgot to pay attention to the temperature. The temperature, of all things! Why did the temp go so far down?"

The local "coil genius," the CA-3, spells it out, "The room is cold, they keep it about 22°C for all their fancy imaging equipment. The table is cold, so the patient can lose a lot of heat through conduction. We don't have the heating blanket underneath, and it's hard to put a Bair Hugger on when they are accessing the femoral artery. Also, the neuroradiologists give a ton of fluid, both contrast medium, and fluid to help float and flush the little coils around. You usually don't think of much volume going through those catheters, but they really lay it on during these procedures. All that stuff adds up to a lot of cold delivery."

"That cold really zoinked us at the end," the CA-2 says. "Just when you really wanted a quick wake up with a quick neuro exam, we have the patient way too cold to extubate and way too cold to do a good exam on."

"Could you get anything, you think?" the instructor asks. "I'll *give* you that she's too cold to extubate.

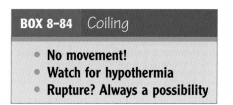

BOX 8–84 *Coiling*
- No movement!
- Watch for hypothermia
- Rupture? Always a possibility

But even if she's intubated, you should still be able at least do a rudimentary neuro exam."

"Is there any other kind?" the CA-3 asks.

"You were expecting maybe cold calorics and counting backwards by 7s?" the CA-2 asks.

"Smart asses, if there were a way to put you on detention, I'd do it," the instructor says.

"OK," the CA-3 says, slapping himself, "sober up. OK, you're right. You could, even if she's intubated, still get her to move the left and right sides."

"That's it," the instructor says. "You don't need anything unbelievably complicated. Just a 'move, not move.' That's plenty enough to tell you if the coil did some badness."

"Good enough for government work," the CA-2 says.

Summary. It's a, pardon the pun, "no brainer" to see that coiling is less invasive than operative clipping. To get to a vessel deep in the brain, a neurosurgeon would have to do a lot of dissection, cranial opening, all kinds of stuff. And even if everything goes well, the surgical retraction alone could cause enough cerebral edema to harm the patient, or at least cause delayed awakening. Then you're stuck: Is the delayed awakening a new neurologic problem? A bleed with subarachnoid hemorrhage? A metabolic problem?

Coiling? A femoral stick, a good deal of fluid, and that's it. A lot less invasive. Complications—yes, they exist. But coiling is now a popular and widespread treatment. So we need to know how to handle these procedures.

In this scenario, the residents did a few things right, a few things wrong—the essence of a great scenario. (If they do everything wrong, then it's too frustrating for the residents, if they do everything right, it's no fun for the instructor and technician.)

Smooth control of blood pressure during induction was essential to prevent rupture of the aneurysm. Tight control of diabetes made sense, but the CA-3's admonition to "avoid hypoglycemia at all costs" was important as well.

In certain cases, patient movement is *not allowed*—retinal cases, for example, where movement can result in eye injury. And in this case, movement was *forbidden*. Movement can cause aneurysm rupture, misplacement of the coil (a coil in the main circulation is a "thrombus-in-waiting"), and it blurs the all-important images. Keep them still! Get that twitch monitor on them and keep the patient paralyzed!

It's easy, when you're distracted with blood pressure considerations, patient movement, and neuroradiol-

ogy complaints, to forget to look at *all* of the vital signs. Can't forget temperature! Not as immediately life-threatening as a lot of things, but it can get you if you get low enough. Coagulopathy, delayed awakening, ventricular ectopy. Hypothermia is no laughing matter.

Which reminds me, did you ever hear the one about. . . . ?

SCENARIO 46. **DNR in the OR: is it really DNR?**
"We're rodding this femur for a pathologic fracture that hasn't happened yet?" the first resident asks.

"Well, yes," the instructor says, "read the preop and that will get you up to speed."

Case: A 40-year-old woman with metastatic breast CA, large met in her left femur. Cachectic. DNR.

"So, she hasn't broken her leg, right?" the second resident says.

"Correct, but the orthopods know it will snap if the barometric pressure changes, so they want to put a rod in it now."

"DNR?"

"Yes," the instructor says, "DNR."

"Um, OK," the second resident says. "So, uh, so in the OR, then, well, what?"

"Take good care of the patient, that's what that means," the instructor says and heads out.

The first resident double checks all the monitors, preoxygenates, and asks, "I think we'll need an A-line for this."

An art trace appears on the screen.

Before the residents can ask for anything else, the patient speaks up, "Doctors, can I talk to you before I go to sleep."

"Sure," the first resident is hopped up and ready to go.

"What is it you want?" the second resident is moving a little slower, still apparently hung up on the implications of the DNR order.

"I know I've got cancer all over, and I'm on about as much MS Contin as someone can take, and I still hurt all the time," she says. "If, in the middle of the case, you know, my heart should stop. Don't be in a big rush to start it again. Do you understand me? I've said goodbye to my kids, and their dad isn't around so it doesn't matter much anyways as far as that goes.

"Maybe, even, I don't know. You give a little too much of this, a little too much of that, you know, it's not like I'm gonna care. Right? And what do I wake up to, anyway? I can't really get around, can't eat. So, you know, just, well, I just want you to know that *whatever* happens here is OK."

"OK," the first resident says, his nervous energy a little abated.

"Got it," the second resident says. "We'll . . . um, OK."

Induction proceeds without incident.

"Give less, she has no protein to bind to anything," the first resident says. "Less, and wait longer, we're sure to get more bang for your buck with everything you give."

Once intubated, and the ventilator is on, the intercom says, "You have no good peripheral access, and the surgeon tells you he anticipates a lot of blood loss."

"OK," the first resident says, "let's go with a central line then."

They go over to a partial-task trainer to practice their central line placement.

After the line is in, they return to the Simulator.

The surgeon (medical student) drapes. Just as the clips go on, the inspiratory pressure alarm on the ventilator goes off. Saturation drops, and the art line drops to 60/40.

"Listen to breath sounds," the first resident says. "This could be a pneumo."

As the second resident puts the stethoscope on the chest, the blood pressure goes to 0.

"I can't hear too well, might be," the second resident says.

"Forget it, give me a 14 gauge, start CPR!" the first resident shouts.

"Wait!"

"Wait what?" the first resident places a needle in the chest (on the Simulator, there is a specific place, on the left side of the chest, where you can "stab" to release a pneumothorax).

On the intercom, "To relieve a pneumothorax, place the needle in the indicated spot on the left." The medical student shows the spot to the resident.

"But she's a DNR!" the second resident says. "You remember what she said. She would just as soon. . . ."

"The hell with that, this is iatrogenic," the first resident shouts. He places the needle and a loud hissing sound escapes.

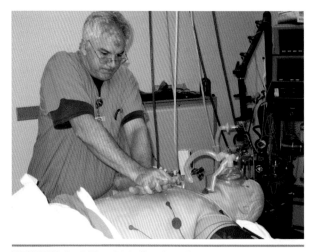

FIGURE 8-113 "To hell with it, that's iatrogenic, I'm starting CPR." What to do with a DNR patient in the OR is a tough ethical question. The Simulator lends itself to exploring such questions. You can set up a scenario with this dilemma, run several residents through, and see how differently people react. Any absolute perfectly correct answer? No. This falls into a gray zone.

The blood pressure returns to normal, saturation improves, and inspiratory pressures go back to normal.

"Cancel CPR, we're OK," the first resident says.

"OK if I start?" the surgeon asks.

At the same time, the two anesthesia residents speak.

"Yes," the first resident says.

"No," the second resident says. Then they look at each other.

"Hey," the second resident says, "we just had a near code there, and we dropped a lung. We should wake her up and see if she's OK before we just go on."

"To hell with that," the first resident snaps back. "Think about what we're doing here. If a butterfly goes past this woman's leg, the femur is going to snap, so the surgeon's had better get this rod in her or her life will be just that much more miserable in her remaining days."

Turning away, the second resident says, "I don't know, maybe we should have just let her go."

"Right, after we drop the lung and give her a tension pneumothorax, we just let her go," the first resident says.

"She's DNR!"

"But we're in the OR!"

"Hey, cheering section up there, can I start?" the surgeon asks again.

"Oh, go ahead," the second anesthesia resident relents.

"All right," the surgeon says, "we're half way into the operation now and I'm going to drill through the center of the femur so we can place this rod."

As the surgeon drills, the end-tidal CO_2 drops, the blood pressure drops, again to 60 systolic. Then the end-tidal CO_2 goes flat.

From the intercom, "The end-tidal CO_2 line is occluded with yellowish fluid."

Multifocal ectopy starts.

"Stop drilling! This is a fat embolus," the second resident says.

Ventricular fibrillation occurs.

"Get the paddles, we have to shock her! 300 asynch!" the first resident shouts.

"Wait!"

"Wait what the hell, you going to do the DNR thing again? This is iatrogenic too!"

The cart comes in, with paddles, the second resident applies the paddles. "Clear, I'm clear, you're clear, everybody clear!"

Shock, shock, shock. No response.

"100% oxygen, hand-ventilate, epi 1 mg now," the first resident is a flurry of activity.

"No," the second resident says. "No way, let her go."

"The f—you say! Give the epi!" the first resident grabs the syringe of epi and gives it.

Resuscitation fails after several more rounds of epi, shocking, and CPR. During the code, the second resident sits in the corner and refuses to participate.

The instructor comes in the room at the end. "Let's finish up in the conference room."

Clinical lessons learned from scenario 46

Debriefing. "Don't say the 'f' word in my direction any more," the second resident fires off.

"Sorry," the first resident says. "Guess I got a little bonkers in there. But still, the whole DNR thing, I mean, come on, we're in the OR, we bring on the code. You can't just stand there."

The instructor nurses a Coke and lets the residents wrestle with the question.

"Sure you can stand there," the second resident says. "You heard her. Mets everywhere. Constant pain. Miserable existence. She doesn't *want* to keep going."

"Well, it's not for us to decide," the first resident says. "In the OR, you're not really a DNR. Think about it. What, you give her Sux and then you say, 'Look, she's not breathing, let's let her go.' That's nuts. *We* gave her the Sux and made her stop breathing. And we did it so we could intubate her. So 'resuscitating' the patient in the OR is just part of the anesthetic.

"Look at it this way. You give too much propofol, her pressure drops. You're not going to give her a little ephedrine to get her pressure up? Sure you would. You made the pressure go down, now you make it go up again."

"Yeah but the pneumothorax was different," the second resident says.

"The hell. I did a procedure. I made the pressure go down. It's my responsibility to get the pressure back up again. Just like as if I'd given too much propofol. What, you're saying a chest tube is too heroic?"

"Well in the end, when that fat embolus occurred, and we went ape with the paddles and the CPR, that was heroic," the second resident says.

"Now wait a minute," the surgeon weighs in. "That was me that made the embolus occur, drilling through the bone. So now I was the one who made the pressure drop. It's my responsibility to get that pressure up now. So I'm sure not going to say, 'Let her go' at that point. We need to fix the complications we cause in the OR. In my book, no one is a DNR in the OR."

All eyes turn on the instructor.

"So, what is it?" the first resident asks.

"Who's right here?" the second resident echoes.

One last drag on that bright red can of sugar, bubbles, and secret recipe, and the instructor puts down the Coke.

"Damn good question."

Summary. Simulation, unlike an Agatha Christie murder mystery, does not always end with a tidy explanation, a neat conclusion, an identified murderer. Sometimes a simulation just "raises the question" and leaves it hanging, for the residents to sort out in their own time and through their own experiences.

The medical aspects of this case lend themselves to a little clearer understanding.

A cachectic patient is sure to be low on intravascular proteins. Hence, whatever drugs you give do have less protein binding, and you get more effect for any given dose. Hence the caution when giving the induction drugs.

After a central line, you should always have a potential pneumothorax on the front of your mind. Major index of suspicion. If things start going haywire (high inspiratory pressures, dropping pressure and sat), rule out pneumothorax first. And if you suspect it, fix it! Under positive-pressure ventilation, it turns into a tension pneumothorax pretty quickly.

During the drilling of bones, a lot of marrow and fat can make its way into the circulation. In this patient, as the drill went through the area of the tumor, the tumor itself could have gotten "ground up" and introduced into the circulation. Tumor embolus, like any other kind of embolus, goes to the right heart and into the pulmonary circulation, cutting off blood supply to the lungs. Hence, end-tidal CO_2 drops, acute right heart failure can set in, and you're off to the CPR races.

And now to the most difficult question—the one that preoccupied the residents the most—What do you do? Do you let her go, as she told you she wanted before the induction? Do you "bring her back" because "no one is a DNR in the OR" (which is the standard thinking)? Do you "bring her back" if it's a "little thing" (a drop in pressure from propofol)? Do you "bring her back" if it's an "anesthesia thing" (the pneumothorax)? Do you "bring her back" if it's a "surgical thing" (the tumor embolus)?

When you bring her back, are you doing her a favor? Are you condemning her to more miserable days of bone pain and despair?

If you don't bring her back, are you risking a lawsuit? (I hate to say this, but you are *always* at risk of a lawsuit.) If you don't bring her back, are you playing God? Is this your right? Are you overstepping your bounds?

Are you right, or are you wrong?

Damn good question.

SCENARIO 47. Kid with a sore, sore throat, epiglottitis

"There's a kid you need to see in the ER," the instructor says. "Now, a little suspension of disbelief here. Child labor laws don't allow us to have a kid in here, so just imagine him a little smaller."

Two anesthesia residents go into an examining room. There, sitting up in a triangular position, head leaning forward, drooling, is a "kid" (a secretary—unfortunately a little tall at 5′11″). Standing next to the "kid" is his mother (a med student).

It takes just a second for the anesthesia residents to readjust their thinking and "make the big guy into a kid."

"Hello, ma'am, we're from the anesthesia department, and we're going to talk to you a little bit, OK?"

"Oh, doctors, you don't know," the mother says. "He's burning up, and, and now he's not even talking, and, and he can't swallow his spit, and, and I don't know what. But I don't have any insurance, so, do I have to fill out something?"

"That's OK," the first anesthesia resident says. "We're going to go to another place to take a closer look at your son's throat, OK? And we'd like you to come along with us, does that sound good?"

"Where are we going?" the mother asks.

"It's right down the hall here," the first anesthesia resident says. "And you know what, Mom. We are going to need some help from you. Can you work with us because this is really important."

"Why?"

"Your son staying calm while we do this is very important," the second resident says. "Calm is the way to go for your son, and the best way for that to happen is for you to be calm too. Are we together on this, Mom?"

"Is this serious?"

"Well, yes, we are concerned, but the main thing is that all of our concern becomes a calm, cool working together," the first resident says.

"Oh, OK. I see."

"Good, then let's all go together," the first resident says.

"Don't we need to get some X-rays or something? Don't I need to do something about the insurance here? I don't have any, you know."

The door opens and the ENT surgeon (medical student) comes in, "Hey, doctors, what's up."

"We're entertaining a diagnosis of epiglottitis," the first resident says. "So Mom and my colleague and you and I are going down the hall here and going to take a good look in this young man's mouth and maybe put a breathing tube in there to help him out. And it would be nice to have you around to help us in case you can provide us the kind of help we might need."

"Got it, I'll get a kit ready," the ENT says. "I'll be ready for just the procedure you might request."

"Maaa,aaaa, aah we, aahaaaah. . . ." the child tries to talk but with all the drooling cannot make himself understood.

"Will he get a shot or anything?" the mother asks.

"*Maaaa, aaaa, aaaah!*" the kid starts making noise and looking alarmed.

"No, no, no, no," the second resident says. "No shots. No shots, no needles. Just a little mask that smells good. Smells like bubble gum, then you take a little nap, that's all."

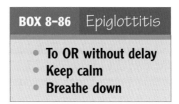

BOX 8-86 Epiglottitis

- **To OR without delay**
- **Keep calm**
- **Breathe down**

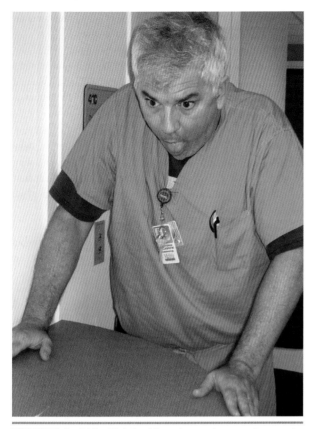

FIGURE 8–114 Epiglottitis patients take up a characteristic "triangular pose" with their two arms propping them up and their head hanging forward. Their tongue may hang out, and they might not be able to swallow their own saliva their throat is so sore. This is airway emergency extraordinaire.

The instructor takes them down into the OR. The "kid" peels off, and in the simulation OR there is a child-sized mannequin.

Mother, the two residents, the ENT, and the child mannequin are all in the OR.

"OK, we're going to just put a little mask on you, let you get a little sleepy," the first resident says.

"Mom," the second anesthesia resident says. "Why don't you stay right here, and we'll all be OK right here. Then once we have a little nap going, then you can step out and I'll even show you the way to go. Sound good?"

"OK, will he be OK?" she asks.

"We are taking good care of him, and we have all the right people and equipment here," the first anesthesia resident says.

The first anesthesia resident puts on the mask, turns on the sevoflurane, and proceeds with an inhalation induction. After a minute, the resident lays the patient down.

"OK, Mom, now we're going to do a few more things, and it would be a good idea for you to step out now. Let's go out in the hallway."

Out in the hallway, the instructor says, "At this point, a nurse takes the mother to the waiting room. You can go back in the OR."

In the operating room, the patient's saturation and vital signs are OK.

"Going to give any muscle relaxant?" the second resident says. "Oh, do we have an IV in? At this point, I'd place an IV."

Over the intercom, "IV in."

"Back to my question, any relaxant?" the second resident asks.

"No, let's keep him breathing spontaneously, then take a look under deep inhalational. Is my ENT friend ready to go if I have trouble?" the first resident asks.

"Kit ready, open, all set," the ENT says. "If you can't intubate, I'll cut."

The first resident picks up a straight blade.

"Wait a minute," the second resident says, "you don't want a straight blade. You'll have to lift the epiglottis with that. I don't think you want to do that, do you?"

"Aaag, right you are." She picks up a curved blade.

She puts the blade in the mouth, intubates, checks the breath sounds, and sees CO_2 on the end-tidal monitor.

"All done, amigos!" the intercom chirps. "Hi ho, hi ho, it's off to the debriefing room we go."

Clinical lessons learned from scenario 47

Debriefing. "But nothing happened," the first resident protests.

"Yeah," the second resident says. "I thought when you came here you'd killed them for sure, and we would run a code and all that cool stuff. Things just went right here. Where's the fun in that?"

"Please, please," the instructor says. "Enough with the fireworks. There's nothing *wrong* if things go *right* here. Simulators aren't just 'code practicers.' Let's go to the DVD."

The DVD includes both the examining room and the OR phases of the exercise.

"I know you did this right, but just for my edification go over your thinking from the word 'go.'"

The first anesthesia resident provides color commentary: "The main thing is that this is an A-number-1 airway emergency. You need to keep the kid calm, gather the horses, especially the ENT horses, and get to the OR ASAP."

"Gotta keep the kid calm," the second resident says. "You have to picture a fiery red, gigantic epiglottis just waiting to completely occlude the airway. And it's so inflamed it could basically get stuck right at the vocal cords, and there you are. No airway. No air in, no air out, and no way José can you intubate. Nightmare city.

"No detour to radiology, no IV, no separation from Mom. Just happy faces and calm demeanor and zippety-do-dah right to the OR, with a trach kit ready to go if the you know what hits the fan."

"What would you see if you got a lateral neck film?" the instructor asks.

"Well, to repeat, I wouldn't go there."

"Humor me."

"You'd see a thumb sign. The epiglottis would look like a big thumb sitting there."

Next, the DVD from the OR plays.

"Why sitting up?" the instructor asks.

"He's sitting up for a reason," the first resident says. "That's the only way air can channel through this area. So don't lay him back until you have to."

"And then, bingo, you got it!" the second resident says.

"Yeah, but not until you reminded me about the blade," the first resident blushes to admit.

"Hey, what are friends for?"

Summary. Epiglottitis is an airway emergency, fortunately not too common, that requires a lot of interpersonal wizardry. Because the great enemy of the tenuous, inflamed airway is *agitation*, the anesthesiologist has to move quickly to the OR but not scare the hell out of child or mother. With good actors (even the wrong size), this whole scene can get practiced in the Simulator.

First, the patient's posture should raise the alarm. Sitting forward, unable to swallow saliva (the throat is so sore, swallowing saliva is like swallowing ground glass), and a pinched, alarmed look on the face. All this says, "Watch out for epiglottitis."

Once you suspect the diagnosis, it's time to move. Go with the clinical picture, don't try to confirm your diagnosis with blood tests or X-rays. Good old-fashioned observation can do all the diagnostic work for you.

In the operating room, keep everyone calm, do an inhalation induction, and once the patient is under anesthesia place an IV. Keep the ENT right nearby because if the patient suddenly occludes (say, when he or she is induced and you lay the patient flat), you won't be able to intubate from above. Stay away from straight blades because that could hit the friable epiglottis and stir up all sorts of trouble.

Students and residents in the Simulator sometimes complain when "everything goes right." But that is one of the virtues of the Simulator—you don't need to kill the patient to make a point. If the residents go through each and every step well—good for them. Successful scenario, nothing wrong with that. And it's worth reviewing a good scenario too. Just as you can review a good tennis shot or a good golf swing, you can also review a good scenario to reinforce the points learned.

Keep such a scenario as a teaching module for other residents.

SCENARIO 48. **Plumbers in the house and the anesthesia machine**

"Hernia?" the first med student says.

"Hernia," the instructor says. "He wants to be asleep. Says he heard about those needles in the back on *Oprah*, you know, how they paralyze people all the time, so he says no way to a spinal. It's a general anesthetic that he wants."

"Got it," the second med student says.

Both the students are finishing a month-long senior elective on anesthesia, so they've done a few cases and are now set to "fly solo" on this simulated case.

"He's in the OR, but you go ahead and check the room out before you begin," the instructor says. "Don't be nervous, the worst you can do is screw up utterly and be a professional and personal failure for the rest of your lives."

"Thanks," the second med student says. "That's encouraging."

In the room, the students do the machine check. While trying to provide positive-pressure ventilation through the bag, they notice a big leak.

"I'm not moving anything," the first student says.

After hunting around, they see that the soda lime CO_2 absorber holder is undone. They push the lever to lock it.

"Still a leak," the second med student says.

After undoing the soda lime holder a second time, they see a granule sitting on the "O" ring.

"That rat bastard has sabotaged us," the first med student says.

"What?" the patient (Simulator, through the speakers) asks.

"I said 'That rare basting has savory juice!' We were talking about a recipe for the grill, sir," the first med student says, then whispers to his colleague, "Damn, forgot the patient is listening."

They continue with their checkout.

Turning on the knobs, they see that the bobbins float freely, nothing stuck. Ventilator works, oxygen cylinders full and work, no hissing when they turn them on (indicating a poor yolk fit). As they continue through their checkout, they hear loud banging and drilling outside their door.

Over the intercom, "They're doing a little construction work, sorry about the noise."

Suction, check. Oxygen analyzer, check and calibrate. Fail-safe system alarm works. All drugs set up. All nice and neat. Airway equipment.

"This light doesn't go on here," the second med student says, trying out the laryngoscope. A little investigative work reveals the batteries are dead. They fix that.

"Should we intubate or use an LMA for this," the first student asks.

"You know what one attending says 'LMA' stands for, don't you?"

"What?"

"'**L**et 'e**M A**spirate."

The surgeon (another med student, pre-scripted for the surgeon's part), walks in. "Hey, good morning. I hope you're going to use an LMA. We've been doing it for all these hernias, and they don't buck or cough at the end like they do with an endotracheal tube. Gotta tell you, makes for the smoothest wake up. That sound good? I'm not telling you what to do, I mean, if you have to tube him, tube him. I'm just telling you kind of how it goes around here. You do what you think is best."

"OK, yeah," the first student says. "We'll use an LMA. Will you be putting some local in the area before we start. A little preemptive analgesia?"

"Sure, I can do that," the surgeon says, then walks out of the room.

"Well," the first student says, "let's go. You give the drugs, and I'll do the LMA."

The instructor talks over the intercom, "Once you've done that, switch places and do it again, so each of you gets to do everything."

"Here we go. 'Sir, you're going to get a little sleepy,'" the first student says.

Propofol 200 mg, then the LMA goes in, they let the patient get back to breathing spontaneously.

"Switch!" the instructor says.

Propofol, then the LMA attempts to go in.

"This isn't going," the second student says. He tries turning the LMA sideways, then tries inserting it backward and flipping it around. No go.

"Try inflating it a little," the first student says. "I've seen them do that sometimes."

With partial inflation of the LMA, it works. The LMA slips in, seal is good, and they are able to let the patient breathe spontaneously on 3% sevoflurane. Drapes go up, and the surgeon starts.

The instructor walks into the room and asks the first med student, "What are all the safety devices we have built into the anesthesia machine to make sure we are delivering oxygen?"

"Well," the first student says, "the most important thing of all is the oxygen analyzer." He taps it, it reads 21%. "Because we're dealing with colorless gases here, we have to always know that the stuff we are actually delivering to the patient is oxygen, and we can only know that if we analyze here, on the inspiratory limb, just before it goes into the patient."

"Good," the instructor encourages, then turns to the second student. "What else?"

The second student has a troubled look on his face, but he can't seem to put his finger on it, so he launches into his answer, "Uh, the bellows, the ventilator bellows, are powered with oxygen. So if there is a hole in the bellows, you will get more oxygen, not less. Wait."

"What?"

"Oh, nothing," he says, and looks at the oxygen flows—2 L oxygen, 2 L air. "Um, oh yeah, the pin system, the . . . the thing where you hook up the cylinder."

"The pin index safety system, on the tanks," the instructor explains. "And what do we have for the oxygen hoses?"

"Diameter index safety system," the second student says. "The hoses have different diameters, so you can't fit the oxygen into the nitrous oxide line." The student continues to look things over, still with a furrowed look on his brow. "Something's, um. . . ."

All the vital signs are OK, even though the sat is a *little* low at 97%. Still, the second student is looking everything over again and again. Outside the room, more banging and drilling and construction sounds.

"What else?" the instructor asks.

The first student pounds down the list, "The oxygen flowmeter is farthest to the right, in a left-to-right flowing system, so if there's a break in the manifold, oxygen will be the last thing cut off.

"The fail-safe system, if the pressure in the oxygen line is below 25 psi, then an alarm goes off. Man, they are loud out there, what are they doing?"

Shrugging, the instructor says, "I think some plumbing stuff."

"OK," the second student goes on, "the oxygen ratio monitor controller, ORMC. If you try to dial in a hypoxic mixture, there is a mechanical deal that doesn't allow it." The second student demonstrates. "And the last thing is the knobs themselves. Oxygen has a fluted handle, and nitrous has a sintered handle. That way you can . . . wait . . . wait. I knew it, I knew something was wrong. Look at that oxygen analyzer. 21%. No way, no way. Look, we've got 2 L of O_2, 2 L of air—we should be at about, what 60%, 65% maybe. Something is wrong here."

He reaches back and turns on the cylinders; goes to 3 L and turns off the air. In a few seconds, the oxygen analyzer goes to 100%. At the same time, the saturation rises to 100% as well.

"Oh man, that's right," the first student says. "You got it, you got it. I missed that. That's right, you have

to check the oxygen analyzer. Hell, I looked right at it, didn't even notice it said 21%, room air."

The instructor goes out into the hallway and comes back in with a boombox. Construction sounds blare out of the speakers. "Here's your construction crew." Simulation done.

Clinical lessons learned from scenario 48

Debriefing. An oxygen analyzer sits on the debriefing table along with a stick model of the oxygen molecule.

"How does the oxygen analyzer work?" the instructor asks.

"Uh. . . ." the students are lost on this.

"Well, here's the deal, doesn't matter how it works," the instructor explains, "so long as it *does* work, and so

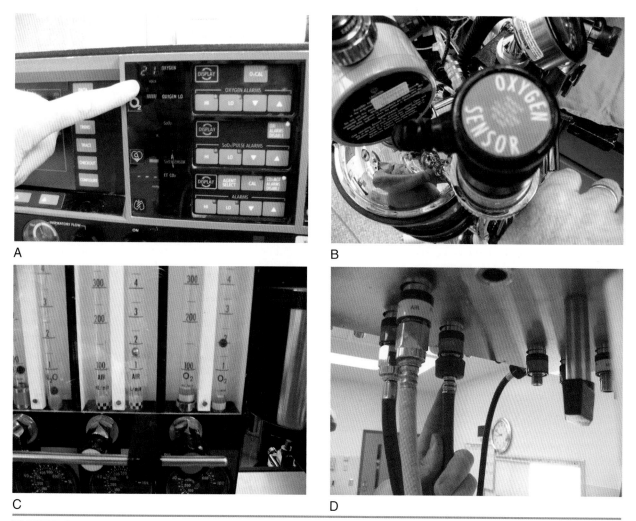

FIGURE 8–115 Something doesn't make sense here. Why would the sensor say 21% oxygen when I'm on 2 liters of O_2 and 2 liters of air. Aha! That's it, a pipeline crossover! In the simulator, you can actually create a pipeline crossover (you would *never* dare do that in the real OR).

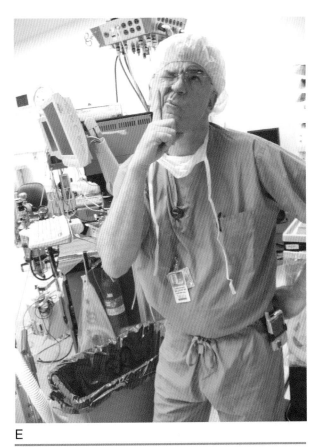

E

FIGURE 8–115 cont'd Hmm. Think, think, think. Just like Winnie the Pooh.

long as you *look* at it, and so long as you *see* and *understand* what you are looking at."

"I can't believe I just blew right past that," the first student says.

"Let's look at that," the instructor says, "let's look at what goes into, I guess we'd call it 'highway hypnosis,' where your eyes are open, you're looking at the road, but the signals just aren't getting into the brain. How does that happen?"

"If there isn't something alarming going on, like the patient's oxygen saturation going down, then I guess I just don't really focus enough," the first student says.

"Why was the patient's saturation OK, anyway?" the instructor asks.

"Young guy, room air, that'll keep the sat at least good. What was it, 97%? You can get that on room air," the first student says. "It's almost too bad he was so healthy—there were no red flags for us to catch."

"So we see that you can have the book stuff down, I mean, come on, you guys got every single safety device we have for delivering oxygen," the instructor continues. "But then, when it boiled right down to it,

you had to make that one little extra leap, that one 'spark of knowledge' that made you *look with eyes that see*."

"How do you teach that?" the first student asks.

"I wish I knew."

"What was with the construction stuff?" the first student asks. "You said they were doing some plumbing work, so how does that give you a pipeline crossover. That's what this was, wasn't it. I mean, if we were at 21% oxygen, then we were getting room air instead of oxygen, right?"

"Right."

"But how did the lines get crossed?" the second student asks. "Those were just plumbers, right. I mean, we didn't have a sewage crossover. God, imagine that. What kind of flowmeters would we need?"

"Aag! Stop!" the instructor says. "God, who hires you people?"

"So what happened?" the second student persists.

"Well, guess who puts in our oxygen lines?" the instructor asks.

"Plumbers?" the first student guesses.

"You got it. Hey, they're just so much piping to the plumbers. And if one gets mixed up with the other, well, then we better find out before the patient crashes."

Summary. Pipeline crossovers are a real danger to anesthesia. Big danger times are during construction or when a place just opens—in effect, construction "just finished." We have to make sure the right gas is in the right line. Dangerous gases, such as hydrocarbons, have even spilled into medical gas lines. Imagine your patient inhaling gasoline!

We have a plethora of monitors to make sure oxygen is getting to the patient, as detailed by the students.

Oxygen analyzer
Oxygen powering the bellows
Fluted handle on the oxygen versus sintered on the
    nitrous
Diameter index safety system
Pin index safety system

Colored lines, green for oxygen tanks and lines (the students didn't mention this)

Oxygen ratio monitor controller

Fail-safe pressure alarm

But all the great alarms and devices are for naught if our *brain is not turned on*. And unfortunately we have no alarm that goes off when our brain is disengaged.

In this scenario, the students clearly knew their stuff. They found several sabotaged elements in the machine, caught the dead batteries in the laryngoscope, debated the merits of the LMA, and did a safe anesthesia. They knew the safety features of the machine. But something was in that second student's bonnet, something was not quite right, and it took him a while to peg it. But he did eventually get it. The oxygen analyzer was not making sense!

Like a good doctor, he went to cylinders, ensuring a good supply of oxygen to the patient.

Don't just look at those numbers. Look at them and *see* them.

SCENARIO 49. **A bad heart, a bad scene, and an intra-aortic balloon pump**

"Doctors," a nurse (secretary from the Simulation Center) says, "could you come to the operating room, please?"

The two senior residents in the hallway shrug their shoulders.

"Sure."

As they walk toward the operating room, the nurse fills them in, "We are having trouble coming off cardiopulmonary bypass. Could you help us out with that?"

"OK."

"And we may need your help with something else too," the nurse adds.

"What's that?"

They enter the operating room, "Well, you'll see."

In the operating room, the lines are tangled beyond belief, pumps are alarming, ventilators are alarming, and the surgeon (a medical student) is yelling bloody murder, "You're killing my patient, you're killing my patient!"

Behind the screen, the anesthesiologist (a Simulation Center secretary) is shouting back, "I can't take this, I can't take this another minute!" As the residents walk in the room, she yells at them, "You take care of this, I'm out of here!" and she runs out.

The two residents are left in the middle of a catastrophe, no lines labeled or clearly going anywhere, the blood pressure at a mean of 50, no report on what's going on, and a furious surgeon.

Turning to her compatriot, the first resident says, "Well, we seem to have a situation here."

"Shall we start with ABC and go from there?" the second resident suggests.

"Do, let's," the first resident replies.

First, they check the ventilator, make sure it's on, and that the chest is rising.

"If this were a heart case, as we are supposing, then we would look in the field and see the lungs rise and fall directly," the first resident says, speaking upward to the intercom.

"Got it," the intercom says.

"Are we on bypass?" the second resident asks. "I'm assuming we crashed and had to go back on bypass."

"That is correct," the surgeon says.

"ACT OK?"

The surgeon (providing the information a perfusionist would give), says "ACT 550."

"OK, good," the first resident says, "let's rest the heart and just give us a little time to straighten things out up here."

Untangling, straightening, and labeling lines takes them about 10 minutes. Once done, the lines look neat and orderly, with one line for drips (the carrier line) and one line for volume. Stopcocks are easily accessible and clearly marked.

A blood gas sits on the anesthesia machine—all is well in the land of metabolism and the "internal milieu."

"OK, now we're ready to come off bypass," the first resident says. "I see that the ventilator is on, and we are ventilating. Are both lungs coming up in the field?"

"Yes," the surgeon says.

"Let's give it a go then," the second resident says.

The intercom helps them jump to the next step, "You attempt to come off, your drips are maxed out, with high-dose epinephrine, a milrinone bolus, and norepinephrine. Blood gases are OK, but you are out of inotropic options."

"Let's get the intra-aortic balloon pump in here," the first resident says.

"You sure we need that?" the surgeon asks.

BOX 8-88	Chaos in the Lines?

- **Untangle, untangle**
- **Volume line**
- **Carrier line**

"Absolutely, the balloon is our friend, and right now we need a friend."

Over the intercom, "Open the first drawer of your anesthesia cart, you will see three drawings of an intra-aortic balloon tracing. Tell me what is right or wrong about each trace. Pretend you are helping the perfusionist to time the balloon correctly."

In the anesthesia cart, there are three traces: one with the balloon inflating early, before the dicrotic notch; one timed correctly, right at the dicrotic notch; and one timed late, well after the dicrotic notch.

The second resident explains, "I would not accept this early inflation pattern. This is inflating so early that the flow of blood out of the aorta would be impeded. Instead of helping the heart, you're hurting it.

"I would not accept this late inflation pattern. This is inflating too late to do you much good. It won't help you unload the heart—that's long gone by the time it inflates—and it doesn't help augment coronary perfusion—for most of diastole, the balloon isn't inflated and isn't helping.

"So, just like *Goldilocks and the Three Bears*," the resident holds up first the late one, then the early one, then the right one, "this one's toooooooo late, and this one's tooooooo early, and this one's juuuuuuuuust right, and so I'll eat it all up. Or at least I'll time the balloon pump with this pattern."

The surgeon speaks, "OK, heart looks good in here, the balloon is helping."

On the monitor, the blood pressure is holding steady at 100/60. (The Simulator monitor cannot recreate the double-humped arterial trace of an intra-aortic balloon pump.)

"Hang the protamine," the surgeon says.

"Protamine hanging," the first resident says. "We'll run it real slow." The residents have the "hunted" look as they glance at the monitors. Just by their look, they seem to be waiting for a protamine reaction to occur.

BP 100/60, dips to 90/55.

"Stopping protamine, going up on the epi," the second resident says. These players aren't taking any chances.

A nurse (Simulator Center secretary) comes in and hands them a blood gas.

"What?" the first resident says. On the blood gas, the hematocrit says 20. "The last 'crit before this was 29? We didn't give that much crystalloid, did we?"

"Any bleeding in the field?" the second resident asks. "Any trouble placing the balloon pump? We could have a retroperitoneal bleed if they stuck

through the back of the femoral artery. Can we get some blood in here?"

"Wait a second," the first resident says. "Let me see the name on that blood gas. It's Varga, Michael, right? Let me see the chart on this patient, what's his name?"

The surgeon clears it up, "This is Micha Vargo."

"Wrong blood gas sample, wrong patient, let's send another gas," the first resident says.

"Repeat 'crit is 28," the intercom announces.

"That's more like it."

"OK, done. Snacky time, go to the debriefing room."

Clinical lessons learned from scenario 49

Debriefing. Nachos with melted cheese and salsa sit on the debriefing table.

"This is living," the first resident says, grabbing a nacho and dipping it in hot sauce. "You simulator people know how to have a good time."

"Hey," the instructor says, "if you don't have fun, no one else is going to have fun *for* you."

"How did we do, professor?" the second resident asks.

"Not bad, you are way smarter than you look. Why don't you tell me what you were thinking as we roll the DVD."

The freaked out anesthesiologist bails out of the room.

"Well," the first resident says, "ideally, you get a bit more of a report than that when you take over a case. But, you know, caca happens. People freak out, or get sick, or pass out, or who knows what; and every now and then, you have to go into a room and just take over in a flash.

"So it's ABC, ABC, ABC. And in a heart case, there is the special consideration that if you're on bypass you want to make sure heparin was given and the ACT is adequate. You don't want to panic on bypass, forget the heparin, and clot off the patient's entire blood volume in the pump, do you? You lose big points when that happens."

"Then once you're sure that the ABCs are taken care of," the second resident picks up the thread, "then you convert chaos into order. Here, the person ahead of us left us a rat's nest of stuff, and who knew what was going where. That's bad in any case, but when you're in a heart case, with lots of hemodynamic troubles, then you *really* need to straighten things out. If you're trying to run in epinephrine, or norepinephrine, and your line is coiled up or kinked or the stopcock is turned the wrong way, then you are not delivering a life-saving drug. You hate to kill someone just because you are untidy with your intravenous lines."

"What about the balloon pump?" the instructor asks.

"You can only pound that stuff out of the heart so much with inotropes. At a certain point, you are just not getting any more out of that poor, flogged heart," the first resident says. "So you need to go with the balloon pump. Yes, the pump can damage the platelets, and yes, the balloon placement can damage the femoral artery, but still, the balloon is the heart's best friend in time of need. You just have to make sure you time it right."

"And you went over that pretty well. What was your big concern with protamine?"

"If you give protamine too fast, you can get the big hurt—pulmonary hypertension, systemic hypotension, pulmonary edema. All the bad things that can happen to your pressure can happen with protamine. So slow is the watchword, and if you suspect a reaction stop the protamine and increase your hemodynamic support."

"How did you catch the blood gas mistake?"

"The most important thing on any study is the *name* on the study, whether it's a chest X-ray or a blood gas or a D-stick," the second resident says. "And you have to go with your suspicion—here's someone who's not bleeding a lot, not getting a ton of crystalloid, and not acting hypovolemic. And this guy dropped his 'crit from 29 to 21 in a short period of time? I don't think so."

"What'd you think of the surgeon, 'You're killing my patient'?"

"Hey," the first resident says, "that's par for the course. We have to deal with that, pure and simple."

Summary. There is a human factor in anesthesia, and you may have to occasionally drop into a middle of a case and take over without knowing anything about the case at all. Anesthesia people have died during cases (!), passed out, freaked out, overdosed on drugs, and had psychotic breaks with reality. (One anesthesiologist turned off the oxygen and told the surgeon, "Bob Barker told me to turn off the oxygen.") So every once in a great while, you have to appear like the knight in shining armor and just save the day.

Like always, start with the ABCs, and pay attention to anything special going on—here, cardiopulmonary bypass. If the area looks disorganized and you can't work with it, take the time to get organized.

In any big case, narrow down to two lines—volume and drips.

Don't mix these two lines; if you do, you might give a whopping load of volume and push in a line of inotrope. Unpleasant surprise! Give volume through the volume line, give drips through the drip line. And make sure your drugs get into the patient! This simple dictum, when ignored, causes disaster. Epi dripping on the floor does the heart *no good whatsoever.*

Anyone working with potentially unstable adults needs to know about intra-aortic balloon pump function. By inflating during diastole the balloon increases (supposedly) coronary flow, and by its rapid deflation the balloon helps unload the heart—just the thing the failing heart needs. And you don't need to wait until your inotropic drip pumps are belching out black smoke before you put the balloon in. Better to put it in when you still have a little wiggle room, rather than wait 'til the patient is almost dead before finally tumbling to the idea of a balloon pump.

The balloon is your friend—remember that.

And while you're remembering that, remember to check all your lab work to make sure the right patient is on that slip of paper. Mr. *Jones'* numbers may be interesting, but correcting them will not help Mr. *Smith.*

SCENARIO 50. **A friend in need, helping diagnose and treat hypoxemia**

"Listen, docs, they are having a terrible time in OR 1 with a lung case. Do you think you can help them out?" a nurse (nursing student) asks.

"Sure," the first resident says.

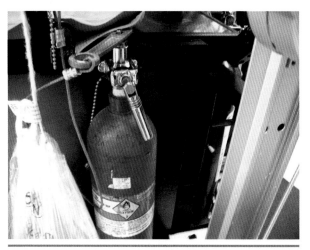

FIGURE 8–116 Check those cylinders every day. You never know when you may have to "go to cylinders" to make sure the patient gets adequate oxygen. There is a reason we check that machine!

"Why not?" the second resident says, "I didn't have anything better to do this afternoon."

In the operating room, an anesthesiologist (medical student) has a patient with a double-lumen endotracheal tube in. The saturation is 85%, and the anesthesiologist definitely has the look of "agita" in his eyes.

"I just can't get this sat up. Can you help me out?"

From across the screen, the surgeon (another medical student) adds her two cents, "Guys, have mercy on me, I can't do this case with the lung going up in my face all the time—please have mercy on me!"

The residents look over the chart—older man with lung CA, hypertension, smoking—a typical case for lung resection.

"God damn it, no kidding, can't you guys help me out," the surgeon is getting more and more exasperated.

"OK, let's take a little time out here, we're just going to delay you for a second while we inflate both lungs for a minute, get the saturation up, then we're going to start from ground zero," the first resident says. He takes the clamp off the left side of the DLT, goes to 100% oxygen (it had been on 50/50 oxygen/nitrous), and hand-ventilates. The oxygen saturation goes up to 100%.

Picking up the fiberoptic, the second resident says, "Let's take a look here and make sure we're in the right place."

In goes the fiberoptic, and the image is put up on a tower, so everyone can see.

"Is this a left-sided tube?" the first resident asks.

"Yes."

"And you put it in the left side?"

"Yes."

"Guess again," the first resident says. On close examination, the bronchial section of the endotracheal tube is going into the right mainstem.

"Oh," the original anesthesiologist says, "that would explain. . . ."

"That would explain why every time I asked you to drop the damned lung, you couldn't do it!" the surgeon yells.

The residents pull the double-lumen way back until it's in the trachea, then they slip the fiberoptic down the bronchial side, use the fiberoptic as a guide—kind of like a Seldinger technique for the lung—and place the double-lumen. Now they pull out, look down the tracheal lumen, and examine the tube.

"I don't see the blue balloon at all," the second resident says. "Pull back a little."

After pulling back, the blue balloon herniates over the carina, obscuring that important landmark.

"Nope, too far," the second resident says. After a short advancement, a crescent of blue is visible just after the carina. "Perfect!"

"Good, now the lung is down just right," the surgeon says.

But even on 100% oxygen, the saturation still dips down to 89%.

"We're going to have to put a little CPAP on this lung that's not getting ventilated," the first resident says.

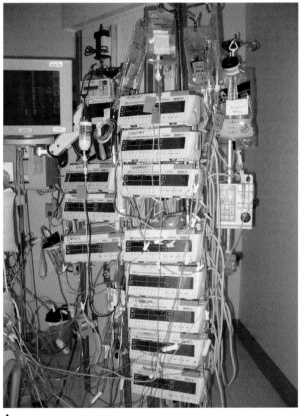

A

FIGURE 8–117 A. AAAG! All these drips, a million inotropes. What's our next option?

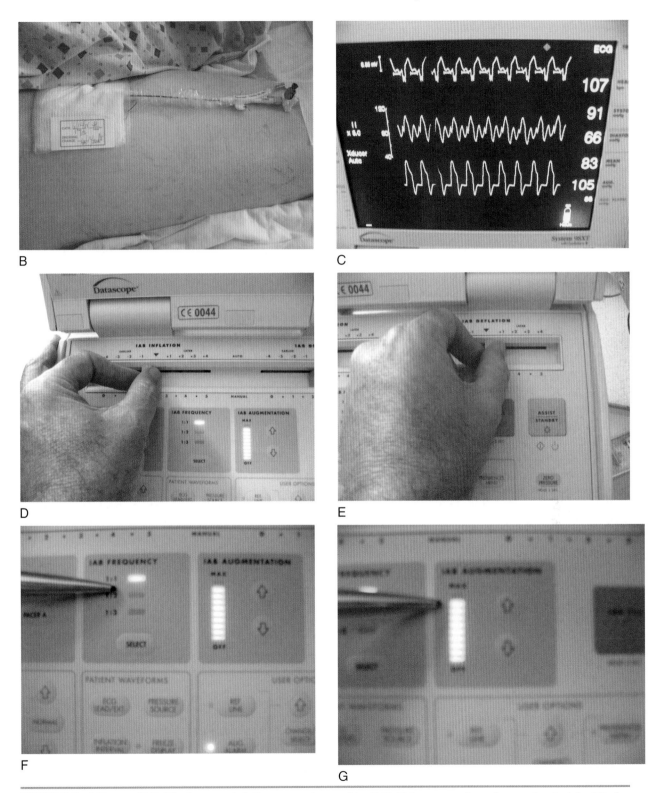

B

C

D

E

F

G

FIGURE 8–117 cont'd **B.** The intra-aortic balloon pump is your friend! **C.** Make sure you know how to time it right. Hit that inflation right in the dicrotic notch to give you the best benefit, both in terms of off-loading and in terms of diastolic augmentation of coronary blood flow. **D–G.** Work those dials. Unless you look at them and work them yourself, you'll never learn it. Remember Confucius' wise words: "I hear and I forget. I see and I remember. I do and I understand."

"How do you do that?" the original anesthesiologist asks.

The second anesthesia resident hooks up a device for delivering CPAP. It hooks up to the oxygen port (used for nasal cannula or mask) on the anesthesia machine.

"Set the flow at 5 L/min, then just adjust this dial," the second resident explains.

"One thing, though," the first resident explains, "you have to look in the field and see that the lung is actually a little bitty, bitty bit inflated. If the lung is just a totally crumpled-up, raisin-like lump, don't kid yourself—you aren't giving any CPAP at all. You're just giving CPAP to the trachea."

Over the intercom, "Any more options if this didn't work?"

The instructor pushes another ventilator into the room.

"Oh, I read about this," the first resident says.

"Where, in the *Enquirer*, where you read all your other stuff?" the second resident snickers.

"No," the first resident says, "in the "Green Hornet." You know—*Anesthesiology*. Somewhere. Here you go."

He hooks up the ventilator to the lung being operated on. Setting the tidal volumes very low—70 cc—PEEP at 0, F_{IO_2} at 1.0, and IMV of 20, the resident turns the ventilator on.

"Hey, the lung's moving here!" the surgeon yells.

"Very much?" the first resident asks.

"Well, no, I guess I can do this," the surgeon admits. "That's fine."

"Works like a charm!" the first resident says, in triumph.

The saturation climbs to 100%.

"Well, what do you know," the second resident says. "Even a blind hog gets an acorn every now and then."

"All done, you little hoggies," the instructor says over the intercom.

Clinical lessons learned from scenario 50

Debriefing. "Oink, oink," the first resident says.

A bag of M&M Chips Ahoy are in the center of the debriefing table.

"Mind if I make a little piggy of myself here?" the second resident asks. "You wouldn't happen to have any milk to wash down these cookies, would you? Not to be too demanding or anything."

Milk appears, and cups.

"Be sure and dip them in the milk first," the instructor says, then demonstrates. "It's mandatory."

All obey. As they pork out, the DVD plays.

"What's the thinking here, when you go into a room to help?" the instructor asks.

Between cookie bites, the first resident says, "Hey, what goes around, comes around. You want to always be there to lend a hand. One day that's you in the meat grinder, and it's good to have someone come around and help you."

"Fair enough," the instructor says. "Let's look at what you did in there."

"First, do whatever you have to do get the saturation up," the second resident says. "When the sat's in the low 80s, that's no time to be going through all your diagnostic gymnastics. Just inflate both lungs, tell the surgeon to take a chill-pill for a second, and get the sat up. Once that's up, you have a little breathing room."

Choking on his cookie, the first resident says, "I like that, breathing room. You're funny. Funny *looking*, that is."

The instructor takes a long breath, then wonders why God has seen fit to put him in a room with such comedic genius. "OK, sat's up, now what?"

"First thing, see if the tube's in the right place," the second resident says. "Here, as you saw, things were going haywire for a simple reason, the tube was completely backward! Every time you did a maneuver to get one side to go down, you were all turned around and making the other side go down. No wonder nothing was going right."

"Remaneuvering a tube once it's been in a while can be tough," the first resident says. "It's all soft, mushy, and flaccid, and may not. . . . No smart comments, you!"

"What?"

"I could read your filthy mind," the first resident continues. "Anyway, the tube is hard to position, so you're best off pulling way back, then using the fiberoptic down the bronchial lumen to guide the tube into place."

On the white board, the instructor lays out the maneuvers in diagrams.

"OK, last thing," the instructor says, "how about fixing the saturation?"

"CPAP to the nonventilated lung—that's the single best thing to do, all the books say," the second resident says. "The little maneuver with the extra ventilator is pretty slick too, though. I mean, you're doing pretty much the same thing—giving that lung a *little something* with which to oxygenate. You don't want that lung to be entirely shut. Pump a little oxygen in there, and let those alveoli help you. Not so much that

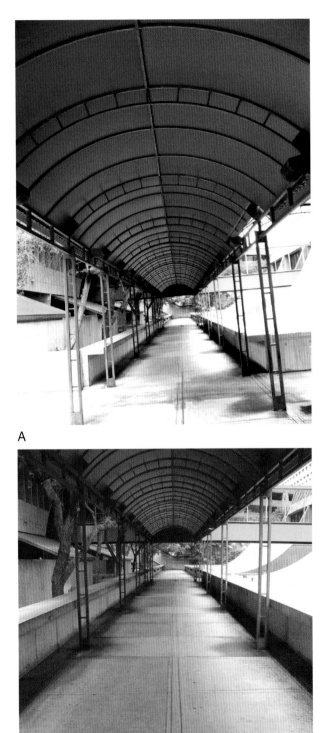

A

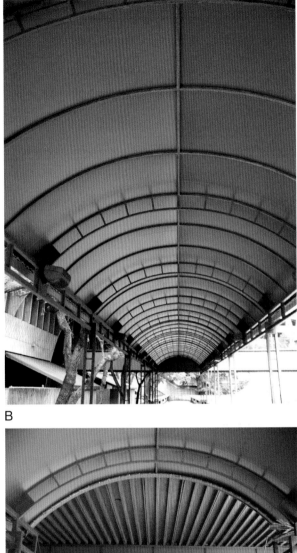

B

C

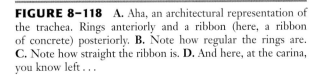

D

FIGURE 8–118 **A.** Aha, an architectural representation of the trachea. Rings anteriorly and a ribbon (here, a ribbon of concrete) posteriorly. **B.** Note how regular the rings are. **C.** Note how straight the ribbon is. **D.** And here, at the carina, you know left . . .

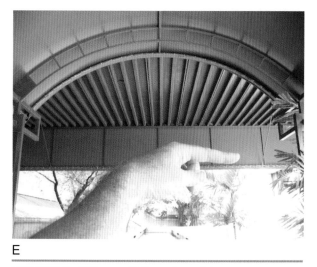

E

FIGURE 8–118 cont'd E. . . . from right.

it gets in the surgeon's face but enough to keep the patient going."

"That ventilator trick was a clinical case, presented in the September 2002 issue of *Anesthesiology*," the instructor says, producing the article for each resident. "Now we live in the era of 'evidence-based medicine.' Any hesitation in applying a technique that's just a 'clinical case' versus waiting for there to be a double-blind placebo controlled multicenter study proving that this technique works?"

The residents mull that one over for a bit. Their mulling does not slow down their pigging out on the cookies, however.

"Tell you the truth," the first resident says. "I kind of hate to admit this, but some of the best tricks I've learned come from those clinical case reports."

"Think about it," the second resident says, "that thing with the extra ventilator makes sense. It's just a little tiny leap in technique from what we normally do. I think it's fair enough to employ a new technique in such a case. Face it, no one's going to do a big study on this. If they do, great, but until then we'll keep scouring the clinical case reports for valuable tips."

"One good anecdote outdoes a dozen obscure and unintelligible studies?" the instructor asks.

"Something like that."

Summary. Double-lumen endotracheal tube cases are like little kids—when they are good, they are very, very good. But when they are bad, they are terrible. But

isolate the lung we must, so you had better know your way around a double-lumen tube.

Of note, the debate about "Univent versus double-lumen tube" is a long and bitter one, with strong opinions on either side. You're best off being comfortable with both.

When things are not going smoothly, first stabilize the patient and then look with a fiberoptic. Relying on auscultation alone is notoriously inaccurate; plus, once the case has started and the patient is on his/her side, it's hard to get your stethoscope in the right place.

Find the carina, by all means find the carina—that is the key. Then position that bronchial balloon so you can just see the rim of it. Not too deep—that may put you past the upper lobe take-off—and not too shallow—that may get you herniating the cuff over the carina and you won't get good lung isolation.

Desaturation under one-lung anesthesia is nerve-wracking. The surgeon will always tell you "this is the worst possible time" for the lung to come up. (It's *always* the worst possible time for them.) CPAP on the lung is your best bet. If you can stand the clutter of a whole other ventilator in your room (what a pain), you can give frequent small breaths to the "nonventilated-but-now-a-little-ventilated lung too."

CONCLUSION OF THE SCENARIOS

This brief foray into scenario-land does not, by any stretch, cover "everything that can happen in anesthesia." And with a little imagination and amateur theatrics, a Simulator instructor could cobble together a host of other clinical "morality plays."

Pheochromocytoma
Dealing with a celebrity who demands special treatment
Handling a SARS case
Bigger mass casualty drills
Airway scenes with different equipment, such as a Light Wand or Bullock scope

The list could go on and on. And the list *should* go on and on. In simulation centers across the nation and across the world, instructors should keep making up a 101, 1001 scenarios, all for the express purpose of teaching their students.

Are scenarios limited?

So long as Simulator teachers have imagination and creativity, the answer to that is "No."

CHAPTER

Bibliography

> *"Order and simplification are the first steps toward the mastery of a subject."*
> —Thomas Mann: *The Magic Mountain* (1924), Chapter 1

So there's a bazillion articles on Simulators, and each article has a bibliography as long as your arm. Where do you start? What do they all mean? Do you pound through each and every one and accrete knowledge like a tree adds growth rings? Is there any theme to them other than, "Simulators are really cool, grab your phone, a credit card, and order before midnight tonight and we'll send you a free Thighmaster"? Is there a way out of this chaos? Yes.

Since 1969 there have been well over 1000 articles published on simulation. The BEME collaboration* (we'll come back to that later) took more than 3 years to identify, collect, read, and evaluate all of these articles. Do not worry—we'll help you through this.

We begin this chapter with a brief description of our general search strategy for articles so you have an idea about how we found all of them. Next we briefly review the current areas of simulation research. Although this chapter focuses on the use of simulators for education, training, and assessment, we provide references for the other areas in case you are interested. The heart of this chapter contains an annotated bibliography separated into interesting themes.

OUR LITERATURE SEARCH

We wanted to provide you with the mother of all simulation bibliographies. So we began the search with references from 1969 when the seminal article about simulation in medical education was published by Abrahamson and then proceed all the way to June 2005. We searched five literature databases (ERIC, MEDLINE, PsychINFO, Web of Science, and Timelit) and employed a total of 91 single search terms and concepts and their Boolean combinations (Table 9–1). Because we know that electronic databases are not perfect and often miss important references, we also manually searched key publications that focused on medical education or were known to contain articles on the use of simulation in medical education. These journals included *Academic Medicine, Medical Education, Medical Teacher, Teaching and Learning in Medicine, Surgical Endoscopy, Anesthesia and Analgesia*, and *Anesthesiology*.

In addition, we also manually searched the annual *Proceedings* of the *Medicine Meets Virtual Reality Conference*, the annual meeting of the Society for Technology in Anesthesia, now the International Meeting on Simulation in Healthcare and the biannual *Ottawa Conference on Medical Education and Assessment*. These *Proceedings* include "gray literature" (e.g., papers presented at professional meetings, doctoral dissertations) that we thought contained the most relevant references related to our review.

---

*Issenberg SB, McGaghie WC, Petrusa ER, Gordon DL and Scalese RJ. Features and uses of high-fidelity medical simulations that lead to effective learning: a BEME systematic review. Medical Teacher 2005;27(1):10–28.

Table 9-1   Search Terms and Phrases.

1. Simulator	47. Curriculum
2. Simulation	48. Community
3. Mannikin	49. Core
4. Human model	50. Optional
5. Virtual reality	51. Elective
6. Full body	52. Integrated
7. Three-dimensional	53. Outcome-based
8. Internal medicine	54. Problem-based
9. Pediatric	55. Multiprofessional
10. Surgery	56. Learning
11. Orthopedic	57. Independent
12. Cardiovascular	58. Large group
13. Endoscopic	59. Lecture
14. Laparoscopic	60. Small group
15. Arthroscopic	61. Instructor
16. Sinus	62. Computer-based
17. Anesthesia	63. Clinical
18. Critical care	64. Peer
19. Emergency	65. Classroom
20. Trauma	66. Hospital
21. Dental	67. Ambulatory
22. Nursing	68. Laboratory
23. Endovascular	69. Clinical skills center
24. Colonoscopy	70. Distance learning
25. Sigmoidoscopy	71. Assessment
26. Intravenous	72. Testing
27. Arterial	73. Evaluation
28. Gastroenterology	74. Grade
29. Multimedia	75. Certification
30. Minimally invasive	76. Validity
31. Suture	77. Reliability
32. Diagnostic	78. Feasibility
33. Ultrasound	79. Skills
34. Forced feedback	80. Procedures
35. Tactile	81. Management
36. Haptic	82. Health promotion
37. Undergraduate	83. Communication
38. Medical school	84. Information
39. Medical student	85. Attitudes
40. Graduate	86. Behavior
41. Resident	87. Decision making
42. Continuing education	88. Patient safety
43. Professional	89. Medical errors
44. Practitioner	90. Team
45. Education	91. Development
46. Training	

We also performed several basic Internet searches using the Google search engine—an invaluable resource to locate those articles you cannot find anywhere else (it reviews every CV on the web—so you are bound to find even the most obscure reference). Our aim in doing all this was to perform the most thorough literature search possible of peer-reviewed publications and reports in the unpublished "gray literature" that have been judged at some level for academic quality.

All of the 91 search terms could not be used within each of the five databases because the databases do not have a consistent vocabulary. Although each database also has unique coverage and emphasis, we did attempt to use similar text word or keyword/phrase combinations in the searches. Thus the essential pattern was the same for each search, but adjustments were made for databases that enabled controlled vocabulary searching in addition to text word or keyword/phrase searching. This approach acknowledges the role of "art" in information science, recognizing that information retrieval requires professional judgment coupled with high-technology informatics—and a whole lot of extra time on your hands. [Ojala M. Information professionals as technologists. Online 2002;26(4)5.]

GENERAL AREAS OF SIMULATION RESEARCH

For the past 36 years, the primary focus of medical simulation research has been to justify its use as a training and assessment method. Nearly all of the articles begin with the obvious comparison of medicine to aviation and clinicians to pilots. Then they spend the rest of the time in a defensive tone justifying simulation as a valid training to the point that you think simulators are the ugly stepsister of books, lectures, small group discussions, and patient rounds. We believe it is time to stop all of this defensive research and start moving forward—let's end the meaningless studies comparing simulators to other unproven methods and begin determining the most effective ways to use simulation for training and assessment. We have an important responsibility, as the current generation of trainers who have seen simulation develop and become integrated with traditional training (we are in a sense *simulation immigrants*). We need to start planning on training the next generations of clinicians who have grown up with simulation (*simulation natives*) and not worry about previous generations of clinicians (*simulation Luddites*) who have looked at simulation as some threat to their unproven, outdated, and *unsafe* "see one, do one, teach one" philosophy. Let us heed the words of Eric Hoffer: "In a time of drastic change, it is the learners who inherit the future. The learned usually find themselves equipped to live in a world that no longer exists."

Simulators for Training and Assessment

How do you categorize the studies? How do you evaluate the effectiveness of the simulation as a training and/or assessment tool? We are in luck. Donald Kirkpatrick devised a very useful system to evaluate the effectiveness of training programs—that has since been modified for direct application to simulation: Donald Kirkpatrick described four levels for evaluating training programs. (Kirkpatrick DI. *Evaluating Training Programs: The Four Levels*, 2nd ed. San Francisco: Berrett-Koehler; 1998). Although originally designed for training settings in varied corporate environments, the concept later extended to health care education. Kirkpatrick's framework for evaluation as adapted for health care education includes all four of these levels. (Freeth D, Hammick M, Koppel I, Reeves S, Barr H. A critical review of evaluations of interprofessional education. http://www.health.ltsn.ac.uk/publications/occasionalpaper02.pdf. Accessed March 10, 2006. Centre for the Advancement of Interprofessional Education, London, 2002.)

> *Level 1: Learners' participation.* This covers learners' views on the learning experience, its organization, presentation, content, teaching methods, and aspects of the instructional organization, materials, quality of instruction.
>
> *Level 2a: Modification of attitudes/perceptions.* Outcomes at this level relate to changes in the reciprocal attitudes or perceptions between participant groups toward the educational intervention.
>
> *Level 2b: Modification of knowledge/skills.* For knowledge this relates to the acquisition of concepts, procedures, and principles; for skills it relates to the acquisition of thinking/problem-solving, psychomotor, and social skills.
>
> *Level 3: Change in behavior.* This documents the transfer of learning to the workplace or willingness of learners to apply new knowledge and skills.
>
> *Level 4a: Change in organizational practice.* This level considers wider changes in the organizational delivery of care attributable to an educational program.
>
> *Level 4b: Benefits to patients.* This level documents any improvement in the health and well-being of patients as a direct result of an educational program.

The higher the level, the greater the impact of simulation's effectiveness on training.

Unfortunately, there are *no* studies at the "Benefits to patients" level, very few at the "change in organization practice"—an example would be the FDA's decision to grant approval for the use of carotid stents only to clinicians who are trained on a Simulator. We demonstrate that there are far more studies in each lower category.

Now that we have everything organized, we will provide a more friendly approach to read the literature by grouping articles into themes and even linking some of these to the Kirkpatrick criteria. Truth to tell, those Kirkpatrick criteria are a little tough to wade through. You feel yourself falling into "education PhD—speak", and not so much "regular old doctor teaching another doctor—speak."

Simulator articles fall into five main "themes."

1. It stands to reason
2. The canary in the mineshaft
3. Gee whiz, golly, I belong too!
4. Halfway to the station
5. Salvation

1. *It stands to reason*: Logic dictates that a Simulator makes sense. You wouldn't want someone flying a plane without flying a "pretend" plane first. You wouldn't want someone manipulating nuclear reactors without practicing first. So, darn it, it just seems inescapable that a Simulator is the way to go in anesthesia too.

Articles from aviation and industry fit into the "it stands to reason" column. Educational theory gives us some "it stands to reason" arguments as well. Teach with a "death-proof" patient—how can you say no to that? Teach with a patient who can "do what you want" at the stroke of a key. Teach in a setting where the learner has to act, to speak, to interact. Teach where the student has an emotional investment. They'll learn better. It just plain "stands to reason."

What would an "anti-Simulator" person say to these "it stands to reason" articles? "Nice. I'm glad a Simulator seems like a good idea. Lots of things seem like good ideas. Has anyone *proven* it's a good idea, or are we to go on a hunch? A hunch with, lest we forget, a half million dollar price tag?"

Articles related to this theme would fall into the Level 1 category—how the learners felt about participating in the simulation experiences—"This was the best learning experience in my career—it sure beats listening to the program director talk about this stuff" and the Level 2a category—did the experience change how they felt about the importance and relevance of the intervention—"I now realize how many things can go wrong and how aware I have to be at all times to prevents mishaps." These are also editorial discussions and descriptive articles about the use of simulators for training and testing and comparing medicine to other high-risk industries—aviation, military.

2. *The canary in the mineshaft*: Miners used canaries to detect poisonous gases. The bird keeled over before the miner did, serving as an "early warning system." Some articles show the Simulator as a "canary in the mineshaft." That was not the *goal* of the articles, but that's what comes through loud and clear.

> "No one in the experiment knew how to treat anaphylaxis."
> "Students routinely fouled up the ACLS protocol."
> "Only a small portion knew how to manage a severe head injury."

Hey, educators! Wake up! *We're not teaching right if our students and residents don't know this stuff!* If no one is recognizing and treating anaphylaxis, then, by God, the Simulator is telling us something. The Simulator is telling us to *teach anaphylaxis better*.

If students are fouling up the ACLS protocol, we should get off our lard butts and *teach that ACLS protocol better*.

If only a small portion know how to manage severe head injury, should we just say—"Oh, no one knows how to manage a severe head injury. What an amusing observation." *No*! Wake up and smell the methane. The Simulator is telling us *something is wrong about how we teach*.

Absent the Simulator, we might *never have known* about these deficiencies. The Simulator acted as the educational equivalent of a canary in the mineshaft, warning us of danger.

3. *Gee whiz, golly, I belong too*! Socrates sat in the marketplace and talked to his students. Attendings sit in the lounge and talk to their residents. The oral tradition in education has a long track record, and no one feels compelled to defend it. Not so the new kid on the block. Computer-run simulators started in the 1960s and, like any "new guy," had to prove themselves. Article after article on simulators say, "Look at our grading methods, they're valid. Look at our reproducibility, see? We're the real thing, honest!" In a way, it's odd. Does any other teaching method go to such great lengths to prove itself?

> Grand Rounds—a test of validity.
> Lectures—a double-blind study of whether they do any good.
> Talking to your resident during the case—gimmick or genuine teaching?

But Grand Rounds, lectures, and plain old talking go way back. They're the air we breathe in academe.

They're a given. Not so and not yet with Simulators. One day maybe. Not yet. So the articles keep rolling out, defending the method, justifying the cost. Don't lock me out. I deserve to be a player in this game. I belong.

4. *Halfway to the station*: Some articles show the Simulator is a great "intermediate teacher."

> Residents did ACLS *on the Simulator*.
> Later, we tested them *on the Simulator*.
> They showed a definite improvement *on the Simulator*.

We presented a head injury patient *in a simulated setting*. We taught this. We taught that. Then we ran another head injury patient *in a simulated setting*. Look at our groovy statistics. By gum, there is a batch of numbers that incontrovertibly proves to any skeptic anywhere that our students did better *in a simulated setting*. So in this fishbowl world of latex, computers, videotapes, and Simulato-faculty, we showed improvement.

Articles related to this theme would fall into the Level 2b category—a measured change in what you know (residents' understanding of crisis resource management principles) and how you do things (residents' ability to apply crisis resource management).

5. *Salvation*: These are the articles that matter, the Holy Grail of Simulator literature. Yes, it's great that there are "it stands to reason" articles. A solid logical base for simulators is comforting. "Canary in the mineshaft" articles help too. We are all looking for better ways to teach. Intellectual honesty demands that we probe for our own weaknesses and failings. If the Simulator can tell me where to shore up my teaching, then thank you Mr. Simulator. "Gee whiz, golly, I belong too" articles merit a place at the table. Simulators are new, they are expensive. We *should ask the hard questions* of so pricey a technology. When scholarly detractors speak up, we should listen. These are not Luddites, throwing their wooden shoes in the looms. These are serious educators who want proof that simulators help. Detractors focus on simulator research. If simulator champions take an "us versus them" approach, the simulator debate sinks into a squabble. If simulator champions take a "let's hear them out" approach, the simulator debate elevates into a living, breathing academic discussion. "Halfway to the station" articles serve as necessary stepping stones. We have to examine simulators in the "in vitro" setting. Lab proof precedes clinical proof, and the simulator is a "lab" of sorts. But "Salvation" articles are the real deal. Pure gold. Precious. Salvation articles show that simulators made a difference in the real

world. Because *someone* trained in the Simulator, someone *else* did better.

A patient didn't have an MI.
A patient didn't have a stroke.
Someone lived, who would have died. And the Simulator made it happen.

How could you ever design a study to prove that?

That explains why "Salvation" articles don't fall out of the sky every day. Truth to tell, that explains why there are no *real* salvation articles. The closest we can come is articles that *suggest* salvation. And they are rare but rare. But oh man do they carry some heft.

Articles related to this theme would fall into the Level 3a category—did resident's actually change their habits after taking a course, and in Level 3b—have any groups changed what they are doing. Finally Level 4—does all this really mean anything important—are patients safer?

So there they are the major themes of simulator articles. Of course, these articles don't neatly plop into their pigeonholes. An article's main idea may be "gee whiz golly, I belong too," but you extract a "canary in the mineshaft" idea. So, this classification system is a little arbitrary and whimsical. But what the heck.

Articles Touching on the Theme "It Stands to Reason"

The articles included in this section say "it stands to reason" that simulators are good things. You read them and you just can't help but blurt it out. "It stands to reason" that a simulator is a good way to teach because you can't hurt a patient while practicing on it. "It stands to reason" that reproducible scenarios that you can "dial in" anytime you want is a good way to train medical professionals.

Then here are the gigantic "leaps of faith" implied by these articles: it stands to reason that it's a better way—pay tons of money to buy one; it stands to reason that it's a better way—pay tons of money and devote hundreds of staff-hours to support one.

In a world of infinite resources and infinite money, we wouldn't even *bring up* these leaps of faith. But that is not the world we live in. So as you read these articles, ask yourself, "OK, so it stands to reason that simulators are good, but just how good, given the cost and time necessary to keep them afloat."

✓ Good ML. Patient simulators for training basic and advanced clinical skills. Med Educ 2003;37(Suppl 1):14–21.
✓ Good ML, Gravenstein JS. Anesthesia simulators and training devices. Int Anesthesiol Clin 1989;27:161–6.

✓ Good ML, Gravenstein JS. Training for safety in an anesthesia simulator. Semin Anesth 1993;12:235–50.

If simulators make so much sense, why is their use so recent? Haven't humans been participating in risky behavior (either to themselves or others) before the Wright Brothers proved powered air flight was possible?

The answer is yes—of course it is. It stands to reason that previous generations of humans must have wanted to practice their skills or to practice protecting themselves. "Historically, whenever the real thing was too expensive, too dangerous, too bulky, too unmanageable, or too unavailable, a *stand-in* was sought."

In a comprehensive review of anesthesia simulators as they were available during the late 1980s and early 1990s, Good and Gravenstein (the original developers of the METI Human Patient Simulator at the University of Florida) provide an example of simulators from antiquity.

The field—warfare. The simulator—a quintain. What's a quintain? A quintain originated from tree stumps upon which soldiers would practice their sword fighting. These were fitted with shields and features to resemble adversaries. By the Middle Ages, quintains were mounted on poles to simulate a joust. It also contained feedback. If the novice failed to attack his "enemy" correctly, a weighted arm on the pole would swing around and smack him on his back. Sometimes, we wish we could do this with some of our students and residents. But alas, we live in a kinder, gentler time.

Good and Gravenstein then cite Andrews, who differentiated between simulators and training devices. Simulator . . . attempts to. . . . [r]epresent the exact or near exact phenomena likely to occur in the real world; are good for *trainee and expert practice* but are *not* necessarily good for *systematic learning* of new skills and knowledge.

Training device . . . systematically presents to the trainee *only the necessary* training stimuli, feedback, reinforcement, remediation, and practice opportunities appropriate to the trainee's learning level and style. It uses fidelity only as necessary to enhance the learning process. These are commonly referred to as task trainers.

Just as in aviation, there is a right blend for simulators and training devices. Much like tackling dummies and practice scrimmages in football, or a punching bag and sparring partner in boxing.

The remainder of the article reviews the educational applications of anesthesia simulators and training devices. The following examples of training devices (task trainers) are listed here along with the original citations for further reading:

Training Devices (Task Trainers)

Lung Model
✓ LOUGHLIN PJ, BOWES WA, WESTENSKOW DR. An oil-base model of inhalation anesthetic uptake and elimination. Anesthesiology 1989;71:278–82.

Gas Man
✓ PHILLIP JH. Gas Man: an example of goal oriented computer-assisted teaching which results in learning. Int J Clin Monit Comput 1986;3:165–73.
✓ TORDA TA. Gas Man. Amaesth Intensive Care 1985;13:111.

Anesthesia Physiologic Model
✓ SMITH NT. Clinical problems and uptake and distribution models. Presented at the Anesthesia Simulator Curriculum Conference, US FDA and Anesthesia Patient Safety Foundation, Rockville MD, September 1989.

Anesthesia Simulator Recorder
✓ SCHWID HA. A flight simulator for general anesthesia training. Comput Biomed Res 1987;2064–75.

Simulators

SIM ONE
See below.

CASE
See below.

GAS
✓ BUCK GH. Development of simulators in medical education. Gesnerus 1991;48:7–28.
✓ GOOD ML, LAMPOTANG S, GIBBY GI, GRAVENSTEIN JS. Critical events simulation for training in anesthesiology. J Clin Monit Comput 1988;4:140.

While there is evidence of using simulators for military training in ancient Rome, their use in medicine did not occur until the mid-sixteenth century. Although it can be argued that Italian physicians such as Mondino de'Luzzi (1275–1326) used "simulators" when he employed cadavers to complement lectures, the idea to use simulation methods to demonstrate rare conditions or a difficult procedure did not occur until the 1540s.

Why then? At the time, many institutions starting to become concerned regarding the safety of women during childbirth. Although physicians (all men) had the knowledge to deliver babies, it was considered a social taboo for a man to perform a task that was the responsibility of the midwives. However, midwives had no formal training and were graduates of the famous "see one, do one, teach one" university. Initial

attempts at formal instruction consisted of lectures with illustrations. This did not affect the infant and mother mortality rates; and more than 100 years later, a father and son physician team from France did something about it—they developed an obstetric simulator.

The Gregoires' Simulator—it was crude by today's standards—human skeletal pelvis contained in a wire basket with oil skin to simulate the genitalia and coarse cloth to simulate the reaming skill. "Real fetuses, likely preserved by some means, were used in conjunction with the manikin." The simulator could reproduce the birth of a child and some complications that would require a trained person to fix.

And yes—there were complaints regarding its validity and transfer to real patients, but for the first time someone said, "it stands to reason we can do a better job and not allow these poor women and children to die."

Over the next two centuries, there were additional obstetric simulators developed in England and the United States—and they appeared to have enjoyed support from lay people and some other physicians. However, some very familiar factors limited their widespread adoption.

- Cost
- Resistance to adopt new methods of instruction
- Skepticism that what was learned from a Simulator could not be transferred to actual practice

You think after 400 years we would have adequately addressed these issues! Even when the majority of students in the late nineteenth century graduated medical school (there was no such thing as residency) without any direct experience with childbirth, available simulators were not adopted, even though "the use of the simulator would provide medical students with at least some experience with birthing techniques and with some of the related complications." But *no*—we would have to wait 80 years before another attempt at simulation for training.

✓ Denson JS, Abrahamson S. A computer-controlled patient simulator. JAMA 1969;208:504–8. [Simulator: SIM-One]

Do not be fooled by the title, the journal, or the year—this article showed the potential of simulators 20 years before the rest of the world would again approach the subject in anesthesia. This simulator was developed under the guidance of Denson, an anesthesiologist, and Abrahamson, a medical educator, both at the University of Southern California; and it was manufactured by Sierra Engineering Company.

Here's what this simulator could do.

- Life-size—6 feet tall, 195 lb on an operating table
- Able to "breath" in normal manner, with carotid and temporal pulses
- Normal blood pressure taken by auscultation
- Eyelid could blink, eyes could dilate and constrict
- Could respond physiologically to four drugs and two gases
- A computer controlled several conditions
  - ○ Cardiac dysrhythmias, "bucking" during intubation
  - ○ Changing blood pressure, pulses, respiratory rate, jaw tension, vomiting
  - ○ Laryngospasm and obstruction of a mainstem bronchus

So what was the purpose of this Simulator, built before Neil Armstrong took his famous walk?

- "a student could learn necessary manual skills before his first examination of a patient"
- "could learn skills in a planned, systematic way"
- "could learn skills in hours or days rather than in months"
- "more time to study of the patients' problems and diseases"
- "saving in instructor time and mental anxiety reduced"
- "greatly reduced *hazard or discomfort* for many patients"

So we had a Simulator that could do many of the things modern simulators can do, and Denson and Abrahamson had identified all of the potential benefits for simulators that we are talking about now! They performed one formal study involving 10 anesthesia residents for endotracheal intubation (the study is described later, in the Halfway to the Station section).

Over the years, Denson and Abrahamsom went on to train many more health care providers, including medical students, interns, inhalation therapists, nurses, nursing students, and ward attendants. In addition to intubation, they trained in ventilator application, induction of anesthesia, intramuscular injection, recovery room care and pulse and respiration measurement (HOFFMAN KI, ABRAHAMSON S. The "cost-effectiveness" of Sim One. J Med Educ 1975;50:1127–8).

Although additional simulators were planned, funding dried up and the culture was not ready for this type of training—the old guard was skeptical of technology, and there was no appreciation of the need to reduce medical errors and improve patient safety,

although Denson and Abrahamson clearly made a case for it. In the words of Abrahamson, the factors that led to Sim-One's demise was "internal administrative problems," which means a lack of university support. As a result "the funding agencies were no longer interested" and there was growing "low esteem the academic world was developing for education." Ouch! (ABRAHAMSON S. Sim One: a patient simulator ahead of its time. Caduceus 1997;13(2):29–41).

What is the legacy of Sim One? As Abrahamson states, "the effectiveness of simulation depends on the instructional method with which the simulation is being compared . . . if there is no alternative training method available (limited patient availability or restrictions on the use of patients), the effectiveness of a simulation device probably depends on the *simple fact that the device provides some kind of learning experience as opposed to none.*" Thus, Abrahamson was saying 30 years ago that it stands to reason we should be using these devices if nothing else exists or if traditional training is too dangerous.

What did they think about this Simulator at the time?

"From an anesthesiologist's point of view, SIM 1 might represent man's most impressive attempt, thus far, to manufacture himself from something other than sperm and ovum."

"The appropriateness of the anesthetist's response to each stress is automatically recorded for his later *bemusement* and education."

"The next phase, Sim II, would appear to be an automated trainer to eliminate the need for a flesh-and-blood instructor, and the obvious finale is to simulate the learner as well."

This is not a community-based practitioner reminiscing about the good-old-days of ether and a biting stick; this was the official response of the Association of University Anesthesiologists! [HORNBEIN TF. Reports of scientific meetings. Anesthesiology 1968;29:1071–7.]

We would have to wait until the late 1980s to pick up from where these pioneers left off.

✓ GABA DM, DEANDA A. A comprehensive anaesthesia simulation environment: re-creating the operating room for research and training. Anaesthesiology 1988;69:387–94.

This article describes the rediscovery of full-body simulators for anesthesia training and introduced Gaba as a player in the wild, wooly world of simulation. You will see his name again and again in this bibliography. Based out of Stanford, home of lots of smart people, it comes as no surprise that Gaba, too, is smart and on a mission to see simulators reach their potential.

Way back in 1988, Gaba laid out how to do a simulation, and he made clear the argument that it just plain "stands to reason" that simulation is a good way to train. He described their setup and how they went through simulations. He argues that a "total simulation" requires the complete capabilities for noninvasive and invasive monitoring. Also, other tasks are performed using standard operating room equipment so the scenario recreates the anesthesiologist's physical as well as mental task environment.

Gaba and DeAnda described a script, actors in the field, "on the fly" decisions by the simulator director, a high-fidelity mannequin—basically all the stuff we do now in the Simulator. He ran 21 people through the Simulator and they all judged the experience as highly realistic. This article did not actually do any kind of study, it just laid out how simulations are done and how much the participants liked it. Finally, Gaba proposed that simulation has "major potential for research, training, evaluation, and certification." Amen to that, Dr. Gaba.

✓ Schwid HA, O'Donnell D. The anesthesia simulator-recorder: a device to train and evaluate anesthesiolgists' responses to critical incidents. Anesthesiology 1990;72:191–7.

Dr. Schwid has shown us that simulators come in all shapes, sizes, types, costs, range of feasibility. This multicenter study evaluated the acceptance of a computer-based anesthesia simulator that uses sophisticated mathematical models to respond to user-controlled interventions, including airway management, ventilation control, and fluid and drug administration (53 different agents).

The Simulator also provided detailed feedback that tracked all of the user's and Simulator's responses—this could be used for formative feedback during training or summative evaluation to determine if the learner has mastered the key critical events. The Simulator was evaluated by 44 residents and attendings at seven institutions. Feedback was very positive, as nearly all participants found the patient's responses to management interventions as realistic and determined it was a good device to test anesthesiologists' responses to critical events. A significant and important finding was that there were no differences in response among any of the institutions—demonstrating the practical transferability of this training device.

It is always tempting to compare this Simulator with the full-body, comprehensive simulator environment developed by Gaba and Good and Gravensein. To do so misses the point! A comprehensive training environment is as much dependent on the faculty facilitator, the debriefing feedback sessions, and the involvement of the "team" as it is on the Simulator.

Schwid's computer-based Simulator and others similar to it have several advantages.

- Greater accessibility to users at any time and place.
- Does not require additional human resources to use (the instructional design and feedback take the place of having an on-site facilitator).
- Allows greater numbers to be trained in fundamental problems-solving skills in a greater number of cases that just is not feasible or possible with a human patient Simulator—numerous studies have demonstrated that problem-solving skills are disease-specific, meaning that a learner's ability to treat hypotension due to tension pneumothorax does not translate into the ability to treat hypotension as a result of an acute myocardial infarction—up to 20 cases per condition may be needed here, which is possible only with computer-based models.

Finally, the two following extreme cases illustrate the use of these devices.

- A resident who consistently fails to treat "patients" correctly on a computer-based Simulator is very likely to have significant problems in the real environment.
- There are always some trainees who perform well on computer simulation but panic or are ineffective in the realistic setting. At least, you know the learner's failure is not the result of a cognitive deficiency—this enables the instructor to focus on communication or team leadership skills.

Anesthesia has consistently looked to aviation as its "model" for training. Well, aviation manufacturers, including Boeing and Airbus, are now "equipping" pilots with computer-based simulators to master prior to attending the full-scale simulator. Rather than compare one simulator type with another, we should focus on the *most effective* methods in the best mix for training.

✓ Gaba DM. Improving anesthesiologists' performance by simulating reality [editorial]. Anesthesiology 1992;76:491–4.

Gaba starts out by discussing a screen-based Simulator study by Schwid. Schwid discovered that residents made errors.

- Missed esophageal intubations.
- Fouled up ACLS protocols.
- Couldn't manage myocardial ischemia, anaphylaxis, or cardiac arrest.

Although Gaba never draws the analogy between the simulation and the aforementioned canaries in the mineshaft, we can see how they fulfill this crucial function. If deadly methane gas had seeped out of the coal deposits, the canaries would suffer a severe case of death, alerting miners to the danger. Maybe simulators should be our "canaries." Instead of waiting for a methane explosion in the mine (a patient catastrophe in the operating room), we should see how the canary's doing (run residents through the Simulator and uncover their weaknesses).

Usually, we analyze cases *retrospectively*, *after* disaster has befallen. This analysis is clouded by incomplete records, failed memories, and, who knows, perhaps a little defensiveness? "I have no idea what went wrong!" So, looking at stuff *after* the fact isn't too good.

We could videotape cases *as* they occur and, in effect, see disasters *during* the fact. Only problem with that is that most of the time nothing happens. We'd be looking at millions of hours of people sitting on a chair. It would be like watching the medical equivalent of C-SPAN. We might save a few patients that way, but we'll kill scores of people with boredom. So, looking at stuff *during* the fact is no good.

How about looking at stuff *before* the fact? Time travel. *Back to the Future* instead of C-SPAN. Only the Simulator can provide that kind of time travel. "It stands to reason" that the Simulator is a good idea. You don't have to wait until a patient is hurt (the retrospective way); you don't have to wade through miles of stultifying tape (the real-time way); you can "create the problems" without patient harm. You do it ahead of time (the prospective way).

Gaba also reviewed the limits of Simulators, including that, despite their sophistication, they can never create a patient with all of the inherent variables seen in clinical medicine—but so long as they are "reasonable" representations of real patients they could be considered valid by experienced anesthesiologists.

Another limitation is that the trainee is never convinced the simulation is 100% real—leading to hypervigilance in which the poor resident is always worried that something bad is going to happen. This would be okay, except that many errors may result, in reality, from the very boredom and fatigue that occur in real practice. At the other end of the spectrum are the smart alecks who believe that they can do whatever they want because no real patient is at risk.

However, this is true in other industries, and they have made successful use of simulation. In medicine, the validation of simulation will be even more difficult than aviation because no two patients are alike (unlike a 747); the effects of training should be measured over years of training and remediation not after a single training session. Gaba summarized his editorial by making the important point: "No industry in which human lives depend in the skilled performance of responsible operators has waited for unequivocal proof of the benefits of simulation before embracing it." I say we embrace it too.

✓ GABA DM. The future vision of simulation in health care. Qual Saf Health Care 2004;13(Suppl 1):i2–10.

In this article, Gaba shows why he is the maven of high-fidelity simulation in health care. He describes a comprehensive framework for future applications of simulations as the key enabling technique for a revolution in health care—one that optimizes safety, quality, and efficiency.

Gaba begins by making the case that simulation addresses current deficiencies of the health care system.

- Places premium on basic science education while leaving clinical training to an unsystematic apprenticeship model
- Emphasizes individual knowledge and skill rather than clinical teams
- Unstructured and minimal continuing education

To address these problems, Gaba proposes that Simulators must be integrated into the fabric of health care delivery at all levels, which is much more complex than piling it on top of the existing system. To do so, he outlines 11 dimensions (and gradients within each) that can take us there. Next, Gaba outlines the various social entities, driving forces, and implementation mechanisms that could forward the agenda of simulation in medicine. Finally, he paints two possible scenarios (he has had lots of practice at developing scenarios) for the fate of simulation in health care.

Optimistic scenario

- Merging of various driving forces
- Emerging proof of the benefits of specific applications of simulation
- Major institutions with dedicated programs to multiprofessional team training

- Public demand for safety in medicine on par to other high-risk industries—liability insurance tied to organizations that embrace simulation as a means to respond to the public demand
- Government support and later demand for simulation training

Pessimistic scenario

- Public becomes more interested in access to care and cost than the quality or safety of care
- Failure reforming the systems of clinical work to match what is being taught in the simulation centers
- Large multicentered trials never materialize owing to lack of funding—thus long-term proof of benefit of simulation never occurs
- Professional organizations focus more on cost of medical care at the expense of increased investment in training
- Simulation centers become liable for trainees who later commit medical errors

Although we certainly take the optimistic view, we know it stands to reason that Simulators will have a significant future in medical training because of the dedication and hard work of individuals who will ensure that it happens.

✓ HELMREICH RL, DAVIES JM. Anaesthetic simulation and lessons to be learned from aviation [editorial]. Can J Anaesth 1997;44:907–12.

This editorial points out that simulators have a lot of potential for serving as tests. All the usual arguments hold—you don't put a patient at risk, you can reproduce the scene. But this editorial goes on to point out a crucial problem with using a Simulator as a "test vehicle." A key problem is the idea of "equifinality"—that is, different techniques can give you the same end result. (*The article does not mention the following example, we made it up just to illustrate the point.*) For example, one anesthesiologist may use epinephrine to achieve a goal, whereas another may use dobutamine to achieve a goal. Both achieve the same goal—better cardiac output. So, in the Simulator, what do you do? Grade someone wrong who uses epinephrine because the "simulator grade book" says you should use dobutamine? The editorial finishes by saying "there is a need to provide opportunities for practice and assessment until the culture supports the fairness of the assessment process." In other words, it "stands to reason" that a Simulator is a good way to test, but we haven't quite gotten there yet.

✓ MURRAY WB, SCHNEIDER AJ, ROBBINS, R. The first three days of residency: an efficient introduction to clinical medicine. Acad Med 1998;73:595–6.

Dr. Murray and the fine folks at Penn State (you can almost smell the chocolate from the Hershey factory) describe the first 3 days of their anesthesia residency. Rather than just shoveling a ton of stuff at their residents, they make the learning more active, using (what else) the Simulator. Result—a questionnaire showed "improvement in the residents' confidence in their ability to carry out clinical tasks."

So, it "stands to reason" that if a Simulator increases the confidence of a resident, a Simulator must be a good thing. A hard-nosed scientific drudge could look at this and say, "This is not rigorous proof." A skeptic could look at it and say, "So what, what difference does that make, a little more confidence?" But I'll bet that to those Penn State residents the added confidence made all the difference in the world when they walked into the OR the first day.

✓ MURRAY DJ. Clinical simulation: technical novelty or innovation in education [editorial]. Anesthesiology 1998;89:1–2.

Dr. Murray is the big cheese in Simulation at Washington University in St. Louis. This is a "do we really need Simulators?" editorial. What did we do in the "B.S. (before simulator) era"? We did residency and did a lot of cases with supervision. We did lectures, one-on-ones with attendings. But why use the past tense? That's what we are doing right now!

So, do we need to throw Simulators into the mix? Yes. You can use Simulators to teach.

- Physiology to medical students
- Crisis management to a "mixed crew"
- Conscious sedation to nurses, techs, and therapists

Murray goes on to say that a lot of different groups need to work in the Simulator. Anesthesiologists alone can't keep the thing humming all the time. A Simulator is a Lamborghini—you bought it, now drive it! Don't let it sit in the garage all day collecting dust. Get that thing on the road.

✓ ISSENBERG SB, MCGAGHIE WC, HART IR. Simulation technology for health care professional skills training and assessment. JAMA 1999;282:861–6.

Dr. Issenberg, who is one of the authors of this book, oversees the development "Harvey," the Cardiology Patient Simulator at the University of Miami. In this Special Communication, Issenberg et al. touch on all the simulation technologies that were available in

1999, laparoscopy simulators to train surgeons, their own mannequin Harvey to train students about 27 cardiac conditions, flat screen computer simulators, and finally anesthesia simulators.

What does Dr. Issenberg have to say about the anesthesia simulators? "The high cost and requirements for accompanying equipment, space, and personnel have resulted in research to justify the installation of such devices." (Hence so many "justification of simulators" articles in this bibliography.) If you look at "intermediate" benefits of simulators, Issenberg points out the following.

> Simulators are highly realistic.
> Training on a simulator can improve the acquisition and retention of knowledge compared with sitting in a lecture hall.
> If ever used as a certification tool, "They allow the examinee to demonstrate clinical skills in a controlled clinical environment while still exhibiting cognitive and language skills."

So, as study after study comes out *hinting* that simulators can make us better practitioners, do we have to wait for proof positive? No.

✓ GORDON JA, WILKERSON WM, SHAFFER DW, ARMSTRONG EG. "Practicing" medicine without risk: students' and educators' responses to high-fidelity patient simulation. Acad Med 2001;76:469–72.

This is a "feel good" qualitative paper about simulators, pure and simple. Altogether, 27 clinical medical students and clerks and 33 educators went through the Simulator and were asked how they feel about it. The medical students were instructed to evaluate and treat two patients: (1) a trauma patient with hypovolemic shock and a tension pneumothorax and (2) a cardiac patient with marginally stable ventricular tachycardia. The educators, on the other hand, were instructed to care for a patient with anaphylaxis. All participants were debriefed in a case discussion afterward and then completed several evaluations to determine who liked the experience.

To get back to the "theme" of this group of articles—It "stands to reason" that an educational method that everyone likes should be an educational method we should use. Everyone likes Simulators. Even better than the statistics (85% loving the Simulator) were the "raw comments" that hammer home just how cool Simulators are.

"I think everyone could benefit from this." "Every medical student should have the opportunity to learn using this Simulator several times each year."

How can you argue with that?

This study also demonstrates the benefit of relatively small sample sizes—you can collect more qualitative data so you know not only what they liked but, more importantly, why they liked it.

✓ GORDON JA, ORIOL NE, COOPER JB. Bringing good teaching cases "to life": a simulator-based medical education service. Acad Med 2004;79:23–7.

Based on their successful pilot studies of positive learner reactions to simulation-based education, Dr. Gordon and his colleagues set out to develop a comprehensive on-campus simulation program at Harvard Medical School. They provide a descriptive case study of how to develop a simulator program in an undergraduate medical curriculum. And when the folks at Harvard give free advice—we listen.

The authors outline several initial steps that are critical to get a simulation program off the ground and make sure it lasts.

- *Step 1*: Interdisciplinary oversight—make sure you have input from all possible stakeholders and include them in the process. This includes education deans, faculty physicians, administrators, educators, and bioengineers.
- *Step 2*: Capital equipment and training—you need money to buy these simulators, and more importantly you need to make sure they maintain close contact with the technical staff of manufacturers to avoid equipment that remains "in the box."
- *Step 3*: Dedicated space allocation—a centralized location available to all students and faculty is important. After that you need no more than 400 square feet to get started.
- *Step 4*: Administration and partnership—give the new program a fancy name to distinguish it as a dedicated on-campus resource: "The MEC Program in Medical Simulation at Harvard Medical School."

The authors provide practical tips on integrating simulation into the existing medical school curriculum by using existing material rather than "reinventing the wheel." Students in every year of medical school can have meaningful education and training using simulation—you don't need to restrict this to junior and seniors in medical school.

However, what separates this program from all others is the development and implementation of a "medical education service" dedicated to providing "education on demand" for any student who wants to use the Simulators. Faculty members and residents provide the instruction so students can use whatever "down time" they have to hone their skills.

This has become very successful, as evidenced by a group of 15 graduating students who wrote to the dean, "the Simulator stands out as the most important educational adventure at Harvard Medical School."

What can be better than that?

✓ GREENBERG R, LOYD G, WESLEY G. Integrated simulation experiences to enhance clinical education. Med Educ 2002;36: 1109–10.

Dr. Greenberg and her faithful minions from the University of Louisville Patient Simulation Center at the Alumni Center for Medical Education (see? what did we tell you about the importance of having an impressive name for your simulation center) combined a high-fidelity Simulator with a standardized patient. The ultimate simulatory experience—first you talk with an actor pretending to have a condition, then you go to the Simulator as if the actor has now "become" the mannequin. Great idea!

First, students meet a patient (SP—standardized patient, the actor) about to have an appendectomy. Next, the student follows the patient into the OR and participates in anesthetizing the patient (Simulator) throughout the procedure. Then the student returns to the waiting room to discuss the procedure with the patient's spouse (SP). Finally, the student examines the patient (SP) 2 weeks later when she presents with a fever. Whew! Faculty like exploring new clinical teaching and testing methods, and the students are more engaged in their education.

This is an educational twist—that it "stands to reason" is a great way to teach. You combine the best of both worlds and give the student a hell of an experience.

✓ EPSTEIN RM, HUNDERT EM. Defining and assessing professional competence. JAMA 2002;287:226–35.

When you think of "medical science" you think of hard data: blood levels of propofol, heart rates that say "beta-blockade achieved," or gastric emptying times. And even in the "softer" realm of medical education, you still look for "hard data": test scores, percentage pass rate of a program, and (in our Simulator world) checklists.

This *JAMA* article takes us even farther into the "soft." What is competence? How do you assess it? Look at their definition of competence and ask yourself, "Just how could I assess competence?" and, not

to be too cagey about it, "Could I use the Simulator to assess competence?"

Competence is "the habitual and judicious use of communication, knowledge, technical skills, clinical reasoning, emotions, values, and reflection in daily practice for the benefit of the individual and the community."

OK, genius, just how in blue blazes do you assess *that*? (For our nefarious purposes, can a couple of hours in the Simulator fill that tall order?) *JAMA* tells us that the three biggies for assessing competence are:

1. Subjective assessments by supervising clinicians.
2. Multiple-choice exams.
3. Standardized patient assessments, that is, the "pretend" patients in the objective structured clinical exam.

Note: Simulators are not mentioned. The million dollar question—Should Simulators be included?

OK, our goal is to assess competence, and we currently have three ways of doing it. Are they any good? (By extension, does a budding Simulationologist see any defects in the current system that the Simulator could fill?)

1. *Subjective assessments by supervising clinicians.* Any problems here? Evaluators often don't see the resident in action—think of the call night, when the attending is not around much. Evaluators have different standards and are subject to bias.
2. *Multiple-choice exams.* Any problems here? Test scores have been inversely correlated with empathy, responsibility, and tolerance—think of a high-scoring resident who is a creep and treats patients like dirt.
3. *Standardized patient assessments.* Any problems here? Yes. Defining pass/fail is difficult. Assessing interpersonal skills may take a lot of exams.

So here we have the current three methods of assessing competence. Look again at the definition of competence and ask yourself if any of these three really hit the nail on the head. Competence is "the habitual and judicious use of communication, knowledge, technical skills, clinical reasoning, emotions, values, and reflection in daily practice for the benefit of the individual and the community."

Does an attending physician's evaluation of a resident assess "the habitual and judicious use of communication, knowledge, technical skills, clinical reasoning, emotions, values, and reflection in daily practice for the benefit of the individual and the community." Not really.

Does a multiple choice exam assess "the habitual and judicious use of communication, knowledge, technical skills, clinical reasoning, emotions, values, and reflection in daily practice for the benefit of the individual and the community." Not really.

Does a standardized patient assessment evaluate "the habitual and judicious use of communication, knowledge, technical skills, clinical reasoning, emotions, values, and reflection in daily practice for the benefit of the individual and the community." Um, *closer*. I think.

This whole world is murky and quasi-scientific. Go ahead, *try* to make a bold and sure statement about assessing competence. "*The best method for assessing competence is the standardized patient assessment!*" Someone asks you, "Prove it." You say, uh, you say . . . what do you say?

So wouldn't it be great if the *JAMA* then said, "So the current methods of assessing competence aren't any good. But putting people through the Simulator fits the bill perfectly!" Well, they didn't. Too bad. But they did say that we need to develop innovative ways to assess professional competence. And, who are we kidding, that is exactly what we're trying to do with our Simulators.

✓ Dillon GF, Boulet JR, Hawkins RE, Swanson DB. Simulations in the United States Medical Licensing Examination (USMLE). Qual Saf Health Care 2004;13(Suppl 1):i41–5.

This is the article we have been waiting for—the people in charge of providing the assessment requirement for a medical license in the United States predicting the inevitable use of simulators in high-stakes examinations.

They provide a current description of the US medical licensing system and explain how all of them use some form of simulation.

- *Step 1*—Focuses on concepts of science basic to the practice of medicine, a computer-delivered examination made up of multiple-choice questions. The simulation is in the form of brief descriptions of patient care situations.
- *Step 2*—Two components: Clinical knowledge (CK)—one-day computerized multiple-choice examination to assess whether an individual possesses the medical knowledge and understanding of clinical science considered essential for the provision of patient care under supervision. Like step 1, the simulation is in the form of brief descriptions of patient care situations. Clinical skills (CS)—one-day 12-station standardized patient-based examination

intended to assess the examinee's data gathering and communication skills directly. The simulations are in the form of actors portraying 12 common, important clinical problems.
- *Step 3*—Two-day examination combining computer-based MCQs and computer-based case simulations intended to assess whether the individual can apply medical knowledge and understanding of biomedical and clinical science essential for the unsupervised practice of medicine. The simulations are in the form of computer-simulated case presentations that unfold according to the responses of the examinee.

The authors, all affiliated with the National Board of Medical Examiners or the Educational Commission of Foreign Medical Graduates acknowledge the use of Simulators, both task trainers and full patient simulators for assessment. Their use in high-stakes testing (for a license) has been limited by their high cost and lack of reliable, valid scoring mechanisms

However, the authors acknowledge that "as the cost of these mannequins declines, and additional . . . studies are completed, they could have a unique role within the licensure process. . . ." Why?

- Simulators can model rare events prone to medical errors with no risks to patients, especially skills that cannot be measured with real patients.
- Real-time responses to therapeutic interventions can be modeled, and thus the management of patient conditions can be assessed.
- It is possible to develop scoring systems based on measurable patient outcomes rather than the judgment of the examiner.
- It is possible to assess joint patient care efforts of a team, including multidisciplinary communication skills.

There—the folks in charge of testing and therefore education and training (testing drives learning) have just stated what we knew all along. Want to go for a ride?

✓ Seropian MA. General concepts in full scale simulation: getting started. Anesth Analg 2003;97:1695–705.

This article is cited later in this book, where we mention, "If you are thinking of starting a simulation center, and you're looking for a good 'how-to' article, this is the one." Dr. Seropian pays most attention to the *person running the Simulator*, not so much the Simulator mannequin itself. It's the *live* component in the Simulator that makes it happen, so Seropian emphasizes the need to "train the trainer," especially in the delicate art of debriefing.

✓ Ohrn MAK, van Oostrom JH, van Meurs WL. A comparison of traditional textbook and interactive computer learning of neuromuscular block. Anesth Analg 1997;84:657–1.

This didn't test a high-fidelity mannequin; rather, it was a test of a flat screen Simulator (majorly cool video game, in effect, teaching neuromuscular blockade). Does this have any relevance to a simulator center? Yes indeed. Any "full service" simulator center would have not just mannequins but all kinds of learning gizmos, including flat screen simulators. It "stands to reason" that we should use all manner of simulation in a simulation center. So, OK, great, does this neuromuscular video game do the trick? Yes.

A group of 23 residents were divided up: Half were taught with textbooks (the same technology used since the Epic of Gilgamesh 5000 years ago), and half were taught with these flat screen computer Simulators (the new technology used since the Epic of Bill Gates just 20 or so years ago). Result: computers taught better, as measured by an exam. Fringe benefit, the residents liked the computer experience more than the textbook one.

You see this again and again and again. No matter what the study, no matter what the technique or result, one thing comes through loud and clear. People *like* this way of learning. If that alone served as justification, there'd be Simulators on every street corner from Miami to Juneau.

Berkenstadt H, Ziv A, Barsuk D, Levine I, Cohen A, Vardi A. The use of advanced simulation in the training of anesthesiolgists to treat chemical warfare casualties. Anesth Analg 2003;96: 1739–42.

Our colleagues in Israel identified another use of simulation training—prepare anesthesiologists to respond to a weapons of mass destruction attack, in this case chemical weapons. Since the early 1990s they have used a curriculum that included lectures, hands-on training with simulated patients undergoing decontamination, and simulated treatment while medical personnel were in full protection gear. However, they acknowledge these courses focused on the logistics of the scenarios and were deficient in providing opportunities for medical personnel to exercise and practice clinical procedures—here comes the use of advanced Simulators to provide these opportunities to respond to chemical attacks. The study included 25 medical personnel divided into multidisciplinary teams of anesthesiologists and intensive care and postanesthesia care nurses. The catch—all trainees had to be in full protective gear, including gas mask, chemical protective gloves, and a multilayered overgarment!

The tasks included the following.

- Airway and breathing resuscitation including intubation on a variety of Simulators (some capable of vomiting)
- Insertion of IV lines

The scenarios included the following.

- Combined head injury and nerve gas intoxication
- Combined chest injury and nerve gas intoxication
- Isolated severe intoxication

Outcome measures included checklists for performance assessment (coordination and communication among team members, leadership in clinical decision making and prioritization) and feedback. They were validated by the input of several experts in anesthesia, intensive care, and trauma management. In addition, there were experts in relevant medical fields from such diverse areas as the Israeli Defense Forces Medical Corps NBC Branch and the National Health Authorities. Participants also completed a postcourse questionnaire gauging their perception of several aspects of the course.

They learned that the medical personnel could actually function with the gas mask, although it did interfere with communication within the medical teams. The chemical protective gloves were found to be the limiting factor in the performance of medical tasks. All 25 participants gave favorable rating to the course. The authors acknowledge that limitations included the lack of pre- and posttesting tools and no quantitative performance evaluations.

This study is important because it demonstrates how existing training and assessment methods can be used to address new needs (response to acts of terrorism) and can be implemented on a national scale. It also highlights the importance of involving all stakeholders in the process of developing outcome measures based on the curriculum. Finally, the study identified two independent variables that affected performance (gas mask—communication; gloves—clinical procedures). This has important implications regarding the assumptions of how prepared medical personnel are.

✓ Berkenstadt H, Gafni N. Incorporating Simulation-Based Objective Structured Clinical Examination (OSCE) into the Israeli National Board Examination in Anesthesiology. Anesth Analg 2006;102:853–8.

No kidding, simulation as an assessment tool has arrived. In Israel, the OSCE, using simulator technology, "has gradually progressed from being a minor part of the oral board examination to a *prerequisite component of the test*."

In Israel, they asked the question, "What should our anesthesia people know before we certify them?" The answers are as follows.

- Trauma
- Resuscitation
- Crisis management in the OR
- Regional anesthesia
- Mechanical ventilation

So, because that's what residents need to *know*, that's what the Israeli board set out to *test*. They create scenarios for each of these areas, put the examinees in the Simulator, videotape and grade their performance, and accredit those who perform well. During the past 2 years, with 104 candidates, the Israeli board used simulation technology as part of their assessment. Most examinees found the exam reasonable to difficult, and most preferred it to the standard oral examinations.

Is Israel the only place doing this?

- In New York, they use a Simulator for "rehabbing" an anesthesiologist with lapsed skills.
- In Heidelberg, they use a Simulator to accredit nurse anesthetists.
- In Rochester, residents have to pass muster in the Simulator before they take overnight call. (Hmm, that sounds like a good idea.)
- Difficult airway management in the Simulator is mandatory at the University of Pittsburgh.

If anyone is still wondering whether the Simulator is coming, we've got news for you. It's already here.

✓ Bond WF, Deitrick LM, Arnold DC, Kostenbader M, Barr GC, Kimmel SR, et al. Using simulation to instruct emergency medicine residents in cognitive forcing strategies. Acad Med 2004;79:438–46.

Emergency medicine residents are at high risk of making thinking errors because of multiple factors, including high-decision density, high levels of diagnostic uncertainty, and high patient acuity at the same time having to deal with a large number of distractions. The way to do this is to instruct clinicians to develop strategies to face these situations. This is called *metacognition*. The problem is that one's ability to handle hypotension due to cardiac arrest does not translate to one's ability to manage hypotension that

results from septic shock. In other words, your problem-solving ability is disease- (context)-specific. However, the authors point out, "but if the resident does not see enough of certain critical problems, he or she may be left with incomplete training."

In an elegant qualitative study (includes an appendix with the survey instrument), the authors put 15 second- and third-year anesthesia residents through a complex case they thought would be mismanaged because *it stands to reason* that learners pay more attention to a case in which they made mistakes than one they performed flawlessly. The patient was a 67-year-old woman with renal failure on dialysis who presented to the emergency department with shortness of breath. The case is embedded with "error traps." For instance, the decision to intubate and use succinylcholine without confirming whether the patient is on dialysis as evidenced by the shunt on her arm. This leads to worsening hyperkalemia and cardiac arrest.

Residents were debriefed on issues such as omission errors and faulty hypothesis generation, given the option to review the videotape of their case, and asked a series of questions related to their experience. Third-year residents appeared to appreciate the global thinking strategies, whereas second-year residents focused more on concrete issues (knowledge gained about succinylcholine). Most residents commented positively on the opportunity to make errors without injuring patients. So when forcing cognitive strategies on your residents—and you need lots of patients to do so—the residents appear to learn from their mistakes. You can't have residents making mistakes on patients, so it stands to reason that you should use Simulators.

✓ Cleave-Hogg D, Morgan PJ. Experiential learning in an anaesthesia simulation centre: analysis of students' comments. Med Teach 2002;24:23–6.

We learn better when we are doing rather than watching or being told something. There is just no better substitute than hands-on experiences. However, Cleave-Hogg and Morgan, at the University of Toronto, pointed out that this is a problem, especially for medical students because:

- Patient safety—Students should not harm patients with hands-on learning.
- Clinical requirements—There are times when you need to act quickly—too fast for the beginning learner.
- Tolerance of faculty—Some faculty are control freaks and just won't allow the lowly student to do anything.

- Case availability—Naturally, real patients often do not offer the right mix of cases for ideal learning.

It stands to reason a method that could address these limitations would offer that all important hands-on experience. Each of the participating 145 fourth-year students was allowed to work through one short case as part of his or her curriculum. The authors asked fourth-year students how they felt regarding their use of Simulators as a learning tool. They had a 100% return rate on the questionnaires (they must have offered pizza). Their comments are in contrast to the Bond study in that most students (88%) valued the cognitive issues over the technical skills (10%) learned. Students in general preferred to have one-to-one feedback rather than getting group feedback. Most importantly, *"they were involved in learning without fear of harming a patient."*

✓ Cooper JB, Barron D, Blum R, Davison JK, Feinstein D, Halasz J, et al. Video teleconferencing with realistic simulation for medical education. J Clin Anesth 2000;12:256–61.

If Simulators are good training tools for individuals and small groups of learners, what about for large groups? If we use additional technology, video-conferencing, it stands to reason we can reach a much broader audience, including places without the facilities and resources of these costly tools. Cooper and colleagues explored the feasibility and success of conducting long-distance clinical case discussions with realistic re-enactments of anesthesia critical events. They set up the equipment to allow two-way audio and visual feedback between the simulation suite and audience. (Details of the technology setup are fully described in the article's Appendix 1).

The audience (which ranged from 50 to 150 people) was initially given information regarding the case from a real "patient" and family; and after a short break they were sent to the OR where the Simulator was in place. Participants on both sides were allowed to ask questions and make comments regarding the case. In fact, when the patient's condition deteriorated, participants were allowed to make suggestions regarding the patient's management. Participants were generally enthusiastic regarding this approach, including 97% who highly rated the educational value of the session. Challenges with the study: A few questioned the cost, and the authors noted the many technical issues that always need to be monitored.

Although not directly studied, the authors believed that the teleconferenced training sessions could enhance the traditional mode of case-based clinical education, and they do acknowledge the "entertainment value of the program." There is nothing wrong with being entertained while learning.

✓ Schwid HA. Anesthesia simulators—technology and applications. Isr Med Assoc J 2000;2:949–53.

Poor Howard. Here he is a full professor, a major element in the Simulator world, and this article in the *IMAJ* misspelled his name at the bottom of every other page in this article. Go figure. It's hard to get the respect you deserve. Professor Schwid's name appears again and again in simulation articles, so keep your eye out for his excellent work from the University of Washington.

This is a review article that lays out all the various kinds of technology available for simulation teaching. Screen-based simulation is, in effect, a high-tech video game where you can study uptake of anesthetic vapors, snake your way through the oxygen flow in an anesthesiology machine, try your hand at neuromuscular blockade pharmacology, or run codes. Mannequin-based simulators win rave reviews from residents (*which jibes with my experience—Author*), and the hunt is on to "prove the effectiveness of simulators."

✓ Eaves RH, Flagg AJ. The U.S. Air Force pilot simulated medical unit: a teaching strategy with multiple applications. J Nurs Educ 2001;40:110–5.

If you can train a learner to manage a single "patient" using a single Simulator, it stands to reason you can train a provider to manage a unit of patients using many Simulators simultaneously. Who has to do this?—nurses, of course!

In this descriptive article Majors Eaves and Flagg from the U.S. Air Force describe the design, development, and implementation of a Simulated Medical Unit (SMU) consisting of 11 patients—nine medium fidelity simulators and two live actors. They point out that recent changes in Department of Defense hospitals have resulted in significant downsizing, with far fewer patients, making it difficult to find clinical experiences to learn skills.

The authors set up a medical ward consisting of patients with:

- Pneumonia
- Fractured tibia-fibula
- Preop and postop appendectomy
- Postop tonsillectomy
- Asthma

- Type 2 diabetes
- Small bowel obstruction

To enhance the realism, nurses were provided expectations of their behavior.

- First priority was safety of patient and staff.
- Each Simulator was to be treated with same care and respect as a live patient (they even had to call them by names).
- Any disregard to the "patient" was met with an incident report—the two words most feared by a nurse.
- All procedures would meet standard of care.
- Teamwork was expected, and peer review was highly encouraged.
- Periodic videotaping for feedback and evaluations was done.

Five nurses spent 3 weeks in the simulated medical unit (SMU) with progressive responsibilities over time.

- Week 1 consisted of learning processes and procedures, especially those unique to the military.
- Weeks 2 and 3 consisted of, for the first few days, an intense review of 15+ basic technical skills; the remaining time was used to build each nurse's organizational skills and critical-thinking abilities as each simulated experience grew from caring for one simulated patient to caring for six to eight simulated patients.
- The final evaluation involved each nurse caring for eight patients (six Simulators, two SPs) in the SMU for 4 hours continuously.

The authors pointed out that this allowed them to see not only a variety of conditions but a variety of presentations of the same condition. It also allowed:

- Practice of prioritizing skills on multiple patients with varying degrees of illnesses
- Practice of the 15+ technical skills on varying patients
- Practice delegating tasks to ancillary help such as medical technicians (Nurses who were not used to delegating quickly fell behind in their tasks and could see the outcome of this.)

The nurses were unanimous in their increased ability to perform at a busy inpatient unit. Although not formally evaluated, when the nurses first took care of real patients the nurses' first preceptors were "amazed" by their ability – their orientation time was cut in half, and they were much more independent than the typical new nurse.

The authors correctly point out the high cost of their exercises (estimated at $1,548,600) and that few organizations would have the resources to develop this type of learning. However, for large organizations who have to train large numbers of personnel in relatively brief periods of time, the "potential costs savings . . . are significant if documentation improves and litigation decreases." What else could an organization want?

✓ HAMMAN WR. The complexity of team training: what we have learned from aviation and its application to medicine. Qual Saf Health Care 2004;13(Suppl 1):i72–9.

We read all the time that the promise of simulation in health care is based in large part on its positive effect in the field of aviation. We cannot imagine a pilot flying a large passenger jet without hours of simulator training and retraining. Aside from the technical marvels of modern flight Simulators, what can we learn from the aviation field about how we train providers to make a safer system with fewer medical errors?

In this article, Hamman drew on his vast experience as an aviation training expert to provide a blueprint of what we can do in medicine to match the aviation industry. First, he notes that most errors in medicine, like aviation, are a result of a breakdown in the team or system rather than an individual. Until the late 1970s, aviation training focused on a pilot's individual skills. In 1978, NASA published its research on the causes of commercial air accidents and concluded that "the majority of disasters resulted not from pilot's lack of technical skill or mechanical failure, but from error associated with breakdowns in communication, leadership, and teamwork." Hamman illustrates this with two examples:

- A delayed commercial flight in Ontario resulted in snow accumulation on the wings that was noticed by several passengers who informed the lead flight attendant. Nothing was reported to the pilot because "the flight attendants did not think it appropriate to say anything to the operating pilot." The plane crashed soon after take off killing 24 passengers.
- Cabin crew of a British Midlands flight did not inform the pilot of flames coming from one of the engines because their training did not prepare them for this crisis event.

Events such as these led to the obvious conclusion that the way pilots and crew had been trained for the previous four decades would no longer suffice in the modern era. Reports such as the Institutes of Medicine's *To Err is Human* have highlighted that the way physicians, nurses, techs have been trained over the last 100 years is entirely inadequate for today's complex health care system.

So what can we learn from aviation?

- Those in charge of hospitals, training programs, and medical school have to accept the challenge of interdisciplinary training as a necessary step to improve the quality and safety of health care. This can change the current situation in which one discipline has no understanding of the contributions of different providers.
- Training cannot occur as a one-step event at the beginning of training but must be a long-term commitment integrated throughout the career of the professional – just as it is in aviation.
- The curriculum should be based on a tasks analysis that leads to specific team-oriented goals and competencies that are appropriate for each phase of a professional's career.
- Simulation should incorporate technical and interdisciplinary team skills in dynamic scenario designs. This should be modeled on the aviation Advanced Qualification Program, which identifies team skills that enhance safety, including awareness of human and system error as well as techniques and skills that minimize their effects.

In summary:

- Individual level – factors that can impair individual performance and increase the likelihood of making mistakes.
- Interpersonal/team level – factors that impair performance both in and out of a complex procedure – communication, cooperation, leadership, decision-making
- Medical system level – factors that impede safe health care delivery and pose a threat to patients

Read this article in full – you will have a clearer picture of where we need to go in medical simulation. Hamman tells us that it will not be easy and will require "much work" but that medicine "should no longer wait." We agree, Captain Hamman.

✓ HOLZMAN RS, COOPER JB, GABA DM, PHILIP JH, SMALL SD, FEINSTEIN D. Anesthesia crisis resource management: real-life simulation training in operating room crises. J Clin Anesth 1995;7:675–87.

Can a successful simulation program developed at Stanford be transferred across the United States to Boston and be just as successful? This article describes the first adoption of Anesthesia Crisis Resource Management (ACRM) outside Stanford and the Kingdom of Gaba. This is important because it demonstrates the possibility and feasibility of simulation training transferability. Once people saw that it could be done in Boston, they started to say, "We can do this too."

Holzman, Cooper, and their Boston colleagues collaborated with Gaba to set up an analogous simulation program including Simulator, mock OR suite, actors, evaluators. They enrolled 68 anesthesiologists of varying levels of experience and 4 nurse anesthetists in ACRM training and evaluated their perception of the experience. As expected, the overall response was very positive, with more junior attendings rating the course higher than senior attendings. They also thought that the course should be taken more often. Senior attendings rated their own performance significantly higher than more-junior anesthesiolgists.

A 6-month follow-up questionnaire from 33 respondents revealed that 8 had been involved in a critical incident since the course and thought that the training prepared them to handle these critical events more effectively. The authors acknowledge that the study did not involve a control group and that an adequate controlled evaluation of participants would be difficult, time-consuming, faculty-intensive, expensive, and need multiple institutions to develop a national standard. That may be true, but in the process they proved that a novel idea borrowed from aviation could be applied to medicine at more than one institution – and it is now routinely performed at hundreds of institutions worldwide.

✓ KURREK MM, FISH KJ. Anaesthesia crisis resource management training: an intimidating concept, a rewarding experience. Can J Anaesth 1996;43:430–4.

This is an early report from the University of Toronto on the early acceptance of Anesthesia Crisis Resource Management (ACRM). The authors sought to obtain the opinions of two groups of practitioners: those who likely had never been trained on Simulators and those who had participated in ACRM workshops at the University of Toronto.

They sent 150 survey questionnaires to a mixture of community and academic anesthesiologists and residents in-training. They received back 59 surveys – a response rate of 39%. This is less than half the minimum response rate of 80% generally considered necessary to avoid bias in the results.

How did this group feel about simulation? They were very supportive of the purchase, training for residents and faculty, willing to spend unpaid time in the Simulator, and thought it had much relevance for anesthesia training. These responses did not vary much between staff and residents. Both staff and residents anticipated much anxiety if trained in a Simulator and did not favor the compulsory use of simulation for recertification.

The authors also sent a survey questionnaire to 36 previous participants in ACRM workshops – 35 were returned (97% response rate – this is excellent). The participants enjoyed all aspects of the course, thought it would be beneficial to anesthesiologists for initial, advanced, and refresher training. They generally thought the course should be taken every 1.5 years.

The authors commented on the perceived level of anxiety of the larger group of inexperienced anesthesiologists as a potential barrier to this group using Simulators because of the fear of Simulators being used for evaluation purposes. It is unfortunate that the authors stated that the evaluation aspect of simulation should be minimized and surmised that "issues of validation and expense make it unlikely that the use of anesthesia simulators will be a viable option for re-certification." *What?* That is probably what pilots first said about flight Simulators.

It stands to reason that all health care providers should feel anxiety when they are going to be tested. How many students make themselves sick with worry and panic over multiple-choice exams? Perhaps the anesthesiologists realized that for the first time in their career someone was going to actually watch their performance – we would all be anxious – but that is not a reason not to do it.

✓ Halamek LP, Kaegi DM, Gaba DM, Sowb YA, Smith BC, Smith BE, et al. Time for a new paradigm in pediatric medical education: teaching neonatal resuscitation in a simulated delivery room environment. Pediatrics 2000;106:E45.

Anesthesia is not the only high-risk, dynamic, stressful area of medicine – how about neonatal resuscitation! Alien fetal and neonatal physiology, tiny anatomy for endotracheal intubation, umbilical vessel catheterization – decisions made by the pediatrician carry lifelong consequences for both patients, mother and infant. Unlike anesthesia, the pediatrician does not have the benefit of a sedated, well monitored patient but most rely on auditory cues such as "crying" (there is no crying under anesthesia), breath and heart sounds, visual cues such as muscle tone and skin color (under anesthesia the patient is draped), and information from the obstetrician, nurse, mother, father, and grandparents among others. The authors make the

case that if Simulators are good for other high-risk industries (aviation) and anesthesia it makes good sense for neonatal medicine – they are right!

Halamek and his colleagues at Stanford developed a course, "NeoSim," that integrates traditional instruction (textbooks, lectures, on-the-job training) with technical and behavioral skills training in a simulated environment. They developed several delivery room crises that included patient problems (meconium aspiration, prenatal depression, hemorrhage, congenital anomalies) with equipment failure and stressful interactions with other delivery room team members. At the time of the study, 38 physicians and nurses had completed the program and overwhelmingly valued the experience. They liked mostly the realistic scenarios, feedback debriefings, and the faculty. Even though many thought the Simulator could have been more realistic, *they nonetheless thought that the entire experience effectively recreated real-life situations that tested their technical and behavioral skills.*

That is the important message – good simulation is *not* about the technology and all the fancy gadgets. It is *how* it is used by the *right* of people – those dedicated to education and training.

✓ Reznek M, Smith-Coggins R, Howard S, Kiran K, Harter P, Sowb Y, et al. Emergency medicine crisis resource management (EMCRM): pilot study of a simulation-based crisis management course for emergency medicine. Acad Emerg Med 2003; 10:386–9.

If CRM works for anesthesia, why not for emergency medicine. Emergency departments are complex, dynamic working environments in which crises can rapidly develop. Reznek and several colleagues at Stanford (where else?) developed the Emergency Medicine Crises Resource Management (EMCRM) course and evaluated participants' perceptions of their training.

The course was modeled after the ACRM textbook (*Crisis Management in Anesthesiology*. New York: Churchill Livingstone; 1994). As with previous iterations of the CRM courses in other disciplines, the participants, comprising 13 emergency medicine residents, gave very positive ratings of the course, their skills as a result of the course, and whether the course would be suitable for initial and refresher training.

This study did not reveal anything new. It just demonstrated that what was once a domain of anesthesia is now being adopted in all high-risk fields of medicine – way to go!

✓ Gaba DM, Howard SK, Fish KJ, Smith BE, Sowb YA. Simulation-based training in anesthesia crisis resource management (ACRM): a decade of experience. Simulation Gaming 2001;32:175–93.

In this review, Gaba and his colleagues provide a 10-year perspective on the development, successful implementation, growth and evaluation, and the ongoing challenges of training health care providers to work as a crew for a larger team. The authors outlined the needs of the course during the late 1980s and early 1990s to address deficiencies in the training of anesthesiologists – these focused on several critical aspects of decision making and crisis management. The team then used aviation training as a model to design and develop the ACRM course that trains not only crews within the same disciplines but also interdisciplinary teams.

Highlights of this successful curriculum, which in large part has been the driving force for the use of high-fidelity simulation, are as follows.

- Expansion of the original 1-day introductory course to a three-stage comprehensive curriculum.
- Expansion and proliferation of the course to scores of institutions worldwide, many of which have made ACRM a required component of the curriculum.
- The decision by the Harvard Risk Management Foundation (the insurer of the Harvard-affiliated hospitals) to provide a different malpractice rate structure for anesthesiologists who have completed the ACRM training.
- Adoption of ACRME principles to other disciplines, such as critical care and emergency medicine, the delivery room, cardiac arrest response teams, and radiology.
- Formation of ACRM instructor training overseen by the three original institutions that introduced ACRM training (Stanford, Boston Center for Medical Simulation, Canadian Simulation Centre in Toronto).
- Numerous studies have demonstrated overwhelmingly positive response to the training by participants.
- A study that demonstrated the possibility of developing reliable technical and behavioral assessment criteria for ACRM competencies.

Ongoing challenges for ACRM include the following.

- High variability in outcome measures that require large numbers of well trained instructors and calibration among centers.
- Biases of simulation testing of simulation-based learning. Are trainees learning and becoming skilled enough to perform well during the simulation or in the real world? Again, we look to aviation, as our belief that transfer does occur.
- Complex skills require ongoing lifelong effort. The real benefits of this training are unlikely to be maximum after a single course but develop through the cumulative experience over many years via a combination of standardized training and experience.
- The workplace must reinforce the work done with the Simulator. Unless the setting in which we practice reinforces what we learn in the simulation centers, their potential cannot be realized. The Institute of Medicine's focus on patient safety, and the need to reduce medical errors, comprise one example that may change the inertia.

The main message is that although it stands to reason that Simulators work it stands to reason even more if the Simulator is guided by a well developed curriculum and not by its technical gadgets.

✓ MORGAN PJ, CLEAVE-HOGG D. A worldwide survey of the use of simulation in anesthesia. Can J Anaesth 2002;49:659–62.

I wonder how they use simulation in Amsterdam or Singapore? Do they face the same challenges of obtaining funding and finding the time to do research? How do they balance their clinical responsibilities with their educational duties? A highly effective way to find this out is to send a survey to as many centers using high-fidelity Simulators and evaluate the results. This is exactly what Drs. Morgan and Cleave-Hogg did.

They searched the WWW and two centers' large database of simulation centers (University of Rochester and Bristol Medical Simulation Center) to identify 158 simulation centers worldwide. They sent a 67-item survey (available at: www.cja.jca.org) designed to capture information regarding the use of Simulators for education, evaluation, and research. They received 60 responses for a rate of 38% (even after a second mailing), which was too low to avoid significant biases in their results. Phone calls to the Center directors would have dramatically increased the response rate (this has been demonstrated in numerous educational studies).

The authors reported primarily quantitative data from the survey.

- About 81% of the centers have dedicated personnel responsible for the operation of the center.

- Most funding (76%) came from the university department, 15% from the government, and 13% from the private sector or other source.
- About 78% used the Simulator for undergraduate training and 85% for postgraduate training (technical skills, rare events, CRM, ACLS, airway).
- Only 15% used the Simulator for assessment.
- About 61% currently engaged in research with more than half citing lack of funding as the primary barrier to research, followed by lack of faculty resources (this is nearly the same for any research in a medical center).

The authors provided a "snapshot" of fewer than half of the identified centers that returned the survey in 2001. The number of simulation centers now numbers several hundred. But what did we learn from this survey? That most centers use Simulators for similar reasons and most face similar challenges. We are more interested in the centers that were outliers. What distinguishes the 15% of centers that use simulation for assessment – how do they do it? What about the simulation centers that do not rely on university or department funding? How did the small number of centers obtain government funding?

We provide a case example to illustrate why these questions are important. The University of Miami's Michael S. Gordon Center for Research in Medical Education has been involved in simulation training, assessment, and research for 40 years. In all this time, the Center has received minimal funding from the university or any department. It has raised through federal, state, and local government sources, national and private foundations, and generous individuals more than $120 million during the past four decades. This Center did not receive the survey but could have offered significant advice from its experience of many successes and a few failures over the past 40 years. There are other centers that were likely missed as well.

The important message is that when you conduct survey studies you do not learn as much if you limit your search to those Centers who mirror your own program. Look for the distractors, the vanguards – there are valuable lessons out there!

✓ OWEN H, PLUMMER JL. Improving learning of a clinical skill: the first year's experience of teaching endotracheal intubation in a clinical simulation facility. Med Educ 2002;36:635–42.

Sometimes "less" is more, and more of "less" is even better. Drs. Owen and Plummer from Flinders University in Adelaide, Australia point out that endotracheal intubation is a fundamental part of airway management, and airway management "is the scaffolding upon which the whole practice of anaesthesia is built." The authors contend that we should not wait until a postgraduate or residency program to hone these skills in learners – it stands to reason these skills can be developed in the undergraduate curriculum.

This article and the training described is unique in two aspects.

- It recognizes that complex clinical skills should be taught to novices in many steps
- Practice on multiple Simulators is better than multiple attempts on a single Simulator.

To address the first issue, Owen and Plummer designed a very practical and straightforward approach to training students about endotracheal intubation. Take a look at their Figure 1 – You see a nice flow-chart that outlines the components of the curriculum.

- Orientation with an intubation video
- Becoming familiar with the equipment
- Observing an expert demonstrating the technique
- Several practice attempts on an "easy" Simulator – emphasizing correct handling of laryngoscope
- Feedback is provided
- Students repeat until they have a satisfactory performance (with more feedback)
- Students are exposed to different and more difficult Simulators to introduce alternate techniques and aids (with more feedback)
- Competence and confidence in endotracheal intubation

To address the second issue – multiple Simulators – the authors recognized that even though human patient Simulators can simulate different airways, it is a waste of valuable resources to have novice students use a full-body Simulator for single tasks. Instead, they identified and use 13 different adult airway trainers in their curriculum to provide the variation critical for learning skills.

Theirs is a good example of maximizing all of a simulation centers' resources with an approach that ensures basic skills in medical students so they are better prepared for postgraduate training. All of you residency directors should be happy with this!

NURSING EDUCATION

It stands to reason that if Simulators offer so much potential to the physicians' disciplines of anesthesia, critical care, and surgery they are just as valuable in nursing education. If one of the primary focuses of medical simulation is interdisciplinary team training, each professional field needs to know what the other is doing.

Enter Drs. Nehring and Lashley from Rutgers, State University of New Jersey College of Medicine. Together and with their colleagues they have written several articles on the use of human patient simulation in nursing education. I list them here so you have easy access.

✓ NEHRING WM, ELLIS WE, LASHLEY FR. Human patient simulators in nursing education: an overview. Simulation Gaming 2001;32:194–204.

This is a well written review of how human patient simulators are used in nursing education. It draws on several examples from the anesthesia field, reviewing the educational, evaluation, and research aspects of using simulation in nursing education.

✓ NEHRING WM, LASHLEY FR, ELLIS WE. Critical incident nursing management using human patient simulators. Nurs Educ Perspect 2002;23:128–32.

The authors describe a unique course, "Critical Incident Nursing Management" (CINM) – a derivation of anesthesia crisis resource management designed by Gaba. CINM is a competency-based method of nursing instruction in which nursing care is taught in the context of critical health incidents (dyspnea in an asthmatic patient).

✓ NEHRING WM, LASHLEY FR. Use of the human patient simulator in nursing education. Annu Rev Nurs Educ 2004;2:163–81.

This is another well written review summarizing the many uses of human patient simulators in nursing education and the authors' personal experience over the past 5 years.

✓ NEHRING WM, LASHLEY FR. Current use and opinions regarding human patient simulators in nursing education: an international survey. Nurs Educ Perspect 2004;25:144–8.

The authors acknowledge the scant literature in nursing education involving human patient simulators (HPSs). As a result, they decided to survey all nursing training programs that had obtained a METI HPS prior to January 2002. They sent out more than 215 surveys and obtained 40 responses (less than 20% response rate). The survey covered demographic data, items on curricular content of HPS use, evaluation of competence, continuing education, and other uses.

What did they learn? The HPS is used in more courses more often in community colleges than in university or simulation center settings. The Simulator was used most often to teach diagnostic skills and critical events. All but three schools reported that faculty was very receptive to the use of Simulators in their curricula. Why were the others not receptive?

- Fear of changing teaching methodology
- Fear technology too advanced
- Perception nursing student level not advanced enough for the technology
- Small number of students that can use the Simulator at one time
- Time needed to learn technology

The authors acknowledge the high cost of Simulation as being a limiting factor to its growth in nursing education. They point out:

- A recent alliance between METI and the National League for Nursing for start-up grants for research
- The need for a system of regional nursing simulation centers to help meet the need to train "competent and confident nurses who have the skills required to work successfully in today's challenging health care environment"

We could not agree more – Nurses have always played critical roles in patient care; and without their full inclusion in simulation-based training we all will suffer!

Additional Articles on Nursing

Fletcher JL. AANA journal course: update for nurse anesthetists—anesthesia simulation: a tool for learning and research. AANA J 1995;63:61–7.

Fletcher JL. AANA journal course: update for nurse anesthetists—ERR WATCH: anesthesia crisis resource management from the nurse anesthetist's perspective. AANA J 1998;66:595–602.

Henrichs B, Rule A, Grady M, Ellis W. Nurse anesthesia students' perceptions of the anesthesia patient simulator: a qualitative study. AANA J 2002;70:219–25.

Kanter RK, Fordyce WE, Tompkins JM. Evaluation of resuscitation proficiency in simulations: the impact of a simultaneous cognitive task. Pediatr Emerg Care 1990;6:260–2.

Lampotang S. Logistics of conducting a large number of individual sessions with a full-scale patient simulator at a scientific meeting. J Clin Monit 1997;13:399–407.

Larbuisson R, Pendeville P, Nyssen AS, Janssens M, Mayne A. Use of anaesthesia simulator: initial impressions of its use in two Belgian university centers. Acta Anaesthesiol Belg 1999;50:87–93.

Lupien AE, George-Gay B. High-fidelity patient simulation. In: Lowenstein AJ, Bradshaw MJ (eds) Fuszard's Innovative Teaching Strategies in Nursing. Sudbury, MA: Jones & Bartlett; 2004. p. 134–48.

March JA, Farrow JL, Brown LH, Dunn KA, Perkins PK. A breathing manikin model for teaching nasotracheal intubation to EMS professionals. Prehosp Emerg Care 1997;1:269–72.

McIndoe A. The future face of medical training—ship-shape and Bristol fashion. Br J Theatre Nurs 1998;8:5, 8–10.

McLellan B. Early experience with simulated trauma resuscitation. Can J Surg 1999;42:205–10.

Monti EJ, Wren K, Haas R, Lupien AE. The use of an anesthesia simulator in graduate and undergraduate education. CRNA 1998;9:59–66.

Morgan PJ, Cleave-Hogg D. A Canadian simulation experience: faculty and student opinions of a performance evaluation study. Br J Anaesth 2000;85:779–81.

Mulcaster JT, Mills J, Hung OR, MacQuarrie K, Law JA, Pytka S, et al. Laryngoscopic intubation: learning and performance. Anesthesiology 2003;98:23–7.

Murray WB, Henry J. Assertiveness training during a crisis resource management (CRM) session using a full human simulator in a realistic simulated environment. Presented at the International Meeting on Medical Simulation, San Diego, 2003.

Nyman J, Sihvonen M. Cardiopulmonary resuscitation skills in nurses and nursing students. Resuscitation 2000;47:179–84.

O'Donnell J, Fletcher J, Dixon B, Palmer L. Planning and implementing an anesthesia crisis resource management course for student nurse anesthetists. CRNA 1998;9:50–8.

Peteani LA. Enhancing clinical practice and education with high-fidelity human patient simulators. Nurse Educ 2004;29:25–30.

Rauen CA. Simulation as a teaching strategy for nursing education and orientation in cardiac surgery. Crit Care Nurse 2004;24:46–51.

Scherer YK, Bruce SA, Graves BT, Erdley WS. Acute care nurse practitioner education: enhancing performance through the use of clinical simulation. AACN Clin Issues 2003;14:331–41.

Seropian MA, Brown K, Gavilanes JS, Driggers B. An approach to simulation program development. J Nurs Educ 2004;43:164–9.

Vandrey CI, Whitman KM. Simulator training for novice critical care nurses. Am J Nurs 2001;101:24GG–LL.

Wilson M, Shepherd I, Kelly C, Pitner J. Assessment of a low-fidelity human patient simulator for acquisition of nursing skills. Nurse Educ Today 2005;25:56–67.

Wong TK, Chung JW. Diagnostic reasoning processes using patient simulation in different learning environments. J Clin Nurs 2002;11:65–72.

Yaeger KA, Halamek LP, Coyle M, Murphy A, Anderson J, Boyle K, et al. High-fidelity simulation-based training in neonatal nursing. Adv Neonatal Care 2004;4:326–31.

Additional Articles on "It Stands to Reason"

Abrahamson S. Human simulation for training in anesthesiology. In: Ray CD (ed) Medical Engineering. Chicago: Year Book; 1974. p. 370–4.

Abrahamson S, Hoffman KI. Sim One: a computer-controlled patient simulator. Lakartidningen 197420;71:4756–8.

Abrahamson S, Wallace P. Using computer-controlled interactive manikins in medical education. Med Teacher 1980;2(1):25–31.

Adnet F, Lapostolle F, Ricard-hibon A, Carli P, Goldstein P. Intubating trauma patients before reaching the hospital—revisited. Crit Care 2001;5:290–1.

Arne R, Stale F, Ragna K, Petter L. PatSim—simulator for practising anaesthesia and intensive care: development and observations. Int J Clin Monit Comput 1996;13:147–52.

Barron DM, Russel RK. Evaluation of simulator use for anesthesia resident orientation. In: Henson L, Lee A, Basford A (eds) Simulators in Anesthesiology Education. New York: Plenum; 1998. p. 111–3.

Barsuk D, Berkenstadt H, Stein M, Lin G, Ziv A. [Advanced patient simulators in pre-hospital management training—the trainees' perspective (in Hebrew).] Harefuah 2003;142:87–90, 160.

Beyea SC. Human patient simulation: a teaching strategy. AORN J 2004;80:738, 741–2.

Block EF, Lottenberg L, Flint L, Jakobsen J, Liebnitzky D. Use of a human patient simulator for the advanced trauma life support course. Am Surg 2002;68:648–51.

Blum RH, Raemer DB, Carroll JS, Sunder N, Felstein DM, Cooper JB. Crisis resource management training for an anesthesia faculty: a new approach to continuing education. Med Educ 2004;38:45–55.

Bond WF, Kostenbader M, McCarthy JF. Prehospital and hospital-based health care providers' experience with a human patient simulator. Prehosp Emerg Care 2001;5:284–7.

Bower JO. Using patient simulators to train surgical team members. AORN J 1997;65:805–8.

Bradley P, Postlethwaite K. Simulation in clinical learning. Med Educ 2003;37(Suppl 1):1–5.

Byrne AJ, Hilton PJ, Lunn JN. Basic simulations for anaesthetists: a pilot study of the ACCESS system. Anaesthesia 1994;49:376–81.

Cain JG, Kofke A, Sinz EH, Barbaccia JJ, Rosen KR. The West Virginia University human crisis simulation program. Am J Anesthesiol 2000;27:215–20.

Chopra V, Engbers FH, Geerts MJ, Filet WR, Bovill JG, Spierdijk J. The Leiden anaesthesia simulator. Br J Anaesth 1994;73:287–92.

Cooper JB, Gaba DM. A strategy for preventing anesthesia accidents. Int Anesthesiol Clin 1989;27:148–52.

Davies JM, Helmreich RL. Simulation: it's a start. Can J Anaesth 1996;43:425–9.

Daykin AP, Bacon RJ. An epidural injection simulator. Anaesthesia 1990;45:235–6.

Denson JS, Abrahamson S. A computer-controlled patient simulator. JAMA 1969;208:504–8.

Doyle D, Arellano R. The virtual anesthesiology training simulation system. Can J Anesth 1994;42:267–73.

Edgar P. Medium fidelity manikins and medical student teaching. Anesthesia 2002;57:1214–5.

Ellis C, Hughes G. Use of human patient simulation to teach emergency medicine trainees advanced airway skills. J Accid Emerg Med 1999;16:395–9.

Euliano TY. Small group teaching: clinical correlation with a human patient simulator. Adv Physiol Educ 2001;25(1–4):36–43.

Euliano TY. Teaching respiratory physiology: clinical correlation with a human patient simulator. J Clin Monit Comput 2000;16:465–70.

Euliano T, Good ML. Simulator training in anesthesia growing rapidly; LORAL model born in Florida. J Clin Monit 1997;13:53–7.

Euliano TY, Mahla ME. Problem-based learning in residency education: a novel implementation using a simulator. J Clin Monit Comput 1999;15:227–32.

Fallacaro MD. Untoward pathophysiological events: simulation as an experiential learning option to prepare anesthesia providers. CRNA 2000;11:138–43.

Fish MP, Flanagan B. Incorporation of a realistic anesthesia simulator into an anesthesia clerkship. In: Henson LC, Lee A, Basford A (eds) Simulators in Anesthesiology Education. New York: Plenum; 1998. p. 115–9.

Flexman RE, Stark EA. Training simulators. In: Salvendy G (ed) Handbook of Human Factors. New York: Wiley; 1987. p. 1012–38.

Forrest F, Bowers M. A useful application of a technical scoring system: identification and subsequent correction of inadequacies of an anaesthetic assistants training programme. Presented at the International Meeting on Medical Simulation, San Diego, 2003.

Freid EB. Integration of the human patient simulator into the medical student curriculum: life support skills. In: Henson LC, Lee A, Basford A (eds) Simulators in Anesthesiology Education. New York: Plenum; 1998. p. 15–21.

Friedrich MJ. Practice makes perfect: risk-free medical training with patient simulators. JAMA 2002;288:2808, 2811–2.

Gaba D, Fish K, Howard S. Crisis Management in Anesthesiology. New York: Churchill Livingstone, 1994.

Gaba DM. Anaesthesia simulators [editorial]. Can J Anaesth 1995;42:952–3.

Gaba DM. Anaesthesiology as a model for patient safety in health care. BMJ 2000;320:785–8.

Gaba D. Dynamic decision making in anesthesiology: cognitive models and training approaches. In: Evans D, Patel V (eds) Advanced Models of Cognition for Medical Training and Practice. Berlin: Springer; 1992. p. 123–47.

Gaba D. Dynamic decision-making in anesthesiology: use of realistic simulation for training. Presented at the Nato Advanced Research Workshop: Advanced Models for Cognition for Medical Training and Practice, Krakow, August 1991.

Gaba D. Human error in anesthetic mishaps. Int Anesthesiol Clin 1989;27:137–47.

Gaba DM. Simulation-based crisis resource management training for trauma care. Am J Anesthesiol 2000;5:199–200.

Gaba DM. Simulator training in anesthesia growing rapidly: CAE model born at Stanford. J Clin Monit 1996;12:195–8.

Gaba DM. Two examples of how to evaluate the impact of new approaches to teaching [editorial]. Anesthesiology 2002; 96:1–2.

Gaba DM, Small SD. How can full environment-realistic patient simulators be used for performance assessment. American Society of Anesthesia Newsletter 1997 (http://www.asahq.org/newsletters/1997/10_97/HowCan_1097.html). Accessed on May 22, 2001.

Gaba DM, Howard SK, Small SD. Situation awareness in anesthesiology. Hum Factors 1995;37:20–31.

Gaba DM, Maxwell M, DeAnda A. Anesthetic mishaps: breaking the chain of accident evaluation. Anesthesiology 1987;66:670–6.

Garden A, Robinson B, Weller J, Wilson L, Crone D. Education to address medical error—a role for high fidelity patient simulation. N Z Med J 2002;22;115:133–4.

Girard M, Drolet P. Anesthesiology simulators: networking is the key. Can J Anaesth 2002;49:647–9.

Glavin R, Greaves D. The problem of coordinating simulator-based instruction with experience in the real workplace. Br J Anaesth 2003;91:309–11.

Good ML. Simulators in anesthesiology: the excitement continues. American Society of Anesthesia Newsletter (1997.http://www.asahq.org/newsletters/1997/10_97/SimInAnes_1097.html).

Goodwin MWP, French GWG. Simulation as a training and assessment tool in the management of failed intubation in obstetrics. Int J Obstet Anesth 2001;10:273–7.

Gordon JA. A simulator-based medical education service. Acad Emerg Med 2002;9:865.

Gordon JA, Pawlowski J. Education on-demand: the development of a simulator-based medical education service. Acad Med 2002;77:751–2.

Grant WD. Addition of anesthesia patient simulator is an improvement to evaluation process. Anesth Analg 2002;95:786.

Gravenstein JS. Training devices and simulators. Anesthesiology 1998;69:295–7.

Grevnik A, Schaefer JJ. Medical simulation training coming of age. Crit Care Med 2004;32:2549–50.

Halamek LP, Kaegi DM, Gaba DM, Sowb YA, Smith BC, Smith BE, et al. Time for a new paradigm in pediatric medical education: teaching neonatal resuscitation in a simulated delivery room environment. Pediatrics 2000;106:E45.

Hartmannsgruber M, Good M, Carovano R, Lampotang S, Gravenstein JS. Anesthesia simulators and training devices. Anaesthetists 1993;42:462–9.

Helmreich RL, Davies JM. Anaesthetic simulation and lessons to be learned from aviation. Can J Anaesth 1997;44:907–12.

Helmreich RL, Chidester T, Foushee H, Gregorich S. Anesthesia crisis resource management: real-life simulation training in operating room crises. J Clin Anesth 1990;7:675–87.

Hendrickse AD, Ellis AM, Morris RW. Use of simulation technology in Australian Defence Force resuscitation training. J R Army Med Corps 2001;147:173–8.

Henrichs B. Development of a module for teaching the cricothyrotomy procedure. Presented at the Society for Technology in Anesthesia Annual Meeting, San Diego, 1999.

Henriksen K, Moss F. From the runway to the airway and beyond: embracing simulation and team training—now is the time. Qual Saf Health Care 2004;13(Suppl 1):i1.

Henry J, Murray W. Increasing teaching efficiency and minimizing expense in the sim lab. Presented at the International Meeting on Medical Simulation, San Diego, 2003.

Henson LC, Richardson MG, Stern DH, Shekhter I. Using human patient simulator to credential first year anesthesiology residents for taking overnight call [abstract]. Presented at the 2nd Annual International Meeting on Medical Simulation, 2002.

Hoffman KI, Abrahamson S. The 'cost-effectiveness' of Sim One. J Med Educ 1975;50:1127–8.

Howells R, Madar J. Newborn resuscitation training—which manikin. Resuscitation 2002;54:175–81.

Howells TH, Emery FM, Twentyman JE. Endotracheal intubation training using a simulator: an evaluation of the Laerdal adult intubation model in the teaching of endotracheal intubation. Br J Anaesth 1973;45:400–2.

Iserson KV, Chiasson PM. The ethics of applying new medical technologies. Semin Laparosc Surg 2002;9:222–9.

Iserson KV. Simulating our future: real changes in medical education. Acad Med 1999;74:752–4.

Jensen RS, Biegelski C. Cockpit resource management. In: Jensen RS (ed) Aviation Psychology. Aldershot: Gower Technical; 1989. p. 176–209.

Jorm C. Patient safety and quality: can anaesthetists play a greater role? Anaesthesia 2003;58:833–4.

Kapur PA, Steadman RH. Patient simulator competency testing: ready for takeoff? Anesth Analg 1998;86:1157–9.

Kaye K, Frascone RJ, Held T. Prehospital rapid-sequence intubation: a pilot training program. Prehosp Emerg Care 2003;7:235–40.

King PH, Pierce D, Higgins M, Beattie C, Waitman LR. A proposed method for the measurement of anesthetist care variability. J Clin Monit Comput 2000;16:121–5.

King PH, Blanks ST, Rummel DM, Patterson D. Simulator training in anesthesiology: an answer? Biomed Instrum Technol 1996;30:341–5.

Kiriaka J. EMS roadshow. JEMS 2000;25:40–7.

Kneebone R. Simulation in surgical training: educational issues and practical implications. Med Educ 2003;37:267–77.

Kofke WA, Rosen KA, Barbaccia J, Sinz E, Cain J. The value of acute care simulation. WV Med J 2000;96:396–402.

Kurrek MM, Devitt JH. The cost for construction and operation of a simulation centre. Can J Anaesth 1997;44:1191–5.

Kurrek MM, Devitt JH, McLellan BA. Full-scale realistic simulation in Toronto. Am J Anesthesiol 2000;122:226–7.

Lacey O, Hogan J, Flanagan B. High-fidelity simulation team training of junior hospital staff. Presented at the International Meeting on Medical Simulation, San Diego, 2003.

Lampotang S, Ohrn MA, van Meurs WL. A simulator-based respiratory physiology workshop. Acad Med 1996;71:526–7.

Lederman L. Debriefing: a critical reexamination of the postexperience analytic process with implications for its effective use. Simulation Games 1984;15:415–31.

Lederman L. Debriefing: toward a systematic assessment of theory and practice. Simulation Gaming 1992;23:145–60.

Lewis CH, Griffin MJ. Human factors consideration in clinical applications of virtual reality. Stud Health Technol Inform 1997; 44:35–56.

Lippert A, Lippert F, Nielsen J, Jensen PF. Full-scale simulations in Copenhagen. Am J Anesthesiol 2000;27:221–5.

Lopez-Herce J, Carrillo A, Rodriguez-Nunez A. Newborn manikins. Resuscitation 2003;56:232–3.

Mackenzie CF, Group L. Simulation of trauma management: the LOTAS experience. http://134.192.17.4/simulati.html:1–10.

Manser T, Dieckmann P, Rall M. Is the performance of anesthesia by anesthesiologists in the simulator setting the same as in the OR? Presented at the International Meeting on Medical Simulation, San Diego, 2003.

Marsch SCU, Scheidegger DH, Stander S, Harms C. Team training using simulator technology in basel. Am J Anesthesiol 2000;74:209–11.

Martin D, Blezek D, Robb R, Camp, LA. Nauss: Simulation of regional anesthesia using virtual reality for training residents. Anesthesiology 1998;89:A58.

McCarthy M. US military revamps combat medic training and care. Lancet 20038;361:494–5.

Meller G. Typology of simulators for medical education. J Digit Imaging 1997;10(Suppl 1):194–6.

Meller G, Tepper R, Bergman M, Anderhub B. The tradeoffs of successful simulation. Stud Health Technol Inform 1997;39: 565–71.

Miller GE. The assessment of clinical skills/competence/ performance. Acad Med 1990;65:S63–7.

Mondello E, Montanini S. New techniques in training and education: simulator-based approaches to anesthesia and intensive care. Minerva Anestesiol 2002;68:715–8.

Morhaim DK, Heller MB. The practice of teaching endotracheal intubation on recently deceased patients. J Emerg Med 1991;9: 515–8.

Mukherjee J, Down J, Jones M, Seig, S, Martin, G, Maze M. Simulator teaching for final year medical students: subjective assessment of knowledge and skills. Presented at the International Meeting on Medical Simulation, San Diego, 2003.

Murray DJ. Clinical simulation: technical novelty or innovation in education. Anesthesiology 1998;89:1–2.

Murray WB, Foster PA. Crisis resource management among strangers: principles of organizing a multidisciplinary group for crisis resource management. J Clin Anesth 2000;12:633–8.

Murray W, Good M, Gravenstein J, Brasfield W. Novel application of a full human simulator: training with remifentanil prior to human use. Anesthesiology 1998;89:A56.

Murray W, Gorman P, Lieser J, Haluck RS, Krummel TM, Vaduva S. The psychomotor learning curve with a force feedback trainer: a pilot study. Presented at the Society for Technology in Anesthesia Annual Meeting, San Diego, 1999.

Murray W, Proctor L, Henry J, Abicht D, Gorman PJ, Vaduva S, et al. Crisis resource management (CRM) training using the Medical Education Technologies, Inc. (METI) simulator: the first year. Presented at the Society for Technology in Anesthesia Annual Meeting, San Diego, 1999.

Norman G. Editorial: simulation—savior or Satan? Adv Health Sci Educ Theory Pract 2003;8(1):1–3.

Norman J, Wilkins D. Simulators for anesthesia. J Clin Monit 1996;12:91–9.

O'Brien G, Haughton A, Flanagan B. Interns' perceptions of performance and confidence in participating in and managing simulated and real cardiac arrest situations. Med Teach 2001;23:389–95.

Olympio MA. Simulation saves lives. ASA Newslett 2001:15–9.

Palmisano J, Akingbola O, Moler F, Custer J. Simulated pediatric cardiopulmonary resuscitation: initial events and response times of a hospital arrest team. Respir Care 1994;39:725–9.

Paskin S, Raemer DB, Garfield JM, Philip JH. Is computer simulation of anesthetic uptake and distribution an effective tool for anesthesia residents? J Clin Monit 1985;1:165–73.

Raemer D. In-hospital resuscitation: team training using simulation. Presented at the 1999 Society for Education in Anesthesia Spring Meeting. Rochester, NY, 1999.

Raemer DB, Barron DM. Use of simulators for education and training in nonanesthesia healthcare domains. American Society of Anesthesia Newsletter 1997. Available at: http://www.asahq.org/newsletter/1997/10_97/UsesOf_1097. html.

Raemer D, Barron D, Blum R, Frenna T, Sica GT, et al. Teaching crisis management in radiology using realistic simulation. In: 1998 Meeting of the Society for Technology in Anesthesia, Orlando, FL, 1998, p. 28.

Raemer D, Graydon-Baker E, Malov S. Simulated computerized medical records for scenarios. Presented at the 2001 International Meeting on Medical Simulation. Scottsdale, AZ, 2001.

Raemer D, Mavigilia S, Van Horne C, Stone P. Mock codes: using realistic simulation to teach team resuscitation management. In: 1998 Meeting of the Society for Technology in Anesthesia. Orlando, FL, 1998, p. 29.

Raemer D, Morris G, Gardner R, Walzer TB, Beatty T, Mueller KB, et al. Development of a simulation-based labor & delivery team course. Presented at the International Meeting on Medical Simulation, San Diego, 2003.

Raemer D, Shapiro N, Lifferth G, Blum RM, Edlow J. Testing probes, a new method of measuring teamwork attributes in simulated scenarios. Presented at the 2001 International Meeting on Medical Simulation, Scottsdale, AZ, 2001.

Raemer D, Sunder N, Gardner R, Walzer TB, Cooper J, et al. Using simulation to practice debriefing medical error. Presented at the International Meeting on Medical Simulation, San Diego, 2003.

Rall M, Gaba D. Human performance and patient safety. In: Miller RD (ed) Miller's Anesthesia, 6th ed. Philadelphia: Elsevier; 2005.

Rall M, Manser T, Guggenberger H, Gaba DM, Unertl K. [Patient safety and errors in medicine: development, prevention and analyses of incidents.] Anasthesiol Intensivmed Notfallmed Schmerzther 2001;36:321–30.

Rall M, Schaedle B, Zieger J, Naef W, Weinlich M. Innovative training for enhancing patient safety: safety culture and integrated concepts. Unfallchirurg 2002;105:1033–42.

Riley R, Grauze A, Chinnery C, Horley R. The first two years of "CASMS," the world's busiest medical simulation center. Presented at the International Meeting on Medical Simulation, San Diego, 2003.

Riley RH, Wilks DH, Freeman JA. Anaesthetists' attitudes towards an anaesthesia simulator: a comparative survey: U.S.A. and Australia. Anaesth Intensive Care 1997;25:514–9.

Rizkallah N, Carter T, Essin D, Johnson C, Steen SN, et al. Mini-sim: a human patient simulator. Presented at the Society for Technology in Anesthesia Annual Meeting, San Diego, 1999.

Robinson B, Little J, McCullough S, Lange R, Lamond C, Levack W, et al. Simulation based training for allied health professionals: physiotherapy respiratory workshop. Presented at the International Meeting on Medical Simulation, San Diego, 2003.

Rubinshtein R, Robenshtok E, Eisenkraft A, Vidan A, Hourvitz A. Training Israeli medical personnel to treat casualties of nuclear, biologic and chemical warfare. Isr Med Assoc J 2002;4:545–8.

Rudolph J, Raemer D. Using collaborative inquiry to debrief simulated crisis events: lessons from action science. Presented at the 2001 International Meeting on Medical Simulation, Scottsdale, AZ, 2001.

Rutherford W. Aviation safety: a model for health care? It is time to rethink the institutions and processes through which health care is delivered if a "culture of safety" is to be achieved. Qual Saf Health Care 2003;12:162–4.

Sanders J, Haas RE, Geisler M, Lupien AE. Using the human patient simulator to test the efficacy of an experimental emergency percutaneous transtracheal airway. Mil Med 1998;163: 544–51.

Sarman I, Bolin D, Holmer I, Tunell R. Assessment of thermal conditions in neonatal care: use of a manikin of premature baby size. Am J Perinatol 1992;9:239–46.

Satish U, Streufert S. Value of a cognitive simulation in medicine: towards optimizing decision making performance of healthcare personnel. Qual Saf Health Care 2002;11:163–7.

Schaefer JJ, Gonzalez RM. Dynamic simulation: a new tool for difficult airway training of professional healthcare providers. Am J Anesthesiol 2000;27:232–42.

Schaivone K, Jenkins L, Mallott D, Budd N. Development of a comprehensive simulation experience: a faculty training project. Presented at the International Meeting on Medical Simulation, San Diego, 2003.

Scherer YK, Bruce SA, Graves BT, Erdley WS. Acute care nurse practitioner education: enhancing performance through the use of clinical simulation. AACN Clin Issues 2003;14:331–41.

Schlindwein M, von Wagner G, Kirst M, Rajewicz M, Karl F, Schochlin J, et al. Mobile patient simulator for resuscitation training with automatic external defibrillators. Biomed Tech (Berl) 2002;47(Suppl 1):559–60.

Schweiger J, Preece J. Authenticity of the METI anesthesia patient simulator: medical students' perception. Crit Care Med 1995;23:432–3.

Schwid HA, O'Donnell D. The Anesthesia Simulator Consultant: simulation plus expert system. Anesthesiol Rev 1993;20:185–9.

Schwid H. An educational simulator for the management of myocardial ischemia. Anesth Analg 1989;68:S248.

Shapiro MJ, Simmons W. High fidelity medical simulation: a new paradigm in medical education. Med Health R I 2002;85:316–7.

Sheplock G, Thomas P, Camporesi E. An interactive computer program for teaching regional anesthesia. Anesthesiol Rev 1993;20:53–9.

Sikorski J, Jebson P, Hauser P. Computer-aided instruction simulating intraoperative vents in anesthesia residents training. Anesthesiology 1983;59:A470.

Skartwed R, Ferguson S, Eichorn M, Wilks D. Using different educational modalities to optimize efficiency in an interdisciplinary simulation center. Presented at the International Meeting on Medical Simulation, San Diego, 2003.

Small S. What participants learn from anesthesia crisis resource management training. Anesthesiology 1998;89:A71.

Small SD, Wuerz RC, Simon R, Shapiro N, Conn A, Setnik G. Demonstration of high-fidelity simulation team training for emergency medicine. Acad Emerg Med 1999;6:312–23.

Smith B, Gaba D. Simulators in clinical monitoring: practical application. In: Lake C, Blitt C, Hines R (eds) Clinical Monitoring: Practical Applications for Anesthesia and Critical Care. Philadelphia: Saunders; 2001. p. 26–44.

Sowb YA, Kiran K, Reznek M, Smith-Coggins R, Harter P, Stafford-Cecil S, et al. Development of a three-level curriculum for crisis resource management training in emergency medicine. Presented at the International Meeting on Medical Simulation, San Diego, 2003.

Stern D. Improving resuscitation team performance using a full body simulator. Presented at the 2001 International Meeting on Medical Simulation, Ft. Lauderdale, FL, 2001.

Taekman J, Andregg B. SimDot: an interdisciplinary web portal for human simulation. Presented at the International Meeting on Medical Simulation, San Diego, 2003.

Taekman J, Eck J, Hobbs G. Integration of PGY-1 anesthesia residents in simulation development. Presented at the International Meeting on Medical Simulation, San Diego, 2003.

Takayesu J, Gordon J, Farrell S, Evans AJ, Sullivan JE, Pawlowski J. Learning emergency medicine and critical care medicine: what does high-fidelity patient simulation teach? Acad Emerg Med 2002;9:476–7 (abstract 319).

Tan G, Ti L, Suresh S, Lee T-L. Human patient simulator is an effective way of teaching physiology to first year medical students. Presented at the International Conference on Medical Simulation, Ft. Lauderdale, FL, 2001.

Tarver S. Anesthesia simulators: concepts and applications. Am J Anesthesiol 1999;26:393–6.

Tarver S. A relational database to improve scenario and event design on the MidSim simulator. Presented at the International Meeting on Medical Simulation, Ft. Lauderdale, FL, 2001.

Tebich S, Loeb R. Using patient simulation to train CA-1 residents' rule-based decision making. Presented at the International Meeting on Medical Simulation, San Diego, 2003.

Thompson W, Pinder M, See J, Chinnery C, Grauze A. Simulation training for the medical emergency team of a metropolitan teaching hospital. Presented at the International Meeting on Medical Simulation, San Diego, 2003.

Underberg K. Multidisciplinary resource management: value as perceived by nurses. Presented at the 2001 International Meeting on Medical Simulation, Scottsdale, AZ.

Underberg K. Nurses' perceptions of a crisis management (malignant hyperthermia) with a full human simulator. Presented at the International Meeting on Medical Simulation, Scottsdale, AZ, 2001.

Vadodaria B, Gandhi S, McIndoe A. Selection of an emergency cricothyroidotomy kit for clinical use by dynamic evaluation on a (METI) human patient simulator. Presented at the International Meeting on Medical Simulation, San Diego, 2003.

Via DK, Kyle RR, Trask JD, Shields CH, Mongan PD. Using high-fidelity patient simulation and an advanced distance education network to teach pharmacology to second-year medical students. J Clin Anesth 2004;16:142–3.

Von Lubitz D. Medical training at sea using human patient simulator. Presented at the International Meeting on Medical Simulation, Scottsdale, AZ, 2001.

Wass V, Van der Vleuten C, Shatzer J, Jones R. Assessment of clinical competence. Lancet 2001;357:945–9.

Watterson L, Flanagan B, Donovan B, Robinson B. Anaesthetic simulators: training for the broader health-care profession. Aust N Z J Surg 2000;70:735–7.

Weinger MB, Gonzalez D, Slagle J, Syeed M. Videotaping of anesthesia non-routine events. Presented at the International Meeting on Medical Simulation, San Diego, 2003.

Weinger MB, Raemer DB, Barker SJ. A new Anesthesia & Analgesia section on technology, computing, and simulation. Anesth Analg 2001;93:1085–7.

Westenskow D, Runco C, Tucker S, Haak S, Joyce S, Johnson S, et al. Human simulators extend an anesthesiology department's educational role. Presented at the Society for Technology in Anesthesia Annual Meeting, San Diego, 1999.

Woods DD. Coping with complexity: the psychology of human behavior in complex systems. In: Goodstein LP, Andersen HB, Olsen SE (eds) Tasks, Errors, and Mental Models. London: Taylor & Francis; 1988. p. 128–48.

Wright M, Skartwed R, Jaramillo Y. Management of a postpartum hemorrhage using the full body human patient simulator. Presented at the International Meeting on Medical Simulation, San Diego, 2003.

Ziv A, Wolpe PR, Small SD, Glick S. Simulation-based medical education: an ethical imperative. Acad Med 2003;78:783–8.

Ziv A, Donchin Y, Rotstein Z. National medical simulation center in Israel: a comprehensive model. Presented at the International Meeting on Medical Simulation, Scottsdale, AZ, 2001.

"It Stands to Reason" Articles in Nonanesthesia Disciplines

Aabakken L, Adamsen S, Kruse A. Performance of a colonoscopy simulator: experience from a hands-on endoscopy course. Endoscopy 2000;32:911–3.

Adrales GL, Chu UB, Witzke DB, Donnelly MB, Hoskins D, Mastrangelo MJ Jr, et al. Evaluating minimally invasive surgery training using low-cost mechanical simulations. Surg Endosc 2003;17:580–5.

Barker VL. CathSim. Stud Health Technol Inform 1999;62:36–7.

Barker VL. Virtual reality: from the development laboratory to the classroom. Stud Health Technol Inform 1997;39:539–42.

Bar-Meir S. A new endoscopic simulator. Endoscopy 2000;32: 898–900.

Baur C, Guzzoni D, Georg O. VIRGY: a virtual reality and force feedback based endoscopic surgery simulator. Stud Health Technol Inform 1998;50:110–6.

Beard JD. The Sheffield basic surgical training scheme. Ann R Coll Surg Engl 1999;81(Suppl):298–301, 307.

Bholat OS, Haluck RS, Kutz RH, Gorman PJ, Krummel TM. Defining the role of haptic feedback in minimally invasive surgery. Stud Health Technol Inform 1999;62:62–6.

Bloom MB, Rawn CL, Salzberg AD, Krummel TM. Virtual reality applied to procedural testing: the next era. Ann Surg 2003; 237:442–8.

Bro-Nielsen M, Tasto JL, Cunningham R, Merril GL. PreOp endoscopic simulator: a PC-based immersive training system for bronchoscopy. Stud Health Technol Inform 1999;62:76–82.

Bro-Nielsen M, Helfrick D, Glass B, Zeng X, Connacher H. VR simulation of abdominal trauma surgery. Stud Health Technol Inform 1998;50:117–23.

Bruce S, Bridges EJ, Holcomb JB. Preparing to respond: Joint Trauma Training Center and USAF Nursing Warskills Simulation Laboratory. Crit Care Nurs Clin North Am 2003;15:149–62.

Burd LI, Motew M, Bieniarz J. A teaching simulator for fetal scalp sampling. Obstet Gynecol 1972;39:418–20.

Cakmak, HK, Kühnapfel U. Animation and simulation techniques for VR-training systems in endoscopic surgery. http://citeseer.nj.nec.com/cakmak00animation.html, 2000.

Caudell TP, Summers KL, Holten J 4th, Hakamata T, Mowafi M, Jacobs J, et al. Virtual patient simulator for distributed collaborative medical education. Anat Rec 2003;270B:23–9.

Chester R, Watson MJ. A newly developed spinal simulator. Man Ther 2000;5:234–42.

Cotin S, Dawson SL, Meglan D, Shaffer DW, Ferrell MA, Bardsley RS, et al. ICTS, an interventional cardiology training system. Stud Health Technol Inform 2000;70:59–65.

Dawson S, Kaufman J. The imperative for medical simulation. Proc IEEE 1998;86:479–83.

De Leo G, Ponder M, Molet T, Fato M, Thalmann D, Magnenat-Thalmann N, et al. A virtual reality system for the training of volunteers involved in health emergency situations. Cyberpsychol Behav 2003;6:267–74.

Dev P, Heinrichs WL, Srivastava S, Montgomery KN, Senger S, Temkin B, et al. Simulated learning environments in anatomy and surgery delivered via the next generation Internet. Medinfo 2001;10:1014–8.

Dev P, Montgomery K, Senger S, Heinrichs WL, Srivastava S, Waldron K. Simulated medical learning environments on the Internet. J Am Med Inform Assoc 2002;9:437–47.

Eaves RH, Flagg AJ. The U.S. Air Force pilot simulated medical unit: a teaching strategy with multiple applications. J Nurs Educ 2001;40:110–5.

Ecke U, Klimek L, Muller W, Ziegler R, Mann W. Virtual reality: preparation and execution of sinus surgery. Comput Aided Surg 1998;3:45–50.

Edmond CV Jr, Wiet GJ, Bolger B. Virtual environments: surgical simulation in otolaryngology. Otolaryngol Clin North Am 1998;31:369–81.

El-Khalili N, Brodlie K, Kessel D. WebSTer: a web-based surgical training system. Stud Health Technol Inform 2000;70:69–75.

Englmeier KH, Haubner M, Krapichler C, Reiser M. A new hybrid renderer for virtual bronchoscopy. Stud Health Technol Inform 1999;62:109–15.

Fellander-Tsai L, Stahre C, Anderberg B, Barle H, Bringman S, Kjellin A, et al. Simulator training in medicine and health care: a new pedagogic model for good patient safety. Lakartidningen 20015;98:3772–6.

Frey M, Riener R, Burgkart R, Proll T. Initial results with the Munich knee simulator. Biomed Tech (Berl) 2002;47(Suppl 1):704–7.

Gordon MS. Cardiology patient simulator: development of an animated manikin to teach cardiovascular disease. Am J Cardiol 1974;34:350–5.

Gordon MS. Learning from a cardiology patient stimulator. RN 1975;38:ICU1, ICU4, ICU6.

Gordon MS, Ewy GA, Felner JM, Forker AD, Gessner IH, Juul D, et al. A cardiology patient simulator for continuing education of family physicians. J Fam Pract 1981;13:353–6.

Gordon MS, Ewy GA, Felner JM, Forker AD, Gessner I, McGuire C, et al. Teaching bedside cardiologic examination skills using "Harvey," the cardiology patient simulator. Med Clin North Am 1980;64:305–13.

Gorman PJ, Lieser JD, Murray WB, Haluck RS, Krummell TM. Evaluation of skill acquisition using a force feedback, virtual reality based surgical trainer. Stud Health Technol Inform 1999;62:121–3.

Grantcharov TP, Rodenberg J, Pahle E, Funch-Jensen PF. Virtual reality computer simulation: an objective method for the evaluation of laparoscopic surgical skills. Surg Endosc 2001;15:242–4.

Grosfeld JL. Presidential address: visions: medical education and surgical training in evolution. Arch Surg 1999;134:590–8.

Gunther SB, Soto GE, Colman WW. Interactive computer simulations of knee-replacement surgery. Acad Med 2002;77:753–4.

Hahn JK, Kaufman R, Winick AB, Carleton T, Park Y, Lindeman R, et al. Training environment for inferior vena caval filter placement. Stud Health Technol Inform 1998;50:291–7.

Hanna GB, Drew Y, Clinch P, Hunter B, Cuschieri A. Computer-controlled endoscopic performance assessment system. Surg Endosc 1998;12:997–1000.

Hanna GB, Drew T, Clinch P, Hunter B, Shimi S, Dunkley P, et al. A micro-processor controlled psychomotor tester for minimal access surgery. Surg Endosc 1996;10:965–9.

Hanna GB, Drew T, Cuschieri A. Technology for psychomotor skills testing in endoscopic surgery. Semin Laparosc Surg 1997;4:120–4.

Hasson HM. Improving video laparoscopy skills with repetitive simulator training. Chicago Med 1998;101:12–5.

Heimansohn H. A new orthodontic teaching simulator. Dent Dig 1969;75:62–4.

Henkel TO, Potempa DM, Rassweiler J, Manegold BC, Alken P. Lap simulator, animal studies, and the Laptent: bridging the gap between open and laparoscopic surgery. Surg Endosc 1993;7:539–43.

Hikichi T, Yoshida A, Igarashi S, Mukai N, Harada M, Muroi K, et al. Vitreous surgery simulator. Arch Ophthalmol 2000;118:1679–81.

Hilbert M, Muller W. Virtual reality in endonasal surgery. Stud Health Technol Inform 1997;39:237–45.

Hilbert M, Muller W, Strutz J. Development of a surgical simulator for interventions of the paranasal sinuses: technical principles and initial prototype. Laryngorhinootologie 1998;77:153–6.

Hochberger J, Maiss J, Hahn EG. The use of simulators for training in GI endoscopy. Endoscopy 2002;34:727–9.

Hubal RC, Kizakevich PN, Guinn CI, Merino KD, West SL. The virtual standardized patient: simulated patient-practitioner dialog for patient interview training. Stud Health Technol Inform 2000;70:133–8.

Iserson KV. Simulating our future: real changes in medical education. Acad Med 1999;74:752–4.

Iserson KV, Chiasson PM. The ethics of applying new medical technologies. Semin Laparosc Surg 2002;9:222–9.

John NW, Phillips N. Surgical simulators using the WWW. Stud Health Technol Inform 2000;70:146–52.

John NW, Riding M, Phillips NI, Mackay S, Steineke L, Fontaine B, et al. Web-based surgical educational tools. Stud Health Technol Inform 2001;81:212–7.

Johnson L, Thomas G, Dow S, Stanford C. An initial evaluation of the Iowa Dental Surgical Simulator. J Dent Educ 2000;64:847–53.

Johnston R, Weiss P. Analysis of virtual reality technology applied in education. Minim Invasive Ther Allied Technol 1997;6:126–7.

Jones R, McIndoe A. Non-consultant career grades (NCCG) at the Bristol Medical Simulation Centre (BMSC). Presented at the International Meeting on Medical Simulation, San Diego, 2003.

Karnath B, Frye AW, Holden MD. Incorporating simulators in a standardized patient exam. Acad Med 2002;77:754–5.

Karnath B, Thornton W, Frye AW. Teaching and testing physical examination skills without the use of patients. Acad Med 2002;77:753.

Kaufmann C, Liu A. Trauma training: virtual reality applications. Stud Health Technol Inform 2001;81:236–41.

Keyser EJ, Derossis AM, Antoniuk M, Sigman HH, Fried GM. A simplified simulator for the training and evaluation of laparoscopic skills. Surg Endosc 2000;14:149–53.

Kneebone R. Simulation in surgical training: educational issues and practical implications. Med Educ 2003;37:267–77.

Kneebone R, ApSimon D. Surgical skills training: simulation and multimedia combined. Med Educ 2001;35:909–15.

Kneebone R, Kidd J, Nestel D, Asvall S, Paraskeva P, Darzi A. An innovative model for teaching and learning clinical procedures. Med Educ 2002;36:628–34.

Knudson MM, Sisley AC. Training residents using simulation technology: experience with ultrasound for trauma. J Trauma 2000;48:659–65.

Krummel TM. Surgical simulation and virtual reality: the coming revolution. Ann Surg 1998;228:635–7.

Kuhnapfel U, Kuhn C, Hubner M, Krumm H, Mass H, Neisus B. The Karlsruhe endoscopic surgery trainer as an example for virtual reality in medical education. Minim Invasive Ther Allied Technol 1997;6:122–5.

Kuppersmith RB, Johnston R, Jones SB, Jenkins HA. Virtual reality surgical simulation and otolaryngology. Arch Otolaryngol Head Neck Surg 1996;122:1297–8.

LaCombe DM, Gordon DL, Issenberg SB, Vega AI. The use of standardized simulated patients in teaching and evaluating prehospital care providers. Am J Anesthesiol 2000;4:201–4.

Ladas SD, Malfertheiner P, Axon A. An introductory course for training in endoscopy. Dig Dis 2002;20:242–5.

Laguna Pes MP. [Teaching in endourology and simulators.] Arch Esp Urol 2002;55:1185–8.

Lucero RS, Zarate JO, Espiniella F, Davolos J, Apud A, Gonzalez B, et al. Introducing digestive endoscopy with the "SimPrac-EDF y VEE" simulator, other organ models, and mannequins: teaching experience in 21 courses attended by 422 physicians. Endoscopy 1995;27:93–100.

Mabrey JD, Gillogly SD, Kasser JR, Sweeney HJ, Zarins B, Mevis H, et al. Virtual reality simulation of arthroscopy of the knee. Arthroscopy 2002;18:E28.

Majeed AW, Reed MW, Johnson AG. Simulated laparoscopic cholecystectomy. Ann R Coll Surg Engl 1992;74:70–1.

Manyak MJ, Santangelo K, Hahn J, Kaufman R, Carleton T, Hua XC, et al. Virtual reality surgical simulation for lower urinary tract endoscopy and procedures. J Endourol 2002;16:185–90.

Marescaux J, Clement JM, Tassetti V, Koehl C, Cotin S, Russier Y, et al. Virtual reality applied to hepatic surgery simulation: the next revolution. Ann Surg 1998;228:627–34.

McCarthy AD, Hollands RJ. A commercially viable virtual reality knee arthroscopy training system. Stud Health Technol Inform 1998;50:302–8.

Medical Readiness Trainer Team. Immersive virtual reality platform for medical training: a "killer-application." Stud Health Technol Inform 2000;70:207–13.

Medina M. Formidable challenges to teaching advanced laparoscopic skills. JSLS 2001;5:153–8.

Medina M. The laparoscopic-ring simulation trainer. JSLS 2002;6:69–75.

Merril GL, Barker VL. Virtual reality debuts in the teaching laboratory in nursing. J Intraven Nurs 1996;19:182–7.

Michel MS, Knoll T, Kohrmann KU, Alken P. The URO Mentor: development and evaluation of a new computer-based interactive training system for virtual life-like simulation of diagnostic and therapeutic endourological procedures. BJU Int 2002;89:174–7.

Molin SO, Jiras A, Hall-Angeras M, Falk A, Martens D, Gilja OH, et al. Virtual reality in surgical practice in vitro and in vivo evaluations. Stud Health Technol Inform 1997;39:246–53.

Munro A, Park KG, Atkinson D, Day RP, Capperauld I. A laparoscopic surgical simulator. J R Coll Surg Edinb 1994;39:176–7.

Munro A, Park KG, Atkinson D, Day RP, Capperauld I. Skin simulation for minor surgical procedures. J R Coll Surg Edinb 1994;39:174–6.

Neame R, Murphy B, Stitt F, Rake M. Virtual medical school life in 2025: a student's diary. BMJ 1999;319:1296.

Neumann M, Mayer G, Ell C, Felzmann T, Reingruber B, Horbach T, et al. The Erlangen Endo-Trainer: life-like simulation for diagnostic and interventional endoscopic retrograde cholangiography. Endoscopy 2000;32:906–10.

Oppenheimer P, Weghorst S, Williams L, Ali A, Cain J, MacFarlane M, et al. Laparoscopic surgical simulator and port placement study. Stud Health Technol Inform 2000;70:233–5.

Owa AO, Gbejuade HO, Giddings C. A middle-ear simulator for practicing prosthesis placement for otosclerosis surgery using ward-based materials. J Laryngol Otol 2003;117:490–2.

Pawlowski J, Graydon-Baker E, Gallagher M, Cahalane M, Raemer DB. Can progress notes and bedside presentations be used to evaluate medical student understanding in patient simulator based programs? Presented at the 2001 International Meeting on Medical Simulation, Scottsdale, AZ.

Pichichero ME. Diagnostic accuracy, tympanocentesis training performance, and antibiotic selection by pediatric residents in management of otitis media. Pediatrics 2002;110:1064–70.

Poss R, Mabrey JD, Gillogly SD, Kasser JR, Sweeney HJ, Zarins B, et al. Development of a virtual reality arthroscopic knee simulator. J Bone Joint Surg Am 2000;82:1495–9.

Pugh CM, Heinrichs WL, Dev P, Srivastava S, Krummel TM. Use of a mechanical simulator to assess pelvic examination skills. JAMA 2001;286:1021–3.

Radetzky A, Bartsch W, Grospietsch G, Pretschner DP. [SUSILAP-G: a surgical simulator for training minimal invasive interventions in gynecology.] Zentralbl Gynakol 1999;121:110–16.

Raibert M, Playter R, Krummell TM. The use of a virtual reality haptic device in surgical training. Acad Med 1998;73:596–7.

Riener R, Hoogen J, Burgkart R, Buss M, Schmidt G. Development of a multi-modal virtual human knee joint for education and training in orthopaedics. Stud Health Technol Inform 2001;81:410–16.

Rogers DA, Regehr G, Yeh KA, Howdieshell TR. Computer-assisted learning versus a lecture and feedback seminar for teaching a basic surgical technical skill. Am J Surg 1998;175:508–10.

Rosen J, Massimiliano S, Hannaford B, Sinanan M. Objective evaluation of laparoscopic surgical skills using hidden Markov models based on haptic information and tool/tissue interactions. Stud Health Technol Inform 2001;81:417–23.

Ross MD, Twombly A, Lee AW, Cheng R, Senger S. New approaches to virtual environment surgery. Stud Health Technol Inform 1999;62:297–301.

Rudman DT, Stredney D, Sessanna D, Yagel R, Crawfis R, Heskamp D, et al. Functional endoscopic sinus surgery training simulator. Laryngoscope 1998;108:1643–7.

Sackier JM, Berci G, Paz-Partlow M. A new training device for laparoscopic cholecystectomy. Surg Endosc 1991;5:158–9.

Sajid AW, Ewy GA, Felner JM, Gessner I, Gordon MS, Mayer JW, et al. Cardiology patient simulator and computer-assisted instruction technologies in bedside teaching. Med Educ 1990;24:512–17.

Sajid AW, Gordon MS, Mayer JW, Ewy GA, Forker AD, Felner JM, et al. Symposium: a multi-institutional research study on the use of simulation for teaching and evaluating patient examination skills. Annu Conf Res Med Educ 1980;19:349–58.

Satava RM. Improving anesthesiologist's performance by simulating reality. Anesthesiology 1992;76:491–4.

Satava RM. The bio-intelligence age: surgery after the information age. J Gastrointest Surg 2002;6:795–9.

Satava RM. Virtual reality and telepresence for military medicine. Comput Biol Med 1995;25:229–36.

Satava RM. Virtual reality surgical simulator: the first steps. Surg Endosc 1993;7:203–5.

Satava RM. Virtual reality, telesurgery, and the new world order of medicine. J Image Guid Surg 1995;1:12–16.

Satava RM, Fried MP. A methodology for objective assessment of errors: an example using an endoscopic sinus surgery simulator. Otolaryngol Clin North Am 2002;35:1289–301.

Schreiner RL, Stevens DC, Jose JH, Gosling CG, Sternecker L. Infant lumbar puncture: a teaching simulator. Clin Pediatr (Phila) 1981;20:298–9.

Schreiner RL, Gresham EL, Escobedo MB, Gosling CG. Umbilical vessel catheterization: a teaching simulator. Clin Pediatr (Phila) 1978;17:506–8.

Schreiner RL, Gresham EL, Gosling CG, Escobedo MB. Neonatal radial artery puncture: a teaching simulator. Pediatrics 1977;59(Suppl):1054–6.

Sedlack RE, Kolars JC. Colonoscopy curriculum development and performance-based assessment criteria on a computer-based endoscopy simulator. Acad Med 2002;77:750–1.

Senior MA, Southern SJ, Majumder S. Microvascular simulator—a device for micro-anastomosis training. Ann R Coll Surg Engl 2001;83:358–60.

Shapiro SJ, Gordon LA, Daykhovsky L, Senter N. The laparoscopic hernia trainer: the role of a life-like trainer in laparoendoscopic education. Endosc Surg Allied Technol 1994;2:66–8.

Shapiro SJ, Paz-Partlow M, Daykhovsky L, Gordon LA. The use of a modular skills center for the maintenance of laparoscopic skills. Surg Endosc 1996;10:816–19.

Shekhter I, Ward D, Stern D, Papadakos DJ, Jenkins JS. Enhancing a patient simulator to respond to PEEP, PIP, and other ventilation parameters. Presented at the Society for Technology in Anesthesia Annual Meeting, San Diego, 1999.

Sherman KP, Ward JW, Wills DP, Mohsen AM. A portable virtual environment knee arthroscopy training system with objective scoring. Stud Health Technol Inform 1999;62:335–6.

Shimada Y, Nishiwaki K, Cooper JB. Use of medical simulators subject of international study. J Clin Monit Comput 1998;14:499–503.

Sica G, Barron D, Blum R, Frenna TH, Raemer DB. Computerized realistic simulation: a teaching module for crisis management in radiology. AJR Am J Roentgenol 1999;172:301–4.

Smith CD, Farrell TM, McNatt SS, Metreveli RE. Assessing laparoscopic manipulative skills. Am J Surg 2001;181:547–50.

Smith CD, Stubbs J, Hananel D. Simulation technology in surgical education: can we assess manipulative skills and what does it mean to the learner. Stud Health Technol Inform 1998;50:379–80.

Smith S, Wan A, Taffinder N, Read S, Emery R, Darzi A. Early experience and validation work with Procedicus VA—the Prosolvia virtual reality shoulder arthroscopy trainer. Stud Health Technol Inform 1999;62:337–43.

Sorid D, Moore SK. Computer-based simulators hone operating skills before the patient is even touched: the virtual surgeon. Comput Graphics 2000;21:393–404.

Stallkamp J, Wapler M. Development of an educational program for medical ultrasound examinations: Ultra Trainer. Biomed Tech (Berl) 1998;43(Suppl):38–9.

Stallkamp J, Wapler M. UltraTrainer—a training system for medical ultrasound examination. Stud Health Technol Inform 1998;50:298–301.

Stone RJ, McCloy RF. Virtual environment training systems for laparoscopic surgery; at the UK's Wolson Centre for Minimally Invasive Surgery. J Med Virtual Reality 1996;1:42–51.

Stredney D, Sessanna D, McDonald JS, Hiemenz L, Rosenberg LB. A virtual simulation environment for learning epidural anesthesia. Stud Health Technol Inform 1996;29:164–75.

Sutcliffe R, Evans A. Simulated surgeries—feasibility of transfer from region to region. Educ Gen Pract 1998;9:203–10.

Sutton C, McCloy R, Middlebrook A, Chater P, Wilson M, Stone R. MIST VR: a laparoscopic surgery procedures trainer and evaluator. Stud Health Technol Inform 1997;39:598–607.

Szekely G, Bajka M, Brechbuhler C, Dual J, Enzler R, Haller U. Virtual reality based surgery simulation for endoscopic gynaecology. Stud Health Technol Inform 1999;62:351–7.

Taffinder N. Better surgical training in shorter hours. J R Soc Med 1999;92:329–31.

Takashina T, Masuzawa T, Fukui Y. A new cardiac auscultation simulator. Clin Cardiol 1990;13:869–72.

Takashina T, Shimizu M, Katayama H. A new cardiology patient simulator. Cardiology 1997;88:408–13.

Takuhiro K, Matsumoto H, Mochizuki T, Kamikawa Y, Sakamoto Y, Hara Y, et al. Use of dynamic simulation for training Japanese emergency medical technicians to compensate for lack of training opportunities. Presented at the International Meeting on Medical Simulation, San Diego, 2003.

Tasto JL, Verstreken K, Brown JM, Bauer JJ. PreOp endoscopy simulator: from bronchoscopy to ureteroscopy. Stud Health Technol Inform 2000;70:344–9.

Taylor L, Vergidis D, Lovasik A, Crockford P. A skills programme for preclinical medical students. Med Educ 1992;26:448–53.

Tendick F, Downes M, Cavusoglu CM, Gantert W, Way LW. Development of virtual environments for training skills and reducing errors in laparoscopic surgery. In: Boger MS, Charles ST, Grundfest WS, Harrington JA, Katzir A, Lome LS, et al (eds) Proceedings of Surgical Assist Systems. Bellingham, WA: SPIE Optical Engineering Press; 1998. p. 36–44.

Thomas WE, Lee PW, Sunderland GT, Day RP. A preliminary evaluation of an innovative synthetic soft tissue simulation module (Skilltray) for use in basic surgical skills workshops. Ann R Coll Surg Engl 1996;78(Suppl 6):268–71.

Tooley MA, Forrest FC, Mantripp DR. MultiMed—remote interactive medical simulation. J Telemed Telecare 1999;5(Suppl 1):S119–21.

Ursino M, Tasto JL, Nguyen BH, Cunningham R, Merril GL. CathSim: an intravascular catheterization simulator on a PC. Stud Health Technol Inform 1999;62:360–6.

Vahora F, Temkin B, Marcy W, Gorman PJ, Krummel TM, Heinrichs WL. Virtual reality and women's health: a breast biopsy system. Stud Health Technol Inform 1999;62:367–72.

Varghese D, Patel H. An inexpensive and easily constructed laparoscopic simulator. Hosp Med 1998;59:769.

Verma D, Wills D, Verma M. Virtual reality simulator for vitreoretinal surgery. Eye 2003;17:71–3.

Wagner C, Schill M, Hennen M, Manner R, Jendritza B, Knorz MC, et al. [Virtual reality in ophthalmological education.] Ophthalmologe 2001;98:409–13 (in German).

Waikakul S, Vanadurongwan B, Chumtup W, Assawamongkolgul A, Chotivichit A, Rojanawanich V. A knee model for arthrocentesis simulation. J Med Assoc Thai 2003;86:282–7.

Walsh MS, Macpherson D. The Chichester diagnostic peritoneal lavage simulator. Ann R Coll Surg Engl 1998;80:276–8.

Wang Y, Chui C, Lim H, Cai Y, Mak K. Real-time interactive simulator for percutaneous coronary revascularization procedures. Comput Aided Surg 1998;3:211–27.

Webster RW, Zimmerman DI, Mohler BJ, Melkonian MG, Haluck RS. A prototype haptic suturing simulator. Stud Health Technol Inform 2001;81:567–9.

Weidenbach M, Wild F, Scheer K, Muth G, Kreutter S, Grunst G, et al. Computer-based training in two-dimensional echocardiography using an echocardiography simulator. J Am Soc Echocardiogr 2005;18:362–6.

Wentink M, Stassen LP, Alwayn I, Hosman RJ, Stassen HG. Rasmussen's model of human behavior in laparoscopy training. Surg Endosc 2003;17:1241–6.

Whalley LJ. Ethical issues in the application of virtual reality to medicine. Comput Biol Med 1995;25:107–14.

Wiet GJ, Stredney D. Update on surgical simulation: the Ohio State University experience. Otolaryngol Clin North Am 2002; 35:1283–8, viii.

Wiet GJ, Stredney D, Sessanna D, Bryan JA, Welling DB, Schmalbrock P. Virtual temporal bone dissection: an interactive surgical simulator. Otolaryngol Head Neck Surg 2002;127:79–83.

Williams CB, Saunders BP, Bladen JS. Development of colonoscopy teaching simulation. Endoscopy 2000;32:901–5.

Wilson MS, Middlebrook A, Sutton C, Stone R, McCloy RF. MIST VR: a virtual reality trainer for laparoscopic surgery assesses performance. Ann R Coll Surg Engl 1997;79:403–4.

Articles Touching on the Theme "The Canary in the Mineshaft"

The next group of articles shows how a Simulator functions as "The Canary in the Mineshaft." The simulator uncovers clinical weaknesses. By extension, then, once you uncover a clinical weakness you can correct the weakness. Correct the weakness, improve the clinician, improve the care for our patients.

In the previous group of articles, the "It Stands to Reason" articles, you had to make a leap of faith to "buy into" Simulators. You had to say, "It stands to reason Simulators are a good thing, so we should lay out a lot of resources to support a Simulator." In this batch of articles, you also have to make a leap of faith. You have to say, "The Simulator functions as a canary in a mineshaft, so it can lead to better patient outcomes."

Simulator as a canary in the mineshaft → better outcome

That's quite a long jump. Instead, we're stuck with a multijump argument.

Teach in the simulator → uncover weakness → correct weakness → achieve better outcome

There's a lot of *implied* benefit and *supposed* improvement—*You hope* that's how it works out in the end. But that, alas, is where we stand right now, at least with these articles. So read on, and see about that valiant canary, braving deadly fumes in the mineshaft.

✓ Barsuk D, Ziv A, Lin G, Blumenfield A, Rubin O, Keiden I, et al. Using advanced simulation for recognition and correction of gaps in airway and breathing management skills in prehospital trauma care. Anesth Analg 2005;100:803–9.

Right now Israel and Denmark are moving toward Simulator scenarios as part of their board certification process, so their views have some heft. ("Ready or not, here we come!" the Simulators seem to be saying to us.)

A group of 72 postinternship doctors were divided into two groups: 36 (non-Simulator-trained) were assessed on two trauma scenarios (one with HPS and one with Sim Man). Their most common airway management mistakes were used to develop a 45-minute additional airway training session for the next group of 36. Those trained in the Simulator did better. Both groups had to go through two scenarios.

- Trauma—The key element was a tension pneumothorax. Hypotension occurred as a second complication.
- Trauma—The key element was severe head trauma with the need to secure the airway. Hypoxemia occurred as a second complication.

In this study, the Simulator came across once again as the canary in the mineshaft. Here, these postinternship doctors, who should know *something*, were making all kinds of mistakes.

- Forgetting to hold cricoid pressure
- Forgetting to hold the endotracheal tube
- Using no medications at intubation, just slamming away

And voila! The Simulator reveals all. Maybe we should call Simulators "truth detectors."

What this study showed was that Simulators are great *intermediate* trainers. *Simulator-trained* people do better in the *Simulator* world. Does that translate into the *real* world? Maybe so, maybe no. For example, several doctors made the mistake of not giving drugs before intubating the Simulator. So you might be tempted to say, "In the real world, with a real patient, they would make the exact same mistake." Well, no. In the real world, the patient would bite down and resist—something the Simulator can't do. The authors noted that there is a need for (1) studies that demonstrate transfer of skills from simulation to reality and (2) to determine the rate of skills degradation over time and decide the correct frequency of training. The appendix in the article includes checklists of specific actions reflecting essential actions for safe treatment and successful outcome of severe chest trauma and severe head trauma.

✓ Berkenstadt H, Kantor GS, Yusim Y, Gafni N, Perel A, Ezri T, et al. Feasibility of sharing simulation-based evaluation scenarios in anesthesiology. Anesth Analg 2005;101:1068–74.

Everything else is globalized, why not anesthesia scenarios? Dr. Berkenstadt and the Tel Hashomer gang snagged four scenarios from Dr. Schwid.

- Esophageal intubation
- Anaphylactic reaction
- Exacerbation of COPD
- Myocardial ischemia

A group of 31 junior anesthesia residents ran through the gauntlet of those four scenarios. They liked them and rated the scenarios as quite realistic. Graders trotted out their checklists, reviewed the videotapes, and passed Solomonic judgment upon the residents. It worked.

Oh, a little sidelight. The Israeli residents did better than the American residents! Dr. Berkenstadt graciously explains this away, saying our two systems are different, and the Israelis maybe had more experience in their home countries before immigrating to Israel. The heck you say! Israel kicked our butt, fair and square.

Now it's time for *us* to whip *our people* into shape. Let me at a resident. I'll teach him a thing or two. I demand a rematch! The World Cup of Simulation. Bring it on!

✓ BYRNE AJ, JONES JG. Inaccurate reporting of simulated critical anaesthetic incidents. Br J Anaesth 1997;78:637–41.

Byrne had previously shown that trainees often misinterpret data presented during a simulated case and make numerous errors when describing their actions. In this study, the authors wanted to determine if these inaccuracies result from trainees—

- Misunderstanding the simulation
- Inability to manage the simulated case
- Inability to remember events accurately

Why wait for real cases to see how trainees react when we have Simulators to serve as the canary? Eleven trainees (3 to 8 years of clinical experience) entered a simulated case using the ACCESS Simulator. The case was a young patient undergoing an ankle repair. They faced two "crises"—an episode of bradycardia followed by an episode of anaphylaxis with bronchospasm and hypotension. The authors evaluated participants' ability to record their actions and their accuracy when documenting the two complications in an incident report.

What happened? For the bradycardia episode, 3 of 11 failed to record the event on their paper chart, and 2 of 11 failed to record their treatment of the arrhyth-

mia. Only 4 of the 11 trainees mentioned bradycardia in the critical incident report, and only 1 of the participants *accurately* documented this event. For the bronchospasm and hypotensive event, the results were worse—none of the trainees mentioned that the arterial pressure had been normal prior to the event, and only 2 of the 11 accurately described the event.

The authors urge caution when studying anesthetic emergencies—previously their diagnosis and treatment was built from the analysis of critical incident forms. This study showed that the information derived from this source may not reflect actual events. How can we solve this dilemma? Byrne offers, "automated recording of monitoring and videotaping of the case would seem to provide the best solution, but this is unlikely to receive widespread acceptance and has significant cost implications." You bet it does . . . there is a high price to pay if our main source of data is full of errors. This time the medical record may also be a canary.

✓ BYRNE AJ, SELLEN AJ, JONES JG. Errors on anaesthetic record charts as a measure of anaesthetic performance during simulated critical incidents. Br J Anaesth 1998;80:58–62.

Byrne and colleagues described "mental workload" as the conscious effort required to carry out a complex task. Experts exert relatively low mental workload while carrying out complex tasks, whereas high mental workload is typical of novices and those who lose control when faced with stressful complicated situations. Anesthesiology often requires one to focus on multiple tasks. Studies in aviation have shown that low mental workload allows an experienced pilot to carry out both primary tasks (highest priority) and secondary tasks (lower priority). Byrne argues that a measure of one's mental workload is his/her ability to carry out secondary tasks.

Rather than use a rater's subjective opinion of residents' ability, Byrne and colleagues used the record chart from a simulated anesthetic case as a reflection of the secondary tasks (the primary task was managing the patient). Ten trainees went through a simulated case using the ACCESS simulator. It involved a 25-year-old woman undergoing ACL repair. All trainees were exposed to the same 25-minute scenario in the same sequence.

- 0–5 minutes—normal baseline
- 5–10 minutes—hypotension
- 10–15 minutes—supraventricular tachycardia
- 15–20 minutes—bronchospasm
- 20–25 minutes—normal baseline

Throughout the case and for a few minutes after the scenario ended, participants completed the record chart to document events and data. The data recorded were the following.

- Heart rate
- Systolic arterial pressure
- Diastolic arterial pressure
- Oxygen saturation
- End-tidal carbon dioxide

What happened? As expected, all trainees treated their "patient" appropriately; however, more than 20% of the values recorded by the participants were in error by more than 25% of the actual values. There was high variability among participants and within the same participant. Two lessons resulted from this study.

- Using the data from patient charts from actual cases may not reflect what actually occurs and may not be accurate indicators of critical incidents. Simulations may be a better method for studying the cause of errors.
- If attention during complex cases is focused on managing the patient and not recording what happens, the use of automated technology to record patient data results in less mental workload and less chance of errors.

It is better to find out that trainees make errors in chart recording during simulated cases rather than waiting for a retrospective investigation of an adverse event.

✓ DeAnda A, Gaba DM. Unplanned incidents during comprehensive anesthesia simulation. Anesth Analg 1990;71:77–82.

DeAnda and Gaba smoked out a few problems while running their Simulators. (This shows what happens when clever people leap into a new field and keep their eyes peeled. They didn't *set out* to study these incidents, but when the incidents happened DeAnda and Gaba were alert to the implications. *Fate favors the prepared mind.*)

Errors during the simulator scenarios were most often human errors—a lot of them document fixation errors. (Damn! I'm forever telling residents to worry about the record at the *end* of the case, when the patient is safely in the hands of the PACU nurse. Take care of the patient *first*!)

What did those silly bunnies do? Forgot to turn the ventilator back on after hand-ventilating, syringe swaps, turning the stopcock the wrong way. You name it, they found a way to mess it up.

The simulator uncovered mistakes galore. This was one overworked canary. When you see the mistakes they made, it does not become such a gigantic leap of faith to think you could:

Run Simulator → see mistakes made → correct mistakes → prevent repeat of mistake → protect patient from harm

✓ Gaba DM, DeAnda A. The response of anesthesia trainees to simulated critical incidents. Anesth Analg 1989;68:444–51.

One of the first studies by Gaba revealed that our residents may not be as good as we presumed. He and DeAnda sent 19 first- and second-year anesthesia residents through five scenarios on their Simulator.

- Endobronchial intubation
- Kinked IV
- Atrial fibrillation with hypotension
- Breathing circuit disconnection
- Cardiac arrest

All of the simulations were videotaped and reviewed. The authors measured the response time to detect and initiate correction of the problems. All kinds of errors were made—here is just a few of the most common.

- Endobronchial intubation: Altogether, 11 of 19 never detected an increase in peak inspiratory pressure; 3 of 19 missed the diagnosis (one was not certain about breath sounds, one thought it was just an artifact, and one did not want to disturb the surgeon!).
- Kinked IV: This took more time to detect (nearly 4 minutes—but was quickly corrected). But . . . six residents did not correct IV access before the next problem.
- Atrial fibrillation with hypotension: Although most (89%) recognized a supraventricular tachycardia, less than half identified it as atrial fibrillation.
- Breathing circuit disconnection: Detection (21 seconds) and correction (53 seconds) occurred quickly, probably because of the alarm that sounded to alert them of the problem.
- Cardiac arrest: Although all participants recognized the lethal dysrhythmia quickly (8 seconds), there was major deviation from standard protocols—8 of the 19 continued anesthetic gases; 6 of the 19 failed to administer epinephrine.

Although second-year residents tended to correct problems faster than the first-year "novices," there was wide variation in each group. Many in the first year did well, and a few second-year residents did poorly. The authors note, "the imperfect behavior of the outliers may be more meaningful than the mean performance of the group."

Not all mines were dangerous, but the canaries identified the ones that were—not all anesthesia residents are dangerous, but the Simulator can identify the ones that may be.

✓ ₁ GARDI T, CHRISTENSEN UC, JACOBSEN J, JENSEN PF, ORDING H. How do anaesthesiologists treat malignant hyperthermia in a full-scale anaesthesia simulator? Acta Anaesthesiol Scand 2001;45:1032–5.

The Danish team is at it again . . . this time they studied 32 teams (1 anesthetist had 9 years' experience; 1 nurse anesthetist had 8 years' experience) from several university and community hospitals. The authors evaluated teams on the ability to correctly diagnose and manage a case of malignant hyperthermia based on national guidelines. The 25- to 30-minute scenario consisted of a "routine" case that gradually evolved to a fulminant syndrome over 15 minutes.

How did the teams do?

● Only 14 of the 32 teams adequately performed hyperventilation—primarily because they switched to manual ventilation rather than leaving the patient on the ventilator and adjusting the settings. Why? Because they were focused on other tasks!
● Most teams did not get around to administering bicarbonate, glucose/insulin, diuretics/mannitol, although they stated they would have if they were just given a little more time—sure!

An important finding in this study was that the cause of undermanagement was more practical than thinking—they knew what to do, they did not execute. The authors concluded that "*practical* training in full-scale simulators can become a useful part of training for complex treatment procedures." *Yes!* These canaries are singing, and we are listening!

✓ HAMMOND J, BERMANN M, CHEN B, KUSHINS L. Incorporation of a computerized human patient simulator in critical care training: a preliminary report. J Trauma 2002;53:1064–7.

It turns out that anesthesiologists are not the only ones who make mistakes. Hammond and his colleagues evaluated eight second-year surgery residents during their critical care rotation. They put the residents through three scenarios on a full-patient Simulator.

● Tension pneumothorax
● Bronchospasm
● Atrial fibrillation with hypotension

Each participant was evaluated on a minimum of 13 preselected tasks. So how did these surgeons do?

● Tension pneumothorax—*No* resident successfully completed this scenario! What happened? Slow listening for breath sounds, failure to check for endotracheal tube position, stop sedation, perform nasotracheal suction, <u>and</u> *no* resident called for assistance until the patient was seriously ill. "Assistance, we don't need no stinking assistance!" say the surgeons.
● Performance during the bronchospasm and atrial fibrillation scenarios improved (or were better if you think as I do that these are easier cases). An unexpected outcome—the fastest successful performance was from the resident with the lowest score!

This study showed that we have problems not only with the training of our residents, especially with tension pneumothorax, but also with our evaluations. How can the resident who saved the patient the fastest have the lowest score? That is the main weakness of a checklist—they reward methodical practice but penalize efficiency—experts always know how to take short cuts. The solution—add a global rating scale, measure decision-making timing.

The authors make an important concluding remark. The true value of the Simulators is less their ability to assess individuals but more their ability to uncover deficiencies in training programs.

✓ JACOBSEN J, LINDEKAER AL, OSTERGAARD HT, NIELSEN K, OSTERGAARD D, LAUB M, ET AL. Management of anaphylactic shock evaluated using a full-scale anaesthesia simulator. Acta Anaesthesiol Scand 2001;45:315–19.

A total of 42 anesthetists in Denmark went through a Simulator session involving an anaphylactic reaction to a drug. Guess what? "Something's rotten in the state of Denmark." (I just had to say that.) Nobody pegged it during the first 10 minutes, and only 6 of 21 teams (the 42 people were divided into 21 two-person teams) ever even considered the right diagnosis. And those people needed hints! Ay Chihuahua, or maybe ay Copenhagen.

Either the Simulator didn't do a good job "conveying" anaphylaxis (the old validity question rears its head again), or no one is teaching anesthesiologists in Denmark to diagnose and treat anaphylaxis. The confounders with anaphylaxis during anesthesia are as follows:

- Is that hypotension just from blood loss to which our friendly surgeon does not admit?
- Is that tachycardia from my "anesthetica imperfecta," and the patient is just light?
- With all the drapes, it's hard to see the skin get flushed.

But the conclusion from this was pretty clear: we need to be better prepared to deal with anaphylaxis because right now we're not. (As you pound through these articles, you can draw whatever conclusion you want. I myself, again and again, see the Simulator as the great "revealer of our teaching inadequacies.")

✓ LINDEKAER AL, JACOBSEN J, ANDERSEN G, LAUB M, JENSEN PF. Treatment of ventricular fibrillation during anaesthesia in an anaesthesia simulator. Acta Anaesthesiol Scand 1997;41:1280–4.

This is one of the earlier studies from Denmark—and this team is not afraid to find out what is wrong with their trainees and are determined to do something about it. The authors point out again that 70% to 80% of accidents in anesthesia are a result of human error. A very serious accident is mismanaging ventricular fibrillation.

A group of 80 anesthetists were divided into 40 teams comprising one anesthetist and one nurse anesthetist. Each session was videotaped; and although participants knew something was going to happen during the simulation—they did not know what "it" would be. Seven minutes into an uncomplicated case of a middle-aged man with a gastric tumor, the patient developed ventricular fibrillation.

Teams were evaluated based on if they followed European Resuscitation Council Guidelines for ventricular fibrillation. How well prepared were these teams for an important "emergency"? It varied . . . widely. *None* of the teams followed the published guidelines. There was wide variation and inconsistency in managing ventricular fibrillation despite said guidelines. Two of the forty teams did not administer any shocks to the patient and 27% of the teams did not give the full three shocks. They committed other mistakes as well.

- Ten percent did not give 100% oxygen.
- Nearly half of the teams (17/40) did not turn off the vaporizer.
- Ten percent continued to administer nitrous oxide.

The authors concluded that better education and training are needed for common skills such as ACLS, and Simulators are well suited for this.

✓ MARSCH SCU, TSCHAN F, SEMMER N, SPYCHIGER M, BREUER M, HUNZIKER PR. Performance of first responders in simulated cardiac arrests. Crit Care Med 2005;33:963–7.

Many of these studies involve "mines" located in the operating room, but what happens during critical events that occur "on the floor" by the "first responders"—because nurses are the ones who actually spend the most time with patients, they are usually the first responders—having to page the resident who is either eating or napping. That is just what Marsch and colleagues did—they enrolled 20 ICU teams, each comprising three nurses and a stand-by resident. Each team responded to a case on the Simulator—a 67-year-old man with an acute myocardial infarction who had just undergone successful angioplasty of the right coronary artery and was being sent to the ICU. The patient soon had a cardiac arrest from pulseless ventricular tachycardia. The teams had to respond.

Although the nurses called the resident promptly to help diagnose the problem faster, there was considerable delay in basic life support (they teach that to babysitters), which resulted in chest compression occurring less that 25% of the time. (As an aside, Dr. Gordon Ewy from University of Arizona is on a crusade—well ahead of the American Heart Association—that in the presence of a cardiac arrest forget about the two breaths, the AED—just go ahead and start compressions—100 per minute—this saves lives!) Back to our story . . . 33% of the teams failed to provide an adequate number of shocks, and 8 of 20 teams failed to give epinephrine.

The authors noted that the first responders failed to build an effective team structure that would ensure effective management of the patient. This may reflect a cultural attitude in which nurses are reluctant to assume a leadership role in the presence of a resident. This was the pervasive attitude in aviation until the 1980s when a couple of plane accidents resulted because flight attendants did not think "it was their place" to bother the pilot about ice on the wings or an engine on fire.

Before they viewed themselves on videotape, the teams thought they had done pretty well. *None* of the participants had realized or recalled unnecessary interruptions in basic life support! We call this the unconscious incompetent. So much for those code flow sheets and incident reports accurately reflecting what happens. But without these important studies, we would not be moving forward.

✓ MORGAN PJ, CLEAVE-HOGG D, DeSOUSA S, TARSHIS J. Identification in gaps in the achievement of undergraduate anesthesia educational objectives using high fidelity patient simulation. Anesth Analg 2003;97:1690–4.

Tweet tweet! The Simulator uncovered the failings and frailties of 165 medical students in this study. What did the simulator unmask?

- Students couldn't manage the airway.
- Students didn't check the blood pressure.
- Students didn't call for help.
- Students didn't do a history/physical.
- Students didn't prepare the airway equipment.

Um, this study begs the question. Just what, precisely, *did* the students do? Did the students *themselves* have a pulse? The authors point out, as we have repeatedly, that residents also make these mistakes. Now that we understand no one is competent, let's do something about it. Morgan and her colleagues have completely overhauled their anesthesia training program for medical students. What more can you ask?

✓ Morgan PJ, Cleave-Hogg D. Evaluation of medical students' performance using the anaesthesia simulator. Med Educ 2000;34:42–5.

Not so much a canary uncovering specific mistakes here ("they blew it on the intubation") as using the Simulator as an overall evaluation tool. Dr. Morgan in Toronto said, "Let's use the simulator on 24 medical students, run them through the gauntlet (RSI—treating hypoxemia, managing hypovolemia, treating anaphylaxis) and see if we can use this as our testing technique." Results were a little muddy, truth to tell. Their "simulator grade" did not correlate with their "clinical grade" (how they were rated on the clerkship by the people who worked with them in the real OR).

Hmmm. Simulator as "grading canary"? This becomes problematic. (Too bad, right when you're on a roll and you think Simulators are perfect in every way, something like this comes along, throwing a wrench in the works, or, more precisely, a wrench in the canary cage.)

✓ Olsen JC, Gurr DE, Hughes M. Video analysis of emergency medicine residents performing rapid sequence induction. J Emerg Med 2000;18:469–72.

This is not a simulation study but a kind of "canary-esque" training study. To uncover intubation errors, Dr. Olsen and his Chicago buddies videotaped emergency medicine residents during intubations. (By

extension to Simulato-land, we use a lot of videotaping to uncover mistakes.) Lo and behold, 45% of the residents don't do the Sellick maneuver right, and 34% don't use the all-important end-tidal carbon dioxide detector to make sure the tube is in the right place.

Once again, to beat the drum:

| Canary uncovers mistake → (no use of end-tidal CO_2 monitor) | Fix mistake → (hey, use the monitor) | Prevent badness (avoid esophageal intubation) |

This canary argument does not seem so far-fetched after all.

✓ Rosenstock C, Ostergaard D, Kristensen MS, Lippert A, Ruhnau B, Rasmussen LS. Residents lack knowledge and practical skills in handling the difficulty airway. Acta Anaesthesiol Scand 2004;48:1014–18.

Denmark again—these guys are the miners of the simulation world. This time they enrolled 36 anesthesia residents, evaluated their knowledge and practice experience regarding difficult airway management, and evaluated their management of a "cannot ventilate, cannot intubate" patient on a Simulator. Surprise!

- Only 17% of the residents passed the written test (>70%); median score was 45% (ouch!). This is knowledge.
- About 97% had difficulty recalling the ASA difficult airway algorithm.
- More than 50% did not know how to oxygenate through a cricothyroid membrane.
- Residents who previously participated in an airway course did not perform any better than those with no previous training.
- About 44% stated they would perform a fiberoptic intubation in a "cannot ventilate, cannot intubate" patient.

What have the Danes done about these results? "The knowledge helped us to define the learning objectives for a new *national compulsory training program for airway management in Denmark.*" *Now*—all residents have to *pass* a 3-day compulsory course in difficult airway management. *Now*—what is the rest of the world waiting for?

✓ Schwid HA, O'Donnell D. Anesthesiologists' management of simulated critical incidents. Anesthesiology 1992;76:495–501.

This article ramps it up a little bit. We're not looking at residents making glitches during *routine* cases, we're looking at much more serious stuff. How do residents and faculty manage *nonroutine* cases?

- Esophageal intubation
- Anaphylaxis
- Myocardial ischemia
- Cardiac arrest

Yegads, I hope but hope that we know how to handle these problems! Here you really *do* want a canary in that mineshaft, detecting errors during critical events that can kill the patient in minutes! Bingo, that's just what the simulator did. That canary keeled over stone-cold dead time after time after time. The simulator pulled back the cover and revealed some whopping inadequacies:

- Residents misjudged esophageal intubations.
- Less than half of everybody (residents *and* faculty) treated anaphylaxis correctly.
- A quarter of all comers treated ischemia correctly (hope I don't get ischemic on their OR table!)
- If your ACLS training was more than 6 months old, *fugetaboudit!* Less than a third knew what they were doing.

I don't know about you, but these findings sure make *me* wake up and smell the coffee.

✓ Schwid HA, Rooke GA, Carline J, Steadman RH, Murray WB, Olympio M, et al. Evaluation of anesthesia residents using mannequin-based simulation: a multiinstitutional study. Anesthesiology 2002;97:1434–44.

Professor Schwid again. Hmm. Why do we think he's the one of "ones to watch" in this Simulator realm? A total of 99 residents at 10 different teaching programs jumped through four flaming hoops.

- Esophageal intubation
- Anaphylaxis
- Bronchospasm
- Myocardial ischemia

The residents were taped and graded. More senior residents did better than junior residents, which generated a nationwide, "Whew!" from anesthesia attendings all across America. (*We must be teaching something, for God's sake.*) Schwid throws down the gauntlet of how to do these kinds of studies.

Checklists. Do you see checklists with simulation studies! That is the "coin of the realm" when it comes to "did the simulatee do right" or "did the simulatee do wrong." You check off whether they gave the nitroglycerin. You check off whether they listened to breath sounds. You check off whether they gave beta blocker. Check, check, check, checkmate.

Check out the checkers. A dizzying array of statistics looked at the people doing the grading. Are they "all on the same page" when it comes to grading? Turns out they were.

Videotape. That's the way to go when it comes to reviewing the scenario. Both for research purposes (the two graders can look at the films separately) and for teaching purposes (the residents can "relive the excitement" and pick up critical learning points).

Something of additional interest pops out of this article. The residents didn't know *bupkis* from bronchospasm. No matter how far along their training, a lot of residents appeared to suffer from adult-onset anencephaly when it comes to the wheezing patient. Are we missing the boat here? Are we not teaching our residents right? Should the beatings increase until our residents get the message? To me, that alone was worth the price of admission on this article. Forget Schwid's elegant design, rigorous mathematics, and large numbers. He uncovered a *glaring defect* in our teaching! Damnation, tomorrow I'm going over bronchospasm with my resident, and I hope you do too!

Additional Articles on the Topic "The Simulator as Canary in the Mineshaft"

Ali J, Adam R, Pierre I, Bedaysie H, Josa D, Winn J. Comparison of performance 2 years after the old and new (interactive) ATLS courses. J Surg Res 2001;97:71–5.

Armstrong-Brown A, Devitt JH, Kurrek M, Cohen M. Inadequate preanesthesia equipment checks in a simulator. Can J Anaesth 2000;47:974–9.

Byrne AJ, Jones JG. Responses to simulated anaesthetic emergencies by anaesthetists with different durations of clinical experience. Br J Anaesth 1997;78:553–6.

DeAnda A, Gaba DM. Role of experience in the response to simulated critical incidents. Anesth Analg 1991;72:308–15.

Kurrek MM, Devitt JH, Cohen M. Cardiac arrest in the OR: how are our ACLS skills? Can J Anaesth 1998;45:130–2.

Mackenzie CF, Jefferies NJ, Hunter WA, Bernhard WN, Xiao Y. Comparison of self reporting of deficiencies in airway management with video analysis of actual performance; LOTAS group: level one trauma simulation. Hum Factors 1996;38:623–35.

Marsch SCU, Muller C, Marquardt K, Conrad G, Tschan F, Hunziker PR. Human factors affect the quality of cardiopulmonary resuscitation in simulated cardiac arrests. Resuscitation 2004;60:51–56.

Morgan PJ, Cleave-Hogg D. Comparison between medical students' experience, confidence and competence. Med Educ 2002;36:534–9.

Moule P. Checking the carotid pulse: diagnostic accuracy in students of the healthcare professions. Resuscitation 2000;44:195–201.

Santora TA, Trooskin SZ, Blank CA, Clarke JR, Scinco MA. Video assessment of trauma response: adherence to ATLS protocols. Am J Emerg Med 1996;14:564–9.

Van Stralen DW, Rogers M, Perkin RM, Fea S. Retrograde intubation training using a mannequin. Am J Emerg Med 1995; 13:50–2.

White JRM, Shugerman R. Performance of advanced resuscitation skills by pediatric housestaff. Arch Pediatr Adolesc Med 1998; 152:1232–5.

Articles Touching on the Theme "Gee Whiz, Golly, I Belong Too"

Picture a new kid trying to enter the "Educational Clubhouse," presently occupied by lectures, textbooks, grand rounds, and clinical work. Those inside the clubhouse have pulled up the rope ladder and said, "No one else allowed in here." The new kid is down below, jumping up and down, saying, "No, really, I want in! I belong too!" That's what this batch of articles addresses—the "Simulator Belongs in the Educational Clubhouse Too."

Now, in all clinical assessments there are three variables—the examiner, the patient, and the student. If we standardize the first two variables, we improve the evaluation such that the student's performance then represents a true measure of his or her clinical competence. Examiner training and the use of reliable evaluation tools allow standardization of the "examiner" component. An inherent feature of Simulators is the ability to standardize many aspects of the "patient" variable in the clinical assessment equation, thus offering a uniform, reproducible experience to multiple examinees. Simulators, however, do not comprise the entire assessment per se but, rather, serve as tools to facilitate standardization and to complement existing evaluation methods. For example, Simulators often serve effectively as one of several tools used in the brief examining stations of an objective structured clinical examination (OSCE).

Assessing Process and Outcome

Numerous assessment criteria are available to evaluate learners, and clerkship directors must choose whether the competence tested relates to a *process* (such as completing an orderly, thorough "code blue" resuscitation) or an *outcome* (such as the status of the "patient" after the cardiac arrest). The following summarizes how one can assess processes and outcomes with Simulators.

Criteria Type	Example
Measure a process	A case-specific checklist to record actions during student suturing on a skin wound simulator
Judge a process	A global rating (with well defined anchor points) that allows an evaluator to observe and judge reliably the quality of suturing performed by a student on a skin wound simulator
Measure an outcome	Observing and recording specific indicators of patient (Simulator) status (alive, cardiac rhythm, blood pressure) after an ACLS code
Judge an outcome	A global rating (with well defined anchor points) that allows an evaluator to observe and judge reliably the quality of the overall patient status after an ACLS code
Combined	Task-specific checklist of cardiac bedside exam; observing and recording correct identification and interpretation of physical findings

✓ ALI J, GANA TJ, HOWARD M. Trauma mannequin assessment of management skills of surgical residents after advanced trauma life support training. J Surg Res 2000;93:197–200.

The purpose of this study was to measure the effectiveness of an Advanced Trauma Life Support (ATLS) course for PGY-1 surgical residents at the University of Toronto. A group of 32 residents were randomly divided into two groups (ATLS trained, not ATLS trained). The outcome measures included eight trauma cases (four pre-ATLS, four post-ATLS).

- Two penetrating torso trauma cases
- Two blunt torso trauma cases
- Two thermal injury
- Two pregnancy trauma

The methods used to measure skills were the following.

- 20-Item checklists for each case
- 5-Point scale rating organizational approach
- 7-Point scale rating adherence to priority
- Global rating of each scenario (honors, pass, borderline, fail)

Pre-ATLS scores were similar in both groups for all outcome measures. The ATLS group scored significantly higher in all scores in all scenarios than the non-ATLS group. There is no big surprise in these outcomes—residents trained in a course should perform better than those not trained. The study did prove that the Simulator should be used, "not only as a tool for training in surgical residency programs but also as a tool for testing trauma resuscitating skills." The major criticism of this study is that none of the outcome measures were formally evaluated for their reliability (Did different raters agree similarly with each resident?), validity (Can the outcome measures discriminate experts from novices?), or feasibility (How much more did the Simulator cost compared to traditional outcome measures used in an ATLS course?).

✓ BLUM RH, RAEMER DB, CARROLL JS, DUFRESNE RL, COOPER JB. A method for measuring the effectiveness of simulation-based team training for improving communication skills. Anesth Anal 2005;100:1375–80.

Although communication skills are probably the most important team behaviors during critical events, they are the most difficult to measure accurately and consistently. Typical assessments employ complex rating forms that require examinees to be videotaped and then reviewed by two or more faculty. These faculty need to be trained and calibrated to use the assessment forms.

Thus, in an effort to develop valid and reliable outcome measures, it is becoming less feasible to do so. Blum and his colleagues in Boston sought to develop a new assessment technique (one that was more feasible) and to determine its validity for measuring communication skills among team members responding to a critical event.

The authors created "probes"—pieces of specific, potentially important information for patient management. The skill of team information sharing (communicating) would be related to the number of team members who became aware of these probes during a scenario. Blum and his colleagues hypothesized that initially there would be a low rate of information-sharing among team members—nearly every simulation study has shown this—but this time it would be quantified (we can stick a score on it). They also hypothesized that any change in team information sharing would correlate with the team members' self-reported change, and there would be an increase in information as trainees advanced from the first scenario to the fifth scenario. They used 22 pilot teams over 8 months to iron out the probes and make revisions—the study included 10 teams (7 faculty, 3 resident/fellow) over a 4 month period.

Teams were randomized to participate in one of two scenarios (respiratory arrest in a complex surgical patient or a trauma patient) as their first and fifth cases. During each scenario, faculty would place the probe with one of the team members. In a postscenario questionnaire, each of the team members was asked about his/her knowledge of the probes.

When they completed the study, they found that a little more than half of the probes were successfully placed, and they were shared an average of 27% of the

time. There was no difference in information sharing from the first to the fifth case.

What accounts for the lack of success? On the surface, this seems like a plausible, practical way to measure information-sharing ability indirectly—how well critical information is shared among team members. However, the probes were highly case-specific.

Respiratory arrest case—probes

- Patient was previously receiving nebulizer treatment.
- Patient was HIV-positive.
- Patient was receiving a morphine infusion for pain control.
- Patient had a steering wheel mark on his chest.

Trauma case—probes

- Patient had received 4 to 5 liters of crystalloid in the emergency department
- Patient had a "shadow" on chest radiograph
- Patient had positive cocaine toxicology
- Patient had received antibiotic (cefoxitin) en route to the OR

These probes are highly specific to the case and would not generalize to other cases. In addition, the probes first had to be placed with a team member—in 33% of the scenarios this was not successful because another team member overheard the faculty member telling about the probe. Reliability is always compromised when testing variables are dependent on another person (no one reacts the same 100% of the time to different individuals). Reliability would increase if the probes were in the form of patient record information (in the chart it stated that the patient was HIV-positive) or data from the simulation itself (steering wheel mark placed on the Simulator's chest).

We agree with the authors that this is a promising area for research—it should be "aimed at improving this methodology and continued measurement of validity and reliability." See that when you fix one corner of the pyramid (feasibility), the other two corners start crumbling away! But we believe probes also belong in the arsenal of assessment techniques for high-fidelity simulations.

✓ BOULET JR, MURRAY D, KRAS J, WOODHOUSE J, MCALLISTER J, ZIV A. Reliability and validity of a simulation-based acute care skills assessment for medical students and residents. Anesthesiology 2003;99:1270–80.

Again, the authors are zooming in on *the* question in Simulation-ness—is the Simulator really a good way to know if people "know their stuff"? Here's the setting. Ask faculty, "What should your people know how to treat? When a patient rolls through the door with *condition X*, your medical students and residents should know how to treat *condition X*. Give us 10 *condition X's*."

Here are the 10 condition X's. (As you look them over, you have to say to yourself, "Yeah, those are reasonable things to ask. These are things you expect to see as a medical student or a resident.")

1. Femur fracture—big bleed, hypotension
2. Myocardial infarction—tachycardia, hypertension, PVCs
3. Pneumothorax—fell off bike, dyspnea, tachycardia, hypoxemia
4. Ectopic pregnancy—bleeding, hypotensive
5. Cerebral hemorrhage—blown pupil, Cushing's triad, unresponsive
6. Ventricular tachycardia—chest pain, unstable
7. Respiratory failure—bronchitis progressing to respiratory insufficiency
8. Asthma—hypoxemia, tachypnea, heading toward respiratory insufficiency
9. Rupturing abdominal aortic aneurysm—abdominal mass, pain, tachycardia
10. Syncope—heart block, hypotension

Hey, that's a pretty good list! I would hope that *any doc* would know how to handle those bad boys. So—40 people jumped in: 24 fourth-year medical students, 10 first-year anesthesia residents, 2 first-year emergency medicine residents, 1 first-year surgery resident, and 3 international medical graduates. (They dropped the international medical graduates.) Each person had to do six of the scenarios. They were videotaped and graded by two faculty and two nurse clinicians. Scoring? The all-pervasive checklist. Seems to be a good thing, as the choice of grader didn't matter much. We live in a binary world, after all, full of 1's and 0's. And that binary system pervades the Simulator grading world. For example, you either *do* intubate or *don't* intubate. Yes/no. 1/0.

Result? Another "whew"—residents did better than medical students. Another result? Few people did well on the cerebral bleed with herniation. (To my mind, not the *purpose* of this study but an extremely important "side result" of the study. As primarily a clinical teacher, I like anything that exposes gaps in our teaching. If a Simulator shows that our residents can't handle cerebral herniation, then we should go back

and teach more about cerebral herniation!) How can this article serve as a resource for Simulator educators? Read and use those 10 scenarios, they're great.

✓ DEVITT JH, KURREK MM, COHEN MM, FISH K, FISH P, MURPHY PM, ET AL. Testing the raters: inter-rater reliability of standardized anaesthesia simulator performance. Can J Anaesth 1997;44:924–8.

We pointed out that if Simulators were to belong in the toolbox of assessments, they have to be reliable—something that is challenging when you have subjective global rating scales and hundreds of checklist items all over the place. This study demonstrates that faculty raters need to be evaluated and debriefed regarding their assessment ability as much as the subjects they are testing. The authors developed two 1-hour scenarios, each with five anesthesia problems (these are included in case you are interested in doing some faculty development).

Scenario 1

1. CO_2 canister leak
2. Sinus bradycardia during peritoneal traction
3. Atelectasis
4. Coronary ischemia
5. Hypothermia

Scenario 2

1. Missing inspiratory valve
2. Hypotension during peritoneal traction
3. Pneumothorax
4. Anaphylaxis
5. Anuria from obstructed catheter

A faculty member familiar with the case and scripted to provide appropriate responses played the role of the trainee (in some instances an incorrect action was taken). Altogether, there were three responses to each problem that were recorded for a total of 30 items to be assessed (2 cases × 5 problems × 3 responses per problem). This session was videotaped and then shown to two board-certified anesthetists who were familiar with the scenario design and construction but were not aware of the programmed responses. They used a specially constructed rating form and reviewed the 30 problems.

Incredibly, there was only one discrepancy between the raters! So the authors successfully completed the first step toward creating the perfect assessment instrument—achieving high reliability. A word of caution: High reliability for a single case with "actors" simulating the trainees does not guarantee high reliability when you have a bunch of young trainees making all sorts of unpredictable mistakes and errors. In other words, when it comes to assessment, you are never safe from the ever-dynamic three-headed monster of validity, reliability, and feasibility.

✓ DEVITT JH, KURREK MM, COHEN MM, FISH K, FISH P, NOEL AG, ET AL. Testing internal consistency and construct validity during evaluation of performance in a patient simulator. Anesth Analg 1998;86:1160–4.

This article looks at the rating system used to evaluate anesthesiologists in a Simulator and sees if it passes the *"duh"* test, that is, the rating system:

● *Reliable*—Do evenly matched residents score similarly on the same exam every time they take it?
● *Valid*—Do more experienced practitioners (attendings) do better than residents?

Eight anesthesiology residents (I wonder if they picked the dumb ones to kind of "hedge their bet") took on 17 university attendings in this "Simulator Super Bowl." It's worth looking at the scenarios, if for no other reason than to steal them for your own Simulator program (same ones as their previous study). They created two separate "five-packs."

Scenario 1

1. CO_2 canister leak
2. Sinus bradycardia with peritoneal retraction
3. Atelectasis
4. Coronary ischemia
5. Hypothermia

Scenario 2

1. Missing inspiratory valve
2. Hypotension during peritoneal retraction
3. Pneumothorax
4. Anaphylaxis
5. Anuria secondary to a kinked Foley

Once again, you have to take your hat off to the scenario designers. These are things we should all know how to fix. The study did produce crystal-clear results—attendings are better than residents and we can grade that easily—the world is thus a well ordered place—the test is valid.

But there's a wrench in the statistical works. To improve the "consistency" and reliability aspect of this study, they had to throw out a few scenarios—sinus bradycardia during peritoneal traction and coronary

ischemia in the first "five-pack" and missing inspiratory valve and hypotension during peritoneal traction in the second "five-pack."

If that makes you wince a little, you're not alone. Throw out some scenarios so "now it's consistent"? Hmm. This may appear to be "cooking the books," but testing organizations do it all of the time. Whenever you are trying to develop a reliable, valid exam, you always put in more items than you ultimately use. Why? Because you do not know if they are good items, ratings, or questions until you try them out with your target population. If you think this is strange, the National Board of Medical Examiners does it all the time. Nearly 25% of the questions on a Step 1, 2, or 3 multiple-choice exam may be thrown out to end up with a good exam. Although it seems tedious (and it is), it is certainly better than developing a new exam and blame poor performance on the residents. Sometimes the exam is just bad.

✓ DEVITT JH, KURREK MM, COHEN MM, CLEAVE-HOGG D. The validity of performance assessments using simulation. Anesthesiology 2001;95:36–42.

The group from Toronto wanted to see if their anesthesia Simulator exam would hold up in "real life" and be able to discriminate the level of training and experience among a large, diverse group of anesthesiologists. In total, 33 university attendings, 46 private practice-based anesthesiologists, 23 senior anesthesia residents, 37 senior medical students, and 3 anesthesiologists who had shown deficiencies and were referred by their hospital or license authorities completed the 1.5-hour scenario on the Simulator in another Super Bowl of Anesthetic Expertise. They plowed through nine problems.

● CO_2 canister leak
● Missing inspiratory valve
● Hypotension from mesenteric traction
● Atelectasis
● Coronary ischemia
● Pneumothorax
● Anaphylaxis (hope none of them were Danish)
● Hypothermia
● Anuria from a kinked Foley

They had to complete all nine problems by the end of 90 minutes. They were evaluated with similarly detailed checklists the authors described in their earlier studies. I'm here to tell you, the order of performance was the following.

1. The pointy headed academic geeks (university attendings)

2. Senior residents
3. Community-practice anesthesiologists
4. Senior medical students

The authors mercifully did not include the "deficient" anesthesiologists in the formal comparison (they ended up between the medical students and the "competent" community anesthesiologists). The study demonstrated that the scoring system was indeed valid. But what about the reliability? Well, this time all items were much more consistent than in previous studies. Why? Probably because there were much larger numbers in this study (NBME uses this method to develop exams). It also showed that the reliability of an exam cannot be taken for granted.

By the way, no doubt the academics puffed out their chests with that, but of course the better-paid private practice types probably just drove away in their Masaratis and said, "To hell with that, I'm flying to my condo in Vail."

✓ Forrest FC, Taylor MA, Postlethwaite K, Apinali R. Use of a high-fidelity simulator to develop testing of the technical performance of novice anaesthetists. Br J Anaesth 2002;88:338–44.

(You'll love this terminology) Twenty-six consultants in anesthesia hobnobbed together in the fantastically named Delphi technique to come up with certain technical tasks that they thought new anesthesia personnel should know. Delphi—like Oracle at Delphi. Just how cool is that? (The Delphi technique—identify 15 to 30 "experts" and obtain consensus opinion about a topic. But calling this the "obtain consensus opinion from experts" technique is as flat and tasteless as a piece of stale Wonder Bread.)

Once all the "oracles had spoken" and rated the importance of technical tasks undertaken during rapid sequence induction and maintenance of general anesthesia, the authors revised their initial list and sent the tasks to the Delphi anesthesia mavens for a second round of review.

Once these were returned, the investigators completed their final rating form and tested it with five novice anesthetists. Five times over 3 months the novices came to the Simulator and "anesthetized" the mannequin.

The idea here is that if the Simulator is a valid tool (to measure the competence of trainees), you should see improvement over the course of the 3 months (assuming the trainees are learning something during their training). Guess what? They did! The novices got better as they got more experienced, and you could see it during the Simulator sessions. This does seem a little "gee whiz, shouldn't that be obvious?" but wait, don't be so judgmental. *Remember*, nothing is so obvious that it does not have to be proven. And for the Simulator to "enter the educational clubhouse" it has to be seen as a "valid way to assess progress."

We strongly suggest reviewing their Table 6 for the impressive, comprehensive rating list of tasks. If you have to develop a rating form for anesthesia, don't reinvent the wheel—take advantage of the Delphi technique. This study resulted in an assessment tool that was high in validity, pretty good in reliability, but not the most feasible (*you* try to get consensus from 26 experts!).

Here, the Simulator did prove to be a "valid way to assess progress." So when the Simulator clamors "Gee whiz, I belong too," we should listen to it. The Simulator does belong.

✓ Gaba DM, Howard SK, Flanagan B, Smith BE, Fish KJ, Botney R. Assessment of clinical performance during simulated crises using both technical and behavioral ratings. Anesthesiology 1998;89:8–18.

This study took on one of the hardest "metrics" imaginable—grading *behavior* and tried to determine whether they could get faculty raters to agree on this. Fourteen teams were created.

On each team, there were four anesthesia providers (one team had four CRNAs, the other teams had four faculty anesthesiologists or four resident anesthesiologists, one team had a mix of faculty and residents). These teams had to take on five crises in a 2.5-hour Simulator session. Two of these crises were videotaped and graded. The teams tackled two significant problems.

1. Malignant hyperthermia
2. Cardiac arrest

Like every study on simulation since the dawn of man, out came the checklists. Independent graders gave points from their checklists (for example, you got points for calling for dantrolene, more points if you mixed it up correctly). This was called the "technical grading," and it went well. Now came the sticky part (and it is still the sticky part today, 8 years later): How do you grade the behavior of the team in a crisis? First you define the behavioral aspects.

- Orientation to case
- Inquiry/assertion
- Communication
- Feedback
- Leadership

- Group climate
- Anticipation/planning
- Workload distribution
- Vigilance
- Reevaluation

Next, you define the 1 to 5 rating scale (poor, substandard, standard, good, outstanding). Thankfully, the investigators had gone all out to provide an illustrative example for each definition (what do we mean by poor performance?).

- Behavior varied over time. At times the team "behaved" well, at times not.
- Behavior varied with persons on the team. In general, "team behavior" mirrored the "team leader's behavior."
- The ability to grade behavior varied. Independent graders have little trouble with the checklist, technical things (dantrolene given, yes or no, there's no wiggle room), but behavior is not so cut-and-dried.

Take-home lesson from this study—looking for a perfect "behavior metric" will prove to be a long struggle.

✓ Gaba D. Two examples of how to evaluate the impact of new approaches to teaching [editorial]. Anesthesiology 2002;96:1–2.

Dr. Gaba tells us in this editorial that it is the *magician*, not the *wand*, that makes the rabbit jump out of the hat. People are quick to point out how much the Simulator itself costs. But Gaba reminds us "the major cost of simulation training is faculty time." Videotape technology is great (that's how golfers review their swing), but that has to be coupled with "expert teaching by motivated faculty."

My take? If you're starting a simulation program, make sure you have a few motivated faculty to make it happen. Send them to Boston for one of those "Teach the Teacher" courses. Fly them to Stanford or St. Louis or Israel or Denmark to watch the real experts in action. When you buy an expensive *wand*, put a lot of money into training your *magician*.

✓ Gordon JA, Tancredi D, Binder W, Wilkerson W, Shaffer DW, Cooper J. Assessing global performance in emergency medicine using high fidelity patient simulator: a pilot study. Acad Emerg Med 2003;10:472.

Twenty-three residents jumped through the flaming hoop of five simulations each. They also did mock oral exams. The residents were at different levels of training, and the purpose of the study was to see if

a Simulator evaluation "made common sense." That is, would the more advanced residents do better than the more junior residents.

Again, someone out there might smack their forehead and say, "Duh, what do you expect!" Well, OK. Good argument. But remember the recurrent theme here. For Simulators to enter the "educational clubhouse" the Simulator better pass the "Duh, what do you expect!" test. The Simulator passed! More senior residents did do better. Conclusion—Simulators once again prove they belong.

✓ Gordon JA, Tancredi DN, Binder WD, Wilkerson WM, Shaffer DW. Assessment of clinical performance evaluation tool for use in a simulator-based testing environment: a pilot study. Acad Med 2003;78(10):S45–7.

The objective structured clinical exam (OSCE) is now 30 years old. Professor Harden and his colleagues at the University of Dundee described its use for testing a variety of surgical skills among medical students. (It took nearly 20 years to be adopted in the United States.) It is an attempt to create a more realistic test than the multiple-choice exam but a test that is still reliable and not dependent on a single rater's opinion. There are many forms and types of OSCEs interpreting an ECG or X-ray, completing a telephone consult, writing a prescription, or communicating and examining a patient. This often is a role-acting test in which the examiner pretends to be a patient, and the examinee has to figure out what's going on and what to do.

For example, an OSCE on myocardial infarction might go like this: *Resident walks in the room; a man is sitting there, clutching his chest, complaining of chest pain and nausea. The resident has to ask questions, order tests, make the diagnosis, and save the day.*

Gordon and his gang asked the question, "If OSCEs have been used for so long with standardized patients (actors)—another form of simulation—can they be used with high-fidelity Simulators serving the role of the patient?" Is examining with *flesh and blood* as good as examining with a Simulator? Answer—yes. How did they come to that conclusion? Once again, they did the "Will the more experienced outperform the less experienced? If so, the test is valid." (Forever, the "Defenders of the Simulator" are proving the Simulator's "validity" as if to say, "We should only use this if we can prove its worth." Has anyone ever asked that question of Grand Rounds? Resident lectures? In-training exams? Should we even be asking Simulators to "prove their validity," or should we "take it on faith" that they are a good thing?) And yes, in both the Simulator exam and the OSCE, the more experienced residents did outdo their junior counterparts.

Flesh and blood test—experience counts. Simulator test—experience counts. Conclusion—we can use the OSCE-Simulator combination as a testing method.

✓ HUMPHRIS GM, KANEY S. Examiner fatigue in communication skills objective structured clinical examinations. Med Educ 2001;35:444–9.

The objective structured clinical examination is the "pretend patient" test. Examiner burnout is a real possibility with these exams. That is, you might expect an examiner to have his/her "wits about him/herself" at the start of the exam, but after a couple hours the examiner might be "running on empty," Not so in this study. Examiners seemed able to "keep up the good work" throughout a complete 2 hours.

Any implication for Simulators? (*The article did not address this point at all; this is my speculation.—Author.*) Yes. Simulator staff should be able to "keep up the good work" for a few hours too. Personal experience shows that you do need breaks after a while, as the Simulator experience requires a lot of concentration and thinking on your feet as the scenario plays out.

✓ MORGAN PJ, CLEAVE-HOGG D, GUEST CB. A comparison of global ratings and checklist scores from an undergraduate assessment using an anesthesia simulator. Acad Med 2001;76:1053–5.

When you're putting residents and medical students through the meat grinder of the Simulator experience, grading gets to be a pain in the neck. Trust me, when you put 15 people through the Simulator in a day, the thought of checking off a million little things can drive you to distraction. The ever-present checklist, seen in study after study, is seen as a kind of "gold standard" of Simulator grading. The other criticism of checklists is that it is possible to score fairly well on a checklist and still not be judged a "competent" anesthesiologist. (Example—resident correctly performs the first nine tasks on a checklist and then misses the tenth. The patient dies—resident score 90%—*no way!*) Other studies demonstrate that experts often score lower on exams using checklists than senior medical students—*how?* Well, the experts know all of the shortcuts to solve the problem and do not need to go through *each* and *every* task.

Can we simplify things? How about a global rating instead of that checklist? Drs. Morgan, Cleave-Hogg, and Guest to the rescue. They went out to compare the reliability of the checklist method with the global rating method. A total of 140 senior medical students each did a 15-minute scenario. They were graded in two ways by five pairs of faculty who had attended an instructional workshop. The 25-point checklist was graded as: 0 = not performed; 1 = performed. A global rating, one-stop shopping. Give the med students a single number grade for their overall performance.

- "1" meant they stunk (clear failure)
- "2" meant they stunk sometimes (borderline failure)
- "3" meant they stunk rarely (borderline pass)
- "4" meant they never stunk (clearly pass)
- "5" meant they smelled quite nice (superior performance)

The global rating correlated with the checklist. The lives of "Simulator graders" just got a lot simpler! Maybe. If you want the best of both worlds, use checklists and a global rating.

✓ MORGAN PJ, CLEAVE-HOGG DM, GUEST CB, HEROLD J. Validity and reliability of undergraduate performance assessments in the anesthesia simulator. Can J Anaesth 2001;48:225–33.

This study reflects a little "salami slicing." It involves the same group of students and raters as the previous study—this time using the data to determine the validity and reliability of their assessment tools. One way to assess validity is to compare students' performance on the Simulator with their ability as determined by written tests and faculty ratings of clinical performance. I guess all of these data could have been included in one big paper—but some of these journals do have word limits and short attention spans.

Altogether, 131 senior students went through one of six 15-minute scenarios that were videotaped and evaluated by a pair of faculty raters. Each scenario had four primary learning objectives that were the focus of the evaluation.

The test showed good reliability for two raters (when a student "stunk," the raters agreed 86% of the time). The test also showed good reliability for a single rater (when two students "stunk," the same rater agreed 77% of the time). The authors determined that to achieve a "gold standard" of 90% you would need to have 2.86 raters (you'll have a hard time finding 0.86 of a person, so go ahead and use three). None of the assessment methods correlated with each other. Performance on the Simulator did not correlate with the written test of clinical ratings (daily operating room performance), and performance on the written test did not correlate with the clinical ratings.

There have been few studies that show good correlation between assessment techniques that assess different competencies. Even the National Board of Medical Examiners new Step 2 CS (standardized patient OSCE) does not correlate well with NBME Step 2 written. Why? Well because you are testing different things. Just because a student can tell you every detail regarding the anatomy of the human airway, it means nothing regarding his ability to intubate that airway.

Although there were limitations acknowledged by the authors in this study and further studies are needed to improve the consistency of items (not raters) in the exam, it is an important contribution in the area of simulator and assessment.

✓ Morgan PJ, Cleave-Hogg D, DeSousa S, Tarshis J. High-fidelity patient simulation: validation of performance checklists. Br J Anaesth 2004;92:388–92.

This is the latest study by Dr. Morgan and her colleagues at the University of Toronto. The study is a model for test development at a medical school. It is not easy and takes many resources—but what a good test you have in the end.

Previous studies (above) from Morgan demonstrated that the test showed good validity and reliability among raters but poor internal consistency (this is a fancy term that means similar test items should be answered correctly or incorrectly by the same test taker). If this is so, you are not supposed to use that item. If you develop enough items and test them, those with poor internal consistency can be revised or thrown out and you use the remaining items for your final examination—you got it!

The authors worked with the school's undergraduate committee to develop 10 case scenarios based on what they considered was appropriate for medical students. The 10 cases were (again—use these and you have a pretty comprehensive curriculum):

- Hypoxemia
- Tachycardia
- Postoperative hypertension
- Postoperative hypotension
- Local anesthetic toxicity
- Total spinal anesthesia
- Difficult intubation
- Hypoxemia following intubation
- Ventricular tachycardia
- Anaphylactic reaction

A group of 135 students went through the 10 scenarios (groups of 10 faced the scenarios with each student responsible for at least one case). Five of the ten scenarios were found to have acceptable internal consistency (difficult intubation, anaphylactic reaction, postoperative hypotension, local anesthesia toxic reaction, hypoxemia following intubation).

Thus, the study team went through a lot of effort for just five items—but they can now confidently state, "these scenarios can be used with confidence to evaluate medical students' performance." How many of us can say that with our tests? Have a look at the appendix in the article, which includes all 10 case scenarios and checklist items. (You will save yourself a lot of work and you will have the benefit of free educational expertise from the University of Toronto.)

✓ Murray D, Boulet J, Ziv A, Woodhouse J, Kras J, McAllister J. An acute care skills evaluation for graduating medical students: a pilot study using clinical simulation. Med Educ 2002;36:833–41.

This is another excellent study from Murray, Boulet, and colleagues about assessment development. By the time they are done, all of the other testing techniques (multiple choice exams) will have to defend their inclusion in the assessment toolbox!

This study used a hemorrhagic-hypotensive scenario based on the educational objectives from Washington University. A group of 43 third-year medical students, 10 fourth-year medical students, and 11 first year ER medicine residents participated. Four raters used the ever-present-in-Simulation-studies checklist. Two raters used a "holistic" (global rating) grading system. The essence of the study was to see if a pick-out-every-detail checklist was any different from an "overall karma" grade. Guess what? Overall karma yielded the same results as that darn checklist. Also, the test showed that more experienced trainees (first-year residents) did better than the medical students. Another "whew" for residency teachers everywhere.

These studies are demonstrating that checklist and global ratings match up pretty well with each other. So which one should you use?—That depends. If you have all of the resources of Washington University or Toronto or National Board, use as many methods as you can; but if resources are limited and training faculty is challenging—think about the global rating. One caution—global ratings are good if you just want to give a "final" grade. But if you want to give feedback to the examinee regarding their poor performance, having that checklist with all blank items would provide real good evidence.

✓ Murray DJ, Boulet JR, Kras JF, Woodhouse JA, Cox T, McAllister J. Acute care skills in anesthesia practice: a simulation-based resident performance assessment. Anesthesiology 2004;101:1084–95.

This is the latest study by Murray, Boulet, and colleagues and one of the most comprehensive and technically sound studies ever carried out on simulation assessment—this is one of those *must-read* articles for those responsible for resident, fellow, student, *anyone* assessment.

The investigators started out by developing six scenarios that could be completed by a resident in a single session. The cases were compared with the topic list by the American Board of Anesthesiologists Content Outline (content validity). The cases were the following.

- Postoperative anaphylaxis
- Intraoperative myocardial ischemia
- Intraoperative atelectasis
- Intraoperative ventricular tachycardia
- Postoperative stroke with intracranial hypertension
- Postoperative respiratory failure

Twenty-eight junior and senior anesthesia residents completed the six cases, which were videotaped. The scoring included three technical ratings and one global (holistic) rating. The technical ratings included the following.

- Traditional checklist of diagnostic and management actions
- Time to key action for the most important three actions
- Key action

Six raters reviewed the videotapes and used different combinations of the scoring methods. What did the investigators demonstrate?

- Senior residents outperformed junior residents over the six cases—*yes*!!
- Some cases were more difficult than others (most difficult was postoperative stroke, easiest was postoperative respiratory failure).
- All of the scoring methods correlated with each other over the six cases (you must use all of the cases to achieve this—you cannot use a single case).
- Raters were pretty consistent between each other, between cases and within cases, demonstrating that the choice of raters had little impact on the performance of the residents (*yes*!—an objective, nonbiased scoring system).

Well, it seems that this team has finally done it—come up with the perfect exam—validity (as determined by matching cases with national objectives and judged to be realistic), reliable (as discussed above), and feasible (these were manageable scenarios over a reasonable time period within the resources of most training programs). *But*, before we begin to pat the backs of the investigators—there are still some questions—and who better to remind of these questions but—Professor Gaba.

In an accompanying editorial Gaba praises the investigators for finally developing a scoring system that is reliable across cases and raters and within cases and raters. But, does good performance on a 5-minute exam mean you are a good anesthesiologist? Gaba reminded us that most problems in anesthesia do not occur during the first 5 minutes (when you are most ready for the problem to occur). In aviation, problems often occur several hours into flight—just as in anesthesia many problems occur several hours into the case (when the resident might be tired or not paying attention). So although this is an extremely important leap for simulation assessment, we are still looking for the perfect test.

✓ WELLER JM, BLOCH M, YOUNG S, MAZE M, OYESOLA S, WYNER J, ET AL. Evaluation of high fidelity patient simulator in assessment of performance of anaesthetists. Br J Anaesth 2003;90:43–7.

Because so many Simulator evaluations depend on videotaped reviews, you need to "evaluate the videotape evaluators." If the Simulator wants to belong in the "educational clubhouse" but the videotape evaluation process is all over the map, maybe Simulators *don't* belong in the educational clubhouse. This study looked at the evaluators. Are they consistent? Do they come up with the same "grade"? How many evaluators do you need? To clarify these questions, take the argument to an absurd endpoint, the rhetorical "reduction ad absurdens."

Five examiners look at a tape of a resident. The examiners opine as follows.

1. This resident stinks. Flunk him.
2. This resident is a genius. Praise him to high heaven.
3. This resident is so-so, no great shakes.
4. What resident?
5. I can't decide. Bring him back next Tuesday.

If such wildly varying opinions happened in a Simulator, then this method has no predictability, no reproducibility, no validity. The Simulator does not belong in the "educational clubhouse." But what did this study show? No such wildly varying opinions.

Three judges looking at videotapes concurred in their assessment. And an *additional* five people looking at the tapes (eight total!) also concurred. So, the Simulator, with its videotape evaluation *does* have predictability, *does* have reproducibility, *does* have validity. Simulation does belong in the educational clubhouse.

Another important point they looked at was, "How many judges do you need?" Let's face it, eight judges all looking at a tape of one resident starts to add up to a lot of personnel hours. So you need, what? Five (still a lot), three? How many? Two. Two judges can provide a reliable assessment. That is doable. So, from a practical standpoint, Simulators again come up as "educational clubhouse-worthy."

✓ Weller JM, Robinson BJ, Jolly B, Watterson LM, Joseph M, Bajenov S, et al. Psychometric characteristics of simulation-based assessments in anaesthesia and accuracy of self-assessed scores. Anaesthesia 2005;60:245–50.

It has been shown that Simulators meet the validity mark.

- Face validity—Nearly everyone judges the Simulator experiences as closer to the real thing than a written test.
- Content validity—You can get consensus opinion regarding what skills should be tested whether you have students or residents.
- Discriminate validity—Experienced practitioners (university) outperform residents (seniors better than juniors) who outperform medical students.

It has been demonstrated by the sheer number of articles in this bibliography that many people are accepting the amount of resources necessary for successful Simulator training and assessment and feasibility challenges are beginning to wane.

That leaves reliability—how consistent is the exam? Many of the articles discussed show evidence for reliability—but how do you achieve the best reliability? That is the focus of this study by Weller and her colleagues at the Wellington Simulation Centre in New Zealand.

- What is the optimal (minimal) number of cases required?
- What is the optimal (minimal) number of raters required?
- What is the optimal test format?
- How accurate is self-assessment?
- What is the interaction of the examinee, rater, and case on the ultimate score?

Whew—that's a lot of questions! But they are up to the task! Twenty-two anesthesia trainees (1 to 5 years experience) went through three highly scripted 15-minute cases (anaphylaxis, oxygen pipe failure, cardiac arrest). They were scored by four raters who reviewed videotapes of their performances.

Through a very complex statistical test called generalizability analysis (I promise we won't discuss that here), the authors learned that you need 10 to 15 cases or 3 to 4 hours to reliably evaluate trainees' ability to manage anesthesia emergencies. They also determined it is more feasible to have one rater score all trainees on a single case and have 15 cases with 15 judges—than to have 4 judges each marking every time in 10 to 12 cases.

Oh—examinees are okay (but not great) in evaluating their own performance. Less experienced trainees tend to overestimate their ability by a greater margin than more experienced trainees—the more you know, the more you realize how much you don't know.

Additional Articles on the Topic "Gee Whiz, Golly, I Belong Too"

Grubb G, Morey JC, Simon R. Sustaining and advancing performance improvements achieved by crew resource management training. Presented at the Ohio State Aviation Psychology Symposium, 2001, pp 1–4.

Grube C, Sinner B, Boeker T, Graf BM. The patient simulator for taking examinations—a cost effective tool? Anesthesiology 2001; 95:A1202.

Henrichs B. The perceptions of student registered nurse anesthetists of the anesthesia patient simulator experience. Presented at Technology for the Next Century, Orlando, FL, 2000.

Henrichs B, Murray D, Kras J, Woodhouse J. Interrater reliability of two scoring systems with the anesthesia simulator. Presented at the International Meeting on Medical Simulation, San Diego, 2003.

Henson LC, Richardson MG, Stern DH, Shekhter I. Using human patient simulator to credential first-year anesthesiology residents before taking overnight call. In: 2nd Annual International Meeting on Medical Simulation, January 2002, abstract A192.

Holcomb JB, Dumire RD, Crommett JW, Stamateris CE, Fagert MA, Cleveland JA, et al. Evaluation of trauma team performance using an advanced human patient simulator for resuscitation training. J Trauma 2002;52:1078–85.

Kurrek M, Devitt J, Cohen M, Szalai J. Inter-rater reliability between live-scenarios and video recordings in a realistic simulator. Presented at the Society for Technology in Anesthesia Annual Meeting, San Diego, 1999.

Mackenzie CF, Jefferies NJ, Hunter WA, Bernhard WN, Xiao Y. Comparison of self reporting of deficiencies in airway management with video analysis of actual performance; LOTAS group: level one trauma simulation. Hum Factors 1996;38:623–35.

Morgan P, Cleave-Hogg D, Byrick R, Devitt J. Performance evaluation using the anesthesia simulator. Anesthesiology 1998;89: A67.

Nadel FM, Lavelle JM, Fein JA, Giardino AP, Decker JM, Durbin DR. Assessing pediatric senior residents' training in resuscitation: fund of knowledge, technical skills, and perception of confidence. Pediatr Emerg Care 2000;16:73–6.

Rogers PL, Jacob H, Rashwan AS, Pinsky MR. Quantifying learning in medical students during a critical care medicine elective: a comparison of three evaluation instruments. Crit Care Med 2001;29:1268–73.

Rosenblatt MA, Abrams KJ; New York State Society of Anesthesiologists, Inc; Committee on Continuing Medical Education and Remediation; Remediation Sub-Committee. The use of a human patient simulator in the evaluation of and development of a remedial prescription for an anesthesiologist with lapsed medical skills. Anesth Analg 2002;94:149–53.

Santora TA, Trooskin SZ, Blank CA, Blarke JR, Scinco MA. Video assessment of trauma response: adherence to ATLS protocols. Am J Emerg Med 1996;14:564–9.

Slagle J, Weinger M, Dinh M-T, Brumer VV, Williams K. Assessment of the intrarater and interrater reliability of an established clinical task analysis methodology. Anesthesiology 2002;96:1129–39.

Tarshis J, Morgan P, Devitt J. Making of student written examinations: interrater reliability. Anesthesiology 1998;88:A68.

Articles Touching on the Theme "Halfway to the Station"

You don't want to look at a high-fidelity simulator as a "partial task trainer," something that teaches you a single skill. We *have* "partial task trainers" (intubation dummies, IV placement models, laparoscopy skill trainers). A Simulator is an "all the tasks integrated together" trainer. But measuring "all the tasks integrated together" is tough. These articles show how the simulator takes you "half way to the station." You *do get better* with the simulator, the burning question always being "Yes, but do you *really get better*, out in the real live world?"

We can't *quite* answer that question with these articles, though we try. We *try* to get all the way to the station, but to be intellectually honest we have to admit this: Simulators only get us half way to the station.

✓ ABRAHAMSON S, DENSON JS, WOLF RM. Effectiveness of a simulator in training anesthesiology residents. J Med Educ 1969;44:515–9.

The paper begins, "the use of simulation in medical education is increasing in frequency and in sophistication." This was written 36 years ago and has been cited in nearly every study since. This study should be read more for historical reasons and to appreciate the vision of the investigators who were clearly ahead of their time. The main focus of the study was to determine if anesthesia residents trained on a Simulator would achieve a predetermined benchmark of competence in less time and with fewer OR trials than residents not "permitted" to use the Simulator.

The authors randomly divided 12 new residents (2 were omitted) into two groups—simulator training versus no Simulator training. The outcomes measures were chart reviews of the resident's cases involving endotracheal intubations. Investigators gave a global rating (+ for acceptable performance, – for unacceptable performance). The residents assigned to Simulator training took fewer trials and days to reach six criteria, although only two of them were statistically significant.

Although the results were not strong, the authors did comment that fewer trials to reach competence meant, "significantly less threat to patient welfare is posed by residents who have trained on the patient simulator." Thus the patient safety movement and high-fidelity Simulator movement was born.

What happened? Medical educators, clinicians, and society were not ready for this yet. The amazing Simulator that was life size, "having a plastic skin, which resembles that of a real human being in color and texture; its configuration is that of a patient lying on an operating table" (sound familiar?), "left arm extended and ready for IV injection, right arm fitted with a blood pressure cuff, and chest wall having a stethoscope taped over location of the heart. It breathes, has a heart beat, synchronized temporal and carotid pulses and blood pressure, opens and closes mouth; blinks it eyes and responds to four IV administered drugs and two gases. The physiological responses to what is done to him are in real time and occur automatically as part of a computer program." Although the Sim One would appear crude and clunky compared to today's models, it was a remarkable engineering achievement that went to waste, as no future models were created. The lessons were the promise of Simulation and what can be achieved through the combined talents of a clinician (Denson), a medical educator (Abrahamson), a psychologist (Wolf), and engineers. (For a fascinating account of the history of this Simulator, see Abrahamson S. Sim One—a patient simulator ahead of its time. Caduceus 1997;13:29–41.)

✓ GOOD ML, GRAVENSTEIN JS, MAHLA ME, WHITE SE, BANNER MJ, CAROBANO RG, ET AL. Can simulation accelerate the learning of the basic anesthesia skills by beginning anesthesia residents [abstract]? Anesthesiology 1992;77:A1133.

This is one of the few abstracts in the bibliography but a very promising study that did not evolve into a full research paper. Nonetheless, 26 beginning anesthesia residents were exposed to lectures, and 26 other beginning residents were taught some basic anesthetic principles (checking the machine, treating hypoxemia, inducing, intubating) in the Simulator. The groups stayed neck-and-neck so long as written exams were done, but during weeks 3 and 8 the Simulator-trained residents were judged "better clinically." The two groups were judged to be equivalent by week 13. So it seems those patients with the traditionally trained group were likely at increased risk for the first 3 months of the residents' training (do not get sick between July and September).

Of note, the Simulator group only had one training session in the Simulator—perhaps a greater difference would have been noted with more frequent early training sessions. So, at least as far as an intermediate assessment of some (let's face it), vital skills, the Simulator seems to be the way to go.

✓ Howard SK, Gaba DM, Fish KJ, Yang G, Sarnquist FH. Anesthesia crisis resource management training: teaching anesthesiologists to handle critical incidents. Aviat Space Environ Med 1992;63:763–70.

This reference is included more because of its originality and influence than its strength in improving skills—in fact the study did not show an improvement in skills—but its description of the design, development, implementation, and evaluation of crisis resource management training have influenced nearly every curriculum and study that have followed. Early on, Howard and Gaba made clear the goals of this type of training.

- Provide trainees with standardized simulated critical events at the touch of a button
- Instruct trainees in the coordinated management of all available resources to *maximize safe patient outcomes* (these guys were interested in patient safety well before the infamous Institute of Medicine report)

The authors provide background about the origins of the course, including a detailed table of 62 critical incidents in anesthesia. In this study, 19 residents and practitioners went through a 2-day course, took written pre- and postcourse exams, and completed course evaluation forms. The course in its original inception was 2 days (1 day for lectures and familiarization with simulation, 1 day for Simulator training on six cases 15 to 30 minutes long and 2 hours of debriefing).

Residents showed an improvement in their knowledge and faculty did not, although they started out much higher. The authors admit they have doubts whether written tests actually mean anything regarding performance, although one needs to know about crises and know how to respond to them before they can show how to respond. *But no skills were evaluated—why?*

The authors argue that any comparison study in which performance is evaluated on a Simulator would automatically benefit the group that trained on the Simulator, and there is no gold standard measure for performance during a crisis. This sounds like a cop-out, and to some extent it is—but we'll give these vanguards some slack because they did boldly go where no anesthesiologist went before. The authors also pointed out that a one-shot course is unlikely to have any real meaningful effect on the skills of clinicians—what is needed is an ongoing lifetime of training in which the entire culture of training and practice adopts the principles of crisis management. Finally, the authors pointed out that "no proof of increased safety has ever been provided for Simulator training or CRM training in aviation." It just stands to reason that this training is important and will ultimately have an effect of patient safety.

✓ Chopra V, Gesink BJ, de Jong J, Bovill JG, Spierdijk J, Brand R. Does training on an anaesthesia simulator lead to improvement in performance? Br J Anaesth 1994;73:293–7.

This is one of the earliest studies (aside from Abrahamson and Sim-One) to evaluate the effect of a Simulator as a training tool. Twenty-eight anesthetists were first evaluated in their ability to manage a case of anaphylactic shock on the Simulator. They were next randomly divided into two groups: One group received Simulator training with a case of anaphylactic shock and the other with a case of malignant hyperthermia. *Four months later* they were evaluated on their ability to manage a case of malignant hyperthermia on the Simulator.

What did they measure?

- Response times of the first treatment step
- Weighted checklist of critical management items
- Deviation from accepted guidelines

What did they find? Perhaps the most baffling conclusion was that "this study shows that anaesthetists trained on a high fidelity anesthesia simulator respond more quickly, deviate less from accepted guidelines, and perform better in handling crisis situations, such as malignant hyperthermia, than those *who are not trained on the simulator*." What? I thought *both* groups were trained on the Simulator. Well, they were—this is an example of poor review during the publishing process. So those trained to respond to malignant hyperthermia on a Simulator performed better on a

Simulator than those trained to respond to another case on a Simulator. We cannot be too hard on the research team because they were one of the first to attempt to study the effect of Simulator training. What is unacceptable is the number of subsequent studies that have not learned from the flaws (or lessons) from this study. We point them out now—so we can move forward.

- This study demonstrates case specificity—clinical ability to respond to a specific clinical case does not translate to ability to respond to a different case even if some of the specific technical skills are similar. The authors evaluated very specific outcomes that were very dependent on the actual case. Had they evaluated more global skills—such as team management, communication skills, leadership skills—the results may have been different. But even these are highly dependent on the specific case. We will see this issue appear again and again.
- The evaluation phase took place 4 months after the training—any training that occurred during the time could have had an impact on the final exam. The authors did not measure this. For example, did any of the anesthetists participate in a real case of malignant hyperthermia? Did they discuss their Simulation experience with their peers?
- The authors do not comment as to why the response times increased after the training—they just took more time to respond! Perhaps they were more reflective, more deliberate and in more control—perhaps.

Despite these flaws, this *is* an important study in the brief history of Simulation training research because it demonstrated that comparison studies (before and after) are possible and feasible.

✓ Byrne AJ, Sellen AJ, Jones JG, Aitkenhead AR, Hussain S, Gilder F, et al. Effect of videotape feedback on anaesthetists' performance while managing simulated anaesthetic crises: a multicentre study. Anaesthesia 2002;57:176–9.

This study began the recent tend to look beyond whether Simulator training is better than no Simulator training by studying the most effective feature of Simulator training—feedback.

Thirty-two anesthetist trainees went through five simulation sessions.

- Hypotension
- Ventricular tachycardia
- Bradycardia
- Anaphylaxis
- Oxygen supply failure

One group received very little feedback about their performance as they went from case to case, and the study group received detailed videotaped feedback regarding their performance for each case. The researcher measured the improvement from the first case to the fifth case in terms of their time to respond to the critical event and the amount of errors on the anesthesia chart (remember: all of the cases are different, and ability on one case does not translate to ability on another case). What do you think happened?

That's right—there was very little difference between the two groups (at least it was not significant). The authors were surprised by the results (but we weren't), but they did have insight as to the reason—the anesthetist had learned how to respond to the crises to which they were exposed, and this case-specific ability does not translate to other cases—not when the skills you are measuring are specific to the clinical case. How can you compare the time it takes to respond to bradycardia (one sign) to the time it takes to respond to anaphylaxis (multiple potential signs). This dilemma has been the focus of serious research during the last couple of years and is reviewed in the "we belong too" section.

This study is important because it was the first multicenter trial to evaluate the effect of Simulator training. While this is a much more valid approach (training programs—regardless of their location should be able to deliver effective training), it introduces the possibility of standardization issues. The authors do not provide any details about how the simulations were calibrated at the multiple centers to ensure the participants were receiving similar training. This is an extremely important factor in the development of our field—we need more transparency in these studies so we can try to replicate a course if it looks good.

✓ Devita MA, Schaefer J, Lutz J, Dongili T, Wong H. Advances in human simulation education: improving medical crisis performance. Crit Care Med 2004;32:S61–5.

This is one of many studies you will be seeing from Devita and colleagues at the WISER Simulation Research Center at the University of Pittsburgh. This center is a state-of-the-art 7000 square foot training institute that houses 10 full-body Laerdal SimMan Simulators. In this study, the team evaluated the effectiveness of a new curriculum aimed at training multidisciplinary teams to respond to critical care scenarios. They point out that most critical codes look like a three-ring circus—internists, nurses, anesthesiologists, all doing their own thing with the most simple of tasks—chest compressions are inadequate. Rather than focus, as most curricula do, on specific procedural skills, they have developed a curriculum that emphasizes communication and teamwork skills—in other words most people know how to perform these skills in isolation but have a hard time during the chaos of life-threatening emergencies.

They have trained more than 200 medical personnel in courses comprising:

- Mandatory precourse web-based tutorials
- Brief didactic session
- Video-recorded simulation session
- Postsimulation debriefing session

They have developed a system that assigns specific tasks for up to eight medical personnel who would typically respond to a critical care event in the hospital. Each participant was exposed to three of the following scenarios.

- Ventricular tachycardia-induced dyspnea
- Acute myocardial infarction and arrhythmia
- Morphine overdose during patient-controlled analgesia
- Acute stroke with mental status changes
- Ventricular fibrillation

By reviewing video recordings of the sessions, they measured the survival status of the "patient" at the end of the simulation session as well as completion of the organization and treatment tasks. All participants, regardless of their profession were awful during the first scenario—the survival rate was 0%—yikes! However, by the third session, the survival rate was more than 80%. By the third training session, nearly every task was completed effectively in an organized manner. The authors nicely summarize the limitations of the study—it did not prove correlation with real patients, interrater agreement, need to measure retention of skills. But hey, the individuals and team appeared to improve their skills, and the authors have just given several good ideas for research projects. Get to it!

✓ Mayo PH, Hackney JE, Mueck JT, Ribaudo V, Schneider RF. Achieving house staff competence in emergency airway management: results of a teaching program using a computerized patient simulator. Crit Care Med 2004;32:2422–7.

Internal medicine interns are the least trained practicing physicians on a typical team yet are often the first ones to respond to in-hospital cardiac arrest codes. Early in their training, they are probably scared,

nervous, and dread the fateful call of their first code. One of the first critical elements is airway management, and it is safe to presume these internists are not very good at this task. The authors wanted to do something about this and developed a mandatory airway training program for interns early in their training.

They divided interns into three groups: group 1—no testing or training; group 2—testing with no training; and group 3—testing with Simulator training. Interns in group 3 were all tested and videotaped after 4 weeks of working with the Simulator. The scenario was an apneic hypotensive patient who's condition worsened to cardiac arrest after not being treated appropriately within 3 minutes. The interns were evaluated by two investigators (who served as nurses).

At the beginning of the study all groups had equally poor airway skills (even though they had all just become certified in ACLS). Group 3 then received intensive training and feedback on airway skills using the Simulator. Four weeks later, all groups were tested again on the Simulator. Group 3 performed significantly better than the other two groups—this is no surprise, as they had received training (but the skills did last 4 weeks). The authors thought it was unethical to deprive the other two groups of training, so they received the same hands-on training as group 3. One of the study authors then followed these interns around for the remainder of the year and evaluated their performance during actual critical cases.

What did he find? A total of 41 of the 50 interns participated in an actual critical case involving airway management skills. This group's performance was judged to be excellent. More than 90% of interns performed all of the predefined airway tasks correctly. This almost sounds like a salvation paper. After training, the interns were judged superior in these key critical skills in scenarios with real patients. Although there are all sorts of problems with the design and methodology of the study, the authors should be commended for attempting long-term follow-up with real patients. What were some of the study's limitations?

- There was no preintervention evaluation of airway skills on real patients—but it makes sense that their improved performance was related to training.
- The study's investigators also served as the residents' evaluators, and this could introduce bias.
- They could not use their videotaped recordings of the participants because their only camera did not capture much of the task (this illustrates the need to

do small pilot studies before engaging in larger trials).

An important issue the authors stress again and again is the limitation of current ACLS courses in that they do not prepare interns in the basic skills they need early in their training.

✓ Schwid HA, Rooke GA, Ross BK, Sivarajan M. Use of a computerized advanced cardiac life support simulator improves retention of advanced cardiac life support guidelines better than a textbook review. Crit Care Med 1999;27:821–4.

This is not a full-body simulator training study; rather, it is a flat-screen computer-based training study. (Again, to tie in with Simulato-land, any simulation center can incorporate some flat-screen computer stations to round out the teaching.)

Do you perform better and retain more skills reading an ACLS textbook or completing a computer-based ACLS simulation program? Nearly a year after ACLS certification, 45 anesthesiology residents, fellows, and faculty were randomly divided to receive booster review either through the American Heart Association ACLS textbook or via the computer-based Anesthesia 3.1.1 Simulator. This training device uses a graphic interface to simulate management of patients with cardiac arrhythmias. Throughout and at the end of the case, feedback is provided such as overall case management including errors made. All participants were evaluated on their ability to respond to a Mega-Code using the MedSIM full-body simulator. The cases included SVT, VF, and second-degree AV blocks.

Those receiving computer-based Simulator training performed significantly better and had higher pass rate than the group who only read textbooks. (In fact, six in the control group never cracked open a book to review, whereas everyone in the Simulator group showed up for training. Why? It was more fun!)

What does that mean to us? Simulator training may lead to better recall. In addition, it demonstrates the utility and feasibility of computer-based training exercises as an important adjunct to Simulator training. Aviation routinely provides a computer-based flight Simulator training program to all pilots prior to their training on the real McCoy.

✓ Schwid HA, Rooke GA, Michalowski P, Ross BK. Screen-based anesthesia simulation with debriefing improves performance in a mannequin-based anesthesia simulator. Teach Learn Med 2001;13:92–6.

A couple of years later, Schwid and his colleagues wanted to repeat the findings of their ACLS study—this time on four critical events in anesthesia. A group of 31 first-year anesthesia residents were randomized into two groups: One group received training covering 10 cases on the computer-based Anesthesia 3.0 Simulator, and the other group read about the proper management of the same cases. The Simulator-trained residents also received individualized written feedback from a faculty member. Three to six months later the residents were evaluated on their ability to manage four cases using the MedSim full-body Simulator (they were videotaped):

- Esophageal intubation
- Anaphylaxis
- Bronchospasm
- Myocardial ischemia

The residents were evaluated on videotape by two faculty members, who used a standardized checklist rating form (see appendix in the article for a copy of the evaluation forms). What do you think happened? You guessed it. The computer Simulator-trained group performed better than the residents who only did some reading. What is the deal?

- More evidence is provided on the utility of computer "microsimulations" for training practical skills.
- The simulator was not the *only* difference—you want to bet that the individual feedback also had something to do with the difference?
- The Simulator-trained group still performed poorly—52.6 points out of 95 (55%). Although their performance was significantly better than that of the "control" group (43.4 points, or 46%), did they achieve an acceptable passing mark? We don't know because the researchers did not set one. Are you comfortable with residents who miss 45% of the tasks? I'm not either.

Many researchers have focused on evaluating the effect of Simulators to train specific tasks rather than the entire management. These are much more feasible studies that allow you to focus training very carefully on one skill and develop tests that are very reliable. The disadvantage is that they have less validity; and because they do not mirror what happens in real situations, you always have to deal with more than one clinical sign/task. However, even the most sophisticated and elaborate full-body simulations are only approximations of reality, and all Simulator training—full-body interactive to part-task trainer—falls within a continuum of fidelity. So we do not exclude these guys. By the way, walk into any state-of-the-art aviation simulation center, and you will see loads of pilots practicing a single skill on a tasks trainer.

We have a training model for crisis management skills—one from aviation that has been adopted for medicine. But do we have a model for training specific individual skills. Yes we do. Anders Ericsson from Florida State University studies the factors that separate the elite performer in sports, chess, and music from the novice and found that it came down to the amount of deliberate practice one engages in can influence their mastery of a skill—what is "deliberate practice."

Deliberate practice involves (1) intense, repetitive performance of intended thinking or doing skills in a focused area (intubation); coupled with (2) rigorous skills assessment; that provides learners (3) specific, informative feedback; that yields increasingly (4) better skills performance in a controlled setting. (See Ericsson KA. Deliberate practice and the acquisition and maintenance of expert performance in medicine and related domains. Acad Med 2004;79(Suppl): S1–12.)

In 1999, our group at the University of Miami was the first in the medical simulation world to recognize the application of deliberate practice in medical skills training. Since then many others have also recognized the value of this model and have begun to incorporate it into their skills training. We next illustrate an article that incorporates features of deliberate practice into their skills training although they did not realize it.

✓ Kovacs G, Bullock G, Ackroyd-Stolarz S, Cain E, Petrie D. A randomized controlled trial on the effect of educational interventions in promoting airway management skill maintenance. Ann Emerg Med 2000;36:301–9.

In this study, the authors evaluated the effect of repetitive practice and feedback on the acquisition of airway management skills. A group of 84 health sciences students were first pretested on their airway management skills with a checklist of key items. The students were then randomized into three groups.

Group 1—no practice sessions, no feedback after evaluation

Group 2—no practice sessions, feedback after each evaluation

Group 3—three practice sessions, with feedback after each practice session and evaluation

All students were evaluated at 16, 25, and 40 weeks after their initial testing session. The students who were allowed to practice performed a minimum of 15 endotracheal intubations (repetitive practice). Group

3 also received close supervision and immediate feedback regarding their skills. Not surprisingly, group 3 achieved much higher competency scores on the airway management tasks than groups 1 and 2. There was no difference in the performances of students in groups 1 or 2. Feedback is not enough—trainees must be allowed to incorporate the feedback they receive into practice. More importantly, the skills of group 3 did not deteriorate over time, whereas those in group 1 did not improve and group 2 showed nonsignificant improvement over group 1. This illustrates the need for ongoing remediation for skills maintenance—think every 2 years is enough for ACLS training?

Too often training programs limit practice time to the convenience of the faculty rather than to the needs of the learner. It would have been nice if the authors included a fourth group that was allowed to practice but received no feedback. But it is a good controlled study illustrating the importance of practice *and* feedback.

Additional "Halfway to the Station" Articles

Ali J, Adam R, Pierre I, Bedaysie H, Josa D, Winn J. Comparison of performance two years after the old and new (interactive) ATLS course. J Surg Res 2001;97:71–5.

Ashurst N, Rout CC, Rocke DA, Gouws E. Use of a mechanical simulator for training in applying cricoid pressure. Br J Anaesth 1996;77:468–72.

Berge JA, Gramstad L, Grimnes S. An evaluation of a time-saving anesthetic machine checkout procedure. Eur J Anaesthesiol 1994;11:493–8.

Bucx MJ, van Geel RT, Wegener JT, Robers C, Stijnen T. Does experience influence the forces exerted on maxillary incisors during laryngoscopy? A manikin study using the Macintosh laryngoscope. Can J Anaesth 1995;42:144–9.

Byrne AJ, Jones JG. Responses to simulated anaesthetic emergencies by anaesthetists with different durations of clinical experience. Br J Anaesth 1997;78:553–6.

Chopra V, Engbers FH, Geerts MJ, Filet WR, Bovill JG, Spierdijk J. The Leiden anaesthesia simulator. Br J Anaesth 1994;73: 287–92.

Curran VR, Aziz K, O'Young S, Bessel C. Evaluation of the effect of computerized training simulator (ANAKIN) on the retention of neonatal resuscitation skills. Teach Learn Med 2004;16: 157–64.

Dalley P, Robinson B, Weller J, Caldwell C. The use of high-fidelity human patient simulation and the introduction of a new anesthesia delivery system. Anesth Analg 2004;99:1737–41.

DeAnda A, Gaba DM. Role of experience in the response to simulated critical incidents. Anesth Analg 1991;72:308–15.

Delson NJ, Koussa N, Hastings RH, Weinger MB. Quantifying expert vs. novice skill in vivo for development of a laryngoscope simulator. Stud Health Technol Inform 2003;94:45–51.

Done ML, Parr M. Teaching basic life support skills using self-directed learning, a self-instructional video, access to practice manikins and learning in pairs. Resuscitation 2002;52:287–91.

Euliano TY. Small group teaching: clinical correlation with a human patient simulator. Adv Physiol Educ 2001;25:36–43.

Euliano TY. Teaching respiratory physiology: clinical correlation with a human patient simulator. J Clin Monit Comput 2000;16:465–70.

Farnsworth ST, Egan TD, Johnson SE, Westenskow D. Teaching sedation and analgesia with simulation. J Clin Monit Comput 2000;16:273–85.

Forrest FC, Taylor MA, Postlethwaite K, Aspinall R. Use of a high-fidelity simulator to develop testing of the technical performance of novice anaesthetists. Br J Anaesth 2002;88:338–44.

From RP, Pearson KS, Albanese MA, Moyers JR, Sigurdsson SS, Dull DL. Assessment of an interactive learning system with "sensorized" manikin head for airway management instruction. Anesth Analg 1994;79:136–42.

Gaba D, Lee T. Measuring the workload of the anesthesiologist. Anesth Analg 1990;71:354–61.

Gaba DM, DeAnda A. The response of anesthesia trainees to simulated critical incidents. Anesth Analg 1989;68:444–51.

Gass DA, Curry L. Physicians' and nurses' retention of knowledge and skill after training in cardiopulmonary resuscitation. Can Med Assoc J 1983;128:550–1.

Goodwin MWP, French GWG. Simulation as a training and assessment tool in the management of failed intubation in obstetrics. Int J Obstet Anesth 2001;10:273–7.

Grant WD. Addition of anesthesia patient simulator is an improvement to evaluation process. Anesth Analg 2002;95:786–7.

Greenberg R, Loyd G, Wesley G. Integrated simulated experiences to enhance clinical education. Med Educ 2002;36:1109–10.

Halamek L, Howard S, Smith B, Smith B, Gaba D. Development of a simulated delivery room for the study of human performance during neonatal resuscitation. Pediatrics 1997;100(Suppl):513–24.

Hosking EJ. Does practicing intubation on a manikin improve both understanding and clinical performance of the task by medical students. Anesth Points West 1998;31:25–8.

Hotchkiss MA, Biddle C, Fallacaro M. Assessing the authenticity of the human simulation experience in anesthesiology. AANA J 2002;70:470–3.

Howard S, Keshavacharya S, Smith B, Rosekind M, Weinger M, Gaba D. Behavioral evidence of fatigue during a simulator experiment. Anesthesiology 1998;89:A1236.

Howard SK, Gaba DM, Smith BE, Weinger MB, Herndon C, Keshavacharya S, et al. Simulation study of rested versus sleep-deprived anesthesiologists. Anesthesiology 2003;98:1345–55; discussion 5A.

Jacobsen J, Jensen PF, Ostergaard D, Lindekaer A, Lippet A, Schultz P. Performance enhancement in anesthesia using the training simulator Sophus (Peanuts). In: Henson LC, Lee AC (eds) Simulators in Anesthesiology Education. New York: Plenum; 1998. p. 103–6.

Kaczorowski J, Levitt C, Hammond M, Outerbridge E, Grad R, Rothman A, et al. Retention of neonatal resuscitation skills and knowledge: a randomized controlled trial. Fam Med 1998;30:705–11.

Kras J, Murray D, Woodhouse J, Henrichs B. The validity of a simulation-based anesthesia acute care skills evaluation. Presented at the International Meeting on Medical Simulation, San Diego, 2003.

Lampotang S. Influence of pulse oximetry and capnography on time to diagnosis of critical incidents in anesthesia: a pilot study using a full-scale patient simulator. J Clin Monit Comput 1998;14:313–21.

Lee SK, Pardo M, Gaba D, Sowb Y, Dicker R, Straus EM, et al. Trauma assessment training with a patient simulator: a prospective randomized study. J Trauma 2003;55:651–7.

Levitan RM, Goldman TS, Bryan DA, Shofer F, Herlich A. Training with video imaging improves the initial intubation success rates of paramedic trainees in an operating room setting. Ann Emerg Med 2001;37:46–50.

Marshall RL, Smith JS, Gorman PJ, Krummel TM, Haluck RS, Cooney RN. Use of a human patient simulator in the development of resident trauma management skills. J Trauma 2001;51:17–21.

Modell JH, Cantwell S, Hardcastle J, Robertson S, Pablo L. Using the human patient simulator to educate students of veterinary medicine. J Vet Med Educ 2002;29:111–6.

Morgan PJ, Cleave-Hogg D. Comparison between medical students' experience, confidence and competence. Med Educ 2002;36:534–9.

Morgan PJ, Cleave-Hogg D, DeSousa S, Tarshis J. Identification in gaps in the achievement of undergraduate anesthesia educational objectives using high-fidelity patient simulation. Anesth Analg 2003;97:1690–4.

Morgan PJ, Cleave-Hogg D, McIlroy J, Devitt JH. Simulation technology: a comparison of experiential and visual learning for undergraduate medical students. Anesthesiology 2002;96:10–6.

Nadel FM, Lavelle JM, Fein JA, Giardino AP, Decker JM, Durbin DR. Teaching resuscitation to pediatric residents: the effects of an intervention. Arch Pediatr Adolesc Med 2000;154:1049–54.

Noordergraaf GJ, Van Gelder JM, Van Kesteren RG, Diets RF, Savelkoul TJ. Learning cardiopulmonary resuscitation skills: does the type of mannequin make a difference? Eur J Emerg Med 1997;4:204–9.

Nyssen AS, Larbuisson R, Janssens M, Pendeville P, Mayne A. A comparison of the training value of two types of anesthesia simulators: computer screen-based and mannequin-based simulators. Anesth Analg 2002;94:1560–5.

Ovassapian A, Yelich SJ, Dykes MH, Golman ME. Learning fibreoptic intubation: use of simulators v. traditional teaching. Br J Anaesth 1988;61:217–20.

Owen H, Plummer JL. Improving learning of a clinical skill: the first year's experience of teaching endotracheal intubation in a clinical simulation facility. Med Educ 2002;36:635–42.

Owen H, Follows V, Reynolds KJ, Burgess G, Plummer J. Learning to apply effective cricoid pressure using a part task trainer. Anaesthesia 2002;57:1098–101.

Riley RH, Wilks DH, Freeman JA. Anaesthetists' attitudes towards an anaesthesia simulator: a comparative survey: U.S.A. and Australia. Anaesth Intensive Care 1997;25:514–9.

St Pierre M, Hofinger G, Buerschaper C, Grapengeter M, Harms H, Breuer G, et al. Simulator-based modular human factor training in anesthesiology: concept and results of the module "communication and team cooperation." Anaesthesist 2004;53:144–52.

Schaefer J, Dongilli T, Gonzalez R. Results of systematic psychomotor difficult airway training of residents using the ASA difficult airway algorithm and dynamic simulation. Anesthesiology 1998;89:A60.

Scherer YK, Bruce SA, Graves BT, Erdley WS. Acute care nurse practitioner education: enhancing performance through the use of clinical simulation. AACN Clin Issues 2003;14:331–41.

Schwid HA, O'Donnell D. Anesthesiologists' management of simulated critical incidents. Anesthesiology 1992;76:495–501.

Schwid HA, O'Donnell D. The anesthesia simulator-recorder: a device to train and evaluate anesthesiologists' responses to critical incidents. Anesthesiology 1990;72:191–7.

Schwid HA, Rooke GA, Carline J, Steadman RH, Murray WB, Olympio M, et al. Anesthesia Simulator Research Consortium: evaluation of anesthesia residents using mannequin-based simulation: a multiinstitutional study. Anesthesiology 2002;97:1434–44.

Tan GM, Ti LK, Suresh S, Ho BS, Lee TL. Teaching first-year medical students physiology: does the human patient simulator allow for more effective teaching? Singapore Med J 2002;43:238–42.

Tweed M, Tweed C, Perkins GD. The effect of differing support surfaces on the efficacy of chest compressions using a resuscitation manikin model. Resuscitation 2001;51:179–83.

Twigg SJ, McCormick B, Cook TM. Randomized evaluation of the performance of single-use laryngoscopes in simulated easy and difficult intubation. Br J Anaesth 2003;90:8–13.

Treloar D, Hawayek J, Montgomery JR, Russell W; Medical Readiness Trainer Team. On-site and distance education of emergency medicine personnel with a human patient simulator. Mil Med 2001;166:1003–6.

Von Lubitz DK, Carrasco B, Gabbrielli F, Ludwig T, Lebine H, Patricelli F, et al. Transatlantic medical education: preliminary data on disease-based high-fidelity human patient simulation training. Stud Health Technol Inform 2003;94:379–85.

Wayne DB, Butter J, Siddal VJ, Fudala MJ, Lindquist LA, Feinglass J, et al. Simulation-based training of internal medicine residents in advanced cardiac life support protocols: a randomized trial. Teach Learn Med 2005;17:210–6.

Weller J, Robinson B, Larsen P, Caldwell C. Simulation-based training to improve acute care skills in medical undergraduates. N Z Med J 2004;117:U1119.

Wik L, Dorph E, Auestad B, Andreas Steen P. Evaluation of a defibrillator-basic cardiopulmonary resuscitation programme for non-medical personnel. Resuscitation 2003;56:167–72.

Wik L, Myklebust H, Auestad BH, Steen PA. Retention of basic life support skills 6 months after training with an automated voice advisory manikin system without instructor involvement. Resuscitation 2002;52:273–9.

Wik L, Thowsen J, Steen PA. An automated voice advisory manikin system for training in basic life support without an instructor: a novel approach to CPR training. Resuscitation 2001;50:167–72.

Wong DT, Prabhu AJ, Coloma M, Imasogie N, Chung FF. What is the minimum training required for successful cricothyroidotomy? A study in mannequins. Anesthesiology 2003;98:349–53.

Wong TK, Chung JW. Diagnostic reasoning processes using patient simulation in different learning environments. J Clin Nurs 2002; 11:65–72.

"Halfway to the Station" Articles in Areas Other than Anesthesia

Agazio JB, Pavlides CC, Lasome CE, Flaherty NJ, Torrance RJ. Evaluation of a virtual reality simulator in sustainment training. Mil Med 2002;167:893–7.

Ahlberg G, Heikkinen T, Iselius L, Leijonmarck CE, Rutqvist J, Arvidsson D. Does training in a virtual reality simulator improve surgical performance? Surg Endosc 2002;16:126–9.

Ali MR, Mowery Y, Kaplan B, DeMaria EJ. Training the novice in laparoscopy: more challenge is better. Surg Endosc 2002;16: 1732–6.

Allen J, Evans A, Foulkes J, French A. Simulated surgery: in the summative assessment of general practice training: results of a trial in the Trent and Yorkshire regions. Br J Gen Pract 1998;48: 1219–23.

Anastakis DJ, Regehr G, Reznick RK, Cusiamano M, Murnaghan J, Brown M, et al. Assessment of technical skills from the bench model to the human model. Am J Surg 1999;177:167–70.

Bergamaschi R, Dicko A. Instruction versus passive observation: a randomized educational research study on laparoscopic suture skills. Surg Laparosc Endosc Percutan Tech 2000;10:319–22.

Blum MG, Powers TW, Sundaresan S. Bronchoscopy simulator effectively prepares junior residents to competency perform basic clinical bronchoscopy. Ann Thorac Surg 2004;78:287–91.

Brehmer M, Tolley D. Validation of a bench model for endoscopic surgery in the upper urinary tract. Eur Urol 2002;42:175–9; discussion 180.

Burdea G, Patounakis G, Popescu V, Weiss RE. Virtual reality-based training for the diagnosis of prostate cancer. IEEE Trans Biomed Eng 1999;46:1253–60.

Chang KK, Chung JW, Wong TK. Learning intravenous cannulation: a comparison of the conventional method and the CathSim Intravenous Training System. J Clin Nurs 2002;11:73–8.

Chaudhry A, Sutton C, Wood J, Stone R, McCloy R. Learning rate for laparoscopic surgical skills on MIST VR, a virtual reality simulator: quality of human-computer interface. Ann R Coll Surg Engl 1999;81:281–6.

Chung JY, Sackier JM. A method of objectively evaluating improvements in laparoscopic skills. Surg Endosc 1998;12:1111–6.

Clancy JM, Lindquist TJ, Palik JF, Johnson LA. A comparison of student performance in a simulation clinic and a traditional laboratory environment: three-year results. J Dent Educ 2002;66: 1331–7.

Colt HG, Crawford SW, Galbraith O 3rd. Virtual reality bronchoscopy simulation: a revolution in procedural training. Chest 2001;120:1333–9.

Crossan A, Brewster S, Reid S, Mellor D. Comparison of simulated ovary training over six different skill levels. In: Proceedings of Eurohaptics 2001 (Birmingham, UK), pp 17–21. Accessed at: www.dcs.gla.ac.uk/~stephen/papers/Eurohaptics2001_crossan.pdf.

Cundiff GW. Analysis of the effectiveness of an endoscopy education program in improving residents' laparoscopic skills. Obstet Gynecol 1997;90:854–9.

Derosis AM, Antoniuk M, Fried GM. Evaluation of laparoscopic skills: a 2-year follow-up during residency training. Can J Surg 1999;42:293–6.

Derosis AM, Bothwell J, Sigman HH, Fried GM. The effect of practice on performance in a laparoscopic simulator. Surg Endosc 1998;12:1117–20.

Derosis AM, Fried GM, Abrahamowicz M, Sigman HH, Barkun JS, Meakins JL. Development of a model for training and evaluation of laparoscopic skills. Am J Surg 1998;175:482–7.

Dobson HD, Pearl RK, Orsay CP, Rasmussen M, Evenhouse R, Ai Z, et al. Virtual reality: new method of teaching anorectal and pelvic floor anatomy. Dis Colon Rectum 2003;46:349–52.

Dorafshar AH, O'Boyle DJ, McCloy RF. Effects of a moderate dose of alcohol on simulated laparoscopic surgical performance. Surg Endosc 2002;16:1753–8.

Eastridge BJ, Hamilton EC, O'Keefe GE, Rege RV, Valentine RJ, Jones DJ, et al. Effect of sleep deprivation on the performance of simulated laparoscopic surgical kill. Am J Surg 2003;186:169–74.

Edmond CV Jr. Impact of the endoscopic sinus surgical simulator on operating room performance. Laryngoscope 2002;112: 1148–58.

Emam TA, Hanna GB, Kimber C, Cuschieri A. Differences between experts and trainees in the motion pattern of the dominant upper limb during intracorporeal endoscopic knotting. Dig Surg 2000;17:120–5.

Engum SA, Jeffries P, Fisher L. Intravenous catheter training system: computer-based education versus traditional learning methods. Am J Surg 2003;186:67–74.

Ewy GA, Felner JM, Juul D, Mayer JW, Sajid AW, Waugh RA. Test of a cardiology patient simulator with students in fourth-year electives. J Med Educ 1987;62:738–43.

Ferlitsch A, Glauninger P, Gupper A, Schillinger M, Haefner M, Gangl A, et al. Evaluation of a virtual endoscopy simulator for training in gastrointestinal endoscopy. Endoscopy 2002;34:698–702.

Francis NK, Hanna GB, Cuschieri A. Reliability of the Dundee endoscopic psychomotor tester (DEPT) for dominant hand performance. Surg Endosc 2001;15:673–6.

Francis NK, Hanna GB, Cuschieri A. The performance of master surgeons on the advanced Dundee endoscopic psychomotor tester: contrast validity study. Arch Surg 2002;137:841–4.

Fraser SA, Klassen DR, Feldman LS, Ghitulescu GA, Stanbridge D, Fried GM. Evaluating laparoscopic skills. Surg Endosc 2003;17:964–7.

Fried GM, Derosis AM, Bothwell J, Sigman HH. Comparison of laparoscopic performance in vivo with performance measured in a laparoscopic simulator. Surg Endosc 1999;13:1077–81.

Gallagher AG, Satava RM. Virtual reality as a metric for the assessment of laparoscopic psychomotor skills: learning curves and reliability measures. Surg Endosc 2002;16:1746–52.

Gallagher AG, Hughes C, McClure N, McGuigan J. A case-control comparison of traditional and virtual reality in laparoscopic performance. Minim Invasive Ther All Techn 2000;9:347–52.

Gallagher AG, McClure N, McGuigan J, Crothers I, Browning J. Virtual reality training in laparoscopic surgery: a preliminary assessment of minimally invasive surgical trainer virtual reality (MIST VR). Endoscopy 1999;31:310–3.

Gallagher AG, Richie K, McClure N, McGuigan J. Objective psychomotor skills assessment of experienced, junior, and novice laparoscopists with virtual reality. World J Surg 2001;25:1478–83.

Gallagher HJ, Allan JD, Tolley DA. Spatial awareness in urologists: are they different? BJU Int 2001;88:666–70.

Gaskin PR, Owens SE, Talner NS, Sanders SP, Li JS. Clinical auscultation skills in pediatric residents. Pediatrics 2000;105:1184–7.

Gerson LB, Van Dam J. A prospective randomized trial comparing a virtual reality simulator to bedside teaching for training in sigmoidoscopy. Endoscopy 2003;35:569–75.

Geyoushi B, Apte K, Stones RW. Simulators for intimate examination training in the developing world. J Fam Plann Reprod Health Care 2003;29:34–5.

Gilbart MK, Hutchison CR, Cusimano MD, Regehr G. A computer-based trauma simulator for teaching trauma management skills. Am J Surg 2000;179:223–8.

Goldiez BF. History of networked simulations. In: Clarke TL (ed) Distributed Interactive Simulation Systems for Simulation and Training in the Aerospace Environment. Bellingham, WA: SPIE Optical Engineering Press; 1995. p. 39–58.

Gor M, McCloy R, Stone R, Smith A. Virtual reality laparoscopic simulator for assessment in gynaecology. Br J Obstet Gynaecol 2003;110:181–7.

Gordon MS, Ewy GA, DeLeon AC Jr, Waugh RA, Felner JM, Forker AD, et al. "Harvey," the cardiology patient simulator: pilot studies on teaching effectiveness. Am J Cardiol 1980;45:791–6.

Grantcharov TP, Bardram L, Funch-Jensen P, Rosenberg J. Impact of hand dominance, gender, and experience with computer games on performance in virtual reality laparoscopy. Surg Endosc 2003;17:1082–5.

Grantcharov TP, Bardman L, Funch-Jensen P, Rosenberg J. Laparoscopic performance after one night on call in a surgical department: prospective study. BMJ 2001;323:1222–2.

Grantcharov TP, Bardram L, Funch-Jensen P, Rosenberg J. Learning curves and impact of previous operative experience on performance on a virtual reality simulator to test laparoscopic surgical skills. Am J Surg 2003;185:146–9.

Haluck RS, Webster RW, Snyder AJ, Melkonian MG, Mohler BJ, Dise ML, et al. A virtual reality surgical trainer for navigation in laparoscopic surgery. Stud Health Technol Inform 2001;81:171–7.

Hamilton EC, Scott DJ, Fleming JB, Rege RV, Laycock R, Bergen PC, et al. Comparison of video trainer and virtual reality training systems on acquisition of laparoscopic skills. Surg Endosc 2002;16:406–11.

Hamilton EC, Scott DJ, Kapoor A, Nwariaku F, Bergen PC, Rege RV, et al. Improving operative performance using a laparoscopic hernia simulator. Am J Surg 2001;182:725–8.

Hanna GB, Cresswell AB, Cuschieri A. Shadow depth cues and endoscopic task performance. Arch Surg 2002;137:1166–9.

Hanna GB, Frank TG, Cuschieri A. Objective assessment of endoscopic knot quality. Am J Surg 1997;174:410–3.

Hasson HM, Kumari NV, Eekhout J. Training simulator for developing laparoscopic skills. JSLS 2001;5:255–65.

Hyltander A, Liljegren E, Rhodin PH, Lonroth H. The transfer of basic skills learned in a laparoscopic simulator to the operating room. Surg Endosc 2002;16:1324–8.

Issenberg SB, McGaghie WC, Gordon DL, Symes S, Petrusa ER, Hart IR, et al. Effectiveness of a cardiology review course for internal medicine residents using simulation technology and deliberate practice. Teach Learn Med 2002;14:223–8.

Johnston R, Bhoyrul S, Way L, Satava R, McGovern K, Fletcher JD, et al. Assessing a virtual reality surgical skills simulator. Stud Health Technol Inform 1996;29:608–17.

Jones DB, Brewer JD, Soper NJ. The influence of three-dimensional video systems on laparoscopic task performance. Surg Laparosc Endosc 1996;6:191–7.

Jones JS, Hunt SJ, Carlson SA, Seamon JP. Assessing bedside cardiologic examination skills using "Harvey," a cardiology patient simulator. Acad Emerg Med 1997;4:980–5.

Jordan JA, Gallagher AG, McGuigan J, McClure N. Randomly alternating image presentation during laparoscopic training leads to faster automation to the "fulcrum effect." Endoscopy 2000;32:317–21.

Jordan JA, Gallagher AG, McGuigan J, McClure N. Virtual reality training leads to faster adaptation to the novel psychomotor restrictions encountered by laparoscopic surgeons. Surg Endosc 2001;15:1080–4.

Jordan JA, Gallagher AG, McGuigan J, McGlade K, McClure N. A comparison between randomly alternating imaging, normal laparoscopic imaging, and virtual reality training in laparoscopic psychomotor skill acquisition. Am J Surg 2000;180:208–11.

Katz R, Nadu A, Olsson LE, Hoznek A, de la Taille A, Salomon L, et al. A simplified 5-step model for training laparoscopic urethrovesical anastomosis. J Urol 2003;169:2041–4.

Kaufmann C, Rhee P, Burris D. Telepresence surgery system enhances medical student surgery training. Stud Health Technol Inform 1999;62:174–8.

Kothari SN, Kaplan BJ, DeMaria EJ, Broderick TJ, Merrell RC. Training in laparoscopic suturing skills using a new computer-based virtual reality simulator (MIST-VR) provides results comparable to those with an established pelvic trainer system. J Laparoendosc Adv Surg Tech A 2002;12:167–73.

Kovacs G, Bullock G, Ackroyd-Stolarz S, Cain E, Petrie D. A randomized controlled trial on the effect of educational interventions in promoting airway management skill maintenance. Ann Emerg Med 2000;36:301–9.

Lingard L, Reznick R, Espin S, Regehr G, DeVito I. Team communications in the operating room: talk patterns, sites of tension, and implications for novices. Acad Med 2002;77:232–7.

MacDonald J, Ketchum J, Williams RG, Rogers LQ. A lay person versus a trained endoscopist. Surg Endosc 2003;17:896–8.

MacDonald J, Williams RG, Rogers DA. Self-assessment in simulation-based surgical skills training. Am J Surg 2003;185:319–22.

Macintosh MC, Chard T. Pelvic manikins as learning aids. Med Educ 1997;31:194–6

Mackay S, Datta V, Chang A, Shah J, Kneebone R, Darzi A. Multiple objective measures of skill (MOMS): a new approach to the assessment of technical ability in surgical trainees. Ann Surg 2003;238:291–300.

Mackay S, Morgan P, Datta V, Chang A, Darzi A. Practice distribution in procedural skills training. Surg Endosc 2002; 16:957–61.

MacMillan AIM, Cuschieri A. Assessment of innate ability and skills for endoscopic manipulations by the advanced Dundee endoscopic psychomotor tester: predictive and concurrent validity. Am J Surg 1999;177:274–7.

Madar J, Richmond S. Improving paediatric and newborn life support training by the use of modified manikins allowing airway occlusion. Resuscitation 2002;54:265–8.

Mahmood T, Darzi A. A study to validate the colonoscopy simulator. Surg Endosc 2003;17:1583–9.

McCarthy A, Harley P, Smallwood R. Virtual arthroscopy training: do the "virtual skills" developed match the real skills required? Stud Health Technol Inform 1999;62:221–7.

McNatt SS, Smith CD. A computer-based laparoscopic skills assessment device differentiates experienced from novice laparoscopic surgeons. Surg Endosc 2001;15:1085–9.

Melvin WS, Johnson JA, Ellison EC. Laparoscopic skills enhancement. Am J Surg 1996;172:377–9.

Monsky WL, Levine D, Mehta TS, Kane RA, Ziv A, Kennedy B, et al. Using a sonographic simulator to assess residents before overnight call. AJR Am J Roentgenol 2002;178:35–9.

Moorthy K, Munz Y, Dosis A, Bann S, Darzi A. The effect of stress-inducing conditions on the performance of a laparoscopic task. Surg Endosc 2003;17:1481–4.

Moorthy K, Smith S, Brown T, Bann S, Darzi A. Evaluation of virtual reality bronchoscopy as a learning and assessment tool. Respiration 2003;70:195–9.

Mossey PA, Newton JP, Stirrups DR. Scope of the OSCE in the assessment of clinical skills in dentistry. Br Dent J 2001;190: 323–6.

Nakajima K, Wasa M, Takiguchi S, Taniguchi E, Soh H, Ohashi S, et al. A modular laparoscopic training program for pediatric surgeons. JSLS 2003;7:33–7.

Neumann M, Friedl S, Meining A, Egger K, Heldwein W, Rey JF, et al. A score card for upper GI endoscopy: evaluation of inter-observer variability in examiners with various levels of experience. Gastroenterology 2002;40:857–62.

Neumann M, Hahn C, Horbach T, Schneider I, Meining A, Heldwein W, et al. Score card endoscopy: a multicenter study to evaluate learning curves in 1-week courses using the Erlangen endo-trainer. Endoscopy 2003;35:515–20.

Neumann M, Siebert T, Rausch J, Horbach T, Ell C, Manegold C, et al. Scorecard endoscopy: a pilot study to assess basic skills in trainees for upper gastrointestinal endoscopy. Langenbecks Arch Surg 2003;387:386–91.

Neumann M, Stangl T, Auenhammer G, Horbach T, Hohenberger W, Schneider I. Laparoscopic cholecystectomy: training on a bio-simulation model with learning success documented using score-cards. Chirurg 2003;74:208–13.

Oddone EZ, Waugh RA, Samsa G, Corey R, Feussner JR. Teaching cardiovascular examination skills: results from a randomized controlled trial. Am J Med 1993;95:389–96.

Ost D, DeRosiers A, Britt EJ, Fein AM, Lesser ML, Mehta AC. Assessment of a bronchoscopy simulator. Am J Respir Crit Care Med 2001;164:2248–55.

O'Toole R, Playter R, Blank W, Cornelius N, Toberts W, Raibert M. A novel virtual reality surgical simulator with force feedback: surgeon vs medical student performance. In: Salisbury JK, Srinivasan MA (eds) Proceedings of the Second Phantoms Users Group Workshop. Dedham, MA: MIT; 1997.

O'Toole R, Playter R, Krumme T, Blank W, Cornelius N, Roberts W, et al. Assessing skill and learning in surgeons and medical students using a force feedback surgical simulator. In: Wells W, Colchester A, Delp S (eds) Proceedings of the International Conference on Medical Image Computing and Computer-Assisted Intervention (MICCAI). Berlin: Springer; 1998. p. 899–909.

O'Toole RV, Playter RR, Krummel TM, Blank WC, Cornelius NH, Roberts WR, et al. Measuring and developing suturing technique with a virtual reality surgical simulator. J Am Coll Surg 1999;189: 114–27.

Paisley AM, Baldwin PJ, Paterson-Brown S. Validity of surgical simulation for the assessment of operative skill. Br J Surg 2001;88:1525–32.

Pearson AM, Gallagher AG, Rosser JC, Satava RM. Evaluation of structured and quantitative training methods for teaching intra-corporeal knot tying. Surg Endosc 2002;16:130–7.

Pedowitz RA, Esch J, Snyder S. Evaluation of a virtual reality simulator for arthroscopy skills development. Arthroscopy 2002; 18:E29.

Peugnet F, Dubois P, Rouland JF. Virtual reality versus conventional training in retinal photocoagulation: a first clinical assessment. Comput Aided Surg 1998;3:20–6.

Pichichero ME, Poole MD. Assessing diagnostic accuracy and tympanocentesis skills in the management of otitis media. Arch Pediatr Adolesc Med 2001;155:1137–42.

Pittini R, Oepkes D, Macrury K, Reznick R, Beyene J, Windrim R. Teaching invasive perinatal procedures: assessment of a high fidelity simulator-based curriculum. Ultrasound Obstet Gynecol 2002;19:478–83.

Powers TW, Murayama KM, Toyama M, Murphy S, Denham EW 3rd, Derossis AM, et al. Housestaff performance is improved by participation in a laparoscopic skills curriculum. Am J Surg 2002;184:626–9; discussion 629–30.

Prystowsky JB, Regehr G, Rogers DA, Loan JP, Hiemenz LL, Smith KM. A virtual reality module for intravenous catheter placement. Am J Surg 1999;177:171–5.

Pugh CM, Youngblood P. Development and validation of assessment measures for a newly developed physical examination simulator. J Am Med Inform Assoc 2002;9:448–60.

Pugh CM, Srivastava S, Shavelson R, Walker D, Cotner T, Scarloss B, et al. The effect of simulator use on learning and self-assessment: the case of Stanford University's E-Pelvis simulator. Stud Health Technol Inform 2001;81:396–400.

Reznek MA, Rawn CL, Krummel TM. Evaluation of the educational effectiveness of a virtual reality intravenous insertion simulator. Acad Emerg Med 2002;9:1319–25.

Reznick R, Regehr G, Macrae H, Martin J, McCulloch W. Testing technical skill via an innovative bench station examination. Am J Surg 1996;172:226–30.

Risucci D, Cohen JA, Garbus JE, Goldstein M, Cohen MG. The effects of practice and instruction on speed and accuracy during resident acquisition of simulated laparoscopic skills. Curr Surg 2001;58:230–5.

Risucci D, Geiss A, Gellman L, Pinard B, Rosser JC. Experience and visual perception in resident acquisition of laparoscopic skills. Curr Surg 2000;57:368–72.

Risucci D, Geiss A, Gellman L, Pinard B, Rosser J. Surgeon-specific factors in the acquisition of laparoscopic surgical skills. Am J Surg 2001;181:289–93.

Rogers DA, Regehr G, Gelula M, Yeh KA, Howdieshell TR, Webb W. Peer teaching and computer-assisted learning: an effective combination for surgical skill training? J Surg Res 2000;92:53–5.

Rosen JM, Soltanian H, Laub DR, Mecinski A, Dean WK. The evolution of virtual reality from surgical training to the development of a simulator for health care delivery: a review. Stud Health Technol Inform 1996;29:89–9.

Rowe R, Cohen RA. An evaluation of a virtual reality airway simulator. Anesth Analg 2002;95:62–6.

Salen P, O'Connor R, Passarello B, Pancu D, Melanson S, Arcona S, et al. Fast education: a comparison of teaching models for trauma sonography. J Emerg Med 2001;20:421–5.

Salvendy G, Root CM, Schiff AJ, Cunningham PR, Ferguson GW. A second generation training simulator for acquisition of psychomotor skills in cavity preparation. J Dent Educ 1975;39: 466–71.

Schijven M, Jakimowicz J. Construct validity: experts and novices performing on the Xitact LS500 laparoscopy simulator. Surg Endosc 2003;17:803–10.

Schijven M, Jakimowicz J. Face-, expert, and referent validity of the Xitact LS500 laparoscopy simulator. Surg Endosc 2002;16:1764–70.

Schijven MP, Jakimowicz, Schot C. The advanced Dundee endoscopic psychomotor tester (ADEPT) objectifying subjective psychomotor test performance. Surg Endosc 2002;16:943–8.

Scott DJ, Bergen PC, Rege RV, Laycock R, Tesfay ST, Valentine RJ, et al. Laparoscopic training on bench models: better and more cost effective than operating room experience? J Am Coll Surg 2000;191:272–83.

Scott DJ, Rege RV, Bergen PC, Guo WA, Laycock R, Tesfay ST, et al. Measuring operative performance after laparoscopic skills training: edited videotape versus direct observation. J Laparoendosc Adv Surg Tech A 2000;10:183–90.

Scott DJ, Young WN, Tesfay ST, Frawley WH, Rege RV, Jones DB. Laparosopic skills training. Am Surg 2001;182:137–42.

Sedlack RE, Kolars JC. Validation of a computer-based colonoscopy simulator. Gastrointest Endosc 2003;57:214–8.

Sedlack R, Petersen B, Binmoeller K, Kolars J. A direct comparison of ERCP teaching models. Gastrointest Endosc 2003;57:886–90.

Semple M, Cook R. Social influence and the recording of blood pressure by student nurse: an experimental study. Nurse Res 2001;8:60–71.

Seymour NE, Gallagher AG, Roman SA, O'Brien MK, Bansal VK, Andersen DK, et al. Virtual reality training improves operating room performance: results of a randomized, double-blinded study. Ann Surg 2002;236:458–63; discussion 463–4.

Shah J, Darzi A. Virtual reality flexible cystoscopy: a validation study. BJU Int 2002;90:828–32.

Shah J, Buckley D, Frisby J, Darzi A. Depth cue reliance in surgeons and medical students. Surg Endosc 2003;17:1472–1474.

Shah J, Montgomery B, Langley S, Darzi A. Validation of a flexible cystoscopy course. BJU Int 2002;90:833–5.

Shah J, Paul I, Buckley D, Davis H, Frisby JP, Darzi A. Can tonic accommodation predict surgical performance? Surg Endosc 2003;17:787–90.

Sherman KP, Ward JW, Wills DP, Sherman VJ, Mohsen AM. Surgical trainee assessment using a VE knee arthroscopy training system (VE-KATS): experimental results. Stud Health Technol Inform 2001;81:465–70.

Smeak DD, Beck ML, Shaffer CA, Gregg CG. Evaluation of video tape and a simulator for instruction of basic surgical skills. Vet Surg 1991;20:30–6.

Sorrento A, Pichichero ME. Assessing diagnostic accuracy and tympanocentesis skills by nurse practitioners in management of otitis media. J Am Acad Nurse Pract 2001;13:524–9.

St Clair EW, Oddone EZ, Waugh RA, Corey GR, Feussner JR. Assessing housestaff diagnostic skills using a cardiology patient simulator. Ann Intern Med 1992;117:751–6.

Stratton SJ, Kane G, Gunter CS, Wheeler NC, Ableson-Ward C, Reich E, et al. Prospective study of manikin-only versus manikin and human subject endotracheal intubation training of paramedics. Ann Emerg Med 1991;20:1314–8.

Strom P, Kjellin A, Hedman L, Johnson E, Wredmark T, Fellander-Tsai L. Validation and learning in the Procedicus KSA virtual reality surgical simulator. Surg Endosc 2003;17:227–31.

Summers AN, Rinehart GC, Simpson D, Redlich PN. Acquisition of surgical skills: a randomized trial of didactic, videotape, and computer-based training. Surgery 1999;126:330–6.

Sung WH, Fung CP, Chen AC, Yuan CC, Ng HT, Doong JL. The assessment of stability and reliability of a virtual reality-based laparoscopic gynecology simulation system. Eur J Gynaecol Oncol 2003;24:143–6.

Suvinen TI, Messer LB, Franco E. Clinical simulation in teaching preclinical dentistry. Eur J Dent Educ 1998;2:25–32.

Taffinder NJ, McManus IC, Gul Y, Russell RC, Darzi A. Effect of sleep deprivation on surgeons' dexterity on laparoscopy simulator. Lancet 1998;352:1191.

Taffinder N, Sutton C, Fishwick RJ, McManus IC, Darzi A. Validation of virtual reality to teach and assess psychomotor skills in laparoscopic surgery: results from randomised controlled studies using the MIST VR laparoscopic simulator. Stud Health Technol Inform 1998;50:124–30.

Torkington J, Smith SG, Rees BI, Darzi A. Skill transfer from virtual reality to a real laparoscopic task. Surg Endosc 2001;15:1076–9.

Torkington J, Smith SG, Rees B, Darzi A. The role of the basic surgical skills course in the acquisition and retention of laparoscopic skill. Surg Endosc 2001;15:1071–5.

Traxer O, Gettman MT, Napper CA, Scott DJ, Jones DB, Roehrborn CG, et al. The impact of intense laparoscopic skills training on the operative performance of urology residents. J Urol 2001;166:1658–61.

Tuggy ML. Virtual reality flexible sigmoidoscopy simulator training: impact on resident performance. J Am Board Fam Pract 1998;11:426–33.

Uchal M, Brogger J, Rukas R, Karlsen B, Bergamaschi R. In-line versus pistol-grip handles in a laparoscopic simulators: a randomized controlled crossover trial. Surg Endosc 2002;16:1771–3.

Uhrich ML, Underwood RA, Standeven JW, Soper NJ, Engsberg JR. Assessment of fatigue, monitor placement, and surgical experience during simulated laparoscopic surgery. Surg Endosc 2002;16:635–9.

Watterson JD, Beiko DT, Kuan JK, Denstedt JD. Randomized prospective blinded study validating acquistion of ureteroscopy skills using computer based virtual reality endourological simulator. J Urol 2002;168:1928–32.

Weghorst S, Airola C, Oppenheimer P, Edmond CV, Patience T, Heskamp D, et al. Validation of the Madigan ESS simulator. Stud Health Technol Inform 1998;50:399–405.

Wentink M, Breedveld P, Stassen LP, Oei IH, Wieringa PA. A clearly visible endoscopic instrument shaft on the monitor facilitates hand-eye coordination. Surg Endosc 2002;16:1533–7.

Westman EC, Matchar DB, Samsa GP, Mulrow CD, Waugh RA, Feussner JR. Accuracy and reliability of apical S3 gallop detection. J Gen Intern Med 1995;10:455–7.

Wilhelm DM, Ogan K, Roehrborn CG, Cadeddu JA, Pearle MS. Assessment of basic endoscopic performance using a virtual reality simulator. J Am Coll Surg 2002;195:675–81.

Woolliscroft JO, Calhoun JG, Tenhaken JD, Judge RD. Harvey: the impact of a cardiovascular teaching simulator on student skill acquisition. Med Teach 1987;9:53–7. Also in: Proc Annu Conf Res Med Educ 1986;25:20–5.

Yoshii C, Anzai T, Yatera K, Kawajiri T, Nakashima Y, Kido M. A new medical education using a lung sound auscultation simulator called "Mr. Lung." J UOEH 2002;24:249–55.

Young TJ, Hayek R, Philipson SA. A cervical manikin procedure for chiropractic skills development. J Manipulative Physiol Ther 1998;21:241–5.

Articles Touching on the Theme "Salvation"

These articles are hard to find, and, truth to tell, there is no absolutely perfect article in this area. What you want to see is, "We proved behind a shadow of a doubt that that the simulator saves lives." Well, you're not going to see that. These articles *hint* at it, *approach* it, and *want* to say it. You judge. *The* article that proclaims true salvation may be a long time in coming.

✓ Schwid H. Computer simulations and management of critical incidents. Acad Med 1994;69:213.

Let the article speak for itself, "After using the simulator the residents stated that they felt better prepared to manage anesthesia-related emergencies and that the simulations caused them to read more about the clinical simulations." Did someone live who might otherwise have died because "they felt better prepared" and they "read more"? This might be a stretch, but I think they just might have.

✓ SHAPIRO MJ, MAREY JC, SMALL SD, LANGFORD V, KAYLOR CJ, JAGMINAS L, ET AL. Simulation based teamwork training for emergency department staff: does it improve clinical team performance when added to an existing didactic teamwork curriculum? Qual Saf Health Care 2004;13:417–21.

This was the first look at real "team simulator training" using nurses, techs, ER residents, and attendings. Of special interest in this study: teams are what actually take care of patients! This study mimics the real world, rather than just how one person performs. Bravo to the people who took on this study.

Guess what? Teams that practiced on the Simulator did better in the (admittedly elusive) area of "team behavior." The killer here is the "metric itself." How in the hell do you measure "team behavior"? I mean, are we wading into the murkiest of subjective waters here? Well, yes. But you have to start measuring team behavior somewhere. So why not here? To dig a little deeper and avoid a complete white-out in the foggy world of behavior assessment, let's look at how they measured team behavior. They looked for specific things—the very things that save or lose a patient's life during a crisis.

- Assigning roles and responsibilities
- Engaging team members in the plan
- Providing situational updates
- Cross-monitoring actions of others
- Conducting event reviews

Hey, wait a minute, this is starting to sound less "touch-feely" and more "this-makes-a-difference"-y. If a team does all those important tasks, then, for example, someone *specific* is told to get, send, and bring back the results of a blood gas, rather than someone just shouting out, "Hey, we need a gas!" Team behavior does make a difference. Well, what do you know, Simulators not only take the *individual* half-way there, they also take the *entire team* half-way there. Simulators teach good team dynamics. Good stuff, that.

✓ HOLZMAN RS, COOPER JB, GABA DM, PHILIP JH, SMALL SD, FEINSTEIN D. Anesthesia crisis resource management: real-life simulation training in operating room crises. J Clin Anesth 1995;7:675–87.

Over a period of 2.5 months, 68 anesthesiologists (a gemisch of attendings and residents at various levels) and 4 nurse anesthetists went into Harvard's simulation center to undergo training in anesthesia crises. The training lasted a few hours per week over a 10-week course. They handled various crises.

Overdose of anesthetic vapors
Oxygen delivery failure

Cardiac arrest
Malignant hyperthermia
Tension pneumothorax
Power failure

Think about it. If you were a program director, wouldn't you want your people to know how to handle those things? I sure would. The result? They loved it!

Debate rages about a Simulator's validity, reliability, worth as an assessment tool. Designing statistically rigid studies to clearly demonstrate improved outcome is nearly impossible. Is there any clear statement we can make about Simulators? Yes. The people who train in Simulators think they're the greatest! How's that for an outcome study you can hang your hat on? If "student reaction" has any place in this great Simulator debate, then hear ye, hear ye—people *like* training in the Simulator. OK, detractors say, people like riding Space Mountain at Disney World too. Maybe we should send our residents to Orlando. Did anything good come of this "groovy experience in the Simulator," or is this all just yummy cotton candy? After 6 months a questionnaire was sent out. Eight of the trainees reported that the Simulator had helped in *real life*. Course participation helped them handle possible malignant hyperthermia, low oxygen pressure, a trauma case, and a subclavian laceration. Four others didn't specify the crisis but said that the course had definitely helped.

Think about it. Could the observations of those eight "Simulation grads" be the Holy Grail? Is this the "Simulation does save lives" everyone has been looking for? Forget, for a moment, the checklists, the validity statistics, the blinded observers. Think about the ultimate goal of all this. Make better clinicians. Save lives. Looks like Simulators might do just that.

✓ WELLER J, WILSON L, ROBINSON B. Survey of change in practice following simulation-based training in crisis management. Anaesthesia 2003;58:471–3.

This is getting very close to where we want to be. In the medical simulation literature, this is about as good as it gets. This is about as close to "Simulators save lives, I'm not kidding" as it gets. Weller and her colleagues run the Wellington Simulation Centre in New Zealand and in a very short time have contributed much to the field of anesthesia simulation. They recognize that although performance on a Simulator is often more reliable and feasible, it requires the great leap of faith that competence on the device predicts performance in the real setting. As an alternative approach, they surveyed 96 anesthesia personnel's own perception of changes in their clinical practice as a result of previous simulation training at their center. A total of 66 of the 96 (69%) responded to the survey (an okay response – you want close to 90% to avoid "survey response bias").

The respondents attended a 1-day crisis management course 3 to 12 months previous to receiving the questionnaire. They were asked to rate the relevance of the course to their practice and the extent to which the training had increased their confidence in crisis management. They were also invited to provide written comments related to their actual experiences since the course.

The respondents rated highly the relevance of the course, perceived a change in their practice as a result of the Simulator training, and found it useful in subsequent crises. The reasons they gave for their increased confidence include the following.

- Opportunity to practice
- Improved teamwork and communication skills
- Greater ability to remain in control and evaluate the crises
- Greater willingness to ask for help

The areas of change they had made to their routine practice include the following (this is level 3 Kirkpatrick!).

- Communication with colleagues
- Working with a team
- Planning for adverse events
- Problem-solving strategies
- Training other colleagues in crisis management

Let's look at the specific crises, because here is the real crux of the matter. Forty-two respondents dealt with a host of critical events—cardiac arrests, major hemorrhage, anaphylaxis, amniotic fluid emboli, air emboli, airway emergencies. Seventy percent of the respondents thought "their management of the crisis was improved as a result of participation in the simulation course." That sentence is it. That sentence is the closest we can come so far to the Golden Fleece, the Holy Grail, the Blue Ribbon of "Simulator Worthiness." "Their management of the crisis was improved as a result of participation in the simulation course." The next step is to see if these changes resulted in improved patient care. We have to be patient, but the day will come. Oh sweet Salvation.

Other articles mention or hint at Salvation from the Simulator.

✓ Jacobsen J, Jensen PF, Osterfaard D, Lindekaer, Lippert A, Schultz P. Performance enhancement in anesthesia using the training simulator Sophus (Peanuts). In: Henson LC, Lee A (eds) Simulators in Anesthesiology Education. New York: Plenum; 1998. p. 103–6.

✓ Olympio MA. Simulation saves lives. In: Newsletter of the American Society of Anesthesiologists. Park Ridge, IL: American Society of Anesthesiologists; October 2001.

REVIEW ARTICLES

Review articles often summarize a number of studies or ideas and may draw conclusions about a particular intervention. These are sometimes called overviews and are often not "systematic." Systematic reviews review a clearly formulated question and use systematic and explicit methods to identify, select, and critically appraise the relevant research; they also collect and analyze data from the studies that are included in the review. A meta-analysis involves the use of statistical techniques in a systematic review to integrate the results of the included studies. Whereas systematic reviews are common in clinical medicine, they are extremely rare in medical education. When they are attempted, the end-product is often disappointing. To illustrate, the Campbell Collaboration supported a systematic review of the literature that evaluated the effectiveness of problem-based learning. The project ended because the investigators could not identify a single study that met their inclusion criteria. Studies in education and training are not as clean as clinical and basic research—but that does not mean we cannot find evidence—it is there if we look carefully.

Barach P, Satish U, Streufert S. Healthcare assessment and performance: using simulation. Simulation Gaming 2001;32:147–55.

Basdogan C, Delp SL, Loan P. Surgical simulation: an emerging technology in emergency medicine. PREEB 1997;6:147–59.

Bond WF, Spillane L. The use of simulation for emergency medicine resident assessment. Acad Emerg Med 2002;9:1295–9.

Buck GH. Development of simulators in medical education. Gesnerus 1991;48:7–28.

Byrne AJ, Greaves JD. Assessment instruments used during anaesthetic simulation: review of published studies. Br J Anaesth 2001;86:445–50.

Collins JP, Harden RM. The use of real patients, simulated patients and simulators in clinical examinations. Med Teach 1998;20:508–21.

Cooper JB, Gaba DM. A strategy for preventing anesthesia accidents. Int Anesthesiol Clin 1989;27:148–52.

Cooper JB, Taqueti VR. A brief history of the development of mannequin simulators for clinical education and training. Qual Saf Health Care 2004;13(Suppl 1):1–8.

Criss EA. Patient simulators: changing the face of EMS education. JEMS 2001;26:24–31.

Forrest FC, Taylor M. High level simulators in medical education. Hosp Med 1998;59:653–5.

Gaba D. Simulators in anesthesiology. Adv Anesth 1997;14:55–91.

Gaba DM. Anaesthesiology as a model for patient safety in health care. BMJ 2000;320:785–8.

Gaba DM, Howard SK, Fish K, Smith BE, Sowb YA. et al. Simulation-based training in anesthesia crisis resource management (ACRM): a decade of experience. Simulation Gaming 2001;32:175–93.

Gaiser RR. Teaching airway management skills: how and what to learn and teach. Crit Care Clin 2000;16:515–25.

Good ML. Patient simulators for training basic and advanced clinical skills. Med Educ 2003;37(Suppl 1):14–21.

Good ML, Gravenstein JS. Anesthesia simulators and training devices. Int Anesthesiol Clin 1989;27:161–8.

Good ML, Gravenstein JS. Training for safety in an anesthesia simulator. Semin Anesthesiol 1993;12:235–50.

Gordon MS, Issenberg SB, Mayer JW, Felner JM. Developments in the use of simulators and multimedia computer systems in medical education. Med Teach 1999;21:32–6.

Gravenstein JS. How does human error affect safety in anesthesia? Surg Oncol Clin N Am 2000;9:81–95, vii.

Grube C, Volk S, Zausig Y, Graf BM. Changing culture—simulator-training as a method to improve patient safety. Presented at the International Meeting on Medical Simulation, Scottsdale, AZ, 2001. Also in: Anaesthesist 2001;50:358–62.

Hotchkiss MA, Mendoza SN. Update for nurse anesthetists. Part 6. Full-body patient simulation technology: gaining experience using a malignant hyperthermia model. AANA J 2001;69:59–65.

Issenberg SB, Gordon MS, Gordon DL, Safford RE, Hart IR. Simulation and new learning technologies. Med Teach 2001;23:16–23.

Issenberg SB, McGaghie WC, Hart IR, Mayer JW, Felner JM, Petrusa ER, et al. Simulation technology for health care professional skills training and assessment. JAMA 1999;282:861–6.

Jevon P. Paediatric resuscitation manikins. Nurs Times 1999;95:55–7.

Lane JL, Slavin S, Ziv A. Simulation in medical education: a review. Simulation Gaming 2001;32:297–314.

Leitch RA, Moses GR, Magee H. Simulation and the future of military medicine. Mil Med 2002;167:350–4.

Lussi C, Grapengeter M, Schuttler J. Simulator training in anesthesia: applications and value. Anaesthesist 1999;48:433–8 (in German).

Mackenzie CF, Jaberi M, Dutton R, Hu P, Xiao Y. Overview of simulators in comparison with telementoring for decision making. Am J Anesthesiol 2000;27:186–94.

McLaughlin SA, Doezema D, Sklar DP. Human simulation in emergency medicine training: a model curriculum. Acad Emerg Med 2002;9:1310–8.

Morgan PJ, Cleave-Hogg D. A worldwide survey of the use of simulation in anesthesia. Can J Anaesth 2002;49:659–62.

Nehring WM, Wlllis WE. Human patient simulators in nursing education: an overview. Simulation Gaming 2001;32:194–204.

Pape M. Realistic manikins simulate patients and help teach healthcare safely. Occup Health Saf 1989;58:38.

Rall M, Manser T, Guggenberger H, Gaba DM, Unertl K. [Patient safety and errors in medicine: development, prevention and analyses of incidents.] Anasthesiol Intensivmed Notfallmed Schmerzther 2001;36:321–30.

Rall M, Schaedle B, Zieger J, Naef W, Weinlich M. Innovative training for enhancing patient safety: safety culture and integrated concepts. Unfallchirurg 2002;105:1033–42.

Schupfer GK, Konrad C, Poelaert JI. [Manual skills in anaesthesiology.] Anaesthesist 2003;52:527–34.

Schwid HA. Anesthesia simulators—technology and applications. Isr Med Assoc J 2000;2:949–53.

Streufert S, Satish U. Improving medical care: the use of simulation technology. Simulation Gaming 2001;32:330–6.

Swank KM, Jahr JS. The uses of simulation in anesthesiology training: a review of the current literature. J La State Med Soc 1992;144:523–7.

Tarver S. Anesthesia simulators: concepts and applications. Am J Anesthesiol 1999;26:939–6.

Treadwell I, Grobler S. Students' perceptions on skills training in simulation. Med Teach 2001;23:476–482.

Vreuls D, Overmayer RW. Human system performance measurements in training simulators. Hum Factors 1985;27:241–50.

Wong AK. Full scale computer simulation in anesthesia training and evaluation. Can J Anaesth 2004;51:455–64.

Wong SH, Ng KF, Chen PP. The application of clinical simulation in crisis management training. Hong Kong Med J 2002;8:13–5.

Ziv A, Small SD, Wolpe PR. Patient safety and simulation-based medical education. Med Teach 2000;22:489–95.

REVIEW ARTICLES IN DISCIPLINES OTHER THAN ANESTHESIA

Ackerman JD. Conference report: medicine meets virtual reality. MD Comput 1999;16(2):40–3.

Ackerman JD. Medicine meets virtual reality 2000. MD Comput 2000;17(3):13–7.

Adamsen S. Simulators and gastrointestinal endoscopy training. Endoscopy 2000;32:895–7.

Ahmed M, Meech JF, Timoney A. Virtual reality in medicine. Br J Urol 1997;80(Suppl 3):46–52.

Akay M. Virtual reality in medicine. IEEE Eng Med Biol Mag 1996;15:14.

Arnold P, Farrell MJ. Can virtual reality be used to measure and train surgical skills? Ergonomics 2002;45:362–79.

Berg D, Berkley J, Weghorst S, Raugi G, Turkiyyah G, Ganter M, et al. Issues in validation of a dermatologic surgery simulator. Stud Health Technol Inform 2001;81:60–5.

Berg D, Raugi G, Gladstone H, Berkley J, Weghorst S, Ganter M, et al. Virtual reality simulators for dermatologic surgery: measuring their validity as a teaching tool. Dermatol Surg 2001;27:370–4.

Champion HR, Gallagher AG. Surgical simulation—a "good idea whose time has come." Br J Surg 2003;90:767–8.

Chinnock C. Virtual reality in surgery and medicine. Hosp Technol Ser 1994;13:1–48.

Coleman J, Nduka CC, Darzi A. Virtual reality and laparoscopic surgery. Br J Surg 1994;81:1709–11.

Cosman PH, Cregan PC, Martin CJ, Cartmill JA. Virtual reality simulators: current status in acquisition and assessment of surgical skills. ANZ J Surg 2002;72:30–34.

Delp SL, Loan JP, Basdogan C, Buchanan TS, Rosen JM, et al. Surgical simulation: an emerging technology for military medical training. In: Military Medicine On-line Today, vol 13. New York: IEEE Press; 1996. p. 29–34.

Delvecchio FC, Preminger GM. Renal surgery in the new millennium. Urol Clin North Am 2000;27:801–12.

Dunkin BJ. Flexible endoscopy simulators. Semin Laparosc Surg 2003;10:29–35.

Emergency Medicine Research Laboratories, University of Michigan. Immersive virtual reality platform for medical training: a "killer-application." In: Westwood JD, Hoffman HM, Mogel GT, Robb RA, Stredney D (eds) Medicine Meets Virtual Reality 2000. Amsterdam: IOS Press; 2000. p. 207–13.

Gerson LB, Van Dam J. The future of simulators in GI endoscopy: an unlikely possibility or a virtual reality? Gastrointest Endosc 2002;55:608–11.

Gessner CE, Jowell PS, Baillie J. Novel methods for endoscopic training. Gastrointest Endosc Clin N Am 1995;5:323–36.

Gladstone HB, Raugi GJ, Berg D, Berkley J, Weghorst S, Ganter M. Virtual reality for dermatologic surgery: virtually a reality in the 21st century. J Am Acad Dermatol 2000;42:106–12.

Gorman PJ, Meier AH, Krummel TM. Computer-assisted training and learning in surgery. Comput Aided Surg 2000;5:120–30.

Gorman PJ, Meier AH, Krummel TM. Simulation and virtual reality in surgical education: real or unreal? Arch Surg 1999; 134:1203–8.

Gorman PJ, Meier AH, Rawn C, Krummell TM. The future of medical education is no longer blood and guts, it is bits and bytes. Am J Surg 2000;180:353–6.

Haluck RS, Krummel TM. Computers and virtual reality for surgical education in the 21st century. Arch Aurg 2000;135: 786–92.

Haluck RS, Krummel TM. Simulation and virtual reality for surgical education. Surg Technol Int 2000;8:59–63.

Haluck RS, Marshall RL, Krummel TM, Melkonian MG. Are surgery training programs ready for virtual reality? A survey of program directors in general surgery. J Am Coll Surg 2001; 193:660–5.

Hamdorf JM, Hall JC. Acquiring surgical skills. Br J Surg 2000;87:28–37.

Higgins GA, Merrrill GL, Hettinger LJ, Kaufmann CR, Champion HR, Satava RM. New simulation technologies for surgical training and certification: current status and future projections. PREEB 1997;6:160–72.

Hochberger J, Maiss J, Magdeburg B, Cohen J, Hahn EG. Training simulators and education in gastrointestinal endoscopy: current status and perspectives in 2001. Endoscopy 2001;33: 541–9.

Hoffman HM. Teaching and learning with virtual reality. Stud Health Technol Inform 2000;79:285–91.

Hoffman HM. Virtual reality meets medical education. In: Satava RM, Morgan K, Sieburg H, Mattheus R, Christensen J (eds) Interactive Technology and the New Paradigm for Healthcare. Amsterdam: IOS Press; 1995. p. 130–6.

Hoffman H, Vu D. Virtual reality: teaching tool of the twenty-first century? Acad Med 1997;72:1076–81.

Hon D. Medical reality and virtual reality. Stud Health Technol Inform 1996;29:327–41.

Hoznek A, Katz R, Gettman M, Salomon L, Antiphon P, de la Taille A, et al. Laparoscopic and robotic surgical training in urology. Curr Urol Rep 2003;4:130–7.

Indelicato D. Virtual reality in surgical training. Dartmouth Undergrad J Sci 1999;1:21–4.

Jackson A, John NW, Thacker NA, Ramsden RT, Gillespie JE, Gobbetti E, et al. Developing a virtual reality environment in petrous bone surgery: a state-of-the-art review. Otol Neurotol 2002;23:111–21.

Kaufman DM, Bell W. Teaching and assessing clinical skills using virtual reality. Stud Health Technol Inform 1997;39:467–72.

Kay CL, Evangelou HA. A review of the technical and clinical aspects of virtual endoscopy. Endoscopy 1996;28:768–75.

Kneebone R. Simulation in surgical training: educational issues and practical implications. Med Educ 2003;37:267–77.

Krummel TM. High-tech training tools available. Bull Am Coll Surg 1998;83:44–5.

Kuo RL, Delvecchio FC, Preminger GM. Virtual reality: current urologic applications and future developments. J Endourol 2001;15:117–22.

Laguna MP, Hatzinger M, Rassweiler J. Simulators and endourological training. Curr Opin Urol 2002;12:209–15.

Lange T, Indelicato DJ, Rosen JM. Virtual reality in surgical training. Surg Oncol Clin N Am 2000;9:61–79, vii.

Lyons J, Miller M, Milton J. Learning with technology: use of case-based physical and computer simulations in professional education. Contemp Nurse 1998;7:35–9.

Macedonia CR, Gherman RB, Satin AJ. Simulation laboratories for training in obstetrics and gynecology. Obstet Gynecol 2003;102: 388–92.

MacIntyre IM, Munro A. Simulation in surgical training. BMJ 1990;300:1088–9.

McClory R, Stone R. Virtual reality in surgery. BMJ 2001;323: 912–5.

Meier AH, Rawn CL, Krummel TM. Virtual reality: surgical application—challenge for the new millennium. J Am Coll Surg 2001;192:372–84.

Meril J, Preminger G, Babayan RK, Roy RT, Merril GT. Surgical simulation using virtual reality technology: design, implementation, and implications. Surg Technol Int 1994;3:53–60.

Mills R, Lee P. Surgical skills training in middle-ear surgery. J Laryngol Otol 2003;117:159–63.

Noar MD. The next generation of endoscopy simulation: minimally invasive surgical skills simulation. Endoscopy 1995;27:81–5.

Ota D, Loftin B, Saito T, Lea R, Keller J. Virtual reality in surgical education. Comput Biol Med 1995;25:127–37.

Pai G. Simulators in clinical surgery. J Audiovis Media Med 1997;20:178–9.

Park A, Witzke DB. Training and educational approaches to minimally invasive surgery: state of the art. Semin Laparosc Surg 2002;9:198–205.

Psotka J. Immersive training systems: virtual reality & education & training. Instruct Sci 1995;23:405–31.

Reznek M, Harter P, Krummel T. Virtual reality and simulation: training the future emergency physician. Acad Emerg Med 2002;9:78–87.

Rosen JM, Soltanian H, Redett RJ, Laub DR. Evolution of virtual reality. IEEE Eng Med Biol 1996;15:16–21.

Rosen JM, Laub DR, Pieper SD, Mecinski AM, Soltanian H, McKenna MA, et al. Virtual reality and medicine: from training systems to performance machines. Presented at the Virtual Reality Annual International Symposium (VRAIS 96), p. 5.

Rosser JC, Gabriel N, Herman B, Murayama M. Telementoring and teleproctoring. World J Surg 2001;25:1438–48.

Rosser JC Jr, Murayama M, Gabriel NH. Minimally invasive surgical training solutions for the twenty-first century. Surg Clin North Am 2000;80:1607–24.

Satava RM. Accomplishments and challenges of surgical simulation. Surg Endosc 2001;15:232–41.

Satava RM. Advanced simulation technologies for surgical education. Am Coll Surg Bull 1996;81:77–81.

Satava RM. Biointelligence age: implications for the future of medicine. Stud Health Technol Inform 2001;81:vii–x.

Satava RM. Cybersurgery: a new vision for general surgery. In: Satava RM (ed) Cybersurgery: Advanced Technologies for Surgical Practice. New York: Wiley; 1998. p. 3–14.

Satava RM. Emerging medical applications of virtual reality: a surgeon's perspective. Artif Intell Med 1994;6:281–8.

Satava RM. Emerging technologies for surgery in the 21st century. Arch Surg 1999;134:1197–202.

Satava RM. Information age technologies for surgeons: overview. World J Surg 2001;25:1408–11.

Satava RM. Laparoscopic surgery, robots, and surgical simulation: moral and ethical issues. Semin Laparosc Surg 2002;9:230–8.

Satava RM. Medical applications of virtual reality. J Med Syst 1995;19:275–80.

Satava RM. Surgical education and surgical simulation. World J Surg 2001;25:1484–9.

Satava RM. Surgical robotics: the early chronicles: a personal historical perspective. Surg Laparosc Endosc Percutan Tech 2002;12:6–16.

Satava RM. Virtual reality. Protocols Gen Surg 1998;1:75–95.

Satava RM. Virtual reality and telepresence for military medicine. Ann Acad Med 1997;26:118–20.

Satava RM. Virtual reality for medical applications. Am J Anesthesiol 2000;27:197–8.

Satava RM. Virtual reality for medical applications. In: Proceedings of the IEEE Enginering Medicine Biology Society Region 8 International Conference, 1997, pp. 19–20.

Satava RM, Ellis SR. Human interface technology: an essential tool for the modern surgeon. Surg Endosc 1994;8:817–20.

Satava RM, Jones SB. An integrated medical virtual reality program: the military application. IEEE Eng Med Biol Mag 1996;15:94–7, 104.

Satava RM, Jones SP. Current and future applications of virtual reality for medicine. Proc IEEE 1998;86:484–9.

Satava RM, Jones SB. Laparoscopic surgery: transition to the future. Urol Clin North Am 1998;25:93–102.

Satava RM, Jones SB. Medical applications of virtual reality. In: Stunney KM (ed) VE Handbook. Hillsdale, NJ: Lawrence Erlbaum Associates; 1999.

Satava RM, Jones SB. Medicine beyond the year 2000. Caduceus 1997;13:49–64.

Satava RM, Jones SB. Preparing surgeons for the 21st century: implications of advanced technologies. Surg Clin North Am 2000;80:1353–65.

Satava R, Jones S. The future is now: virtual reality technologies. In: Tekian A, McGuire C, McGaghie W (eds) Innovative Simulations for Assessing Professional Competence: From Paper and Pencil to Virtual Reality. Chicago: University of Illinois; 1999. p. 179–93.

Satava RM, Jones SB. Virtual environments for medical training and education. PREEB 1996;6:139–146.

Satava RM, Jones SB. Virtual reality environments in medicine. In: Mandall EL, Bashook PG, Dockery JL (eds) Computer-Based Examinations for Board Certification. Evanston, IL: American Board of Medical Specialties; 1996. p. 121–31.

Satava RM, Cuschieri A, Hamdorf J. Metrics for objective assessment of surgical skills workshop: metrics for objective assessment. Surg Endosc 2003;17:220–6.

Shah J, Mackay S, Vale J, Darzi A. Simulation in urology—a role for virtual reality? BJU Int 2001;88:661–5.

Smith SG, Torkington J, Darzi A. Objective assessment of surgical dexterity using simulators. Hosp Med 1999;60:672–5.

Spicer MA, Apuzzo ML. Virtual reality surgery: neurosurgery and the contemporary landscape. Neurosurgery 2003;52:489–97; discussion 496–7.

Stewart D. Medical training in the UK. Arch Dis Child 2003;88:655–8.

Stone RJ. The opportunities for virtual reality and simulation in the training and assessment of technical surgical skills. In: Surgical Competence: Challenges of Assessment in Training and Practice. London: Royal College of Surgeons of England; 1999. p. 109–25.

Torkington J, Smith SG, Rees BI, Darzi A. The role of simulation in surgical training. Ann R Coll Surg Engl 2000;82:88–94.

Vanchieri C. Virtual reality: will practice make perfect? J Natl Cancer Inst 1999;91:207–9.

Wantman A. Can simulators be used to assess clinical competence? Hosp Med 2003;64:251.

Wysocki WM, Moesta KT, Schlag PM. Surgery, surgical education and surgical diagnostic procedures in the digital era. Med Sci Monit 2003;9:RA69–75.

ARTICLES THAT DESCRIBE THE DEVELOPMENT OF SIMULATORS/SIMULATIONS: ENGINEERING ISSUES

Anderson JH, Raghavan R. A vascular catheterization simulator for training and treatment planning. J Digit Imaging 1998;11(Suppl 1):120–3.

Anne-Claire J, Denis Q, Patrick D, Christophe C, Philippe M, Sylvain K, et al. S.P.I.C. pedagogical simulator for gynecologic laparoscopy. Stud Health Technol Inform 2000;70:139–45.

Arne R, Stale F, Ragna K, Petter L. PatSim—simulator for practising anaesthesia and intensive care: development and observations. Int J Clin Monit Comput 1996;13:147–52.

Asano T, Yano H, Iwata H. Basic technology of simulation system for laparoscopic surgery in virtual environment with force display. Stud Health Technol Inform 1997;39:207–15.

Avis NJ, Briggs NM, Kleinermann F, Hose DR, Brown BH, Edwards MH. Anatomical and physiological models for surgical simulation. Stud Health Technol Inform 1999;62:23–9.

Aydeniz B, Meyer A, Posten J, Konig M, Wallwiener D, Kurek R. The "HysteroTrainer"—an in vitro simulator for hysteroscopy and falloposcopy: experimental and clinical background and technical realisation including the development of organ modules for electrothermal treatment. Contrib Gynecol Obstet 2000;20:171–81.

Barnes SZ, Morr DR, Oggero E, Pagnacco G, Berme N. The realization of a haptic (force feedback) interface device for the purpose of angioplasty surgery simulation. Biomed Sci Instrum 1997;33:19–24.

Basdogan C, Ho CH, Srinivasan MA. Simulation of tissue cutting and bleeding for laparoscopic surgery using auxiliary surfaces. Stud Health Technol Inform 1999;62:38–44.

Basdogan C, Ho CH, Srinivasan MA, Small SD, Dawson SL. Force interactions in laparoscopic simulations: haptic rendering of soft tissues. Stud Health Technol Inform 1998;50:385–91.

Baumann R, Glauser D, Tappy D, Baur C, Clavel R. Force feedback for virtual reality based minimally invasive surgery simulator. Stud Health Technol Inform 1996;29:564–79.

Berkley J, Weghorst S, Gladstone H, Raugi G, Berg D, Ganter M. Fast finite element modeling for surgical simulation. Stud Health Technol Inform 1999;62:55–61.

Bernardo A, Preul MC, Zabramski JM, Spetzler RF. A three-dimensional interactive virtual dissection model to simulate transpetrous surgical avenues. Neurosurgery 2003;52:499–505; discussion 504–5.

Blezek DJ, Robb RA, Camp JJ, Nauss LA, Martin DP. Simulation of spinal nerve blocks for training anesthesiology residents. Proc SPIE 1997;3262:45–51.

Bockholt U, Ecke U, Muller W, Voss G. Realtime simulation of tissue deformation for the nasal endoscopy simulator (NES). Stud Health Technol Inform 1999;62:74–5.

Bockholt U, Muller W, Voss G, Ecke U, Klimek L. Real-time simulation of tissue deformation for the nasal endoscopy simulator (NES). Comput Aided Surg 1999;4:281–5.

Brown J, Montgomery K, Latombe JC, Stephanides M. A microsurgery simulation system. In: Medical Image Computing and Computer-Assisted Interventions (MICCAI), Utrecht, The Netherlands, October 2001 (www.citeseer.nj.nec.com/brown01 microsurgery.html).

Carter DF. Man-made man: anesthesiological medical human simulator. J Assoc Adv Med Instrum 1969;3:80–6.

Christensen UJ, Andersen SF, Jacobsen J, Jensen PF, Ording H. The Sophus anaesthesia simulator v. 2.0: a Windows 95 control-center of a full-scale simulator. Int J Clin Monit Comput 1997;14:11–6.

Dang T, Annaswamy TM, Srinivasan MA. Development and evaluation of an epidural injection simulator with force feedback for medical training. Stud Health Technol Inform 2001;81:97–102.

Dawson SL, Cotin S, Meglan D, Shaffer DW, Ferrell MA. Designing a computer-based simulator for interventional cardiology training. Catheter Cardiovasc Interv 2000;51:522–7.

De S, Srinivasan MA. Thin walled models for haptic and graphical rendering of soft tissues in surgical simulation. Stud Health Technol Inform 1999;62:94–9.

Downes M, Cavusoglu MC, Gantert W, Way LW, Tendick F. Virtual environments for training critical skills in laparoscopic surgery. Stud Health Technol Inform 1998;50:316–22.

Dubois P, Rouland JF, Meseure P, Karpf S, Chaillou C. Simulator for laser photocoagulation in ophthalmology. IEEE Trans Biomed Eng 1995;42:688–93.

Dumay AC, Jense GJ. Endoscopic surgery simulation in a virtual environment. Comput Biol Med 1995;25:139–48.

Edmond CV Jr, Heskamp D, Sluis D, Stredney D, Sessanna D, Wiet G, et al. ENT endoscopic surgical training simulator. Stud Health Technol Inform 1997;39:518–28.

Euliano TY, Caton D, van Meurs W, Good ML. Modeling obstetric cardiovascular physiology on a full-scale patient simulator. J Clin Monit 1997;13:293–7.

Feinstein DM, Raemer DB. Arterial-line monitoring system simulation. J Clin Monit Comput 2000;16:547–52.

Gorman P, Krummel T, Webster R, Smith M, Hutchens D. A prototype haptic lumbar puncture simulator. Stud Health Technol Inform 2000;70:106–9.

Henrichs B. Development of a module for teaching the cricothyrotomy procedure. Presented at the Society for Technology in Anesthesia Annual Meeting, San Diego, 1999.

Hiemenz L, Stredney D, Schmalbrock P. Development of the force-feedback model for an epidural needle insertion simulator. Stud Health Technol Inform 1998;50:272–7.

Hill JW, Holst PA, Jensen JF, Goldman J, Gorfu Y, Ploeger DW. Telepresence interface with applications to microsurgery and surgical simulation. Stud Health Technol Inform 1998;50:96–102.

Hsieh MS, Tsai MD, Chang WC. Virtual reality simulator for osteotomy and fusion involving the musculoskeletal system. Comput Med Imaging Graph 2002;26:91–101.

Hunter IW, Jones LA, Sagar MA, Lafontaine SR, Hunter PJ. Ophthalmic microsurgical robot and associated virtual environment. Comput Biol Med 1995;25:173–82.

Hutter R, Schmitt KU, Niederer P. Mechanical monitoring of soft biological tissues for application in virtual reality based laparoscopy simulators. Technol Health Care 2000;8:15–24.

John NW, Thacker N, Pokric M, Jackson A, Zanetti G, Gobbetti E, et al. An integrated simulator for surgery of the petrous bone. Stud Health Technol Inform 2001;81:218–24.

Jones R, Pinnock C. The development of the epidural simulator training apparatus (ESTA). Presented at the International Meeting on Medical Simulation, San Diego, 2003.

Kelsey R, Botello M, Millard B, Zimmerman J. An online heart simulator for augmenting first-year medical and dental education. In: Proceedings of the AMIA Symposium, San Antonio, TX, 2002, pp. 370–4.

Kesavadas T, Joshi D, Mayrose J, Chugh K. A virtual environment for esophageal intubation training. In: Westwood JD, Hoffman HM, Robb RA, Stredney D (eds) Medicine Meets Virtual Reality. Amsterdam: IOS Press; 2002. p. 221–7.

Kim KH, Kwon MJ, Kwon SM, Ra JB, Park H. Fast surface and volume rendering based on shear-warp factorization for a surgical simulator. Comput Aided Surg 2002;7:268–78.

Kizakevich PN, McCartney ML, Nissman DB, Starko K, Smith NT. Virtual medical trainer: patient assessment and trauma care simulator. Stud Health Technol Inform 1998;50:309–15.

Kuppersmith RB, Johnston R, Moreau D, Loftin RB, Jenkins H. Building a virtual reality temporal bone dissection simulator. Stud Health Technol Inform 1997;39:180–6.

Larsen OV, Haase J, Ostergaard LR, Hansen KV, Nielsen H. The Virtual Brain Project—development of a neurosurgical simulator. Stud Health Technol Inform 2001;81:256–62.

Larsson JE, Hayes-Roth B, Gaba DM, Smith BE. Evaluation of a medical diagnosis system using simulator test scenarios. Artif Intell Med 1997;11:119–40.

Lathan C, Cleary K, Greco R. Development and evaluation of a spine biopsy simulator. Stud Health Technol Inform 1998;50:375–6.

Mabrey JD, Cannon WD, Gillogly SD, Kasser JR, Sweeney HJ, Zarins B, et al. Development of a virtual reality arthroscopic knee simulator. Stud Health Technol Inform 2000;70:192–4.

Meglan DA, Raju R, Merril GL, Merril JR, Nguyen BH, Swamy SN, et al. The teleos virtual environment tool kit for simulation-based surgical education. Stud Health Technol Inform 1996;29:346–51.

Montgomery K, Stephanides M, Schendel S. Development and application of a virtual environment for reconstructive surgery. Comput Aided Surg 2000;5:90–7.

Montgomery K, Thonier G, Stephanides M, Schendel S. Virtual reality based surgical assistance and training system for long duration space missions. Stud Health Technol Inform 2001;81:315–21.

Muller W, Bockholt U. The virtual reality arthroscopy training simulator. Stud Health Technol Inform 1998;50:13–9.

Muller W, Bockholt U, Lahmer A, Voss G, Borner M. VRATS—Virtual Reality Arthroscopy Training Simulator. Radiologe 2000;40:290–4.

Neumann M, Hochberger J, Felzmann T, Ell C, Hohenberger W. Part 1. The Erlanger endo-trainer. Endoscopy 2001;33:887–90.

Oppenheimer P, Gupta A, Weghorst S, Sweet R, Porter J. The representation of blood flow in endourologic surgical simulations. Stud Health Technol Inform 2001;81:365–1.

Oppenheimer P, Weghorst S, MacFarlane M, Sinanan M. Immersive surgical robotic interfaces. Stud Health Technol Inform 1999;62:242–8.

O'Toole RV 3rd, Jaramaz B, DiGioia AM 3rd, Visnic CD, Reid RH. Biomechanics for preoperative planning and surgical simulations in orthopaedics. Comput Biol Med 1995;25:183–91.

Ottensmeyer MP, Ben-Ur E, Salisbury JK. Input and output for surgical simulation: devices to measure properties in vivo and a hepatic interface for laparoscopy simulators. Stud Health Technol Inform 2000;70:236–42.

Petty M, Windyga P. A high level architecture-based medical simulation system. Simulation 1999;73:281–7.

Pieper S, Delp S, Rosen J, Fisher SS. A virtual environment system for simulation of leg surgery. Proc SPIE 1996;1457:188–96.

Playter R, Raibert M. A virtual surgery simulator using advanced haptic feedback. Minim Invasive Ther Appl Technol 1997;6:117–21.

Popp HJ, Schecke T, Rau G, Kasmacher H, Kalff G. An interactive computer simulator of the circulation for knowledge acquisition in cardio-anesthesia. Int J Clin Monit Comput 1991;8:151–8.

Ra JB, Kwon SM, Kim JK, Yi J, Kim KH, Park HW, et al. Spine needle biopsy simulator using visual and force feedback. Comput Aided Surg 2002;7:353–63.

Radetzky A, Nurnberger A. Visualization and simulation techniques for surgical simulators using actual patient's data. Artif Intell Med 2002;26:255–79.

Riding M, John NW. Force-feedback in Web-based surgical simulators. Stud Health Technol Inform 2001;81:404–6.

Rosen J, MacFarlane M, Richards C, Hannaford B, Sinanan M. Surgeon-tool force/torque signatures—evaluation of surgical skills in minimally invasive surgery. Stud Health Technol Inform 1999;62:290–6.

Rosenberg LB, Stredney D. A haptic interface for virtual simulation of endoscopic surgery. Stud Health Technol Inform 1996;29:371–87.

Schwid HA. A flight simulator for general anesthesia training. Comput Biomed Res 1987;20:64–75.

Stansfield S, Shawver D, Sobel A. MediSim: a prototype VR system for training medical responders. Presented at the IEEE Virtual Reality Annual International Symposium (VRAIS), 1998. pp. 198–205.

Stefanich L, Cruz-Neira C. A virtual surgical simulator for the lower limbs. Biomed Sci Instrum 1999;35:141–5.

Stredney D, Wiet GJ, Yagel R, Sessanna D, Kurzion Y, Fontana M, et al. A comparative analysis of integrating visual representations with haptic displays. Stud Health Technol Inform 1998;50:20–6.

Suzuki N, Hattori A, Ezumi T, Uchiyama A, Kumano T, Ikemoto A, et al. Simulator for virtual surgery using deformable organ models and force feedback system. Stud Health Technol Inform 1998;50:227–33.

Sweet R, Porter J, Oppenheimer P, Hendrickson D, Gupta A, Weghorst S. Simulation of bleeding in endoscopic procedures using virtual reality. J Endourol 2002;16:451–5.

Syroid N. Design, implementation, and performance of a respiratory gas exchange simulator. Presented at the 2001 International Meeting on Medical Simulation, Ft. Lauderdale, FL, 2001.

Szekely G, Brechbuhler C. Virtual reality based surgery simulation for endoscopic gynaecology. PREEB 2000;9:310–33.

Tanaka H, Nakamura H, Tamaki E, Nariai T, Hirakawa K. Brain surgery simulation system using VR technique and improvement of presence. Stud Health Technol Inform 1998;50:150–4.

Tanner G, Angers D, Van Ess D, Ward C. ANSIM: an anesthesia simulator for the IBM PC. Comput Methods Programs Biomed 1986;23:237–42.

Tendick F, Downes M. A virtual environment testbed for training laparoscopic surgical skills. PREEB 2000;9:235–55.

Thomas G, Johnson L, Dow S, Stanford C. The design and testing of a force feedback dental simulator. Comput Methods Programs Biomed 2001;64:53–64.

Thurfjell L, Lundin A, McLaughlin J. A medical platform for simulation of surgical procedures. Stud Health Technol Inform 2001;81:509–14.

Tsai MD, Hsieh MS, Jou SB. Virtual reality orthopedic surgery simulator. Comput Biol Med 2001;31:333–51.

Tseng CS, Lee YY, Chan YP, Wu SS, Chiu AW. A PC-based surgical simulator for laparoscopic surgery. Stud Health Technol Inform 1998;50:155–60.

Van Meurs WL, Beneken JEW, Good ML, Lampotang S, et al. Physiologic model for an anesthesia simulator. Anesthesiology 1993;79:A1114.

Van Meurs WL, Good ML, Lampotang S. Functional anatomy of full-scale patient simulators. J Clin Monit 1997;13:317–24.

Von Lubitz DK, Van Dyke Parunak H, Levine H, Beier KP, Freer J, Pletcher T, et al. The VIBE of the burning agents: simulation and modeling of burns and their treatment using agent-based programming, virtual reality, and human patient simulation. Stud Health Technol Inform 2001;81:554–60.

Voss G, Bockholt U, Los Arcos JL, Muller W, Oppelt P, Stahler J. LAHYS TOTRAIN·intelligent training system for laparoscopy and hysteroscopy. Stud Health Technol Inform 2000;70:359–64.

Wade L, Siddall V, Gould R. A simple device for simulating left subclavian vein placement of a triple lumen catheter with the METI HPS-010 adult mannequin. Presented at the International Meeting on Medical Simulation, San Diego, 2003.

Weale AR, Mitchell DC. A do-it-yourself vascular anastomosis simulator. Ann R Coll Surg Engl 2003;85:132.

Weidenbach M, Trochin S, Kreutter S, Richter C, Berlage T, Grunst G. Intelligent training system integrated in an echocardiography simulator. Comput Biol Med 2004;34:407–25.

Weidenbach M, Wick C, Pieper S, Quast KJ, Fox T, Grunst G, et al. Augmented reality simulator for training in two-dimensional echocardiography. Comput Biomed Res 2000;33:11–22.

Weingartner T, Hassfeld S, Dillmann R. Virtual jaw: a 3D simulation for computer assisted surgery and education. Stud Health Technol Inform 1998;50:329–35.

Westenskow DR. Humidification of a simulator's expired gases for respiratory rate monitoring. Presented at the 2001 International Meeting on Medical Simulation, Scottsdale, AZ, 2001.

Witzke DB, Hoskins JD, Mastrangelo MJ Jr, Witzke WO, Chu UB, Pande S, et al. Immersive virtual reality used as a platform for perioperative training for surgical residents. Stud Health Technol Inform 2001;81:577–83.

Ziegler R, Fischer G, Muller W, Gobel M. Virtual reality arthroscopy training simulator. Comput Biol Med 1995;25:193–203.

USING SIMULATORS (AS A DEPENDENT VARIABLE) TO EVALUATE NONHUMAN ENGINEERING ISSUES (INDEPENDENT VARIABLE: USE OF NEW INSTRUMENT, ANESTHETIC AGENT) RATHER THAN TESTING ON HUMANS

Agutter J, Drews F, Syroid N, Westneskow D, Albert R, Strayer D, et al. Evaluation of graphic cardiovascular display in a high-fidelity simulator. Anesth Analg 2003;97:1403–13.

Anastakis DJ, Hamstra SJ, Matsumoto ED. Visual-spatial abilities in surgical training. Am J Surg 2000;170:469–71.

Dyson A, Harris J, Bhatia K. Rapidity and accuracy of tracheal intubation in a mannequin: comparison of the fibreoptic with the Bullard laryngoscope. Br J Anaesth 1990;65:268–70.

Eyal R, Tendick F. Spatial ability and learning the use of an angled laparoscope in a virtual environment 2001. Stud Health Technol Inform 2001;81:146–52.

Feinstein DM, Raemer DB. Arterial-line monitoring system simulation. J Clin Monit Comput 2000;16:547–52.

Gorman PJ, Lieser JD, Marshall RL, Krummel TM. End user analysis of a force feedback virtual reality based surgical simulator. Stud Health Technol Inform 2000;70:102–5.

Hanna GB, Shimi SM, Cuschieri A. Task performance in endoscopic surgery is influenced by location of the image display. Ann Surg 1998;227:481–4.

Holden JG, Flach JM, Donchin Y. Perceptual-motor coordination in an endoscopic surgery simulation. Surg Endosc 1999;13:127–32.

Kain ZN, Berde CB, Benjamin PK, Thompson JE. Performance of pediatric resuscitation bags assessed with an infant lung simulator. Anesth Analg 1993;77:261–4.

Keller C, Brimacombe J, A FR, Giampalmo M, Kleinsasser A, Loeckinger A, et al. Airway management during spaceflight: a comparison of four airway devices in simulated microgravity. Anesthesiology 2000;92:1237–41.

Lovell A, Tooley M, Lauder G. Evaluation and correction for haemodynamic drug modelling in a paediatric simulator. Presented at the International Meeting on Medical Simulation, San Diego, 2003.

Merry AF, Webster CS, Weller J, Henderson S, Robinson B. Evaluation in an anaesthetic simulator of a prototype of a new drug administration system designed to reduce error. Anaesthesia 2002;57:256–63.

Michels P, Gravenstein D, Westenskow DR. An integrated graphic data display improves detection and identification of critical events during anesthesia. J Clin Monit 1997;13:249–59.

Murray WB, Good ML, Gravenstein JS, van Oostrom JH, Brasfield WG. Learning about new anesthetics using a model driven, full human simulator. J Clin Monit Comput 2002;17:293–300.

Nathanson MH, Gajraj NM, Newson CD. Tracheal intubation in a manikin: comparison of supine and left lateral positions. Br J Anaesth 1994;73:690–1.

Passmore PJ, Read OJ, Nielsen CF, Torkington J, Darzi A. Effects of perspective and stereo on depth judgements in virtual reality laparoscopy simulation. Stud Health Technol Inform 2000;70:243–5.

Raemer D, Puyana J, Lisco S, O'Connell T. Market testing a simulated continuous blood gas analysis monitor in realistic simulation scenarios. Presented at the 2001 International Meeting on Medical Simulation, Scottsdale, AZ.

Santamore DC, Cleaver TG. The sounds of saturation. J Clin Monot Comput 2004;18:89–92.

Seehusen A, Brett PN, Harrison A. Human perception of haptic information in minimal access surgery tools for use in simulation. Stud Health Technol Inform 2001;81:453–8.

Smith B, Howard S, Weinger M, Gaba D. Performance of the pre-anesthetic equipment checkout: a simulator study. Presented at the Society for Technology in Anesthesia Annual Meeting, San Diego, 1999.

Sowb YA, Loeb R, Smith B. Clinician's response to management of the gas delivery system. Presented at the Society for Technology in Anesthesia Annual Meeting, San Diego, 1999.

Taffinder N, Smith SG, Huber J, Russell RC, Darzi A. The effect of a second-generation 3D endoscope on the laparoscopic precision of novices and experienced surgeons. Surg Endosc 1999;13:1087–92.

Thoman WJ, Gravenstein D, van der Aa J, Lampotang S. Autoregulation in a simulator-based educational model of intracranial physiology. J Clin Monit Comput 1999;15:481–91.

Thoman WJ, Lampotang S, Gravenstein D, van der Aa J. A computer model of intracranial dynamics integrated to a full-scale patient simulator. Comput Biomed Res 1998;31:32–46.

Thurfjell L, Lundin A, McLaughlin J. A medical platform for simulation of surgical procedures. Stud Health Technol Inform 2001;81:509–14.

Trochin S, Weidenbach M, Pieper S, Wick C, Berlage T. An enabling system for echocardiography providing adaptive support through behavioral analysis. Stud Health Technol Inform 2001;81:528–33.

Wanzel KR, Hamstra SJ, Anastakis DJ, Mataumoto ED, Cusiamano MD. Effect of visual-spatial ability on learning of spatially-complex surgical skills. Lancet 2002;359:230–1.

Westenskow D, Bonk R, Sedlmayr M. Enhancing a human simulator with a graphic display of physiology. Presented at the Society for Technology in Anesthesia Annual Meeting, San Diego, 1999.

Wiklund ME. Patient simulators breathe life into product testing. MDDI Medical Device & Diagnostic Industry, June 1999 (www.devicelink.com/mddi/archive/9/06/contents.html).

Via D. Eye tracking system improves evaluation of performance during simulated anesthesia events. Presented at the 2001 International Meeting on Medical Simulation, Scottsdale, AZ.

Conclusion

May the road rise up to meet you,
May the wind be ever at your back.
May the sun shine warm upon your face and the rain fall softly on your fields.
And until we meet again, may God hold you in the hollow of his hand.

Irish blessing

The quantum physics professor is conducting magic shows in his September years, entertaining grandkids and doing charity benefits. "Watch, kids, watch the magic wand!" Jimmy the Magnificent whirls his wand around the hat, then reaches deep, deep into the black top hat.

In the front row, a tow-haired, freckled kid drops open his mouth. He doesn't notice it, but as he leans forward his cup of root beer is leaning forward too, spilling onto the ground. Jimmy the Magnificent pulls out—a Palm Pilot? "Ooops! That's not what I wanted!"

The root beer-spilling kid says, "Caaa-aaa."

Jimmy the Magnificent whirls his wand around the other way. "Abracadabra!"

A Blackberry combination cellphone Internet-access device?

"Ooops!" Jimmy the Magnificent says, "here you, you there, in the front row, reach in your pocket and pull me out some fairy dust."

Now dropping the root beer cup entirely, the kid reaches in his pocket and pulls out, well, nothing. "It's . . ." he stammers, "there's nothing there."

"No problem kid, fairy dust is invisible, just sprinkle it on my wand, quick, before the fairy dust blows away!"

He obeys, sprinkling the fairy dust over the magic wand. It's supposed to be invisible, but the kid thinks he sees a little glint of light for just a second. Maybe *some* fairy dust you can see, for just a little bit.

Jimmy the Magnificent balances the wand in his hand, cocks his head back a little and closes his eyes. "Uh huh," Jimmy says, "Yep. Yep. That's just right, it's got the feel now. That was just the right amount."

Round and round the wand goes, first one way, then the other. Into the hat goes Jimmy's hand, and this time—out comes a big white rabbit, so big you could hardly believe it could even fit in there! Oh man! *No one* at school will believe this, I mean this is way better than that stuff on TV cause that's all mirrors and computer stuff but this is *real*. That's a real rabbit, and that wand had *my* fairy dust on it—*no one* else's made that rabbit pop right out, well, get pulled out, of the hat.

At the end of the show, Jimmy the Magnificent is packing up his stuff. His wand rolls off the table and falls onto the ground. The tow-haired, freckled kid had just emerged from the bathroom across the room. He sees the wand.

"Hey, Mister! Mister Magician!" the kid shouts. He runs across the room, picks up the wand, and hands it to Jimmy the Magnificent. "Don't forget your magic!"

Jimmy picks up the wand, points it at the kid's chest. "Don't worry," Jimmy says, "the magic's right there—in your heart."

INDEX

Note: Page numbers followed by f refer to illustrations of medical equipment and procedures; page numbers followed by b refer to boxed material.